CHILD AND ADOLESCENT CLINICAL PSYCHOPHARMACOLOGY

rth Edition

Child and Adolescent Clinical Psychopharmacology
Fourth Edition

Wayne Hugo Green, M.D.
New York University Child Study Center
New York, New York

Wolters Kluwer Health | Lippincott Williams & Wilkins

Philadelphia · Baltimore · New York · London
Buenos Aires · Hong Kong · Sydney · Tokyo

Publisher and Executive Editor: Charles W. Mitchell
Senior Managing Editor: Lisa Kairis
Project Manager: Jennifer Harper
Senior Manufacturing Manager: Benjamin Rivera
Associate Director of Marketing: Adam Glazer
Design Coordinator: Terry Mallon
Production Services: Laserwords Private Limited, Chennai, India
Printer: R.R. Donnelley, Crawfordsville

530 Walnut Street
Philadelphia, PA 19106 USA
LWW.com

3rd edition, © 2001 Lippincott Williams & Wilkins
2nd edition, © 1995 Williams & Wilkins
1st edition, © 1991 Williams & Wilkins

Library of Congress Cataloging-in-Publication Data

Green, Wayne H.
  Child and adolescent clinical psychopharmacology / Wayne Hugo
  Green.—4th ed.
    p. ; cm.
  Includes bibliographical references and index.
  ISBN-13: 978-0-7817-5950-2
  ISBN-10: 0-7817-5950-1
  1. Pediatric psychopharmacology. I. Title.
  [DNLM: 1. Mental Disorders—drug therapy. 2. Adolescent.
3. Child. 4. Psychopharmacology—methods. 5. Psychotropic Drugs
—therapeutic use. WS 350.2 G798c 2007]
RJ504.7.G74 2007
615'.78'083—dc22

                              2006027373

Care has been taken to confirm the accuracy of the information presented and to describe generally accepted practices. However, the authors, editors, and publisher are not responsible for errors or omissions or for any consequences from application of the information in this book and make no warranty, expressed or implied, with respect to the currency, completeness, or accuracy of the contents of the publication. Application of this information in a particular situation remains the professional responsibility of the practitioner.

The authors, editors, and publisher have exerted every effort to ensure that drug selection and dosage set forth in this text are in accordance with current recommendations and practice at the time of publication. However, in view of ongoing research, changes in government regulations, and the constant flow of information relating to drug therapy and drug reactions, the reader is urged to check the package insert for each drug for any change in indications and dosage and for added warnings and precautions. This is particularly important when the recommended agent is a new or infrequently employed drug.

Some drugs and medical devices presented in this publication have Food and Drug Administration (FDA) clearance for limited use in restricted research settings. It is the responsibility of the health care provider to ascertain the FDA status of each drug or device planned for use in their clinical practice.

To purchase additional copies of this book, call our customer service department at (800) 638-3030 or fax orders to (301) 223-2320. International customers should call (301) 223-2300.

Visit Lippincott Williams & Wilkins on the Internet: at LWW.com. Lippincott Williams & Wilkins customer service representatives are available from 8:30 am to 6 pm, EST.

10 9 8 7 6 5 4 3 2 1

To my parents
Albert George Green
and
Mildred Hugo Green
and my uncle and aunt,
Alfred John Green
and
Ada May Green

Contents

Preface

It is now 15 years since the publication of the first edition of *Child and Adolescent Clinical Psychopharmacology*. Three major trends in child and adolescent psychopharmacology since the last edition are striking. First, after a period of major enthusiasm with the newer medications, in particular the Selective Serotonin Reuptake Inhibitors (SSRIs) and the Atypical/Second Generation Antipsychotics (SGAs), and the increased number of prescriptions of these drugs written for children and adolescents, there has been a rather significant retrenchment, replete with FDA Black Box and Bold Print warnings. It is important to note that although the SSRIs and SGAs are widely prescribed for many different psychiatric disorders in children and adolescents, almost all these prescriptions are for off-label/non FDA-approved indications. The only currently approved FDA indications for using SSRIs in children and adolescents are for fluoxetine in patients diagnosed with Major Depressive Disorder (MDD; ages $\geq$ 8 years) or Obsessive-Compulsive Disorder (OCD; ages $\geq$ 7 years), sertraline in OCD (ages $\geq$ 6 years), and fluvoxamine in OCD (ages $\geq$ 8 years); there are no FDA-approved uses for SGAs in patients < 18 years of age. Thus, most of the findings that have contributed to the markedly increased caution recommended in administering these drugs have been the result of studies conducted in children and adolescents after the initial marketing and reports of adverse events. This has been in large part due to the longer-term experience in the use of these drugs in greater numbers of children and adolescents. The treatment-related adverse events associated with these drugs, which were not immediately apparent because of their rarity and the lack or sufficient numbers of patients to detect statistically significant adverse effects, or the length of time necessary for adverse effects to appear, became of marked concern. Meta-analyses of data from many studies have also been important in elucidating some of these findings. Although overall safer than the drugs they have tended to supercede, with time it has became apparent that many of these drugs have their own problems.

All antidepressants are now required to have a Black Box Warning added to their labeling stating, "Warning: Suicidality in Children and Adolescents— Antidepressants increased the risk of suicidal thinking and behavior (suicidality) in short-term studies in children and adolescents with major depressive disorder (MDD) and other psychiatric disorders" (The full warning is printed at the beginning of the chapter on antidepressants.) The subsequent decrease of up to 20% in the prescription of antidepressants to adolescents that was reported

(Rosack, 2005) is likely related to this. The recent Special Double Issue on SSRIs of the Journal of Child and Adolescent Psychopharmacology (Volume 16, Numbers 1 and 2, 2006) included nine articles focused on adverse events, in particular the risk of suicidality, associated with the use of SSRIs in children and adolescents.

Some of the atypical antipsychotics have been found to cause increased risk of metabolic syndrome, Type II diabetes, and significant weight gain; increases in serum prolactin levels; and adverse cardiovascular effects such as a prolonged QTc interval. In addition, the FDA has directed manufacturers of atypical antipsychotic drugs to add a Black Box Warning that elderly patients with dementia-related psychosis treated with atypical antipsychotic drugs are at increased risk of death 1.6 to 1.7 times that seen in placebo-treated patients. Atypical antipsychotic drugs are not approved for treatment of patients with dementia-related psychoses.

The FDA has also directed that a Black Box Warning be added to the labeling of amphetamine products stating "Amphetamines have a high potential for abuse. Administration of amphetamines for prolonged periods of time may lead to drug dependence, particular attention should be paid to the possibility of subjects obtaining amphetamines for non-therapeutic use or distribution to others and the drugs should be prescribed or dispensed sparingly. Misuse of amphetamine may cause sudden death and serious cardiovascular adverse events." The FDA has received reports of sudden death associated with unusual amphetamine dosing in children with structural cardiac abnormailites. The FDA does not recommend general use of amphetamines in children or adults with structural cardiac abnormalities. One manufacturer of mixed amphetamine salts notes for its extended release product, "Its misuse is associated with serious cardiovascular adverse events and may cause sudden death in patients with preexisting cardiac structural abnormalities."

Magnesium pemoline preparations and nefazodone hydrochloride have been withdrawn from the market because of serious adverse events.

It is clear that practitioners of child and adolescent psychopharmacology must remain vigilant in monitoring their patients for adverse effects and educating them and their caregivers about such adverse effects. Polypharmacy continues to be widely used and has the potential to contribute further to adverse effects because of known and unknown adverse drug interactions.

The second trend has been an increasing number of new drug formulations to increase duration of action and eliminate or significantly decrease the need for multiple daily doses. There have been newly introduced extended release forms of amphetamine, methylphenidate, and dexmethylphenidate preparations. A daily methylphenidate transdermal delivery system has recently been approved. Fluoxetine is available as a capsule to be taken weekly. Duloxetine hydrochloride, a recently introduced antidepressant, is available only as a delayed release capsule. Extended release stimulant preparations are especially helpful in that many children and adolescents can be freed from the stigma of having to take medication in school. Overall, decreasing the number of doses of medication per day is thought to increase compliance in taking medication as prescribed.

Thirdly, already approved drugs have been approved for additional indications or use in different age populations. Examples include several mood stabilizers/antiepileptic drugs and Second Generation Antipsychotics have been approved for the additional indications of treatment of acute manic or mixed episodes associated with Bipolar I Disorder. Two SSRIs, escitalopram and paroxetine, are now approved to treat Generalized Anxiety Disorder, although not in children and adolescents. Fluoxetine is now approved for treating depression in patients $\geq$ 8 years old and OCD in patients $\leq$ 7 years old.

All of the above issues are covered more fully under the specific drugs in the text that follows.

I again thank my colleagues for their positive responses to the earlier editions of the book and their enthusiasm for yet another addition.

Wayne Hugo Green, M.D.

Preface to the First Edition

This book is written with the conviction that proper psychiatric treatment of children and adolescents will, on some occasions, necessitate the use of psychopharmacotherapy. It is not intended to suggest that psychopharmacotherapy is warranted for most patients in this age group.

Most children and adolescents seen in private practices and in mental hygiene clinics do not require medication. Indeed, medication is not appropriate for many patients of this age group seen on inpatient psychiatric services.

Clinicians who administer psychoactive medication to children and adolescents will almost certainly encounter individuals with strong viewpoints on this treatment. Some are convinced that drugs are the answer to a child's or adolescent's problem. Others are equally certain that drugs are an anathema and ought to be avoided at all costs.

In this second, antidrug group, two lines of reasoning seem to appear with regularity in a significant minority of cases.

Some health and educational professionals working with children and adolescents maintain that in the face of compelling psychological explanations for a mental disorder, or for significant contributions to it, drugs should not be used. This group argues that drugs may have inimical effects and, further, that psychotherapy alone should be able to do the job.

A few professionals, but more often parents and relatives, offer a variation on this theme. They believe drugs should be avoided because the drugs will make their children "zombies" or "dope them up" or "make them become drug addicts later on."

The author's point of view is that the etiology of virtually all psychiatric disorders is multiply determined. Each individual case must be fully assessed and evaluated for the potential benefits and risks of administering a specific medication. In those cases where potential benefits appear to significantly outweigh risks, usually a trial of medication is indicated.

Still, extreme caution is required in employing psychoactive medications. The long-term effects of psychoactive medications on the maturation and development of children and adolescents are at best only partially known, and many of their known untoward effects are potentially harmful.

But when a mental illness is delaying or disrupting the maturation and development of a patient, effective medication may aid considerably in bringing about more normal development and socialization. The medication often will augment the patient's ability to respond to other treatment modalities as well.

The clinician must successfully negotiate among these conflicting viewpoints and objectives in order to undertake a clinical trial of a psychoactive drug in a reasonably favorable or at least dispassionately neutral atmosphere.

Time and reality are two extremely important factors often overlooked by critics of psychopharmacotherapy. In deciding about medication, it is essential to employ a realizable goal, not some unattainable ideal.

For example, a latency-age child is diagnosed with a conduct disorder and attention deficit hyperactivity disorder. School officials threaten to suspend the child, with eventual placement in a special education class for children with behavioral problems.

In many such cases, an argument can be made that the child's problems are primarily psychological, that they could be helped by tutoring and individual and family therapies, and that medication should be withheld.

However, the realities of the case and the time frame for behavior change may call for trying medication. It may be exceedingly difficult to engage and work with the parents and the child. The child's symptoms may not have responded to the initial evaluation and intervention. The attitude of the school officials may be that the child's behavior must improve quickly.

In a situation such as this, if psychopharmacotherapy is likely to significantly hasten the therapeutic response to other treatments, or to prevent the patient from being removed from the regular classroom, the author recommends a trial of medication, unless other compelling factors are involved.

This book provides a framework for making an informed decision to undertake a clinical trial of a psychoactive medication and guides the clinician through the myriad issues involved in that decision.

Wayne Hugo Green, M.D.

SECTION I

General Principles

CHAPTER 1

Introduction

This book will review selected topics and most drugs used in child and adolescent psychopharmacology from a practical, clinically oriented perspective. It is intended primarily for clinicians actively engaged in treating children and adolescents with psychoactive medications. These include child psychiatrists, pediatricians, family physicians, residents in child and adolescent psychiatry, residents in general psychiatry, pediatric residents, and other health care professionals who may prescribe drugs to patients in this age group. In addition, other clinicians and mental health personnel who work with children receiving psychoactive medication may wish to review the medications their patients are receiving, as may some parents/caregivers of such children.

The first part of the book focuses rather intensively on the general principles of psychopharmacotherapy for children and adolescents. The reader is presented with a clinically useful way of thinking about psychopharmacotherapy, beginning with the initial clinical contact and continuing through the psychiatric evaluation, psychodynamic formulation, diagnosis, and development of the treatment plan. For those cases in which psychoactive medication is recommended as a part of the treatment plan, the necessary medicolegal responsibilities of the clinician in introducing and explaining the purpose of medication to the relevant caretakers and the patient, steps to obtain informed consent and assent to administer medication, ways of maximizing the chances of the legal guardian's and patient's acceptance of a trial of the medication and cooperation with its administration, and the necessary documentation of these facts in the clinical record are reviewed. Following this, the entire process of administering medication is discussed. This begins with a consideration of which drug to choose for the initial trial of medication and subsequent medications, should the first choice(s) not result in adequate clinical improvement. Examples of algorithms, which are often helpful in medicating complicated clinical cases, are also included. The necessary documentation of target symptoms and any baseline behavioral ratings that will be useful in assessing clinical response or the development of untoward effects and the baseline physical and laboratory assessments to be selected are then discussed. This part of the book ends with a detailed presentation of the principles of administering psychoactive medication from the initial dose, through titration and determining the optimal dose, to maintenance therapy, duration of treatment, and issues in terminating medication. These principles are generalizable and provide clinical guidelines for selecting and administering any psychoactive medication to children and adolescents.

The second portion of the book begins with a short chapter discussing the history of child psychopharmacology and some issues concerning psychopharmacological research in children and adolescents. The purpose of this review is to remind the reader where the information that follows is placed in the history of child psychopharmacology and of the importance of research and a critical assessment of the presented data for informed clinical practice.

After these brief introductory comments, the remainder of Section II focuses on specific psychopharmacological agents that are presently the most important in the clinical practice of child and adolescent psychiatry. These drugs are presented by their class. Many specific psychoactive medications are presently used to treat diverse psychiatric disorders or symptoms across psychiatric diagnoses (e.g., lithium for its antiaggressive effects), and this method of organization avoids repeating similar information under several diagnoses. Equally important, as we learn more about the etiopathogenesis of psychiatric disorders, it becomes increasingly useful, both scientifically and clinically, to think about how drugs affect basic neurotransmitter and psychoneuroendocrine functioning across diagnoses. Drugs may affect one or more neurotransmitter systems. For example, the atypical or second-generation antipsychotics have a very complex mixture of pharmacologic properties. They primarily influence not only the dopamine and serotonin systems as antagonists but also the noradrenergic and cholinergic systems and have antihistaminic and other properties (Stahl, 2000). Likewise, a specific neurotransmitter system may be important in one or more diagnostic categories. For example, there appears to be a relationship between the serotonergic system's functioning and aggressive or violent behavior and self-destructive behavior among various diagnostic groups (Linnoila et al. 1989 Mann et al. 1989). Several books devoted solely to the behavioral pharmacology of serotonin have been published (e.g., Bevan et al. 1989 Coccaro and Murphy, 1990 and Brown and van Praag, 1991).

As might be expected in a clinically oriented book, the standard, often older, psychopharmacological treatments established by investigational and clinical studies as both efficacious and safe for use in children and adolescents and approved by the U.S. Food and Drug Administration (FDA) for advertising as such are still included. The literature reviews determining the efficacy of these treatments, however, are kept to a minimum, because comprehensive reviews are readily available elsewhere. (For the interested reader, a list of such additional readings is given in Chapter 3 of Section II.)

It is important to note that currently most first line drugs, with the exception of the stimulants, prescribed to treat psychiatric disorders in children and adolescents are off-label/not FDA approved for the age or indication or both, although they are FDA approved for older individuals, usually adults, and for a more limited range of indications. This is because these newer drugs are often more effective, have fewer or less serious untoward/adverse effects or both, than older FDA-approved drugs. In particular, the selective serotonin reuptake inhibitor (SSRI) antidepressants and the atypical/second-generation antipsychotics are currently more frequently prescribed for non-FDA–approved indications in children and adolescents than the FDA-approved drugs. It is also interesting to note that the tricyclic antidepressants, which have been surpassed by the SSRIs in the total number of prescriptions written, are not approved for use in treating depression in children under age 12, but fluoxetine, an SSRI has approval for use in children aged 7 years and older. Medications that appear to be likely candidates for eventual FDA approval (if the necessary studies were funded and carried out) or which are beginning to be used in standard practice are emphasized. Because reviews of these medications are usually less readily available and some studies are very recent, relevant studies are summarized here. Although this emphasis on the literature of studies of drugs used for non-FDA–approved or off-label indications over FDA-approved drugs may seem paradoxical, it is deliberate and reflects current clinical practice. This is because a major difficulty occurs when patients do not respond with sufficient amelioration of symptoms to FDA-approved pharmacological treatments currently available, or even more importantly, no FDA-approved drug is approved for the treatment indication, or untoward effects prevent the drug's use in adequate doses. When the patient's symptoms prevent him or her from functioning in a psychosocial environment that will facilitate normal growth, maturation, and development, many clinicians use FDA-approved drugs for non-FDA–approved indications to treat their patients. Although this book does not proselytize for the use of medication for non-FDA–approved uses, it does present the clinician with possible alternative treatments for patients who are resistant to standard pharmacological treatments. In fact, the use of many of these medications for off-label indications is medically accepted in standard clinical practice, for example, the use of methylphenidate preparations in children under 6 years of age. As with FDA-approved treatments, the physician must consider, perhaps even more carefully, the risks versus the potential benefits of using any medication for non-FDA–approved indications. Medicolegal and some practical issues of using drugs for non-FDA–approved indications are considered in appropriate sections of the book.

The author emphasizes that no book can substitute for a careful reading of the FDA-approved labeling (manufacturer's labeling/package insert) which contains additional information on all FDA-approved medications discussed in this book, unless it reprints them verbatim. No drug should be prescribed without the physician's having read and become familiar with its labeling information; to do so is a disservice to one's patient and renders one vulnerable to professional liability. This information, however, focuses on the drug's use for indications approved by the FDA and for many psychotropic drugs, there is little about the drug's use for nonapproved indications in children and adolescents.

The package insert for many drugs is reprinted verbatim in the current *Physicians' Desk Reference* (PDR, 2006) and its supplements. The reader is reminded that the PDR, although convenient, includes products primarily marketed by their trade names. Once exclusive manufacturing rights have expired and the drug is marketed primarily or solely as a generic preparations, the PDR usually lists the drug with only the company of manufacture and dose forms available without giving detailed prescribing information. How this affects the prescribing practices of physicians to whom the PDR is distributed free of charge would be interesting to study. To obtain such information about older drugs such as chlorpromazine (Thorazine) or imipramine (Tofranil), one has to consult a source such as *Drug Information for the Health Care Professional, Volume 1* (Thompson Healthcare, 2005), a current psychopharmacology textbook, or the web.

CHAPTER 2

General Principles of Psychopharmacotherapy with Children and Adolescents

PSYCHIATRIC DIAGNOSIS AND PSYCHOPHARMACOTHERAPY

Psychopharmacotherapy should always be part of a comprehensive treatment plan arrived at after a thorough psychiatric evaluation that results in a diagnosis, or at least a working diagnosis. It is scientifically indefensible to initiate treatment without first attempting to formulate as clear an understanding of the clinical picture as possible. This will enable clinicians to institute the most appropriate and rational treatment(s) available in their therapeutic armamentaria for the situation at hand.

Current Psychiatric Diagnostic Nomenclature

A major difficulty with the official American Psychiatric Association (APA) nomenclature, the *Diagnostic and Statistical Manual of Mental Disorders*, Fourth Edition, Text Revision (DSM-IV-TR) (APA, 2000), and indeed with most current psychiatric nomenclatures, is that etiology is not usually taken into account in formulating a diagnosis. One reason for this is that, at our present state of knowledge, we do not know the etiologies of many conditions. Hence, we are often treating specific constellations of behavioral symptoms without adequately understanding their biological and genetic underpinnings and how they interact with their psychosocial and physical environments. For example, autistic disorder is not etiologically homogeneous but has a multitude of causes.

Theoretically, for a given psychiatric disorder, drugs may be effective by correcting the condition(s) leading to it or by influencing events somewhere along the usually complex pathways between the hypothesized abnormality(ies) and its subsequent psychological and/or behavioral consequences. Therefore, some psychoactive drugs may be effective in several dissimilar disorders because they influence or modify neurotransmitters and psychoneuroendocrine events in the brain along or near the end of these interacting, partially confluent, or final common pathways.

Other psychoactive drugs appear to exert their therapeutic effects through entirely different mechanisms in different diagnostic entities—for example, imipramine in depression, attention-deficit/hyperactivity disorder (ADHD), and enuresis.

Some patients with a specific diagnosis (e.g., ADHD, autistic disorder, or schizophrenia) will not have a satisfactory clinical response or will be refractory to a specific drug—even one known to be highly effective in statistically significant double-blind studies—or will even have a worsening of symptoms. This may reflect differences in genetic makeup or other biologically determined conditions, psychosocial environments, and/or internalized conflicts and the contributions each makes to the etiopathogenesis of each patient's psychiatric disorder.

Although diagnostic issues are not discussed specifically in this book, it is emphasized that an accurate diagnosis may be of critical importance in choosing the correct medication. For example, Bowden and Sarabia (1980), Carlson and Strober (1978), and Horowitz (1977) reported on a total of 17 adolescents with bipolar manic-depressive disorder who were initially misdiagnosed as having schizophrenia. Most of the patients with bipolar disorder who were diagnosed incorrectly were treated with antipsychotics and either failed to show clinical improvement or responded poorly. When they were later correctly diagnosed as having manic-depressive disorder and were treated with lithium carbonate, the patients showed remarkable improvements or complete remissions of their psychoses. Horowitz (1977) noted that the presence of mood disturbance with marked lability and prominent elevations and depressions, grandiosity and flight of ideas, and pressured speech, hyperactivity, and distractibility predicted lithium-responsive manic-depression (bipolar disorder) even when massive alterations of thinking and hallucinations were present. Therefore, at times the lack of expected clinical response to a medication should suggest to the clinician the possibility of an incorrect diagnosis and that a careful diagnostic reconsideration should be undertaken.

Other unfortunate clinical consequences may result from incorrect diagnoses. For example, antidepressants may precipitate an acute psychotic reaction when given to some individuals with schizophrenic disorder. Stimulant medications, too, may precipitate psychosis when given in sufficient doses to some children or adolescents with borderline personalities or unrecognized schizophrenia.

Wender (1988) noted that clinical experience suggested that some children diagnosed with ADHD were treated with stimulants and rapidly developed tolerance to them but were actually suffering from a major depressive disorder and that they responded to treatment with tricyclic antidepressants with remarkable improvement.

Changing diagnostic criteria may also complicate matters. For example, some of the controversy regarding the efficacy of stimulants in the mentally retarded may have resulted from diagnostic issues. Until the publication of DSM-II (APA, 1968) there was no specific APA diagnosis for what was commonly known as the hyperactive child. There were various labels for this condition, including *hyperactive child, hyperkinetic syndrome, minimal brain dysfunction (MBD)*, and *minimal cerebral dysfunction*. One influential definition of MBD was that of the Minimal Brain Dysfunction National Project on Learning Disabilities in Children in 1966. This report defined MBD to designate children of near average, average, or above average general intelligence with certain learning and/or behavioral disabilities ranging from mild to severe, which are associated with deviations of function of the central nervous system. These deviations may manifest themselves by various combinations of impairment in perception, conceptualization, language, memory, and control of attention, impulse, or motor function. These aberrations may arise from genetic variations, biochemical irregularities, perinatal insults or other illnesses or injuries sustained during the years, which are critical for the development and maturation of the central nervous system, or from other unknown organic causes (Clements, 1966, p. 53).

Mental retardation was considered evidence of more than "minimal" dysfunction, and the various etiologies were thought to be biological. Because of this concept, children with mental retardation were excluded from the possibility of receiving a codiagnosis of MBD, hyperactive child, or an equivalent diagnosis, and some clinicians may not have tried stimulant medication in their patients who had even mild mental retardation.

The situation changed with the publication of DSM-II, which noted that "in children, mild brain damage often manifests itself by hyperactivity, short attention span, easy distractibility, and impulsiveness" (APA, 1968, p. 31). It also suggested that unless there are significant interactional factors (e.g., between child and parents) that appear to be responsible for these behaviors, the disorder should be classified as a nonpsychotic organic brain syndrome and not as a behavior disorder, such as hyperkinetic reaction of childhood or adolescence. DSM-II conceptualized hyperkinetic reaction of childhood as a reactive disorder secondary to internalization of interpersonal conflicts with resulting characteristic symptoms. There was no other available category for a child or adolescent of normal intelligence who exhibited such symptoms as his or her natural baseline of behavior, unless one assumed some degree of brain damage.

In DSM-III (APA, 1980a), the diagnosis of attention-deficit disorder with hyperactivity (ADDH) was based on the presence of a specific constellation of symptoms, and no etiology was hypothesized. Hence, children of any intelligence could exhibit such features. DSM-III additionally notes that mild or moderate mental retardation may predispose one to the development of ADDH and that the addition of this diagnosis to the severely and profoundly retarded child is not clinically useful because these symptoms are often an inherent part of the condition.

DSM-III-R redefines ADDH somewhat, renames it (ADHD), and refines its relation with mental retardation. It notes that many features of ADHD may be present in mentally retarded people because of the generalized delays in intellectual development. DSM-III-R (APA, 1987), DSM-IV (APA, 1994), and DSM-IV-TR (APA, 2000) note that a mentally retarded child or adolescent should be additionally diagnosed with ADHD only if the relevant symptoms significantly exceed those that are compatible with the child's or adolescent's mental age.

DIAGNOSIS AND TARGET SYMPTOMS

In making the decision about which psychoactive medication to select initially, two major issues should be addressed: diagnosis and target symptoms. Both are important and are often interrelated. It is important to make the most accurate diagnosis possible using the available data and to identify and quantify target symptoms in order to choose an efficacious drug and to assess the results of medication. The target symptoms must be of sufficient severity and must interfere so significantly with the child's or adolescent's current functioning and future maturation and development that the potential benefits of the drug will justify the risks concomitant with its administration.

The initial medication may be chosen with respect to either diagnosis or target symptoms or both. Sometimes the decision is not difficult, because the same medication is appropriate for both the target symptoms and the diagnosis. For example, antipsychotics are the drugs of first choice for treating schizophrenia and are appropriate for most of the significant target symptoms (e.g., hallucinations, thought disorder, and delusions). The symptom "hyperactivity," however, is present in numerous childhood psychiatric disorders, but all hyperactivity is not the same (Fish, 1971). The clinician should be fully aware of the diagnosis in treating this symptom. Hyperactivity in a youngster with ADHD would be expected to respond favorably to the administration of a stimulant, whereas a schizophrenic youngster who is in relative remission but exhibits marked hyperactivity would have a risk of having his or her psychotic symptoms reexacerbated if stimulant medication were used. Stimulant drugs, the drugs of choice in ADHD, are sometimes considered to be relatively contraindicated in schizophrenia and may cause worsening of psychotic symptoms. More recently, however, clinicians have prescribed stimulants to psychotic children who are being maintained on antipsychotic medication but have the remaining symptoms of hyperactivity, distractibility, and inattention, with resulting further clinical improvement.

Medication can also be prescribed to treat specific diagnoses. Lithium, for example, has a certain specificity for treatment of mania in patients diagnosed with bipolar disorder, manic, but also appears to have an antiaggressive action that cuts across various diagnoses. Lithium has been used effectively to treat aggression directed against others or self-injurious behavior in children and adolescents diagnosed with conduct disorder, mental retardation with disturbance of behavior, and autistic disorder.

SPECIAL ASPECTS OF CHILD PSYCHOPHARMACOTHERAPY

Maturational/Developmental Issues

Physiologic Factors

The relation between biological developmental issues and psychopharmacotherapy has been emphasized in the 1987 book *Psychiatric Pharmacosciences of Children and Adolescents* (Popper, 1987b). Children and adolescents may require larger doses of psychoactive medication per unit of body weight compared to adults to attain similar blood levels and therapeutic efficacy. It is usually assumed that two factors explain this situation: more rapid metabolism by the liver and an increased glomerular filtration rate in children compared to that in adults. The latter suggests a greater renal clearance for some drugs, including lithium, which helps in explaining the fact that therapeutic dosages of lithium in children usually do not differ from those in adults (Campbell et al. 1984a).

Teicher and Baldessarini (1987) pointed out that children may respond to drugs differently compared to adults because of pharmacodynamic factors (drug-effector mechanisms) that are caused by developmental changes in neural pathways or their functions (e.g., Geller et al. [1992] reported that prepubescent subjects treated with the tricyclic antidepressant nortriptyline reported almost no anticholinergic adverse effects; especially noteworthy was the lack of any prominent dry mouth frequently reported by adults) or because of pharmacokinetic factors caused by developmental changes in the distribution, metabolism, or excretion of a drug.

Jatlow (1987) has noted that, although the rapid rate of drug disposition may decrease gradually throughout childhood, there may be an abrupt decline around puberty. Drug disposition usually reaches adult levels by middle to late adolescence. Clinically, this would indicate that the clinician should be especially alert to possible changes in pharmacokinetics during the time period around puberty and be ready to adjust dose levels if necessary. When they are available, it may be useful to obtain plasma concentration levels if there appears to be a change in the clinical efficacy of a drug as a child matures into an adolescent.

Puig-Antich (1987) summarized some of the evidence that catecholamine (norepinephrine, epinephrine, and dopamine) systems are not fully anatomically developed and operationally functional until adulthood. The relatively high prevalence of ADHD in younger children and its spontaneous improvement in many children over time may reflect maturational changes in catecholamine function. Interestingly, both the fact that younger children respond to stimulant medication differently from older adolescents and adults with respect to affect or mood and do not report elation, excitation, or euphoria and the fact that mania and euphoria are relatively rare in childhood may also be explained by the immaturity of the catecholamine systems (Puig-Antich, 1987); they can also be considered to result from developmental pharmacodynamic factors.

Similarly, the pharmacokinetics of many drugs change over the course of life. Children and younger adolescents may differ from older adolescents and adults, as the elderly may again differ from those who are middle-aged. For example, children and adolescents under 15 years of age treated with clomipramine had significantly lower steady-state plasma concentrations for a given dose compared to adults (PDR, 1990). Rivera-Calimlim et al. (1979) reported that children and adolescents 8 to 15 years of age required larger doses of chlorpromazine than adults to attain similar plasma concentrations.

There may also be differences between acute and chronic pharmacokinetics. For example, Rivera-Calimlim et al. (1979) reported a decline in plasma chlorpromazine levels in most of their child and adolescent patients who were on a fixed dose and suggested it might be due to autoinduction of metabolic enzymes for chlorpromazine during long-term treatment, as had been previously reported in adults.

A clear relationship between plasma concentrations and clinical response to imipramine was noted for prepubescent subjects and older adults with endogenous depression but not for adolescents and young adults (Burke and Puig-Antich, 1990). The authors hypothesized that the relatively poor clinical efficacy of tricyclic antidepressants in postpubescent adolescents and young adults compared with the clinical response of prepubescent children and older adults is secondary to a negative effect of increased sex hormone levels on the antidepressant action of imipramine.

Herskowitz (1987) reviewed the developmental neurotoxicity of pharmacoactive drugs. Developmental neurotoxicity is concerned with stage-specific, drug-induced biochemical or physiologic changes, morphologic manifestations, and behavioral symptoms. For example, stimulant medication may adversely affect normal increases in height and growth, at least temporarily, in some actively growing children and adolescents. Some psychoactive drugs taken during early pregnancy have significant potential for damaging the fetus (e.g., lithium may cause cardiac malformations).

Cognitive/Psychological/Experiential Factors

The maturation and development of the central nervous system as well as the life experiences accumulating since infancy determine much of the specific level of functioning of a given child or adolescent. Although detailed knowledge of these factors is essential to evaluate any child or adolescent psychiatrically, this book addresses only their specific relevance to psychopharmacotherapy.

In general, the younger the patient, the less the verbal facility available to convey information to the clinician and, reciprocally, the less the cognitive ability available to understand information the clinician wishes to impart. Part of the psychiatric evaluation leading to a decision that psychotropic medication is indicated will provide the clinician with an assessment of the level of the patient's ability to communicate his or her emotional status and of his or her cognitive/linguistic ability to understand the proposed treatment and reliably report the effect of the treatment.

In the very young child or the child with no communicative language, the clinician can only observe behavioral effects of medication directly or learn of them as reported by others. The younger the child, the fewer the compliments or complaints about the beneficial or adverse effects. Also, the young child has less-differentiated emotions and more limited experience with feelings and emotions and with communicating them to others than older children. In addition, some chronically depressed or anxious children may not have had a sufficiently recent normal emotional baseline with which they can compare their present mood. Such children may experience a depressed mood as their normal, usual state of being and, therefore, do not have a normal baseline frame of reference upon which to draw in describing how they feel.

The younger the child, the less accurate his or her time estimates. Until approximately 10 years of age, concepts of long periods of time are often not easily understood. It can be very useful and at times essential to use concrete markers of time in discussing time concepts and chronology of events with children. For example, the clinician may enquire whether something occurred before or after the last birthday, specific holidays (e.g., Christmas, Thanksgiving, or Halloween), specific events (e.g., separation or divorce of parents, when the family moved to another home, an operation, a relative's death, or the birth of a sibling), the seasons or weather (e.g., winter, snow, cold, or summer, hot), or the school year (e.g., specific teacher's name or grade, or Christmas, spring or Easter, or summer vacation).

Concepts such as concentration, distractibility, and impulsivity may be beyond the understanding of some early latency-age children. Different children may use different words or expressions to mean the same concept. It is important to be certain that a child knows the meaning of a specific word and not assume an understanding because the child responds to a question. If there is any doubt, ask what something means or explain it in another way. It can be very useful to ask the same thing in several different ways.

In the final analysis, once the patient's psychopathology and his or her developmental experiential factors are taken into account, it is the quality of the relationship between the clinician and the child or adolescent that becomes paramount in determining the usefulness of information shared.

Relationship to the Patient's Family or Caregivers

Diagnosis, Formulation, and Development of the Treatment Plan

A complete psychiatric assessment, including appropriate psychological tests, resulting in a working diagnosis and comprehensive treatment plan; appropriate physical and laboratory examinations; and baseline behavioral measurements should be completed as minimum prerequisites before the initiation of psychopharmacotherapy. The treatment plan should be developed in conjunction with either the parent(s) or the primary caretaker and should include participation of the child or adolescent as appropriate to his or her understanding. Treatment with psychoactive drugs should always be part of a more comprehensive treatment regimen and is rarely appropriate as the sole treatment modality for a child or adolescent.

At variance with this traditional wisdom, however, are the results of several studies comparing the treatment of hyperactive children with stimulant medication alone versus stimulant medication combined with other interventions, such as cognitive training, attention control, social reinforcement, and parent training. A review of these studies concluded that "the additional use of various forms of psychotherapies (behavioral treatment, parent training, cognitive therapy) with stimulants has not resulted in superior outcomes than medication alone" (Klein, 1987, p. 1223). One possible factor contributing to this result is that in several studies children who were treated with methylphenidate alone showed improvement in social behavior. Following this course of treatment, adults—both parents and teachers—related to the children more positively (Klein, 1987). The Multimodal Treatment Study Group of Children with Attention-Deficit/Hyperactivity Disorder (MTA) Cooperative Group also found that stimulant medication was the most important factor in improving ADHD symptoms. This is further discussed in Chapter 4 (MTA Cooperative Group, 1999a, 1999b).

It seems clinically unlikely, however, that all the difficulties of ADHD children are secondary to the target symptoms that improve with methylphenidate. Those difficulties that result from other psychosocial problems, including psychopathological familial interactions and long-standing maladaptive behavioral patterns, would be expected to benefit from additional interventions; until it is possible to differentiate those children whose difficulties arise from their attention deficit *per se* from children whose symptoms are of multidetermined origin, a comprehensive treatment program is recommended for all children.

The legal guardian/caregiver and the child or adolescent patient, to the degree appropriate for the patient's age and psychopathology, should participate in formulating the treatment plan. The use of medication, including expected benefits and possible short- and long-term adverse effects, should be reviewed with the caregivers/parents and patient in understandable terminology. It is essential to carefully assess the attitude and reliability of the persons who will be responsible for administering the medication. Unless there is a positive or at least honestly neutral attitude toward medication and some therapeutic alliance with the parents, it will be difficult or infeasible to make a reliable assessment of drug efficacy and compliance. Likewise, to store and administer medication safely on an outpatient basis requires a responsible adult, especially if there are young children in the home or if the patient is at risk of suicide.

It should be explained to parents that, even if medication helps some biologically determined symptoms (e.g., in some cases of ADHD), the disorder's presence may have caused psychological difficulties in the child or adolescent as well as disturbances in familial and social relationships. Controlling or ameliorating the biological difficulty does not usually correct the long-standing internalized psychological or interpersonal problems and long-standing maladaptive patterns of behavior immediately. Resolving these difficulties will take time and may often require concomitant individual, group, family, or other therapeutic intervention.

Compliance

Compliance is an issue of particular importance in child and adolescent psychiatry. Because the parents or other caretakers are usually interposed between the physician and patient, compliance is somewhat more complex than in adult psychiatry, in which the patient usually relates directly to the physician.

Obviously, for psychopharmacotherapy to be effective in the disorder for which it is prescribed, the drug should be taken following the prescribed directions. Erratic compliance or running out of medication may cause the patient to undergo what is in effect an abrupt withdrawal of medication. Withdrawal syndromes may sometimes be confused with adverse effects, worsening of the clinical condition, or inadequate medication levels. In some cases, such as when an antipsychotic is used, the patient is at increased risk for an acute dystonic reaction if the physician starts at the optimal dose after the drug has been discontinued for several days or more. In addition, when medication is stopped, it may sometimes require a higher dose of medication to regain the same degree of symptom control. For example, Sleator et al. (1974) found that 7 of 28 hyperactive children who showed clinical worsening during a month-long placebo period after having received methylphenidate for 1 to 2 years required an increase in dose to regain their original clinical improvement. Hence, it is very important to emphasize to parents that running out of medication is to be avoided.

Many factors may interfere with compliance. Some parents will at times withhold medication if their child appears to be doing well, or, conversely, increase the medication without the physician's approval if behavior worsens, or even administer the drug to the child as a punishment.

When parents or legal guardians seek treatment for their children primarily because of pressure from others such as a school, a child welfare agency, or a court, there may be considerable resistance to both treatment and medication. Some of these parents may delay filling the prescription, lose it, or simply not fill it. Other parents consider it something to be done when convenient, especially if they have to travel any distance to get the prescription filled. If money is involved, even the amount necessary for travel to the pharmacy or to pay for the medication, some families, especially those on public assistance or very limited budgets, may have to delay purchasing the medication for legitimate financial reasons. These issues may come into play each time the prescription is renewed; additionally, it is common in many clinics for parents to miss appointments, including those when medication is to be renewed.

At times, some children and adolescents, both outpatients and inpatients, may actively try to avoid ingesting medication. Their techniques include pretending to place the pill in their mouths and later discarding it, and placing the pill under the tongue or between teeth and the cheek when swallowing and later spitting it out. Compliance in these cases may be improved if the person administering the medication observes it in the mouth and watches the patient swallow it. Crushing the medication may be helpful in some cases, but one must be certain that absorption rates will not be so significantly altered as to cause decreased clinical efficacy or adverse or toxic effects. If available, switching to a liquid form of the drug may be indicated for some patients.

Another factor that influences compliance, particularly in older children and adolescents, is related to adverse effects. For example, if they feel "funny" or different or if they develop a stomachache, they may be more reluctant to take medication. Adolescents may be especially sensitive to adverse effects affecting their sexual functioning. The more responsible a child or adolescent is for administering his or her own medication, the more likely, in general, that unpleasant, adverse effects will interfere with compliance. Akathisia is a particularly unpleasant adverse effect which Van Putten and Marder (1987) found increased the likelihood of non-compliance in adults receiving antipsychotics. Richardson et al. (1991) reported that children and adolescents who developed parkinsonism while receiving neu-roleptics were very aware of the symptoms and described them as "zombie-like" and a reason for noncompliance with outpatient treatment. Sheard (1975) noted that individuals treated for aggressive behavior may tolerate adverse effects poorly and discontinue treatment to avoid them. It is likely that these and other adverse effects would have similar influences on children and adolescents.

Noncompliance may be lessened sometimes if an adequate, understandable explanation of the simple pharmacokinetics of the drug is given to parents and patients when initially discussing medication. For example, the importance of keeping blood levels fairly constant by taking the medication as prescribed can be emphasized and reviewed again if lack of compliance becomes important. Conversely, when parents continue to sabotage treatment consciously, unconsciously, because of their own psychopathology, or for other reasons, and this behavior seriously interferes with the psychiatric treatment of a child or adolescent, it may be necessary to report the patient to a government agency as a case of medical neglect and request legal intervention. Likewise, it may be necessary to discontinue medication if compliance is very poor or so unacceptably erratic as to be potentially dangerous.

Explaining Medication to the Child or Adolescent

The clinician should discuss the medication with the child or adolescent as appropriate to the patient's psychopathology and ability to understand. Giving the patient an opportunity to participate in his or her treatment is helpful for many reasons.

The patient can feel like an active partner in the treatment. This can alleviate feelings of passivity (i.e., that treatment is something over which the patient has no control). Letting the patient know that he or she should pay attention to the effects of the medication in order to report them to the therapist, that the patient will be listened to, and that the information the patient conveys will be considered seriously in regulating the medicine also helps the therapeutic relationship. The patient can also be informed that although medication may provide some relief or help, it cannot do everything, and he or she must still contribute effort toward reaching the treatment goals. This can be particularly important during adolescence, when issues of autonomy and control over one's own body are normal developmental concerns.

Because the patient is experiencing firsthand the disorder being treated, in many cases valuable information necessary for regulating the medication can be obtained directly. Some fairly young children can express whether the medicine makes them feel better, more calm, or quiet; less mad or less like fighting; happier or sadder; less afraid, upset, nervous, or anxious; or worse, sleepy, tired, more bored, "madder," or harder to get along with; and so on. Although parents or caretakers can provide much useful information, they may be unaware of some information that the patient can provide if time is taken to learn the words or expressions that the child uses to communicate feelings and experiences.

Adverse effects should be explained so that the child or adolescent understands them. The patient's awareness that adverse effects may be transient (e.g., that tolerance for sedation may develop) or reversible with dose reduction may be helpful in gaining cooperation during the titration period. Foreknowledge also increases the sense of control and can decrease fear of some adverse effects. For example, if an acute dystonic reaction is a possibility, it is important to realize how frightening this can be to some patients (and their parents). Discussing beforehand that if this reaction occurs, medicine will help, and the condition will go away can make the experience less frightening. Also, if a rapidly effective oral medication such as diphenhydramine, an antihistamine with anticholinergic properties, is made available and patients and parents are aware of what is happening, the medication may be administered earlier in the process, frequently aborting a potentially more severe reaction.

Children who ride bicycles and adolescents who drive a car, motor bike, or motorcycle, or operate potentially dangerous machinery should be cautioned if a medication may cause sedation or other impairment. They should be told to wait until they are sure how they are reacting to the medication before engaging in these activities. Similarly, if an adolescent is likely to use alcohol or other psychoactive drugs, he or she should be warned of possible additive or other adverse effects. Drugs like monoamine oxidase inhibitors are too risky to recommend except in very cooperative patients who are able to follow the necessary strict dietary restrictions to avoid a potential hypertensive crisis.

Medicolegal Aspects of Medicating Children and Adolescents

Medicolegal issues usually involve concerns about the clinician's clinical competence. Although it may be obvious, these issues arise primarily when something goes wrong. Incidentally, that "wrong something" may have nothing to do with the clinician's specific treatment or competence but may, for example, be an outcome that displeases the patient or guardian. Even then, for a medicolegal issue to arise, someone who has become aware of it must decide to pursue the matter legally.

The importance of these issues is that the clinician's relationship with the patient and his or her family or caretakers can either increase or decrease the likelihood of legal proceedings. As a general rule, the better the quality of the relationship and rapport between the physician and the patient and his or her family, the less the likelihood for legal proceedings to occur. Parents who are angry at their child's physician, who feel neglected or not cared about, are more likely to institute legal proceedings. Taking time to explain what the medicine may and may not do is important; no medication can be guaranteed to be clinically effective and safe for every patient.

If there is a risk that a depressed patient may attempt suicide but the patient is not hospitalized, this should be discussed with all concerned parties. The patient may be asked to commit verbally or in writing to a contract to contact the clinician before any attempt to take his or her own life. Legal guardians should be informed of and concur with the decision that their child or ward will not be hospitalized and that, although there is a risk, the degree of risk is acceptable to avoid hospitalization. The guardians should be asked to provide more formal supervision until the depression improves sufficiently. If such measures are carried out and documented and a working rapport established, the risk of legal action and/or liability will be lessened should a suicide attempt, successful or otherwise, occur.

The clinician should make a genuine effort to establish a working rapport with parents who have consented under duress to the treatment of their child or adolescent (e.g., if their child has been removed from their care by a governmental agency because of abuse or neglect or where medication may be a prerequisite for remaining in a particular educational program), although this is frequently difficult.

Holzer (1989) noted that most, if not all, malpractice claims occur in cases with either an unexpected clinical outcome or an event that is perceived by the patient (or parents) as avoidable or preventable. The aspects of psychopharmacotherapy that have potential for medicolegal implications parallel this book's entire section on general principles of psychopharmacotherapy. Lawsuits are most frequently brought if something is omitted or if something goes wrong that could reasonably have been prevented. It should be emphasized that proper documentation in the clinical record is essential. If this is not done, the clinician's position is precarious if legal difficulties arise. Particular areas of concern are discussed later.

For a comprehensive overview of malpractice issues in psychiatric practice, see the chapter on this topic in Nurcombe and Partlett's *Child Mental Health and the Law* (1994).

Issues Concerning Diagnosis and Implications for Drug Choice and Premedication Workup

The areas of major concern are making a correct psychiatric diagnosis and being aware of any coexisting medical conditions. Taking accurate medical and psychiatric histories, including previous medications and the patient's response to them as well as adverse effects and allergic reactions, is essential. Nurcombe (1991) notes that if adverse reactions to a drug or drug interactions occur that could have been predicted by taking an accurate and adequate history, the physician may be held liable. History taking must be followed by a proper premedication workup; if the patient has a medical condition, the physician must consider how the psychotropic medication would affect that condition and whether there may be interactions with other medications the patient is taking. Some examples of this include the following: (a) making an incorrect diagnosis and prescribing the wrong medication, or failing to detect or recognize coexisting conditions that would contraindicate the chosen medication; (b) prescribing a drug that will interact adversely with another medication the patient is taking or a drug to which the patient has previously been allergic; or (c) failing to perform a baseline and serial electrocardiograms (ECGs) or to monitor serum levels when tricyclics are used because of possible cardiotoxicity.

Issues Concerning Informed Consent

The treatment plan should be discussed and agreed to by the legal guardian and the patient as appropriate for his or her age and understanding. The diagnosis and the risks and benefits of the proposed treatment and alternative treatment possibilities should be reviewed. To give informed consent, a patient (or legal guardian) must be mentally competent, have sufficient information available, and not be coerced. Adolescents 12 years of age and older should participate formally in developing their treatment plans and in giving informed "assent." If this is not possible, it should be so stated in the clinical record. It is wise to have both the legal guardian and, when appropriate, the patient sign the treatment plan and/or an informed consent ("assent" for underage individuals) for medication. If this is not done, at a minimum the clinician must document the discussion of the treatment plan and the response of the patient and legal guardian in the clinical record.

Nurcombe (1991) recommends that the following be discussed:

a. The nature of the condition that requires treatment.
b. The nature and purpose of the proposed treatment and the probability that it will succeed.
c. The risks and consequences of the proposed treatment. [It should be noted, e.g., if the proposed medication is an off-label use and that possible rare or long-term treatment-emergent adverse events or unknown drug interactions may occur, especially for newer drugs where there is relatively little clinical experience. Also newer, post-initial drug marketing adverse events must be explained clearly and not minimized which could be interpreted as misleading in order to obtain consent, for example, the recent warning for all antidepressant drugs that they increased suicidal thinking and behavior in short-term studies in children and adolescents with major depressive and other psychiatric disorders should not be downplayed. Another example would be to discuss possible prolactin increase, weight gain, and onset of type 2 diabetes with risperidone.]
d. Alternatives to the proposed treatment and their attendant risks and consequences.
e. Prognosis with and without the proposed treatment (p. 1132).

Popper (1987a) adds that it should be explicitly stated that there may be unknown risks in taking the medication, especially when using novel psychopharmacological treatments or treatments in which risks versus benefits are uncertain.

Involuntary medication of patients occurs primarily in emergency rooms and in inpatient wards. This is usually permissible in a true emergency, but Nurcombe (1991) cautions that even involuntary commitment to a hospital for psychiatric treatment permits involuntary medication only in narrowly defined circumstances. Administering medication forcibly without judicial approval in a nonemergency situation may be considered battery. Physicians should become thoroughly familiar with their state laws and local hospital policies governing these matters.

Issues Concerning the Administration of Medication

Issues that concern the administration of medication include justification for the decision to use medication in treating the psychiatric condition (risks vs. benefits), rationale for the initial drug chosen, and administration of the drug by the appropriate route, usually orally, and in a clinically efficacious dose. If a patient is suicidal, the prescribing physician should ascertain to the best of his or her ability and document that only sublethal amounts of medication are accessible to the patient. It is best to have a responsible adult, usually a parent, have control of the medication—keeping it where the patient does not have access to it and dispense it to the patient as directed. The medication should be completely or nearly finished before more is prescribed. The clinician must monitor the medication adequately for the duration of the therapy and should either discontinue the medication or attempt to do so at appropriate intervals, or document in the clinical record the reasons for the decision not to follow this protocol.

Examples of behavior that may increase medicolegal risk include failing to prescribe medication for a condition for which most practitioners would; prescribing a medication without personally evaluating the patient (e.g., based on another physician's report); prescribing an inappropriate drug for the diagnosis (e.g., amphetamines to a drug abuser); using an unsatisfactory rationale to justify the choice of drug, administering an inappropriate dosage for the disorder (e.g., subtherapeutic levels); or administering medication by an inappropriate route (e.g., continuing to give medication intramuscularly when it is no longer indicated or necessary). A patient's use of prescribed medication to attempt or successfully complete a suicide may also result in legal action.

Off-label Prescribing/Deviating from a Manufacturer's Labeling of a Drug

This book discusses many uses of psychoactive medications that are different from those formally recommended by the manufacturer or approved by the U. S. Food and Drug Administration (FDA) for advertising as safe and effective. Many of these off-label uses are medically accepted, but others are not yet common medical practice. Deviating from the usual clinical practice may increase the risk of legal action. Although legally permissible, using FDA-approved drugs for non-FDA–approved indications and using FDA-approved drugs for approved indications in children below the age limit for which they are approved may increase the potential for liability. Similarly, not adhering to the recommendations of the drug manufacturer (in the package insert or as reprinted in the *Physicians' Desk Reference* [PDR])—for example, exceeding recommended dosages—should alert the clinician to carefully document the rationale for doing so. In general, however, clinicians are on solid ground if they have assessed the risk/benefit ratio for prescribing a medication for a non-FDA–approved indication and have documented a scientifically reasonable rationale for choosing a particular drug over other possible treatments in the medical record.

It should be clear that the preceding discussion of off-label use applies primarily to situations where data were lacking at the time of application for approval by the FDA and subsequent research and clinical practice support a rationale for their use. Most frequently, there were insufficient data to determine efficacy and safety in the pediatric age-group or the drug was being used for a diagnosis not initially studied. It should be clear that ignoring specific safety recommendations contained in the package insert that are based on verifiable data is an entirely different situation and is not condoned.

In clinical practice, standard treatments and off-label (non-FDA–approved) but clinically accepted treatments that may be efficacious with less risk almost always should be tried before less clinically accepted or riskier medications. Concurrence of a consultant and appropriate psychopharmacological references supporting such use may be helpful when the off-label use is not commonly accepted (Nurcombe, 1991). As a general principle, the more novel the treatment or uncertain the risk/benefit ratio, the more severely disabling the condition should be for which it is used.

Issues Concerned with Documenting Ongoing Appropriate Attention to Medication and Related Matters in the Clinical Record

The patient's clinical record should reflect continued appropriate monitoring of the medication's efficacy; monitoring for the presence or absence of adverse effects, including tardive dyskinesia; results of laboratory tests or other procedures (e.g., ECG) performed at appropriate intervals to monitor adverse effects; justifications for increases or decreases in dosage or changes in times of administration; decisions to employ a drug holiday or discontinue medication; and consequences of discontinuing medication, including any change in symptomatology, reexacerbation of symptoms, rebound effects, or withdrawal syndromes such as a withdrawal dyskinesia.

When patients are hospitalized, it is important for the clinician to address in the medical record not only his or her own observations of the patient but also those of other professionals who have reported or recorded behaviors or symptoms that may indicate adverse effects of medication (e.g., unsteadiness of gait reported by a nurse or falling asleep in class reported by a teacher).

Most authorities recommend that children and adolescents who are receiving psychoactive medication should have it discontinued or at least tapered down periodically, typically within 6 months to at most 1 year, to ascertain whether it is still needed or whether a lower dose might be sufficient. That this has been done should be documented in the chart, and if the clinician delays this tapering excessively, the reason should be clearly explained in the chart (e.g., the previous attempt resulted in a severe relapse of symptoms that were difficult to control in a schizophrenic adolescent or a clinical decision has been reached to delay an attempt to lower or discontinue medication until the completion of the school year because functioning has been marginal although somewhat improved with medication). Decisions such as these should also be discussed with the parents and the patient and their agreement documented as part of the treatment plan.

The reviews of Nurcombe (1991) and Nurcombe and Partlett (1994) of medicolegal aspects of the entire practice of child and adolescent psychiatry, including specific court cases and decisions, are recommended to the interested reader. Popper (1987a) has written an interesting chapter on ethical considerations of the relationship between obtaining consent for the use of medication from parents and children and adolescents and incomplete or unknown medical knowledge of the risks and long-term effects of psychoactive medication used during childhood and adolescence.

BASELINE ASSESSMENTS PRIOR TO INITIATION OF MEDICATION

All patients should have a complete medical history and physical and neurologic examinations. These examinations are essential to identify any organic factors contributing to the psychiatric symptomatology and any coexisting medical abnormalities. In addition, all drugs may cause adverse physical and psychological effects; hence, a baseline examination prior to the initiation of psychopharmacotherapy should be mandatory.

Although there is considerable information available for stimulant medications, relatively little information is available concerning the long-term adverse effects of psychoactive drugs on the growth and development of children and adolescents. Because of this fact as well as the potential medicolegal ramifications, particularly when drugs are used for non-FDA–approved indications, it is recommended that the premedication workup be reasonably comprehensive. The reader who wishes a more detailed review of laboratory tests and diagnostic procedures applicable to general psychiatry than that provided in the subsequent text is referred to the helpful book by Rosse et al. (1989).

Physical Examination

The physical examination should include recording baseline temperature, pulse and respiration rates, and blood pressure. Height and weight should be entered on standardized growth charts, such as the National Center for Health Statistics Growth Charts (Hamill et al. 1976), so that serial measurements and percentiles may be plotted over time. In their recent review, Correll and Carlson (2006) have indicated that the relative potency of atypical/second generation antipsychotic drugs in inducing weight gain and increasing the risk for developing the metabolic syndrome is approximately: clozapine = olanzapine ≫ risperidone ≥ quetiapine > ziprasidone ≥ aripiprazole.

Laboratory Tests and Diagnostic Procedures

The following are frequently recommended premedication laboratory tests and diagnostic procedures. Some of these tests may have already been done as a part of the pediatric/medical evaluation that should be a part of any comprehensive psychiatric evaluation. These tests will be addressed more specifically under each class of medications or, if appropriate, for specific drugs when they are discussed. Obviously, the premedication workup will be influenced by and should be modified to accommodate any particular abnormal findings in the medical history or examination, such as renal, thyroid, and cardiac abnormalities, or by any initial abnormal laboratory results themselves.

Laboratory tests routinely or frequently recommended as part of a comprehensive, complete, pediatric examination, and/or premedication workup include the following:

1. Complete blood cell count (CBC), differential, and hematocrit
2. Urinalysis
3. Blood urea nitrogen (BUN) level
4. Serum electrolyte levels for sodium (Na^+), potassium (K^+), chloride (Cl^-), calcium (Ca^{2+}), and phosphate (PO_4^{3-}), and carbon dioxide (CO_2) content
5. Liver function tests: aspartate aminotransferase (AST) or serum glutamic oxaloacetic transaminase (SGOT), alanine aminotransferase (ALT) or serum glutamic pyruvic transaminase (SGPT), alkaline phosphatase, lactic dehydrogenase (LDH), and bilirubin (total and indirect)

6. Blood glucose especially when second-generation antipsychotics will be pre-scribed as they can cause metabolic syndrome and cause or exacerbate type 2 diabetes, The American Diabetes Association has published, in collaboration with the APA, a protocol for monitoring adult patients who will be treated with second generation antipsychotics. Fasting plasma glucose and a fasting lipid profile are recommended (American Diabetes Association and American Psychiatric Association, 2004)

7. Lipid profile: hyperlipidemia with elevated triglyceride and cholesterol serum levels have been reported as an adverse effect of some second generation antipsychotics. Sheitman et al. (1999) reported an increase of almost 40% in serum triglycerides in adults taking olanzapine

8. Serum lead level determination in children under 7 years of age and in older children when indicated

9. If substance abuse (alcohol or drugs) is suspected, screening of urine and/or blood is usually indicated

Other laboratory tests may be recommended prior to using specific psychoactive medications.

Pregnancy/Pregnancy Test

Because drugs may have known or unknown adverse effects on the developing fetus, a serum beta human chorionic gonadotropin test for pregnancy should be considered for any adolescent capable of becoming pregnant, at a time as close to beginning the medication as convenient and reasonable. A related issue is that, if an adolescent is considered to be at significant risk for becoming pregnant despite birth control counseling, certain medications (e.g., lithium) should not be prescribed if at all possible, as the embryo would usually be exposed to the drug before pregnancy was detected.

Risk versus benefit must be carefully considered for both the patient and the (potential) embryo/fetus if a woman is on medication and has unprotected sexual relations or attempts to become pregnant. As is also well known, pregnancies do occur at times even with "protected" sex. Once pregnancy is verified, serious concerns about teratogenic risk to the embryo/fetus arise. "A pregnant woman should not take any drug unless it is necessary for her own health or that of her fetus" (Friedman and Polifka, 1998, p. ix). Additional concerns occur when mothers who are taking medication wish to breast-feed their infants, as some drugs and/or their metabolites are secreted in breast milk.

Discussion of these very important issues on a drug-by-drug basis is beyond the scope of this book. In addition to the package insert, the reader who needs more information is referred to an excellent overview of the management of pregnant psychiatric patients on medication and a compendium of psychiatric drugs with their known risks and teratogenic effects, and the risks related to breast feeding (Friedman and Polifka, 1998).

Thyroid Function Tests

There is a strong association between clinical thyroid disease and psychiatric dis-orders, particularly mood disorders (Esposito et al. 1997). Thyroid function tests (thyroxine [T_4], triiodothyronine resin uptake [T_3RU], and thyroid-stimulating hormone or thyrotropin) are recommended prior to the use of tricyclic antidepressants and lithium. Abnormal thyroid function can aggravate cardiac arrhythmias that may occur as an adverse effect of tricyclic antidepressants (PDR, 1995). Lithium has been reported to cause hypothyroidism with lower T_3 and T_4 levels and elevated I_{131} uptake.

Kidney Function Tests

Many drugs are excreted at least partially through the kidney and in the urine. Because of reported adverse effects of lithium carbonate on the kidney, baseline evaluation of kidney function should be determined. Jefferson et al. (1987) suggest that a baseline serum creatinine and urinalysis are usually adequate and that more extensive testing (e.g., creatinine clearance, 24-hour urine volume, and maximal urine osmolality) is not practical or necessary for most patients.

Prolactin Levels

Prolactin is a polypeptide protein hormone synthesized and secreted by lactotrophs of the anterior pituitary gland. Prolactin stimulates breast tissue development and production of milk and lactation. Prolactin secretion is controlled by the tuberoinfundibular dopamine pathway and the inhibitory action of dopamine on D_2 receptors located on the surface of pituitary lactotrophs (Ayd, 1995; Stahl, 2000). Drugs that antagonize dopamine D_2 receptors, that is, with D_2 blocking action such as antipsychotics and cocaine, as well as drugs that may indirectly influence dopaminergic function such as fluoxetine, therefore have the capability of causing elevated prolactin levels (hyperprolactinemia) that have been associated with inhibition of gonadotropin secretion, with galactorrhea and amenorrhea in women and with gynecomastia, decreased testosterone level, and impotence in men (Kane and Lieberman, 1992). In their recent review, Correll and Carlson (2006) have indicated that the relative potency of antipsychotic drugs in inducing hyperprolactinemia is approximately: risperidone > haloperidol > olanzapine > ziprasidone > quetiapine > clozapine > aripiprazole.

The long-term clinical implications/effects of hyperprolactinemia on the general maturation and development of children and adolescents, and, in particular, on their endocrine and central nervous systems, are unknown. Because of this, a baseline prolactin level may be useful prior to initiating treatment with a drug known to affect prolactin secretion.

Wudarsky et al. (1999) reported prolactin levels in 35 subjects (22 males, 13 females; mean age, 14.1 ± 2.3 years, age range 9.1 to 19 years) diagnosed with schizophrenia ($N = 32$) or psychotic disorder not otherwise specified (NOS) ($N = 3$) before age 13 who were treated with haloperidol, olanzapine, and/or clozapine for 6 weeks. Reference normal plasma prolactin values used for this study were as follows: adult range (combined male and female), 1.39 to 24.2 ng/mL; mean for adult males, 5.6 ng/mL (range, 1.61 to 18.77 ng/mL), and for adult females, 7.97 (range, 1.39 to 24.2). Conventional normal reference values for prepubescent males are 4.0 ± 0.5 ng/mL and for prepubescent females, 4.5 ± 0.6 ng/mL.

Mean baseline prolactin levels were measured after a mean washout period of 3 weeks and were below normal limits. Prolactin levels during the sixth week were significantly elevated from baseline for all three drugs (haloperidol, 9.0 ± 4.2 ng/mL vs. 47.8 ± 30.6 ng/mL [$P < .001$]; clozapine, 9.0 ± 3.4 ng/mL vs. 11.2 ± 4.0 ng/mL

[$P < .007$]; olanzapine, 10.0 ± 4.7 ng/mL vs. 23.7 ± 7.7 ng/mL [$P < .003$]). The mean plasma prolactin level for the 10 subjects on haloperidol was above the upper limit of normal (ULN), and 9 subjects had levels above the ULN. The mean plasma prolactin value for the 15 subjects on clozapine, although significantly elevated from baseline, remained within the ULN, and plasma prolactin levels remained within the normal range for all 15 subjects. The mean plasma prolactin level for the 10 subjects on olanzapine was above the ULN, and 7 of the subjects had plasma prolactin levels above the ULN. The authors noted that plasma prolactin levels usually returned to baseline values within a few days after medication was discontinued but persisted for up to 3 weeks in a few cases. When compared with adults, these younger subjects had more robust increases in plasma prolactin levels on haloperidol and olanzapine but not clozapine, perhaps because of a greater number or sensitivity of dopamine receptors in the tuberoinfundibular systems of children and adolescents. The authors called for additional studies of prolactin response to various medications in this age-group and the effects of hyperprolactinemia on their development and maturation (Wudarsky et al. 1999).

Saito et al. (2004) conducted a prospective study of 40 subjects (22 males, 18 females; mean age, 13.4 years, age range 5 to 18 years) that examined the change in prolactin levels from baseline to a mean of 11.2 weeks of treatment with risperidone ($N = 21$), olanzapine ($N = 13$), or quetiapine ($N = 6$). Primary diagnoses were schizophrenia/psychosis ($N = 14$); mood disorder ($N = 14$); disruptive behavior disorder ($N = 9$); intermittent explosive disorder ($N = 1$); pervasive developmental disorder NOS ($N = 1$); and eating disorder NOS ($N = 1$); 80% of the subjects were taking two or more psychotropic medications. The authors hypothesized that, because of risperidone's relatively high affinity for D_2 receptors in the pituitary, children and adolescents receiving risperidone would develop hyperprolactinemia to a greater extent than those subjects receiving olanzapine and quetiapine. Baseline prolactin levels were drawn before beginning the atypical antipsychotic in 17 (43%) subjects and within 1 week after beginning treatment in 23 (57%). The reference range for normal was 3.9 to 25.4 ng/mL for all children, 4.1 to 18.4 ng/mL for males, and 3.4 to 24.1 ng/mL for females. Baseline prolactin levels, pubertal status, and gender were not significantly different among the three groups. Hyperprolactinemia was present in 53% of the subjects at end point. A greater percentage of subjects receiving risperidone (15/21 or 71%) had elevated prolactin levels (group mean end-point level 46.8 ± 33.3 mg/mL) than subjects receiving olanzapine (5/13 or 38%) with a group mean end-point level of 24.5 ± 17.8 ng/mL or subjects receiving quetiapine (1/6 or 17%) with a group mean end-point level of 16.7 ± 10.1 ng/mL. The end-point level of risperidone was significantly higher than that of olanzapine ($P = .008$) and that of quetiapine ($P = .027$). Prolactin levels in the olanzapine and quetiapine groups were not significantly different from each other. Regarding end-point prolactin levels, there were no significant gender differences, and postpubertal females did not have significantly different levels from the entire group. In addition, end-point prolactin levels were not associated with changes in weight. Interestingly, 25% (seven women and three men) of the entire group reported sexual adverse effects: breast tenderness ($N = 4$), irregular menses ($N = 3$), decreased libido ($N = 3$), erectile dysfunction ($N = 3$), galactorrhea, and amenorrhea ($N = 1$); the authors suggested that this rather high level resulted from their asking specific questions rather than recording only spontaneous reports. There was no association between the drug taken and sexual side effects; five of these subjects were on risperidone; three were on olanzapine; and two were on quetiapine. The authors also noted that the lower incidence of hyperprolactinemia in their study compared to that of Alfaro et al. (2002) is likely because the doses they employed were only approximately one half those used in the Alfaro et al. study. This study also suggested that children and adolescents may be more likely than adults to develop hyperprolactinemia at a specific dose of atypical antipsychotic.

Pappagallo and Silva (2004) reviewed the literature through 2003 on the effect of atypical antipsychotic drugs in children and adolescents. They identified 14 studies with a total of 276 subjects. The authors concluded that, of the atypical antipsychotics, risperidone has been more frequently associated with hyperprolactinemia and clozaril, the least; however, they noted that aripiprazole, which has been recently approved, has partial D_2 agonist properties and may result in smaller increases in prolactin levels; to date, studies in adults have shown no significant prolactin elevations; values in children and adolescents had not been reported. The authors note that there is some evidence that prolactin levels may decrease over time without dose reduction. When prolactinemia is present, the authors suggest that other possible causes, including oral birth control pills, opiates, and pregnancy, be considered. If the increase in prolactin is mild and adverse effects associated with prolactin are not troublesome, one can elect to continue to administer the medication with close monitoring of clinical effects and periodic prolactin levels. It is noted that data which elucidate the long-term effects of hyperprolactinemia on the physical and emotional development of such children and adolescents are not yet available.

Croonenberghs et al. (2005) conducted an international multisite 1-year open-label trial of risperidone with 504 patients (419 males, 85 females; mean age 9.7 ± 2.5 years, range 4 to 14 years). Mean serum prolactin levels at baseline were 7.7 ± 7.1 ng/mL for boys (ULN 18 ng/mL) and 10.1 ± 8.1 ng/mL for girls (ULN 25 ng/mL). Prolactin levels rose rather sharply and peak average prolactin levels occurred at week 4 in both boys and girls and were above normal limits for both (boys, 28.2 ± 14.2 ng/mL and girls, 35.4 ± 19.1 ng/mL). Prolactin levels then gradually decreased until by the ninth month of treatment they were again within normal limits for both and remained there for the duration of the study although they remained higher than baseline. The following adverse effects, which could possibly be related to hyperprolactinemia, were noted: mild to moderate gynecomastia in 25 subjects (22 men, 3 women); menstrual disturbances in 6 subjects; galactorrhea in 1 patient and moderately severe menorrhagia in 1 patient. However, as these symptoms can occur in normal populations, it is impossible to assess the added risk attributed by risperidone as there is no control group.

Electrocardiogram

Many psychiatric medications may have adverse effects on the cardiovascular system, on both the electroconductivity of the heart, as evidenced by the ECG, and on hemodynamics (e.g., blood pressure). A baseline ECG is recommended as part of the complete physical examination of every child prior to prescribing psychoactive medication; it should be mandatory in any person with a history of, or clinical findings suggestive of, cardiovascular disease. ECGs are noninvasive and relatively inexpensive. It is not rare to detect an unsuspected cardiac abnormality.

The American Heart Association has issued useful guidelines regarding the cardiovascular monitoring of children and adolescents receiving psychotropic drugs (Gutgesell et al. 1999 [note that the reprint of this article in the *Journal of the American Academy of Child & Adolescent Psychiatry* appears to have inadvertently omitted the anticonvulsants from Table I]). Although helpful, these guidelines are conservative; for example, they state that no ECG monitoring is necessary when prescribing alpha-2-adrenergic agonists such as clonidine and guanfacine, while Kofoed et al. (1999) present data supporting a cogent argument that pretreatment ECGs are necessary to assist in distinguishing drug-induced changes from variability unrelated to the drug effects of clonidine. In addition, the list of psychotropic agents included in the guidelines is not up to date; all the atypical antipsychotics as well as the newer antidepressants are missing.

It also frequently occurs that if the response to a particular drug is not clinically satisfactory, it is discontinued and another drug is prescribed or another drug may be added to the initial drug. In some such cases the new drug or combination of drugs would make an ECG necessary for optimal clinical practice.

A baseline ECG should be recorded prior to the administration of tricyclic antidepressants to determine any preexisting conduction or other cardiac abnormality because clinically important cardiotoxicity may occur, especially at higher serum levels. The ECG should be monitored with dose increases and periodically thereafter if tricyclics are used (this is discussed in detail in Chapter 7 under "Tricyclic Antidepressants and Cardiotoxicity").

Most of the antipsychotics, both standard and atypical, may cause ECG changes, including prolongation of the QTc interval. Lithium may also cause cardiac abnormalities, and an ECG is recommended prior to initiating therapy. Carbamazepine may also prolong the QTc interval.

Polypharmacy may also cause drug/drug interactions; of particular importance are interactions where one drug may affect the metabolism of a second drug (e.g., by inhibiting metabolism by the cytochrome P450 enzyme system). For example, two sudden deaths were reported when clarithromycin, which inhibits the cytochrome P450 enzyme system, and pimozide, which is metabolized by the P450 enzyme system, were administered simultaneously, giving rise to the possibility that their interaction was a contributing or causal factor.

Electroencephalogram

An electroencephalogram (EEG) may be considered for patients to whom antipsychotics, tricyclic antidepressants, or lithium will be administered, because all these drugs have been associated with either lowered threshold for seizures or other EEG changes. This group would include patients who have a history of seizure disorder, who are on an antiepileptic drug for a seizure disorder, or who may be at risk for seizures (e.g., following brain surgery or head injury).

Blanz and Schmidt (1993) reported a significant increase in pathologic EEG findings (short biphasic waves) in child and adolescent patients receiving clozapine. Similarly, Remschmidt et al. (1994) reported EEG changes in 16 (44%) of 36 adolescents being treated with clozapine. Baseline EEG and periodic monitoring of EEG while on clozapine should be mandatory.

Baseline Behavioral Assessment

Clinical Observations

Baseline observations and careful characterizations of both behavior and target symptoms must be recorded in the clinical record. These should include direct observations by the clinician in the waiting room, office, playroom, and/or ward, as well as those reported by other reliable observers in other locations, such as the home and school. It is important to include usual eating and sleeping patterns, because these may be altered by many drugs. These observations should be described both qualitatively and quantitatively (amplitude and frequency), and the circumstances in which they occur should be noted in the clinical record.

It is also essential to record an accurate baseline rating in the clinical record before beginning psychopharmacotherapy in children or adolescents who have existing abnormal movements or who are at risk of developing them (e.g., patients diagnosed with autistic disorder or severe mental retardation and/or patients who will be treated with antipsychotics). This documentation is necessary both to follow the patient's clinical course and to be able to differentiate among recrudescence of preexisting involuntary movements, stereotypies, and mannerisms and any subsequent withdrawal dyskinesias or new stereotypies that may occur when medication, particularly an antipsychotic, is discontinued. The availability of these longitudinal data becomes even more critical if the treating physician changes. Although the baseline data can be documented in the clinician's records, the use of a rating scale such as the Abnormal Involuntary Movement Scale (AIMS) (Rating Scales, 1985) that assesses abnormal movements is strongly recommended.

To be able to assess the efficacy of a specific medication, a baseline observation period, with reasonably stable or worsening target symptoms, is necessary. Other than in emergency situations (e.g., a violent, physically assaultive, and/or severely psychotic individual), observation of the patient for a minimum of 7 to 10 days is recommended before initiating pharmacotherapy. For inpatients, this will permit assessment of the combined effects of hospitalization and a therapeutic milieu and the removal of the identified patient from his or her living situation on the patient's psychopathology and symptoms. For outpatients, this observation period will give the clinician an opportunity to see the effect of the clinical contact and assessment on the symptom expression of the patient and the psychodynamic equilibrium of the family. During this observation period, some children and adolescents, both inpatients and outpatients, will improve enough that psychopharmacotherapy will no longer be indicated. Unfortunately, because of the high cost of inpatient hospitalization and pressure by various managed care organizations, patients are often medicated before there is time to assess their responses to the inpatient environment.

Rating Scales

Rating scales are an essential component of psychopharmacological research. They provide a means of recording serial qualitative and quantitative measurements of behaviors, and their interrater reliability can be determined. Two of the most influential publications concerning rating scales and psychopharmacological research in children are the *Psychopharmacology Bulletin's* special issue *Pharmacotherapy of Children* (1973) and its 1985 issue featuring "Rating Scales and Assessment Instruments for Use in Pediatric Psychopharmacology Research" (Rating Scales, 1985).

Although rating scales are valuable in nonresearch settings, they tend to be used less in clinical practice. Perhaps those most frequently used are the various

TABLE 2.1 ● **Conners Parent-Teacher Questionnaire**

INSTRUCTIONS: Listed below are items concerning children's behavior or the problems they sometimes have. Read each item carefully and decide how much you think this child has been bothered by this problem at this time: **Not at All, Just a Little, Pretty Much**, or **Very Much**. Indicate your choice by circling the number in the appropriate column to the right of each item.

Answer All Items	Not at All	Just a Little	Pretty Much	Very Much
1. Restless (overactive)	0	1	2	3
2. Excitable, impulsive	0	1	2	3
3. Disturbs other children	0	1	2	3
4. Fails to finish things he starts (short attention span)	0	1	2	3
5. Fidgeting	0	1	2	3
6. Inattentive, distractible	0	1	2	3
7. Demands must be met immediately; frustrated	0	1	2	3
8. Cries	0	1	2	3
9. Mood changes quickly	0	1	2	3
10. Temper outbursts (explosive and unpredictable behavior)	0	1	2	3
	None	Minor	Moderate	Severe
How serious a problem do you think this child has at this time?	0	1	2	3

Modified from Department of Health, Education, and Welfare, Health Services and Mental Health Administration, National Institutes of Health.

Conners rating instruments: Conners Teacher Questionnaire (CTQ), Conners Parent-Teacher Questionnaire, Conners Parent Questionnaire (CPQ) (*Psychopharmacology Bulletin*, 1973). The abbreviated Conners Parent-Teacher Questionnaire (CPTQ), reproduced as Table 2.1, is useful in helping to identify patients who have ADHD and to record serial ratings that provide good periodic estimates of the clinical efficacy of medication in the classroom and home environments. The CPTQ can be completed in a short time because it has only 11 items. The first 10 items are common to the CTQ and the CPQ; the eleventh item is an overall estimate of the degree of seriousness of the child's problem at the time of the rating; that item is not included in the following discussion of scoring. A total score of 15 on the first 10 items has been widely used in research as the cut-off for two standard deviations above the mean, and subjects scoring 15 or more points have been considered hyperactive (Sleator, 1986). The mean value of the 10 items of the CPTQ yields a score comparable to factor IV, the hyperactivity index, of the CTQ, and a 0.5-point or more decrease in the mean (or a decrease of 5 points in the total score on the first 10 items of the CPTQ) generally indicates that medication is effecting a meaningful improvement (Greenhill, 1990).

The AIMS (Table 2.2) is a 12-item scale designed to record in detail the occurrence of dyskinetic movements. Abnormal involuntary movements are rated

(text continues on page 29)

TABLE 2.2 ● Abnormal Involuntary Movement Scale (AIMS)

INSTRUCTIONS: Complete Examination Procedure before making ratings. MOVEMENT RATINGS: Rate highest severity observed. Rate movements that occur upon activation one less than those observed spontaneously

		(Circle One)				
FACIAL AND ORAL MOVEMENTS:	1. **Muscles of Facial Expression** (e.g., movements of forehead, eyebrows, periorbital area, cheeks; include frowning, blinking, smiling, grimacing)	0	1	2	3	4
	2. **Lips and Perioral Area** (e.g., puckering, pouting, smacking)	0	1	2	3	4
	3. **Jaw** (e.g., biting, clenching, chewing, mouth opening, lateral movement	0	1	2	3	4
	4. **Tongue** Rate only increase in movement both in and out of mouth, NOT inability to sustain movement	0	1	2	3	4
EXTREMITY MOVEMENTS:	5. **Upper** (arms, wrists, hands, fingers) Include choreic movements (i.e., rapid, objectively purposeless, irregular, spontaneous), athetoid movements, (i.e., slow, irregular, complex, serpentine). Do NOT include tremor (i.e., repetitive, regular, rhythmic)	0	1	2	3	4
	6. **Lower** (legs, knees, ankles, toes) e.g., lateral knee movement, foot tapping, heel dropping, foot squirming, inversion and eversion of foot	0	1	2	3	4
TRUNK MOVEMENTS:	7. **Neck, shoulders, hips** (e.g., rocking, twisting, squirming, pelvic gyrations	0	1	2	3	4

GLOBAL JUDGMENTS:	8. **Severity of abnormal movements**		
		None, normal	0
		Minimal	1
		Mild	2
		Moderate	3
		Severe	4
	9. **Incapacitation due to abnormal movements** Rate only patient's report	None, normal	0
		Minimal	1
		Mild	2
		Moderate	3
		Severe	4
	10. **Patient's awareness of abnormal movements** Rate only patient's report	No awareness	0
		Aware, no distress	1
		Aware, mild distress	2
		Aware, moderate distress	3
		Aware, severe distress	4
DENTAL STATUS:	11. **Current problems with teeth and/or dentures**	No	0
		Yes	1
	12. **Does patient usually wear dentures?**	No	0
		Yes	1

(continued)

TABLE 2.2 ● *(Continued)*

EXAMINATION PROCEDURE

Either before or after completing the Examination Procedure observe the patient unobtrusively, at rest (e.g., in waiting room).

The chair to be used in this examination should be a hard, firm one without arms.

1. Ask patient whether there is anything in his/her mouth (gum, candy, etc.) and if there is, to remove it.
2. Ask patient about the current condition of his/her teeth. Ask patients if he/she wears dentures. Do teeth or dentures bother patient now?
3. Ask patient whether he/she notices any movements in mouth, face, hands, or feet. If yes, ask to describe and to what extent they currently bother patient or interfere with his/her activities.
4. Have patient sit in chair with hands on knees, legs slightly apart, and feet flat on floor. (Look at entire body for movements while in this position.)
5. Ask patient to sit with hands hanging unsupported. If male, between legs, if female and wearing a dress, hanging over knees. (Observe hands and other body areas.)
6. Ask patient to open mouth. (Observe tongue at rest within mouth.) Do this twice.
7. Ask patient to protrude tongue. (Observe abnormalities of tongue movement.) Do this twice.
8. Ask patient to tap thumb, with each finger, as rapidly as possible for 10–15 seconds; separately with right hand, then with left hand. (Observe facial and leg movements.)[a]
9. Flex and extend patient's left and right arms (one at a time). (Note any rigidity and rate on DOTES.)
10. Ask patient to stand up. (Observe in profile. Observe all body areas again, hips included.)
11. Ask patient to extend both arms outstretched in front with palms down. (Observe trunk, legs, and mouth.)[a]
12. Have patient walk a few paces, turn, and walk back to chair. (Observe hands and gait.) Do this twice.[a]

DOTES = Dosage and Treatment Emergent Symptoms Scale (Guy, 1976).
Code: 0 = None; 1 = Minimal, may be extreme normal; 2 = Mild; 3 = Moderate; 4 = Severe.
[a]Activated movements.
Modified from Department of Health, Education, and Welfare. Public Health Service. Alcohol, Drug Abuse, and Mental Health Administration, National Institute of Mental Health.

on a 5-point scale from 0 to 4, with 0 being none, 1 being minimal or extreme normal, 2 being mild, 3 being moderate, and 4 being severe. If a procedure is used to activate the movements (e.g., having the patient tap his or her thumb with each finger as rapidly as possible for 10 to 15 seconds separately with the right and then the left hand), movements are rated one point lower than those occurring spontaneously. Seven of the items rate abnormal involuntary movements in specific topographies: four items concern facial and oral movements, two items concern extremity movements, and one item concerns trunk movements. Three items are global ratings: two by the clinician concern the overall severity of the abnormal movements and the estimated degree of incapacity from them and a third records the patient's own degree of awareness of the abnormal movements. Using the AIMS will also make it less likely that an area that should be assessed will be omitted inadvertently and will also provide quantitative ratings for following the clinical course. Having a baseline and subsequent AIMS ratings available is most helpful to the initial treating physician in assessing any changes in baseline abnormal involuntary movements increases, decrements, or changes in topography during the course of active treatment with psychoactive medication, as well as during periods of withdrawal from medication. These ratings are often essential to differentiate preexisting abnormal involuntary movements from withdrawal dyskinesias. Such ratings are even more helpful when other physicians may assume the treatment of the patient at a future time.

Medicating the Patient: Selecting the Initial and Subsequent Medications

In general, it is recommended that a drug approved by the FDA—for the patient's age, diagnosis, and target symptoms—be chosen initially unless other, off-label drugs which are equally or more clinically effective and safer regarding adverse effects are available and are regularly used in the practice of child and adolescent psychopharmacology (e.g., the atypical antipsychotics). Factors such as selecting the drug with the least risk of serious adverse effects; known previous response(s) of the patient to psychotropic medication; the responses of siblings, parents, and other relatives with psychiatric illnesses to psychotropic medication; family history (e.g., a history of Tourette's disorder); and the clinician's previous experience in using the medication should also be weighed in choosing the initial and, if necessary, subsequent drugs.

Recently, the Texas Children's Medication Algorithm Project published algorithms for the treatment of childhood major depressive disorder (Hughes et al. 1999) and childhood ADHD with and without common comorbid disorders (Pliszka et al. 2000a, 2000b) diagnosed by DSM-IV (APA, 1994) criteria. The algorithms and guidelines for their use were developed using expert consensus methodology based on scientific evidence, when available, and clinical experience and opinion, when necessary, with the goal of synthesizing research and clinical experience for clinicians in the public health sector and thereby increasing the quality and consistency of their treatment strategies.

Three of the Texas Children's Medication Algorithms are reproduced in Figures 2.1, 2.2, and 2.3 as examples of the current state of the art in child and adolescent psychopharmacology. To fully appreciate the thinking behind these and before using them, the complete publications should be read carefully. Algorithms serve only as a guide, and many clinicians will modify them to suit the individual clinical needs of their patients. Note that in Figure 2.2, magnesium pemoline, is no longer an option as all drug companies manufacturing and distributing this drug in the United States have stopped doing so because the risk of acute hepatic failure is considered greater than the potential benefits. Therefore, clinicians will skip this stage and proceed directly to stage 4. In the ADHD with comorbid tic disorder, the authors administer a stimulant and alpha-agonist together, which some clinicians would not feel comfortable about, given the controversy about coadministering methylphenidate and clonidine. Psychotherapeutic and psychosocial interventions, which are important to varying degrees with different patients, are not specifically integrated with these algorithms but remain essential components of any comprehensive treatment program.

Generic Versus Trade Preparations

There has been controversy in the literature on the merits of brand-name drugs, usually the initial, patented preparations of a medication, and generic preparations, which typically enter the market after exclusive patent rights expire and cost considerably less than the brand-name product. Although the active ingredients in the various preparations should be pharmaceutically equivalent, the inert ingredients and the manufacturing processes may vary; therefore, the bioavailability of a drug may be significantly different among various preparations.

(text continues on page 34)

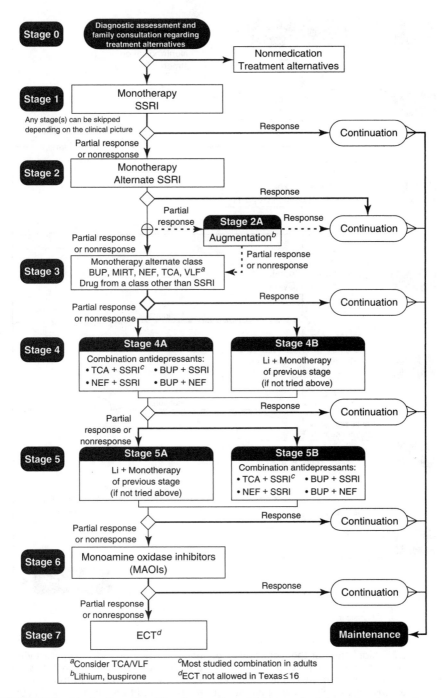

FIGURE 2.1   Medication algorithm for treating children and adolescents who meet DSM-IV criteria for major depressive disorder. SSRI, selective serotonin reuptake inhibitor; BUP, bupropion; MIRT, mirtazapine; NEF, nefazodone; TCA, tricyclic antidepressant; VLF, venlafaxine; ECT, electroconvulsive therapy. (Adapted from Crismon et al. 1999).

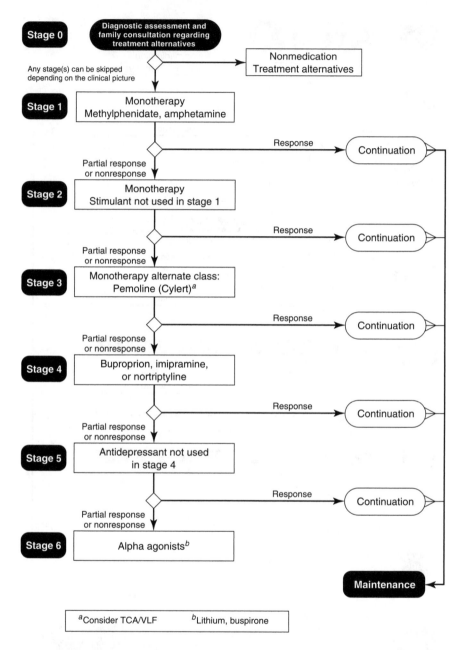

FIGURE 2.2   Algorithm for the medication treatment of attention-deficit/hyperactivity disorder without comorbid psychiatric disorder. Note, since this algorithm was published, pemoline has been withdrawn from the market. [a]Plus liver function monitoring and substance abuse history. [b]Cardiovascular side effects. (Adapted from Pliszka et al. 2000a; Pliszka SR, Greenhill LL, Crismon ML, et al. Texas Consensus Conference Panel on Medication Treatment of Childhood Attention-Deficit/Hyperactivity Disorder. The Texas children's medication algorithm project: report of the Texas consensus conference panel on medication treatment of childhood attention-deficit/hyperactivity disorder. Part I. *J Am Acad Child Adolesc Psychiatry* 2000a;39:908–919.)

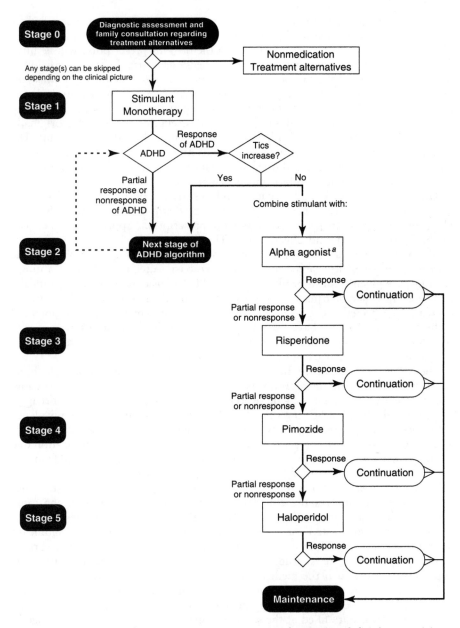

FIGURE 2.3 Algorithm for the medication treatment of attention-deficit/hyperactivity disorder (ADHD) with comorbid tic disorder. [a]Caution: cardiovascular side effects. (Adapted from Pliszka et al. 2000a; Pliszka SR, Greenhill LL, Crismon ML, et al. Texas Consensus Conference Panel on Medication Treatment of Childhood Attention-Deficit/Hyperactivity Disorder. The Texas children's medication algorithm project: report of the Texas consensus conference panel on medication treatment of childhood attention-deficit/hyperactivity disorder. Part I. *J Am Acad Child Adolesc Psychiatry* 2000a;39:908–919.)

Many states now permit substitution of generic drugs for drugs prescribed by the brand name under specified conditions. New York State, for example, requires all prescription forms to have imprinted on them "This prescription will be filled generically unless prescriber writes 'daw' [dispense as written] in the box below." New York State publishes a book, *Safe, Effective and Therapeutically Equivalent Prescription Drugs*, listing approved preparations of various prescription drugs. Pharmacists are directed to "substitute a less expensive drug product containing the same active ingredients, dosage form and strength" as the drug originally prescribed, if available (New York State Department of Health, 1988, p. iii). The book recognizes the differences in bioavailability among products. For example, for chlorpromazine it does not authorize substitution of oral solid immediate-release products because of potential bioequivalence problems.

The FDA Center for Drug Evaluation and Research publishes a book, *Approved Drug Products with Therapeutic Equivalence Evaluations* (the "Orange Book"), which lists drugs, both prescription and nonprescription, approved by the FDA on the basis of safety and effectiveness. The list gives the FDAs evaluations of the therapeutic equivalence of prescription drugs that are available from multiple sources. It classifies drug preparations into two basic categories: A and B ratings. A ratings are given to drug products that the FDA considers to be therapeutically equivalent to other pharmaceutically equivalent products for which there are no known or suspected bioequivalence problems or for which actual or potential problems are thought to have been satisfactorily resolved. B ratings are given to drug products that the FDA does not at this time consider to be therapeutically equivalent to other pharmaceutically equivalent products.

The 1988 FDA "Orange Book," for example, rates preparations of chlor-promazine for oral administration as "BP," indicating that there are potential bioequivalence problems among these preparations. Oral preparations of nortripty-line are rated "BD," indicating that there have been documented bioequivalence problems when a pharmaceutically equivalent drug from another source was sub-stituted. Dubovsky (1987) reported a case of severe nortriptyline intoxication due to changing from a generic to a trade preparation, which seemed to result from the significantly greater bioavailability of the trade preparation.

These comments are not a recommendation for any preparation over any other but are meant to inform the clinician that different preparations of the same medication of the same strength may have different bioavailabilities and that when they are substituted for one another, there is a potential for significant clinical repercussions. If prescriptions are written that may be filled with various generic preparations, it is prudent for the physician to inform the patient or responsible adult that if the medication is different when refilled, to inform him or her and to note any changes in symptoms or feelings after switching to a new preparation. Although changes in manufacturer may occur at times even when prescriptions are filled at the same pharmacy, the likelihood of a change in manufacturer increases when different pharmacies are used. If a patient runs out of medication while traveling and must obtain the drug(s) from a new source, a change of manufacturer may be more likely. Hence, it is worthwhile to remember to ascertain that a patient has sufficient medication before going to summer camp or traveling.

Standard (FDA-approved) and Nonstandard (Off-label) Treatments

In this book, those treatments that have been approved by the FDA for advertising and interstate commerce will be considered standard treatments. This implies that the drug has demonstrated clinical efficacy and that its use is substantially safe. The FDA's legal authority over how marketed drugs are used, the dosages employed, and related matters is limited to regulating what the manufacturer may recommend and must disclose in the package insert or labeling. "The prescription of a drug for an unlabeled (off-label) indication is entirely proper if the proposed use is based on rational scientific theory, expert medical opinion, or controlled clinical studies" (American Medical Association, 1993, p. 14).

Over the past four decades, a substantial body of clinical and investigational data has accumulated on using FDA-approved drugs to treat children below the recommended age (e.g., imipramine to treat major depressive disorder in children under 12 years of age), using FDA-approved drugs to treat children and adolescents for non-FDA–approved (off-label) indications (e.g., lithium to treat aggressive conduct disorder in any age-group and tricyclic antidepressants to treat ADHD), and using drugs before they were approved by the FDA for any indication (investigational drugs) to treat psychiatric disorders in children and adolescents (e.g., clomipramine and fluvoxamine maleate).

Selective serotonin reuptake inhibitor (SSRI) antidepressants and atypical antipsychotics are at present the most clinically important FDA-approved drugs used for nonapproved (off-label) indications in children and adolescents, although some SSRIs are approved for some indications in this age-group. There is a growing consensus among child psychiatrists that the benefit/risk ratio of their use for non-FDA–approved indications is often preferable to that of some currently approved medications (e.g., a decreased risk of developing tardive dyskinesia). This will be discussed in more detail in the specific drug section of the book.

Drug Interactions

Many psychoactive drugs have significant interactions with other medications. It is essential to be aware of any drug, prescription or otherwise, that the patient may be taking concurrently and to evaluate the potential interaction.

As part of the medical history, enquiries should be made about all medications, including those prescribed by other physicians; over-the-counter drugs; dietary supplements; and herbal preparations used even occasionally by the patient; and, as appropriate, alcohol and illicit or recreational drug use. Parents or caretakers and patients, as appropriate to their age and mental abilities, should be instructed to inform any physician who may treat them of the psychoactive medication(s) currently being taken. Similarly, patients whom the clinician is treating with psychoactive medication should be instructed to report at the next appointment whenever another physician prescribes any other medication for them or if they take any other drugs, over the counter or illicit, on their own initiative.

If substance abuse is known or suspected, screening of urine and/or blood for toxic substances may be indicated.

Drug interactions are discussed for each of the classes of psychoactive drugs. An attempt has been made to emphasize the most important interactions and those interactions most likely to be encountered by the physician who is treating psychiatrically disturbed children and adolescents.

It is beyond the scope of this book to review all possible drug interactions. It is the prescribing physician's responsibility to attempt to determine any other drugs his or her patient is taking and to assess any potentially adverse interactions of the medications before prescribing a new medication. The package insert, current PDR, current *Drug Interactions and Side Effects Index, Drug Facts and Comparisons, Drug Interactions in Psychiatry* (Ciraulo et al. 1989), or other suitable reference should be consulted. When appropriate and with the patient's consent, any other physicians treating the patient should be contacted so that a comprehensive treatment regimen that addresses both the psychiatric and the medical disorders of the patient safely may be mutually developed.

Regulating the Medication

Selecting the Initial Dosage

It is recommended in most cases that the treating physician initially prescribe a low dose, which will be either ineffective or inadequate for most patients. Although this cautious approach may lengthen the time necessary to reach a therapeutic dose, it is worthwhile for several reasons. First, pharmacokinetics vary not only among various age-groups but also among individuals of a specific age. For genetic and other reasons, some individuals, e.g., slow metabolizers, may be highly sensitive and responsive to a given medication whereas others, e.g., rapid metabolizers, may be relatively resistant or nonresponsive. By beginning with a low dose, the physician will avoid starting at a dose that is already in excess of the optimal therapeutic dose for a few patients, and those children and adolescents who are good responders at low dosages of medication will not be missed. If the initial dose is too high, the therapeutic range for these low-dose responders will not be explored and only adverse effects, which may at times even be confused with worsening of target symptoms, will be seen. Hence, a potentially beneficial medication may be needlessly excluded. For example, first, with stimulants a worsening of behavior may occur when optimal therapeutic doses for a specific patient have been exceeded. Second, with some drugs (e.g., methylphenidate), there is no significant relationship between the serum level and clinical response. Third, excessive initial dosage may also cause behavioral toxicity, particularly in younger children. Behavioral toxicity may occur before other adverse effects and includes symptoms such as worsening of target symptoms, hyperactivity or hypoactivity, aggressiveness, increased irritability, mood changes, apathy, and decreased verbal productions (Campbell et al. 1985). Fourth, some adverse effects of the drug may be eliminated or minimized; for example, acute dystonic reactions of antipsychotics and some adverse effects of lithium carbonate appear to be related in many cases to both serum levels and the rapidity of increase in serum level, and sedation may be less of a problem if dosage is increased gradually (Green et al. 1985).

The primary exceptions to gradual titration occur when an emergency situation exists, most often where there is danger or potential danger for injury to self, others, or property, and acute agitation or psychosis must be controlled as soon as possible.

Timing of Drug Administration

Scheduling Dosages

Times chosen for administration of the drug and the number of times the drug is administered per day should be related to the pharmacokinetics of the drug; for example, stimulants are most frequently given around breakfast and lunch, whereas antipsychotics may initially be given three or four times daily to reduce the risk of sedation and acute dystonic reactions. Once dosage has been stabilized, it may be clinically more convenient and may sometimes increase compliance if medications that have longer half-lives are administered only once or twice daily. Over the past decade, the number of long-active, controlled, sustained, or extended-release preparations of drugs has increased significantly. Prescription of such has likewise increased with increased convenience to the patient. This has been especially helpful in that many school children taking stimulant medication for ADHD no longer need to take it in school.

Pharmacokinetics and developmentally determined pharmacodynamic factors must still take precedence over convenience. For example, it may be possible to give the entire daily dose of an antipsychotic at bedtime to children and adolescents, whereas because younger children metabolize tricyclic antidepressants differently compared to adolescents and adults and they may be more sensitive to cardiotoxic effects, it is recommended that these drugs continue to be administered to children and younger adolescents in divided doses.

Drug Holidays

Because of the adverse effects of medications and their known and unknown effects on the growth, maturation, and development of children and adolescents, it is universally agreed that it is prudent to use medication in as low a dose and for as short a time as is clinically expedient. For some children, "drug holidays" may be a useful means of minimizing the cumulative amount of medication taken over time. The feasibility and type of drug holidays vary with the diagnosis and the severity of the disorder.

When stimulant medication is needed primarily to improve behavior (increase attention span and decrease hyperactivity and sometimes conduct problems) for classroom functioning, as with some ADHD children, it is often possible to withhold medication on weekends and on school holidays and vacations, including the entire summer. This is particularly important if there appears to be evidence of any suppression of height and weight percentiles, because there may be catch-up or compensatory growth following discontinuation of stimulant medication.

Sometimes parents find that their hyperactive child is not a serious management problem without medication at home but that difficulties arise when the child accompanies them on a shopping excursion or goes to a birthday party. In cases like this, when the parents' judgment can be trusted and medication is not used as a punishment, an understanding with the parents and child that medication may be used occasionally on weekends or vacations in situations that are particularly difficult for the child may be therapeutically indicated.

There is reasonable concern about the possibility of the development of an irreversible tardive dyskinesia in children and adolescents who receive long-term therapy with antipsychotic medication. There is some evidence that the development of tardive dyskinesia may be associated with both the total amount of antipsychotic drug ingested and the duration of treatment, although constitutional vulnerabilities to developing tardive dyskinesia also appear to play an important role (Jeste and Wyatt, 1982). Consequently, possible means of reducing the total amount of an antipsychotic drug ever taken may be clinically important in reducing the likelihood of developing tardive dyskinesia.

Newton et al. (1989) compared 6-week periods of haloperidol daily and 6-week periods of haloperidol with repeated weekly 2-day drug holidays in a crossover experiment with seven older adult patients with schizophrenia. Serum haloperidol levels were reduced by approximately 25% during holiday periods, with no significant change in mental status, severity of psychiatric symptoms, or scores on scales rating movement disorders.

Similarly, Perry et al. (1989) reported on 52 child outpatients aged 2.3 to 7.9 years diagnosed with infantile autism, full syndrome, who were treated with haloperidol for 6 months. The subjects were assigned on a random basis in a double-blind protocol to receive haloperidol continuously (daily) or discontinuously (5 days/week with 2 contiguous days of placebo). There was no significant clinical difference between the groups, and in both groups, children who had symptoms of irritability, angry and labile affect, and uncooperativeness responded best. The incidence of adverse effects, including tardive and withdrawal dyskinesia, did not vary significantly between the two groups.

Dosage Increases

Changes in medication level should be based on the clinical response of the patient, and the rationale for each change should be documented in the clinical record. Knowledge of the characteristic time frame of response for a particular drug and diagnosis should influence these decisions. Therefore, the clinician may increase dosage once or twice weekly in some cases, when using stimulants or neuroleptics. On the other hand, the clinical efficacy of antidepressants may not be fully apparent for several weeks when used to treat a major depressive disorder. Once the total daily dose of an antidepressant has reached a level that is usually associated with clinical response, increasing the dose because of a failure to respond during the first 2 or 3 weeks of treatment is not psychopharmacologically sound practice unless serum drug levels are being monitored and are thought to be in the subtherapeutic range.

Titration of Medication

The goal of the clinician is to achieve meaningful therapeutic benefits for the patient with the fewest possible adverse effects. Here again it is recommended that risks versus benefits be assessed. To do so scientifically, however, it is necessary to explore the dose range of a patient's response. Unless there are extenuating circumstances, it is usually advisable to continue raising the dose level until one of the following events occurs:

1. Entirely adequate symptom control is established.
2. The upper limit of the recommended dosage (or higher level if commonly accepted) has been reached.
3. Adverse effects that preclude a further increase in dose have occurred.
4. After a measurable improvement in target symptoms, a plateau in improvement or a worsening of symptoms occurs with further increases in dose.

Unless this procedure is followed, an injustice may be done to the patient. This occurs most frequently when there is some behavioral improvement and the treating clinician stabilizes the dosage at that point. Further significant improvement that might have occurred had a higher dose been given is missed. It is recommended that the next higher dose be explored. If there is significant additional improvement, the therapist, in consultation with the patient and his or her parents, can make a judgment regarding whether the benefits outweigh the risks from the additional dosage.

Determining the Optimal Dose

Once the titration of the therapeutic dose to maximum clinical benefit has been achieved for a specific patient, the lowest possible dose that produces those desired effects should be determined. This is considered the optimal dose for a specific patient. In clinical practice, this may sometimes require a compromise, and amelioration of target symptoms to an acceptable degree may occur only when some adverse effects are also present.

In those cases in which either no significant therapeutic benefit occurs or adverse effects prevent the employment of a clinically meaningful therapeutic dose, trial of a different medication must be considered. If there is a partial but meaningful clinical response, some clinicians would consider adding an additional medication (polypharmacy) rather than discontinuing the drug and administering another. Whatever the case, clinicians should not continue to prescribe medication in doses that do not result in significant clinical improvement.

Adverse Effects (Side Effects)

All drugs, including placebos, have adverse effects, or side effects. Actually, if one excludes allergic and idiosyncratic reactions, many adverse effects are as much a characteristic of the pharmacologic makeup of a specific drug and are as predictable as the drug's therapeutic effects. Individual patients may vary as much in their experience of adverse effects of a drug as in their therapeutic responses to it. Adverse effects are important not only because of the immediate problematic effects they cause but also because they may be intimately related to issues of compliance, as discussed in the preceding text.

It is sometimes useful to think of adverse effects as the "unwanted effects" of the drug for the specific patient and therapeutic indication. For a different patient and situation, an adverse or side effect will actually become the desired therapeutic action of the drug. For example, sedation, which may be an adverse effect when a benzodiazepine is prescribed for anxiolysis, is the desired result when a benzodiazepine is prescribed as a soporific. Similarly, appetite suppression is usually an undesired effect of stimulants prescribed for ADHD but the action of choice when used in treating exogenous obesity.

Many adverse effects are related to dose or serum levels, but others are not. They may occur almost immediately (e.g., an acute dystonic reaction) or be delayed for years (e.g., tardive dyskinesia). They may be life threatening or fatal, or relatively innocuous. There is also evidence that the adverse effects of a specific drug may differ according to the age and/or diagnosis of the subjects. For example, haloperidol produced excessive sedation in hospitalized school-age aggressive-conduct-disordered children on doses of 0.04 to 0.21 mg/kg/day (Campbell et al. 1984b) but not in preschoolers with autistic disorder on doses of 0.019 to 0.217 mg/kg/day (Anderson et al. 1984).

A thorough knowledge of the most important and frequent adverse effects of the medications considered is essential and will often play a decisive role in which medication is selected and/or when dosage is scheduled. For example, if a schizophrenic youngster has insomnia, the clinician may select a low-potency antipsychotic drug and adjust the dosage schedule so that any sedation will aid the child in falling asleep. As an added benefit, the risk of an acute dystonic reaction is lower than if a high-potency antipsychotic drug had been chosen.

Likewise, the management of adverse effects is a vital component of pharmacotherapy. In clinical practice, careful attention to adverse effects and flexibility about the time and amounts of specific doses may enable one to obtain a satisfactory clinical result with a minimal or acceptable level of adverse effects that is not possible if a fixed dosage schedule is used, as in some research protocols. Therefore, one can adjust medication levels slowly and in small increments or divide doses unequally over the day (e.g., giving more in the morning, more before bed, or the entire daily dose at bedtime).

The clinician must remember that the ability to understand adverse effects and verbalize unusual sensations, feelings, or discomfort not only varies among individual children but is developmentally determined. Younger children spontaneously report adverse effects less frequently than older children. Hence, the younger the child, the more essential it becomes for caretakers to be actively looking for adverse effects and for the physician to ask the patient about adverse effects using language appropriate to the child's level of understanding.

Many psychotropic drugs may cause treatment-emergent sexual dysfunction–related adverse effects which are of significant concern to adolescents, especially those who may be sexually active. As many adolescents are uncomfortable in discussing such matters and do not spontaneously report them, it is particularly important for the clinician to routinely ask about such symptoms in a nonjudgmental, nonthreatening way.

It is essential that the clinician examine the patient frequently for the development of adverse effects during the period when the medication is being regulated, at regular intervals during maintenance therapy, and during scheduled periodic withdrawals of the medication. For example, with antipsychotic drugs, one should look particularly for sedation and extrapyramidal side effects, the development of abnormal movements, and, during drug withdrawal periods, any evidence of a withdrawal dyskinesia. Completion of the AIMS, as described earlier, is recommended as an aid in quantifying and following abnormal movements over time.

Monitoring of Serum Levels of Drugs and/or of Their Metabolites

Morselli et al. (1983) and Gualtieri et al. (1984a) reviewed the pharmacokinetics of psychoactive drugs used in child and adolescent psychiatry and the clinical relevance of determining their serum or blood levels. Determining the blood or plasma levels of drugs and/or their metabolites is most useful when accurate measurements of all significant active metabolites of a drug are available and there is a known relationship between the clinical effects of the drug and serum concentration (Gualtieri et al. 1984a).

Clinically, the monitoring of serum levels is useful to verify compliance and to be certain that adequate therapeutic serum levels are available (i.e., that values fall within the therapeutic window) and thereby avoid discontinuing a trial of medication before clinically effective serum levels have been reached or, conversely, avoid inadvertently reaching toxic serum levels.

School-aged children often have more efficient physiologic systems for drug metabolism and excretion than adults. As a result, doses comparable to those administered to adults, either on a total daily dose or on a dose-per-unit-weight basis, may result in subtherapeutic serum levels in children and younger adolescents. This could be one factor contributing to the clinical observation that children with schizophrenia, as a group, appear to show less dramatic clinical improvement than adolescents and adults when administered neuroleptics (Green, 1989). It will be necessary to measure antipsychotic serum levels to determine if this lack of improvement is due to subtherapeutic levels in some cases, because some children may also show clinical improvement at lower serum levels than adults (Rivera-Calimlim et al. 1979).

Meyers et al. (1980) reported the case of a 13-year-old prepubescent boy diagnosed as having schizophrenia who required a dose of haloperidol of at least 30 mg/day to reach therapeutic serum neuroleptic levels. Monitoring serum levels of antipsychotic drugs may therefore yield clinical information that is, at times, extremely useful. If a child or adolescent does not have a satisfactory response to usual doses of antipsychotic drugs, serum neuroleptic levels should be determined, if available, before deciding to discontinue the drug.

In addition to age-related differences in pharmacokinetics, remarkable interindividual variations occur. For example, Berg et al. (1974) reported that a 14-year-old girl with bipolar manic-depressive disorder required up to 2,400 mg of lithium daily to maintain serum lithium levels of 1 mEq/L. Her father had the same disorder and also required unusually high doses of lithium to reach therapeutic levels.

Currently, regular determinations of serum levels should be considered mandatory when lithium carbonate, antiepileptic drugs, or tricyclic antidepressants are used in treating children and adolescents. In current practice, for example, monitoring of drug and metabolite serum levels is of considerable practical importance in the use of the tricyclic antidepressants. This monitoring is needed because there is minimal correlation between the dose and serum level, and serum levels are correlated significantly with the clinical response and/or potentially serious adverse effects (e.g., cardiotoxicity). For example, Puig-Antich et al. (1987) have emphasized that they found no predictors of total maintenance plasma levels, including dosage, in their prepubertal subjects treated with imipramine for major depressive disorder. They also reported that positive therapeutic response to imipramine in prepubertal children was strongly correlated with serum levels over 150 ng/mL.

Similarly, Biederman et al. (1989b) reported that desipramine serum levels varied an average of 16.5-fold at four different dose levels in 31 children and adolescents diagnosed with attention-deficit disorder. These authors, however, found no significant linear relationship between the total daily dose or weight-corrected (mg/kg) daily dose and the steady-state serum desipramine level and any outcome measure, including clinical improvement. There was a tendency for serum desipramine levels in subjects who were rated very much or much improved on the Clinical Global Improvement Scale to average 60.8% higher than in unimproved subjects.

Morselli et al. (1983) also emphasized that monitoring drug plasma levels of haloperidol, chlorpromazine, imipramine, and clomipramine is particularly helpful in optimizing long-term treatment with these agents.

On the other hand, a detailed review of the pharmacokinetics and actions of methylphenidate concluded that "blood MPH [methylphenidate] levels are not statistically related to clinical response, nor are they likely to prove clinically helpful until this lack of correlation is understood" (Patrick et al. 1987, p. 1393).

Serum levels are also mandatory when antiepileptic drugs are being used for control of seizures, although this use is not reviewed in this book. When antiepileptic drugs are used for other psychiatric indications, such as control of aggression or as mood stabilizers, effective serum levels are thought to be in the same range as when they are used to control seizures. Monitoring of serum levels (both drug and significant metabolites) will become increasingly important for other drugs used in child and adolescent psychiatry as their determinations become more readily available and correlations with clinical efficacy and adverse effects are established.

Length of Time to Continue Medication

Children and adolescents are immature, developing individuals progressing toward adulthood. Because of concerns about long-term adverse effects such as tardive and withdrawal dyskinesias and growth retardation as well as our inadequate knowledge of other long-term adverse effects of psychopharmacological agents on their biological and psychological maturation, there is virtually unanimous agreement that medication should be given for as short a period as possible.

The vicissitudes of the natural courses of psychiatric illnesses in children and adolescents are often not predictable for specific individuals. It is to be hoped, especially when there is a significant psychosocial etiologic factor, that medication will augment the child's response to other therapeutic interventions and enhance his or her social and academic functioning, maturation, and development. Once real gains are made and internalized, the cycle of failures broken, and the maladaptive patterns replaced with more appropriate ones, it may be possible to discontinue the drug and maintain therapeutic gains. Even in chronic conditions with strong biological underpinnings, such as pervasive developmental disorder, schizophrenia, and depression, the clinical course may spontaneously vary so that in some patients psychoactive medication may be reduced or even discontinued.

Periodic Withdrawal/Tapering of Medication

It is usually considered mandatory to discontinue psychotropic medications (or to attempt to do so) in child and adolescent patients on a regular basis, certainly no less frequently than every 6 months to 1 year. There may be occasional exceptions to this (e.g., the long-term prophylactic use of lithium carbonate or an antidepressant to prevent recurrences of mood disorders or not withdrawing an antipsychotic in a child or adolescent being treated for schizophrenia who has experienced serious relapses during prior withdrawal attempts). Whenever medication is continued beyond 6 to 12 months, it is important to document the clinical reasons for doing so in the medical record.

Discontinuation/Withdrawal Syndromes

Rapidly metabolized drugs such as methylphenidate and amphetamines may be discontinued abruptly. However, with these drugs, which have short half-lives, there may be some rebound effect during routine daily administration of the drug as serum levels decline during late afternoon or evening.

To minimize the likelihood of developing withdrawal syndromes, it is recommended that most medications be gradually reduced rather than stopped abruptly.

The clinician should continue to complete the AIMS in patients who had preexisting abnormal movements prior to the initiation of medication that may have been masked or ameliorated or who are otherwise at risk for developing abnormal movements following withdrawal. If a withdrawal dyskinesia emerges upon discontinuing an antipsychotic drug, effort should be made to keep the patient off antipsychotics. Any abnormal movements should continue to be recorded on the AIMS.

Gualtieri et al. (1984b) reported both physical withdrawal symptoms (e.g., decreased appetite, nausea and vomiting, diarrhea, and sweating) and acute behavioral deterioration in approximately 10% of children and adolescents after their withdrawal from long-term treatment with antipsychotics. Both types of withdrawal symptoms ceased spontaneously within 8 weeks. It is extremely important that the clinician recognize that such symptoms may be expected withdrawal effects and that they are not necessarily a return of premedication symptoms. The symptoms must be monitored qualitatively and quantitatively over a sufficient period to see if they diminish, as would be expected with a withdrawal syndrome, or if they indicate that the underlying psychiatric disorder still requires medication for symptom amelioration.

When tricyclics are withdrawn abruptly or too rapidly, some children experience a flu-like withdrawal syndrome resulting from cholinergic rebound. This characteristically includes gastrointestinal symptoms such as nausea, abdominal discomfort and pain, vomiting, and fatigue. Tapering the medication down over a 10-day period rather than abruptly withdrawing it will usually avoid this effect or significantly diminish the withdrawal syndrome. The clinician is cautioned that in patients with poor compliance, who in essence may undergo periodic self-induced acute withdrawals, the withdrawal syndrome may be confused with adverse effects, inadequate dose levels, or worsening of the underlying psychiatric disorder.

A withdrawal or discontinuation syndrome has also been identified for the SSRIs. Rosenbaum et al. (1998) reviewed the literature on discontinuation-emergent symptoms in adults taking SSRIs and noted that dizziness, headache, nausea, vomiting, diarrhea, movement disorders, insomnia, irritability, visual disturbances, lethargy, anorexia, tremor, electric shock sensations, and lowered mood have all been reported following SSRI discontinuation. There appeared to be a relationship between half-life and the development of discontinuation-emergent symptoms. Patients abruptly discontinued from drugs with longer half-lives, for example fluoxetine, developed fewer clinically significant effects than patients who abruptly discontinued drugs with short half-lives, for example paroxetine or sertraline.

Similarly, it is recommended that the alpha-adrenergic agonists, clonidine hydrochloride and guanfacine hydrochloride, be tapered gradually to reduce the likelihood of a hypertensive reaction and other symptoms, such as headache, nervousness, and agitation. This is more important for clonidine, as its half-life is significantly shorter than that of guanfacine.

In significant numbers of cases, after an initial treatment period of varying duration, medication may no longer be required or adequate symptom control can be maintained on a lower maintenance dose. For example, Sleator et al. (1974) administered a 1-month-long period of placebo to 28 of 42 hyperactive children who had been treated with methylphenidate for between 1 and 2 years. Eleven of the 28 were able to continue performing adequately behaviorally and academically without medication. Seventeen of the 28 showed worsening during the placebo period; of the 17, 10 functioned well when their initial dose was resumed, whereas 7 needed an increase in dose to maintain their original gains.

In contrast, over time, higher doses may be required occasionally to maintain gains. This may reflect a worsening of the psychiatric disorder *per se* or a developmental/maturational effect, as in a child with autistic disorder who becomes both stronger and more aggressive as he or she enters adolescence. In other cases, the need for increased medication may be a consequence of an individual's normal physiologic maturation altering the drug's pharmacokinetics and/or normal or excessive weight gain.

Specific Drugs

CHAPTER 3

Introduction

Child psychopharmacology is a relatively new field. The 1937 publication by Charles Bradley reporting the effects of administering racemic amphetamine sulfate (Benzedrine) to 30 children 5 to 14 years of age with various behavioral disturbances is usually considered to mark the beginning of the modern era of child psychopharmacology.

More than 20 years later, the first book concerned exclusively with psychopharmacologic research in child psychiatry, *Child Research in Psychopharmacology,* evolved out of the 1958 Conference on Child Research in Psychopharmacology sponsored by the National Institute of Mental Health (Fisher, 1959). The book contains an annotated list of 159 references of studies of the effects of psychopharmacologic agents administered to children with psychiatric problems, beginning with Bradley's 1937 publication. Interestingly, M. Molitch and coworkers also published, in 1937, three papers concerning the use of amphetamine sulfate in children, including two placebo-controlled studies (Molitch and Eccles, 1937; Molitch and Poliakoff, 1937; Molitch and Sullivan, 1937). Two of the studies found that amphetamine sulfate improved scores of children on intelligence tests, and one reported that 86% of 14 enuretic boys who had not responded to placebo were dry when given increasing doses of amphetamine sulfate and reverted to bedwetting within 2 weeks after the drug was discontinued.

In the 1950s the classes of drugs currently most important in general psychiatry were introduced: the antipsychotics (chlorpromazine and other compounds), the antidepressants, and lithium carbonate. The benzodiazepines, in particular diazepam and chlordiazepoxide, were introduced into clinical psychiatric practice in the early 1960s. Then in the late 1980s and throughout the 1990s, the selective serotonin reuptake inhibitor (SSRI) antidepressants and the atypical antipsychotics, now referred to as second generation antipsychotics, began to be introduced. Because of increased difficulties in conducting psychopharmacologic research and in obtaining FDA approval of the safety and efficacy of psychoactive drugs in children and younger adolescents, the investigation and introduction into clinical practice of psychoactive drugs in children have always lagged somewhat behind that for adults. Weiner and Jaffe (1985) have written a brief but interesting overview of the earlier history of child and adolescent psychopharmacology.

Texts focusing entirely or significantly on child and adolescent psychopharmacology include those by Aman and Singh (1988); Bezchlibnyk-Butler and Virani (2004); Campbell et al. (1985); Gadow (1986a, 1986b); Klein et al. (1980); Kutcher

(1997, 2002); Martin et al. (2003); Riddle (1995a, 1995b); Rosenberg et al. (2002); Rosenberg et al. (1994); Walsh (1998); Weiner (1985); Werry (1978); and Werry and Aman (1999). The reader who wishes an in-depth review of major issues of the past decade, spanning the entire field of psychopharmacology, is referred to *Neuropsychopharmacology: The Fifth Generation of Progress,* Davis et al. (2002).

In most instances, reviews of the literature establishing the clinical efficacy and safety of earlier FDA-approved treatments for the psychiatric disorders of children and adolescents are not included in this book. Readers who wish to review the research data establishing these standard treatments will find such information to be accessible in the texts cited above.

Section II of this book summarizes the standard treatments but also focuses in greater detail on research into new and not yet approved uses of drugs in child and adolescent psychiatry and reviews these studies. Some knowledge of psychopharmacologic research principles and techniques is essential to critically evaluate the data that appear in the psychiatric literature and to make informed clinical decisions about whether a trial of a particular drug is warranted for a particular patient.

Most important psychopharmacologic research designs include comparison of the drug being investigated with either placebo or a drug approved as a standard treatment for the psychiatric disorder in question. Hence it is important to have a basic understanding of placebos.

PLACEBOS

According to the *Oxford English Dictionary* (OED) (1989), the English word *placebo* was directly adopted from the Latin word meaning "I shall be pleasing or acceptable." By 1811 it was defined in *Hooper's Medical Dictionary* (OED, 1989) as "an epithet given to any medicine adapted more to please than benefit the patient." In 1982 the OED added the following definition of *placebo*, which fairly accurately described its current use in psychopharmacologic research: "A substance or procedure which a patient accepts as a medicine or therapy but which actually has no specific therapeutic activity for his condition or is prescribed in the belief that it has no such activity." Although placebos are often comprised of substances thought to be inert, in psychopharmacologic research, placebos may also contain active ingredients chosen to simulate adverse effects of the drug to which the placebo is being compared. The purpose of this is to keep all participants "blind" by making it more difficult for patients and observers to distinguish between drug and placebo based solely on the drug's adverse effects.

Placebos play a crucial role in clinical psychopharmacologic research by providing nonspecific treatment effects for comparison with the drug under investigation. These nonspecific psychological and physiologic changes are not drug specific and may be measured by rating scales (Prien, 1988). These changes include both beneficial and adverse effects produced by the expectations the patient or observers have about the drug, natural fluctuations in the clinical course of the disease, and spontaneous alterations in the patient's condition that may have nothing to do with the illness under consideration; effects of the relationship among the patient, therapist, and other medical staff; and other unknown effects.

Because of these nonspecific effects, even "inert" placebos have side effects. These may commonly include such symptoms as fatigue, tiredness, anxiety, muscle aches, nausea, diarrhea, constipation, dry mouth, dysmenorrhea, and behavioral changes such as increased or decreased aggressiveness, impulsiveness, attention span, or irritability. These are often symptoms that might appear periodically in the general population. It is the difference in incidence and severity of these unwanted effects between placebo and drug that is important.

The most methodologically sound use of a placebo for testing a new medication is a double-blind, randomized, parallel-groups design (Prien, 1988). Stanley (1988) has written an interesting article concerning ethical and clinical considerations in the use of placebos that evaluated such factors as withholding medication during a placebo period and whether treatment may be ethically withheld in a placebo-controlled trial when a known treatment is available.

Head-to-head studies compare a new drug to a drug already recognized as effective and safe. This strategy/design can avoid the ethical conundrum of denying treatment to patients who would have been assigned placebo in a placebo-controlled study and is important when delay of treatment known to be effective for a given diagnosis could result in serious harm to the patient. Prien (1988) offered six alternative study designs for use when it is not possible to use a double-blind, randomized, parallel-groups design and discussed some of their limitations. White et al. (1985) edited a fascinating book concerning the theory, ethics, use in research and clinical practice, and mediating mechanisms of placebos.

EVALUATING RESEARCH STUDIES

Efficacy and safety are determined by a statistically significant benefit with acceptable adverse effects of the new medication compared with placebo. Statistics, however, inform us about groups of patients, not individuals. Hence if etiologically dissimilar groups are subsumed under the same diagnosis, a few patients may truly benefit, but their improvement could be so diluted by the larger majority who did not benefit that the drug might show no statistically significant benefit. Some researchers now note whether there are strong individual responders in a drug study even when there is no statistical difference between experimental and control groups. Therefore individual case reports, studies of relatively small numbers, and open studies should not be summarily dismissed.

In evaluating the literature on child and adolescent psychopharmacology, it is important to remember that a drug that is statistically and significantly better than another drug or placebo does not necessarily mean that the drug is the optimal treatment for a given condition or for a specific child or adolescent. The drug may be effective only in certain environments (e.g., a laboratory) and cannot be generalized to more ordinary circumstances, or it may improve only certain symptoms but not affect other major target symptoms to a clinically meaningful degree, or the overall improvement may be relatively modest with significant symptoms or deficits remaining. For example, Sprague and Sleator (1977) found that 0.3 mg/kg of methylphenidate produced optimal enhancement of learning short-term memory tasks in hyperkinetic children in the laboratory, but 1 mg/kg of methylphenidate produced the maximum improvement of social behavior in the classroom as shown by ratings on the Abbreviated Conners Rating Scale. Another example is that although children with autistic disorder have shown statistically significant improvements with several drugs, the degree of their improvement is typically modest, with marked residual deficits remaining, and at present no drug is satisfactory for treatment of this condition (Green, 1988).

In evaluating research, diagnostic criteria and the diagnostic heterogeneity/ homogeneity of the sample, and both the severity of the patients included and the clinical setting in which the drug was given, must be evaluated. Therefore until the formalization by DSM-III (1980) of diagnostic distinctions between schizophrenia with childhood onset and autistic disorder (or their equivalents), both were subsumed under the diagnosis of schizophrenia, childhood type; many studies included diagnostically heterogeneous samples or the composition of the sample could not be determined, rendering interpretation of the studies difficult or impossible (Green, 1989).

Gadow and Poling (1988) provide another relevant example. They noted that stimulant medication is not commonly prescribed for the mentally retarded in residential facilities where most of the residents are usually severely or profoundly retarded. They pointed out that some reviews of the use of stimulants in the mentally retarded falling into these diagnostic categories suggested that stimulants might not be useful in treating behavior disorders in the retarded and could even exacerbate attention deficit in these patients. They noted that the large majority of mentally retarded individuals are not in institutions and that they are prescribed stimulants for management of disturbed behavior, particularly hyperactivity, much more frequently and with more favorable results than one might expect from reading the literature. In fact, these authors concluded that stimulants were highly effective in diminishing conduct problems and hyperactivity for some mentally retarded individuals, whatever their IQs.

As psychiatric nosology and diagnosis become more refined and the etiopatho-geneses of more homogeneous subgroups are delineated, more focused research may be undertaken, and more specific and rational psychopharmacology will inevitably follow.

SPECIFIC DRUG TREATMENTS

In this section of the book, psychopharmacologic agents are organized and dis-cussed by class rather than according to the psychiatric diagnoses for which they are treatments. The rationale for this organization is related to several of the issues discussed in the first part of the book. At the present time most diagnoses are based on phenomenology (i.e., constellations of clinical symptoms) rather than on any basic understanding of the etiopathogenesis of the condition. Therefore. a given drug may be used to treat several psychiatric diagnoses. Hence repetition of facts under each diagnostic category and extensive cross-referencing are avoided.

Each class of drugs is introduced with some general comments, including indications for use, contraindications, interactions with other drugs, and the most common untoward effects. The basic pharmacokinetics, including approximations of time of peak serum levels and the drug's serum half-life, major metabolites, and excretion, are discussed. Unless otherwise noted, all dosage recommendations are for oral administration.

Specific drugs of each class are reviewed individually. Traditional or standard, FDA-approved treatments are discussed but additionally, many treatments not approved for advertising by the FDA but reported to be efficacious in the literature and used clinically by practitioners are discussed as well.

Most of the studies cited in this book either illustrate a particular point or provide the reader with some of the evidence for using off-label treatments. This evidence ranges from convincing to merely suggestive of a possible alternative for a seriously disturbed patient who has not responded satisfactorily to any prior treatment attempts. Excellent and extensive literature reviews of the standard psychopharmacologic treatments discussed later are readily accessible in the additional earlier texts on child and adolescent psychopharmacology referenced earlier in this chapter.

Although always important, informed consent, preferably written, is particularly important if FDA-approved drugs are used for nonapproved indications. If standard approved treatments for a seriously disabling disorder have been tried with little or no success, a clinical trial of a nonapproved or even an investigational medication is much more easily justified. The physician has the responsibility to become thoroughly familiar with the official package labeling information provided by the manufacturer of the drug or the relevant entry in the latest edition and supplements of the *Physicians' Desk Reference* (PDR, 2006) before prescribing any drug.

Table 3.1 lists the most common psychiatric diagnoses in children and younger adolescents for which psychopharmacotherapy may be therapeutically indicated and the medications that have been used in treating that disorder. Whenever a specific drug or class of drugs is generally preferred for a particular condition, an attempt has been made to rank them in order of usual preference if possible; however, for some diagnoses there are many drugs for which there is no clear order of preference. The listing of a medication indicates that it is discussed or reports of interest are summarized in the text; such a listing does not necessarily imply that the drug is a recommended treatment.

TABLE 3.1 ●   DSM-IV Diagnoses in Childhood and Adolescence for Which Psychopharmacotherapy May be Therapeutically Indicated and Drugs Discussed in the Text

Attention-Deficit/Hyperactivity Disorder
Methylphenidate preparations
Amphetamine preparations
Atomoxetine
Clonidine
Guanfacine
Fluoxetine
Clomipramine
MAOIs
Bupropion
Venlafaxine
Haloperidol
Tricyclic antidepressants

Bipolar Disorder/Mania
Lithium
Valproic acid

(continued)

TABLE 3.1 ● *(Continued)*

Carbamazepine
Risperidone

Conduct Disorder (Severe, Aggressive)
Atypical/Second Generation Antipsychotics
Haloperidol; Other First Generation Antipsychotics
Methylphenidate
Lithium
Buspirone
Propranolol
Valproic Acid
Carbamazepine
Trazodone
Clonidine
Molindone

Encopresis
Lithium

Enuresis
DDAVP
Imipramine
Benzodiazepines
Carbamazepine
Amphetamines
Clomipramine
Desipramine

Generalized Anxiety Disorder (Overanxious Disorder of Childhood in DSM-III-R)
Benzodiazepines
Diphenhydramine
Fluoxetine
Buspirone
Hydroxyzine

Intermittent Explosive Disorder
Propranolol

Major Depressive Disorder
Antidepressants
Lithium augmentation
Lithium for prophylaxis

Manic Episode
Lithium
Valproic acid
Atypical/Second Generation Antipsychotics

TABLE 3.1 ● *(Continued)*

Mental Retardation (with Severe Behavioral Disorder and/or Self-Injurious Behavior)
Atypical/Second Generation Antipsychotics
Haloperidol
Chlorpromazaine
Lithium
Propranolol
Naltrexone

Obsessive-Compulsive Disorder
Sertraline
Fluoxetine
Paroxetine
Fluvoxamine
Clomipramine
Clonazepam

Panic Disorder
Sertraline
Paroxetine
Alprazolam
Clonazepam
Tricyclic Antidepressants

Pervasive Developmental Disorders
Risperidone and Other Atypical/Second Generation Antipsychotics
Haloperidol
Fluphenazine
Naltrexone
Methylphenidate Preparations
Amphetamines Preparations
Clomipramine
Buspirone
Clonidine

Post-Traumatic Stress Disorder
Sertraline
Propranolol

Schizophrenia
Atypical/Second Generation Antipsychotics
First Generation Antipsychotics

(continued)

TABLE 3.1 ● *(Continued)*

Selective Mutism
Fluoxetine
Sertraline

Separation Anxiety Disorder
Fluoxetine
Chlordiazepoxide
Alprazolam
Buspirone
Clomipramine
Imipramine
Clonazepam

Sleep Disorders
Primary Insomnia
Benzodiazepines
Diphenhydramine
Hydroxyzine
Clonidine

Circadian Rhythm Sleep Disorder
Benzodiazepines
Diphenhydramine
Hydroxyzine

Sleep Terror Disorder
Diazepam
Alprazolam
Imipramine
Carbamazepine

Sleepwalking Disorder
Diazepam
Imipramine

Tourette's Disorder
Haloperidol
Pimozide
Clonidine
Desipramine
Guanfacine
Bupropion
Nortriptyline
Fluoxetine

CHAPTER 4

Sympathomimetic Amines and Central Nervous System Stimulants

Note: The U.S. Food and Drug Administration (FDA) has directed that a Black Box Warning be added to the labeling of amphetamine products stating that "Amphetamines have a high potential for abuse. Administration of amphetamines for prolonged periods of time may lead to drug dependence, particular attention should be paid to the possibility of subjects obtaining amphetamines for non-therapeutic use or distribution to others and the drugs should be prescribed or dispensed sparingly. Misuse of amphetamine may cause sudden death and serious cardiovascular adverse events." It is noted specifically for Adderall XR that "Its misuse is associated with serious cardiovascular adverse events and may cause sudden death in patients with preexisting cardiac structural abnormalities." The FDA has received reports of sudden death associated with unusual amphetamine dosing in children with structural cardiac abnormalities. The FDA does not recommend general use of amphetamines in children or adults with structural cardiac abnormalities.

INTRODUCTION

Sympathomimetic amines and central nervous system stimulants are commonly referred to as stimulants. Two of these agents, methylphenidate (MPH) and amphetamines are the drugs of choice for treating attention-deficit/hyperactivity disorder (ADHD). Magnesium pemoline, which also falls into this category of drugs, was withdrawn from the market in 2005 by manufacturers because the increased risk of acute hepatic failure was unacceptable. Atomoxetine, a selective norepinephrine reuptake inhibitor (SNRI) is also approved by the FDA to treat ADHD; however, head-to-head comparisons suggest that stimulants are more effective than atomoxetine in improving hyperactivity, impulsivity, and inattention in such subjects (Starr and Kemner, 2005; Wigal et al. 2005; National Medical Association, FOCUS presentation, 2005; this is reviewed in Chapter 7 under the section "Atomoxetine versus Stimulants in the Treatment of Attention-Deficit/ Hyperactivity Disorder in Children and Adolescents").

The most useful recent comprehensive review of the use of stimulants in treating ADHD is "Practice Parameter for the Use of Stimulant Medications in the Treatment of Children, Adolescents, and Adults" (Greenhill et al. 2002).

Bradley's (1937) report on the use of racemic amphetamine sulfate (Benzedrine) in children having behavioral disorders is usually cited as the beginning of child psychopharmacology as a discipline. Since this initial report, more research has been published on the stimulants and on ADHD than on any other childhood disorder. Double-blind, placebo-controlled studies have consistently found that stimulants are significantly superior to placebo in improving attention span and in decreasing hyperactivity and impulsivity. Although most of the earlier studies were in children, two double-blind studies have confirmed the clinical efficacy of MPH in treating adolescents diagnosed with attention deficit disorder (ADD) who also had ADD as children (Klorman et al. 1988a, 1988b). Since then, many more studies on the use of stimulants in adolescents and adults have been published.

Several investigators have reported that MPH also improved academic performance and/or peer interactions (e.g., Pelham et al. 1985, 1987; Rapport et al. 1994). Whalen et al. (1987) reported on 24 children between 6 and 11 years of age who were diagnosed with ADD or ADDH and who received either placebo, 0.3 mg/kg MPH daily, or 0.6 mg/kg MPH daily, in random order so that all children received each dosage level for a total of 4 days. The authors reported that all children showed decrements in negative social behaviors when rated during relatively unstructured outdoor activities at the 0.3 mg/kg level, compared with placebo. The youngest 12 children showed further improvement in social behavior at the higher dose.

Rapport et al. (1994) evaluated the acute effects of four dose levels (5, 10, 15, and 20 mg) of MPH on classroom behavior and academic performance of 76 children diagnosed with ADHD in a double-blind, placebo-controlled, within-subject (crossover) protocol. Compared with baseline, the subjects showed a nearly linear increase in normalization of behavior as the dose of MPH increased. On the Abbreviated Conners Teacher Rating Scale, scores improved in 16% and normalized in 78% of the subjects. Attention, measured by on-task behavior, improved in 4% and normalized in 72% of the subjects. Academic efficiency, measured by the percentage of academic assignments completed correctly, improved in 3% and normalized in 50% of the subjects. Hence there are several different clinically significant subsets of children: those who improve in all domains, those who improve in the behavioral and attention domains but do not improve in the academic domain and require additional interventions (e.g., tutoring), those who show behavioral improvement but no significant improvement in attention or academic ratings, and a fourth subset who do not benefit from MPH in any of the three domains.

In a double-blind, placebo-controlled study of 40 children (age range, 6 to 12 years; mean, 8.6 ± 1.3 years) who were diagnosed with ADHD and treated with MPH, DuPaul et al. (1994) found that subjects ($N = 12$) who had additional internalizing symptoms such as anxiety or depression and who had high scores on the internalizing scale of the Child Behavior Checklist (CBCL) were significantly less likely to benefit from MPH at three different doses (5, 10, and 15 mg) in school, as evidenced by teachers' ratings and in the clinic setting compared with subjects with borderline ($N = 17$) or low ($N = 11$) scores on the CBCL. There was a significant deterioration in functioning on MPH among some children. In particular, 25% of the subjects in the high internalizing group were rated on the Teacher Self-Control Rating Scale as showing a worsening in classroom behavior, compared with 9.1% in the low and none in the borderline internalizing groups. On the same scale, however, 50% of the high, 93.75% of the borderline, and 72.7% of the low internalizing groups were rated as improved or normalized.

ADHD and conduct disorder may frequently coexist; in fact, DSM-IV-TR (APA, 2000) notes that if either diagnosis is present, the other diagnosis is commonly found. Psychostimulants also reduce some forms of aggression present in children diagnosed with ADDH (Allen et al. 1975; Klorman et al. 1988b). Amery et al. (1984) compared dextroamphetamine and placebo in ten boys diagnosed with ADDH with a mean age of 9.6 ± 1.6 years. Dextroamphetamine was administered in doses of 15 to 30 mg/day. The authors reported that scores on the Thematic Apperception Test Hostility Scale and Holtzman Inkblot Test Hostility Scale, and observations of overt aggression in a laboratory free play situation, were reduced significantly ($P < .05$) during a 2-week period on dextroamphetamine, compared with a similar period on placebo. These data are important, as ADHD and conduct disorder frequently coexist, and stimulants are often not considered in treating children whose conduct disorders are the primary consideration.

Approximately 75% of children with ADHD treated with stimulants will show favorable responses (Green, 1995). Among these favorable responses, there will be a spectrum. Some children will respond extremely well; others will benefit but to a lesser degree. Also, some children with ADHD (or an earlier equivalent diagnosis) will respond favorably to one stimulant drug but less favorably, not at all, or unfavorably to another. For example, Arnold et al. (1976) conducted a double-blind crossover study of D-amphetamine, L-amphetamine, and placebo in 31 children with minimal brain dysfunction (MBD). Both isomers were statistically superior to placebo and did not differ significantly from each other. Interestingly, of the 25 children with positive responses, 17 responded well to both isomers, 5 responded favorably to the d-isomer only, and three responded favorably to the L-isomer only (Arnold et al. 1976).

In a double-blind crossover study, Elia et al. (1991) compared MPH, dextroamphetamine, and placebo in treating 48 males (age range, 6 to 12 years; mean, 8.6 ± 1.7 years) with a history of hyperactive, inattentive, and impulsive behaviors that interfered with functioning both at home and at school. Following a 2-week baseline period, subjects were assigned randomly for 3-week periods during each week of which the dosage was increased, unless untoward effects prevented it, to one of three regimens: (a) MPH doses were given at 9 AM and 1 PM: subjects weighing < 30 kg received during week 1, 12.5 mg; week 2, 20 mg; and week 3, 35 mg. Subjects weighing 30 kg or more received during week 1, 15 mg; week 2, 25 mg; and week 3, 45 mg. The actual mean dosage for all subjects for week 1 was 0.9 mg/kg; week 2, 1.5 mg/kg; and week 3, 2.5 mg/kg. (b) Dextroamphetamine doses were given at 9 AM and 1 PM: subjects weighing < 30 kg received during week 1, 5 mg; week 2, 12.5 mg; and week 3, 20 mg. Those weighing 30 kg or more received during week 1, 7.5 mg; week 2, 15 mg; and week 3, 22.5 mg. The actual mean dosage for all subjects during week 1 was 0.4 mg/kg; week 2, 0.9 mg/kg; and week 3, 1.3 mg/kg. (c) Placebo dosage was held at the preceding week's level, increased to a lower dosage than mandated by the next level, or decreased because of untoward effects in 19 subjects (40%), including seven on MPH, seven on dextroamphetamine, and five on both drugs. The authors reported that 38 (79%) subjects responded to MPH and that 42 (88%) responded to dextroamphetamine; overall, 46 (96%) of the 48 subjects had a positive clinical response to one or both stimulants as rated on the Clinical Global Impressions (CGI) Scale and, in particular, for restless and inattentive behaviors. Eight subjects did not respond to MPH, four did not respond to dextroamphetamine, and two did not respond to either drug. Elia et al. (1991) distinguished between behavioral nonresponse and untoward effects, which few investigators have done. They noted that, although behavioral nonresponse to stimulants is rare, when a wide range of doses is given, most subjects had some untoward effects. During week 2 or 3 of treatment, untoward effects required that for 19 (40%) of the subjects, the dose be only partially increased in 15 (6 on MPH, 4 on dextroamphetamine, and 5 on both), held constant in 2 (one on each medication), and decreased in 2 subjects receiving dextroamphetamine. When behavioral nonresponders were combined with subjects having untoward effects, the rate of nonresponse was similar to that reported in the literature. The authors noted that making a definitive clinical decision regarding improvement was often difficult because behavioral improvements had to be balanced against untoward effects, and different symptoms responded independently to dosage, setting, and subject (Elia et al. 1991).

Wender (1988) notes that the development of tolerance to the therapeutic effects of stimulant medication is unusual and that when it occurs, it progresses gradually over a period of 1 or 2 years. If this occurs, a trial of another stimulant is suggested, because complete cross-tolerance among the stimulants does not occur (Wender, 1988). There is a suggestion that the efficacy of stimulants typically decreases with age (Taylor et al. 1987).

Gadow and Poling (1988) reviewed the literature on the use of stimulants in the mentally retarded and concluded that stimulants are highly effective in reducing symptoms of hyperactivity and conduct disorder in some individuals, regardless of the degree of their retardation.

Normal prepubertal boys and college-aged men reacted similarly to patients diagnosed with ADHD when given single doses of dextroamphetamine; they exhibited decreased motor activity and generally improved attentional performance (Rapoport et al. 1978a, 1980a). Hence earlier teachings that stimulants have a paradoxical effect in hyperactive children are incorrect, and a positive response to stimulant medication cannot be used to validate the diagnosis of ADHD.

METHYLPHENIDATE AND ATTENTION-DEFICIT/ HYPERACTIVITY DISORDER

In 1999, the landmark studies of the authoritative Multimodal Treatment Study Group of Children with Attention-Deficit/Hyperactivity Disorder (MTA) Cooperative Group were published (MTA Cooperative Group, 1999a, 1999b). Its 14-month randomized, multisite, clinical trial of four different treatment strategies for 579 children, aged 7 to 9.9 years, diagnosed with attention-deficit/hyperactivity disorder (ADHD) combined type reaffirmed the treatment efficacy of the stimulants, especially MPH. Four types of treatment were compared: (a) medication management, (b) intensive behavioral treatment, (c) combined medication and intensive behavioral treatment, and (d) standard community care by community providers. All four groups improved, but for most ADHD symptoms children in the medication and combination groups improved significantly more than those in the intensive behavior treatment and standard community care groups. Core ADHD symptoms improved equally with the combined treatment or with medication alone; however, the combined therapy may have provided modestly better

TABLE 4.1 ● **Some Pharmacokinetic Properties of Stimulant Drugs**

Drug	Principal metabolite(s)	Peak serum levels	Serum half-life	Principal route(s) of excretion
Methylphenidate (Ritalin)	Liver →75% ritalinic acid, which is pharmacologically inactive	1.9 h (range, 0.3–4.4 h); Ritalin S-R, 4.7 h (range, 1.2–8.2 h)	2–2.5 h	Kidney excretes 70% to 80%, primarily as ritalinic acid, in 24 h
Dextroamphetamine sulfate (Dexedrine)	Liver P-hydroxylation, N-demethylation, deamination, and conjugation	2 h for tablet; 8–10 h for spansule	6–8 h in children, 10–12 h in adults	May be excreted unchanged by kidney. Amount varies according to urinary pH—from 2% to 3% in very alkaline urine, to 80% in acidic urine.

outcomes for non-ADHD symptoms (e.g., oppositional and aggressive symptoms) and positive functioning (MTA Cooperative Group, 1999a, 1999b).

PHARMACOKINETICS OF STIMULANTS

The stimulants undergo some metabolism in the liver and are primarily excreted by the kidneys. Table 4.1 gives the site of metabolism, main metabolic products, time of peak plasma levels, serum half-lives, and routes of excretion of methylphenidate and dextroamphetamine.

STANDARD STIMULANT PREPARATIONS COMPARED WITH LONG-ACTING OR SUSTAINED-RELEASE FORMS

Sustained-release preparations make once-daily dosage possible. One early report found the clinical efficacy of sustained-release MPH to occur approximately 1 hour later and to be less than the standard-release form of MPH on several important measures of disruptive behavior in two studies of 22 boys with ADHD (Pelham et al. 1987). These authors thought that if once-daily dosage was necessary, then slow-release dextroamphetamine would often be preferable to sustained-release MPH. Birmaher et al. (1989) noted that the maximum serum level takes longer to develop when sustained-release tablets are administered and that peak serum levels are lower compared with those for an equivalent dose of standard MPH. These authors suggested that the relative inefficacy of sustained-release MPH could result from differences in pharmacokinetics or absorption, or from tachyphylaxis.

Some subsequent studies, however, have reported significantly different results. Pelham et al. (1990) administered standard MPH, 10 mg every morning and noon; sustained-release MPH, 20 mg every morning; dextroamphetamine spansule (long-acting), 10 mg every morning; pemoline (pemoline has subsequently been withdrawn from the market), 56.25 mg every morning; and placebo in random order for 3 to 6 days. Each double-blind, placebo-controlled, crossover study involved 22 boys, ages 8.08 to 13.17 years, diagnosed with ADHD. Midday placebos were given during the periods when long-acting drugs were administered. Subjects were rated on measures of social behavior and classroom performance, and on a continuous performance task. All four medication conditions had similar time courses, with effects evident between 1 and 9 hours after ingestion, and they were significantly, and approximately equally, better than placebo. The effects of the three long-acting preparations were as great, or almost as great, at 9 hours as at 2 hours after ingestion. Only 15 (68%) of the 22 patients improved sufficiently for the authors to recommend that they continue to receive stimulant medication. For these 15 patients, dextroamphetamine spansules were recommended for 6, pemoline for 4, sustained-release MPH for 4, and standard MPH for 1. The clinical implications of this study are potentially very important because they suggest that the great majority (i.e., 14 [93.3%] of 15 children with ADHD) derive more overall benefit from long-acting forms than from standard-release forms of stimulants. At the time of the study, it was estimated that approximately 90% of children receiving medication for ADHD were prescribed MPH, and, of these, only approximately 10% received the sustained-release form.

Fitzpatrick et al. (1992) compared the efficacy of standard and sustained-release MPH, and a combination of the two forms, in a double-blind, placebo-controlled study of 19 children (17 males and 2 females; age range, 6.9 to 11.5 years) diagnosed with ADD. Dosage of sustained-release MPH was 20 mg/day for all patients. Patients weighing < 30 kg and > 30 kg received 7.5 and 10 mg, respectively, in the morning and at noon, when on standard MPH only, and 5 and 7.5 mg, respectively, in the morning and at noon, when receiving standard MPH in combination with sustained-release MPH. Patients were rated on several scales by parents, teachers, and clinicians. All three active drug conditions were significantly better than placebo and were approximately equivalent in efficacy.

These studies, in which the medications were administered for relatively short periods, have relatively small numbers of subjects and need to be replicated with larger populations. They do, however, alert the clinician to the likelihood that sustained-release preparations are more efficacious than thought initially and they may be the preferred dosage forms for most children with ADHD.

Since the preceding studies, several new stimulant preparations with increased duration of action have appeared on the market. Adderall, which is a preparation of four amphetamine salts, has a duration of action that increases significantly with increases in dose and is compared to MPH and reviewed later under the discussion of amphetamines; Adderall XR, a longer acting form of Adderall has also been released. Extended-release forms of MPH in tablet, capsule, and Concerta, an extended-release MPH preparation that uses an osmotic delivery system combined with a semipermeable membrane to achieve a reported 12-hour duration of effect, have all been marketed. These drugs are further discussed later.

CONTRAINDICATIONS FOR STIMULANT ADMINISTRATION

Known hypersensitivity to the medication and glaucoma are significant contraindications.

Stimulants may cause stereotypies, tics, and psychosis *de novo* in sensitive individuals or if given in high enough doses. Stimulants are relatively contraindicated in children and adolescents with a history of schizophrenia or other psychosis, pervasive developmental disorders, or borderline personality organization, because they appear to worsen these conditions in some cases. However, stimulants have been given to some patients with these diagnoses with beneficial results. If the patients are also being treated simultaneously with antipsychotic medication, the risk may be diminished.

There is controversy over whether the stimulants should be given to children and adolescents with tic disorder, Tourette's disorder, or a family history of such. Their use in pervasive developmental disorders and in Tourette's disorder or with tic disorders is discussed in greater detail later.

Stimulants may aggravate symptoms of marked anxiety, tension, and agitation, and are contraindicated when these symptoms are prominent (PDR, 2005, p 2353). Stimulants also have the potential to cause hypertensive crises when used with monoamine oxidase inhibitors (MAOIs). They should not be used concomitantly with an MAOI or within 14 days of an MAOI's being discontinued.

Stimulants have a potential to be abused. They should not be prescribed to patients who have a history of drug abuse or when there is a likelihood that family members or friends would abuse the medication. In some cases in which the family is unreliable but stimulants are the drug of choice, it is worthwhile to attempt to work out a way to dispense and store all the stimulant medication at school, because, for most children, coverage during the time in school is the foremost consideration.

Magnesium pemoline was withdrawn from the market in 2005 because its potential risks were greater than its potential benefits. Reports of acute hepatic failure, some of which were fatal and others which necessitated liver transplants were the reason for this. The reader who wishes to have information regarding magnesium pemoline may consult the prior edition of this book.

INTERACTIONS OF STIMULANTS WITH OTHER DRUGS

Stimulants should not be administered with MAOIs or until at least 14 days after MAOIs were last ingested, to avoid possible hypertensive crises.

In combination with tricyclic antidepressants, the actions of both may be enhanced.

Stimulants potentiate sympathomimetic drugs (including street amphetamines and cocaine) and may counteract the sedative effect of antihistamines and benzodiazepines.

Lithium may inhibit the stimulatory effects of amphetamines.

Amphetamines may act synergistically with phenytoin or phenobarbital to increase anticonvulsant activity.

Many other drug interactions, which are less likely to be encountered in child and adolescent psychiatry than those mentioned in the preceding text, may occur.

Methylphenidate and Clonidine

On July 13, 1995, a National Public Radio broadcast reported that sudden deaths had occurred in three children taking a combination of MPH and clonidine. The ramifications of this are discussed in Chapter 9 in the section "Interactions of Clonidine Hydrochloride with Other Drugs."

ADVERSE EFFECTS OF STIMULANTS

There is some evidence that, overall, the untoward effects of MPH occur less frequently and with less severity than those from dextroamphetamine (Conners, 1971; Gross and Wilson, 1974). Gross and Wilson (1974) noted that side effects were infrequently severe enough to necessitate immediate discontinuation of the medication (1.1% of 377 patients for MPH and 4.3% of 371 patients for dextroamphetamine).

The most frequent and troublesome immediate untoward effects include insomnia, anorexia, nausea, abdominal pain or cramps, headache, thirst, vomiting, lability of mood, irritability, sadness, weepiness, tachycardia, and blood pressure changes. Many of these symptoms diminish over a few weeks, although the cardiovascular changes may persist.

Since 1972, disturbances in growth—decrements in both height and weight percentiles—have been reported for both MPH and dextroamphetamine, and the long-term untoward consequences of these effects have been of particular concern (Safer et al. 1972). There has been controversy about the significance of these changes. Mattes and Gittelman (1983) reported significant decreases in height and weight percentiles over a 4-year period. A subsequent controlled study found a significant reduction in growth velocity during the period when stimulants are actively administered (Klein et al. 1988). Despite this adverse effect on growth during the active treatment phase, it appears that an accelerated rate of growth or growth rebound occurs once the stimulant is discontinued and that there is usually no significant compromise of ultimate height attained (Klein and Mannuzza, 1988). It seems likely, however, that some children are at greater risk for growth suppression than others, and serial heights and weights of any child receiving stimulant medication should be plotted carefully on a growth chart (e.g., the National Center for Health Statistics Growth Chart) (Hamill et al. 1976).

Vincent et al. (1990) reported no significant deviations from expected height and weight growth velocities in 31 adolescents diagnosed with ADHD who had received MPH continuously for a minimum of 6 months to a maximum of 6 years after their 12th birthdays. Mean age at the beginning of the study was 12.9 ± 0.8 years. The mean daily dose was 34 ± 14 mg or 0.75 ± 0.29 mg/kg and did not differ significantly with age or sex. The results suggested that early adolescent growth is not significantly adversely affected by MPH.

Faraone et al. (2005) reported on the long-term effects of extended-release mixed amphetamine salts extended release (MAS XR) on growth in 568 children (mean age 8.7 ± 1.8 years, age range, 6 to 12 years; 78% male, 73% white, 12% black, 9% Hispanic), in a multicenter, open-label study. Subjects received doses of 10 to 30 mg/day for a period of 6 to 30 months. Based on the Centers of Disease Control norms, subjects experienced decreases in weight, body mass index (BMI) and height percentiles over the period of study; these decrements were greatest for the heaviest and tallest children; these deficits occurred primarily during the first year and decreases in weight, BMI, and height were not significant during the second year on medication. The height deficit was significant for subjects whose baseline heights were greater than the 25th percentile ($P = .001$ for the second quartile and $P < .0001$ for the third and fourth quartiles). The height loss was only 1.2 percentile points for the shortest children at baseline, whereas the tallest children at baseline experienced a 10 percentile decrease in height at the end of the study. The authors noted that monitoring growth parameters was essential but that for most children, the decreases caused by MAS XR was not likely to be of clinical concern.

Charach et al. (2006) followed up 79 subjects, age range 6 to 12 years, who were diagnosed with Attention-deficit/Hyperactivity Disorder by DSM-III-R criteria (APA, 1980a) and maintained on stimulant medication, annually for up to 5 years to determine the long-term effects of stimulants on their heights and weights. Subjects were taking various preparations of amphetamine and MPH, which were converted to an equivalent daily dose of MPH in mg/kg/day based on their potency. Small but statistically significant effects were found. Based on a statistical model, patients receiving >1.5 mg/kg/day of MPH show a decrease in expected weight gain after 1 year and subjects receiving >2.5 mg/kg/day have a decrease in expected height after 4 years on medication; the higher the dose, the greater the decrease in expected weight or height. Regular monitoring of height and weight is indicated for children and adolescents administered stimulants as a long-term treatment.

A few children treated with stimulants may develop a clinical picture resembling schizophrenia. This condition occurs most frequently when untoward effects such as disorganization are misinterpreted as a worsening of presenting symptoms and the dosage is further increased until prominent psychotomimetic effects occur. It may also occur when stimulants are administered to children with borderline personality disorders or schizophrenia, conditions in which stimulants are usually contraindicated. In most such cases, the psychotic symptomatology improves rapidly after discontinuation of the drug (Green, 1989).

Some parents express concern that treatment with stimulants will predispose their child to later drug abuse or addiction. Most available evidence indicates that this is not the case. Although drug abuse itself is of major concern in our culture, children diagnosed with ADHD who have been treated with stimulants appear to be at no greater risk for drug or alcohol abuse as teenagers and adults than controls (Weiss and Hechtman, 1986).

For children (6 to12 years of age) taking OROS MPH in doses up to 54 mg daily, the most frequent adverse events were headache (14%), upper respiratory tract infection (8%), abdominal pain (7%), vomiting (4%), loss of appetite (4%), insomnia (4%), increased cough (4%), and pharyngitis (4%). The most frequent adverse events for adolescents taking OROS MPH in doses up to 72 mg daily, were headache (9%), accidental injury (6%), and insomnia (5%) (PDR, 2006).

REBOUND EFFECTS OF STIMULANTS

Rebound effects may occur beginning approximately 5 hours after the last dose of MPH. Behavioral symptoms of rebound are often identical to those of the ADHD being treated and, in some cases, may even exceed baseline levels prior to administration of stimulants.

Rapoport et al. (1978a) reported that normal children who received dextroamphetamine experienced behavioral rebound approximately 5 hours after a single acute dose. Symptoms included excitability, talkativeness, overactivity, insomnia, stomachaches, and mild nausea.

STIMULANTS' RELATIONSHIP TO TICS AND TOURETTE'S DISORDER

Stimulants can exacerbate existing tics and precipitate tics and stereotypies *de novo*. Because of this, manufacturers state its use is contraindicated in patients with motor tics, a diagnosis of Tourette's disorder or a family history of Tourette's. There is some disagreement among experts regarding whether stimulants should be given to persons with tics, Tourette's disorder, or a family history of either condition.

In a study of 1,520 children diagnosed with ADDH and treated with MPH, Denckla et al. (1976) reported that existing tics were exacerbated in 6 cases (0.39%), and tics developed *de novo* in 14 cases (0.92%). After the discontinuation of MPH, all 6 of the tics that had worsened returned to their premedication intensity, and 13 of the 14 new tics completely remitted.

Shapiro and Shapiro (1981) reviewed the relationship between treating ADDH with stimulants and the precipitation or exacerbation of tics and Tourette's syndrome (TS). They also noted that they had treated 42 patients for symptoms of both MBD and TS with a combination of MPH and haloperidol. Dosage of MPH ranged from 5 to 60 mg/day and was individually titrated for each patient. The authors also used MPH (dose range, 5 to 40 mg/day) in 62 additional patients with TS to counteract the untoward effects of haloperidol, such as sedation, amotivation, dysphoria, cognitive impairment, and dullness. Shapiro and Shapiro (1981) concluded that the evidence suggests that stimulants do not cause or provoke TS, although high doses of stimulants can cause or exacerbate tics in predisposed patients. Clinically, they noted that tics seemed less likely to be exacerbated by stimulants in patients who were also taking haloperidol for TS; when tics did increase in intensity, they remitted within 3 to 6 hours, the approximate duration of the usual clinical effects of MPH.

Lowe et al. (1982) reported on a series of 15 patients diagnosed with ADDH who were treated with stimulant medications, including MPH, dextroamphetamine, and pemoline. These patients subsequently had tics develop *de novo*, or had existing tics worsen, sometimes into full-blown cases of Tourette's disorder. Nine subjects had existing tics; eight had family histories of tics or Tourette's disorder. Twelve of the 15 cases eventually required medication for control of the tics. The authors considered the presence of Tourette's disorder or tics to be a contraindication to stimulant medication and that stimulants should be used with great caution in the presence of a family history of tics or Tourette's disorder. They also considered the development of tics after treatment with stimulants sufficient reason to discontinue the use of stimulant medication.

Lowe et al. (1982) noted that the early clinical signs of Tourette's disorder may be difficult to differentiate from ADDH. Shapiro and Shapiro (1981) noted that approximately 57% of children with tics or TS had concomitant minimal brain disorder (MBD), although most children with MBD do not develop either tics or TS.

Comings and Comings (1984) investigated the relationship between TS and ADDH. They found that ADDH was present in 62% of 140 males < 21 years of age diagnosed with TS. A study of their family pedigrees suggested that the TS gene could be expressed as ADDH but without tics. The authors thought that their data implied that patients diagnosed with ADDH and treated with stimulants who subsequently developed tics had ADDH as a result of the TS gene and probably would have developed tics or TS even if they had not received stimulants. It is unclear whether stimulant medication might hasten the expression of such symptoms.

Gadow et al. (1992) treated 11 boys, aged 6.1 to 11.9 years (mean, 8.3 ± 1.96 years), diagnosed with comorbid tic disorder and ADHD, with MPH. The drug was administered under double-blind conditions; each subject was assigned to random 2-week periods of placebo and MPH in doses of 0.1, 0.3, and 0.5 mg/kg/day.

The authors noted that MPH significantly decreased hyperactive and disruptive behaviors in class and reduced physical aggression on the playground. Vocal tics were also significantly reduced in the lunchroom and classroom. Based on this and other studies cited in their report, the authors concluded that MPH is a safe and effective treatment for some children with comorbid ADHD and tic disorder over a short-term period; however, they cautioned that a risk of protraction or irreversible worsening of tics may exist for some individuals and that the consequences of long-term treatment of such patients are unknown.

Gadow et al. (1995) conducted a double-blind, placebo-controlled, 8-week study in which 34 prepubertal children, 31 males and 3 females, 6.08 to 11.9 years of age, diagnosed by DSM-III-R (APA, 1987) criteria with attention-deficit/hyperactivity disorder (ADHD) and comorbid chronic motor tic disorder or Tourette's disorder were treated with placebo and MPH in doses of 0.1, 0.2, and 0.5 mg/kg given twice daily (usually before leaving for school and at noon) for 2 weeks for each condition. Most children were additionally diagnosed with opposition defiant or conduct disorder. Tics were rated on five different scales by one of the authors and on the Global Tic Rating Scale by parents and teachers.

All 34 subjects responded with dramatic clinical improvement in hyperactivity and inattentive, disruptive, oppositional, and aggressive behaviors when treated with MPH. Teachers noted significant improvement in symptoms on the 0.1 mg/kg dose. There were no statistically or clinically significant adverse effects on the severity of tics with MPH treatment, but in the classroom, there was an increased frequency of motor tics on the 0.1 mg/kg/dose compared with placebo and in the physician's 2-minute motor tic count on the 0.5 mg/kg/dose. Teachers rated vocal tics as significantly less frequent on all three doses of MPH than placebo. The authors concluded that MPH was a safe and effective treatment for most children diagnosed with comorbid ADHD and tic disorder. They also cautioned that it can be extremely difficult to determine whether MPH or natural fluctuations are responsible for observed changes in the frequency or intensity of tics and that MPH is reported to have a negative effect on tics in some children (Gadow et al. 1995).

Gadow et al. (1999) continued to follow prospectively the 34 children who participated in their 1995 study at 6-month intervals for an additional 2 years of open treatment with MPH. There was no significant change in mean group scores rating severity or frequency of motor or vocal tics during the 2-year maintenance period compared with baseline or double-blind placebo ratings. Direct observations in the simulated classroom were almost identical at baseline, during the double-blind placebo protocol and the 2-year follow-up. Although there was no evidence that MPH maintenance therapy for up to 2 years exacerbated vocal or motor tics for their subjects as a group, the authors cautioned that their results do not rule out the possibility of this occurring in specific individuals. Behavioral improvements in ADHD symptomatology were maintained during the 2-year follow-up; however, behavioral problems associated with oppositional defiant and conduct disorders did not maintain their gains. Over the 2-year period there was a significant increase of approximately 10 beats/minute in heart rate, which was not felt to be clinically significant, and slightly less weight gain (0.72 kg) and less height gain (0.67 cm) than expected, both of which are so small as to not be of concern for most children.

Castellanos et al. (1997) conducted a 9-week, double-blind crossover, placebo-controlled treatment protocol (in three separate cohorts) with a total of 20 males (mean age 9.4 ± 2.0 years, range 6 to 13 years) diagnosed with comorbid ADHD and Tourette's disorder comparing methylphenidate (MPH), dexedrine (DEX), and placebo at various doses. Doses of stimulants were quite high at the upper range (e.g., 45 mg/dose [90 mg/day] for MPH and 22.5 mg/dose [45 mg/day] for DEX). Efficacy was determined by ratings on the Tourette Syndrome Unified Rating Scale and the Conners teachers' hyperactivity ratings. Medication was administered at breakfast and lunch daily. Because of the three separate cohorts, only a summary of the overall findings will be given here. Target ADHD behaviors of all subjects improved on teachers' ratings on stimulants, and there was no significantly greater improvement at the higher doses. At the lowest dose (12.5 or 15 mg/dose for MPH and 5 or 7.5 mg/dose for DEX), there was no significant change of tic severity. At highest drug doses, tic severity was significantly increased but DEX increased the severity significantly more than MPH or placebo. Of particular clinical interest was the finding that the increases in tics that occurred at higher doses of MPH tended to diminish over time and return to placebo levels when MPH was maintained or increased; this occurred in 17 of the 20 subjects. This diminution in tic severity also occurred with DEX but less significantly (in 9 of 20 subjects, $P < .01$). The authors concluded that stimulants (usually MPH is preferred) at the lowest effective dose should be considered as a possible treatment for children with comorbid ADHD and Tourette's disorder.

To further investigate whether treatment with MPH causes tics *de novo* or worsens preexisting tics in children diagnosed with ADHD, Law and Schachar (1999) conducted a 1-year-long randomized, placebo-controlled, prospective study of 91 such children who had never received medication for ADHD or tics. Inclusion criteria included the following: presence of at least 8 of the 14 DSM-III-R (APA, 1987) criteria for the diagnosis of ADHD in either the school or the home setting and a minimum of 5 such criteria in the other setting; ADHD symptoms beginning before age 7 and of at least 6 months' duration; Full Scale Intelligence Quotient (FSIQ) > 80 (based on the Block Design and Vocabulary subtests of the (WISC-III) (Wechsler, 1974); and no primary anxiety of affective disorder. Exclusion criteria were as follows: severe motor or vocal tic disorder or Tourette's disorder, as it was assumed that MPH would exacerbate such tics, but subjects with mild to moderate tics were permitted, as the authors assumed the risk of their worsening would be less and they would be more easily managed if they did occur.

Subjects were recruited from 302 consecutive referrals to an ADHD program in an urban pediatric hospital. Admission criteria were met by 105 children, and 91 elected to participate in the study. Mean age was 8.35 ± 1.55 years. Of the 46 randomly assigned to the MPH group, 11 (23.9%) had preexisting tics; of the 45 randomly assigned to the placebo group, 16 (35.6%) had preexisting tics. Study medication was begun at doses of 5 mg at breakfast and at noon on schooldays; the use of weekend and holiday medication was decided by the caregiver. Medication was increased by 10 mg weekly (each dose increased by 5 mg) until a target dose of 0.7 mg/kg/day was achieved or untoward effects precluded further increase. If families elected to switch to the alternative medication, which was an option, another blinded titration to reach the target goal was performed. Tics were rated on a 10-point scale: 0 = no tics, 1 to 3 = mild tics, 4 to 6 = moderate tics, and 7 to 9 = severe tics.

If tics developed during the treatment, the current dose of medication was continued for 1 week. If the tic did not diminish, medication was decreased by 5-mg amounts until the tic was rated as mild or disappeared. In most cases of mild tic, parents and children elected to continue with the protocol, as the clinical improvement outweighed the impact of mild tics. During the 1-year protocol,

27 (60%) of the subjects on placebo requested to change to the alternative medication because of inadequate clinical improvement; none switched because of onset of a tic disorder. No patient receiving MPH elected to switch medications. At the end of 1 year for a total of 72 subjects, there remained 18 subjects in the placebo group; the MPH group was increased by the 27 subjects who switched from placebo and decreased by one subject because of follow-up difficulties.

The mean dose of MPH at the end of dose titration was 0.5 mg/kg/day. The target of 0.7 mg/kg/day was not reached for many subjects because of untoward effects, both physiologic (insomnia, dizziness, decreased appetite, headache, and daytime drowsiness) and behavioral (staring and preoccupations), and development or worsening of tics. Because of the switches from placebo to MPH, the final distribution of subjects whose tics predated the study's onset was 21 (29.2%) of the 72 subjects in the MPH group and 6 (33.3%) of the 18 subjects in the placebo group.

By the end of the study, 10 (19.6%) of the 52 subjects with *no preexisting tics* who received MPH and 2 (16.7%) of the 12 subjects remaining in the placebo group had developed clinically significant tics that were of moderate intensity or worse, including one child in the MPH group who developed Tourette-like symptoms. There was no significant difference in the development of tics *de novo* between the groups ($P = .59$). The 12 subjects who developed tics were managed by maintaining the dose of MPH at the level when tics emerged in eight cases, reducing the MPH dose in three cases, and adding clonidine in one case. Among the 27 subjects with preexisting tics, 7 (33.3%) of the 21 receiving MPH had worsening of their tics, including 1 boy who developed Tourette-like symptoms; 2 (9.2%) experienced no change in their tics; 5 (23.8%) experienced improvement; and 7 (33.3%) had complete remission of their tics. Of the six such patients in the placebo group, two (33.3%) had worsening of tics and four had complete remission of their tics. Hence in both the MPH group and the placebo group, 66.7% (14/21 and 4/6) of the subjects with preexisting tics experienced improvement or no change in their tics, and tics worsened in 33.3% of the subjects (7/21 and 2/6). There was no significant difference between the groups ($P = .70$).

Tics *de novo* developed throughout the 1-year treatment in both groups. In the MPH group, 20 subjects developed new tics: 12 (60%) within 4 months, 6 (30%) between 4 and 8 months, and 2 (10%) between 8 and 12 months. In the placebo group, 9 subjects developed new tics: 1 (11.1%) within 4 months, 5 (55.6%) between 4 and 8 months, and 3 (33.3%) between 8 and 12 months. Only 12 of these 29 subjects who developed new tics were reported to still have tics at the end of the study, illustrating both the waxing and waning natural course of tics as well as the response to decreasing the dose of MPH in some cases. Law and Schachar (1999) concluded that titration of MPH to an optimal average maintenance dose of 0.5 mg/kg/day does not cause tics *de novo* or worsen preexisting tics of moderate severity or less, more often than placebo in children being treated for ADHD for up to 1 year.

Sverd (2000) recently reviewed the use of methylphenidate (MPH) to treat children with comorbid ADHD and tic disorders. Sverd concluded that the literature supports that ADHD is genetically related to Tourette's disorder in a substantial proportion of cases, that stimulants cause tics *de novo* or exacerbation of tics relatively infrequently, and that MPH may be safely used to treat children diagnosed with ADHD and comorbid tic disorder.

Currently, a conservative approach would consider the stimulants relatively contraindicated in treating children and adolescents with tics or Tourette's disorder, and a reason for caution in the presence of family history of such. In fact, two manufacturers of MPH products state that it is contraindicated in patients with motor tics or with a family history or diagnosis of Tourette's disorder. A review of the relevant literature, however, suggests that if risks and benefits are carefully assessed, it is reasonable to attempt a trial with MPH or amphetamine (there are more data for MPH) in such patients if they are carefully monitored.

STIMULANT DRUGS APPROVED FOR USE IN CHILD AND ADOLESCENT PSYCHIATRY

The stimulants are the most frequently prescribed psychiatric drugs during childhood. In 1977 more that half a million children were being treated with MPH in the United States alone (Sprague and Sleator, 1977). By 1987 it was conservatively estimated that in the United States, 750,000 youth were being treated with medication for hyperactivity or inattentiveness (Safer and Krager, 1988). In Baltimore County, 6% of all public elementary school students were receiving such medication; MPH accounted for 93% of the drugs prescribed, and other stimulants accounted for another 6% (Safer and Krager, 1988). Because MPH is the most commonly prescribed drug for ADHD, it will be used to illustrate the use of the stimulants, despite its having appeared on the scene considerably later than dextroamphetamine sulfate.

Methylphenidate Hydrochloride (Ritalin, Ritalin LA, Ritalin-SR, Methylin, Methylin ER, Metadate, Metadate ER, Concerta, Daytrana)

Note: There is a boxed warning concerning Drug Dependence that the FDA has directed manufacturers of methylphenidate products to include in the package insert: (name of methylphenidate product) should be given cautiously to patients with a history of drug dependence or alcoholism. Chronic, abusive use can lead to marked tolerance and psychological dependence with varying degrees of abnormal behavior. Frank psychotic episodes can occur, especially with parenteral abuse. Careful supervision is required during drug withdrawal from abusive use since severe depression may occur. Withdrawal following chronic therapeutic use may unmask symptoms of the underlying disorder that may require follow-up.

Pharmacokinetics of Methylphenidate Hydrochloride

Administration of MPH with meals does not appear to adversely affect its absorption or pharmacokinetics and may diminish problems with appetite suppression (Patrick et al. 1987).

An improvement of target symptoms can be seen in as few as 20 minutes after a therapeutically effective dose is given (Zametkin et al. 1985). Peak blood levels occur between 1 and 2.5 hours after administration (Gualtieri et al. 1982), and the serum half-life is approximately 2.5 hours (Winsberg et al. 1982). Patrick et al. (1987) have reviewed the pharmacokinetics of MPH in detail. The major metabolite produced in the liver is ritalinic acid, which is pharmacologically inactive. Between 70% and 80% of the radioactivity of radiolabeled MPH, > 75% of which is ritalinic acid, is recovered in the urine within 24 hours.

Because of these pharmacokinetics, the most frequent times to administer standard/immediate-release preparation MPH to children and adolescents are before leaving for school and during the lunch hour. This dosage schedule usually ensures adequate serum levels during school hours, which is the foremost consideration for most students.

Concerta was designed to have a 12-hour duration of effect and to be administered once daily in the morning. It is a new MPH product that uses osmotic drug delivery technology to provide for the delivery of MPH at a controlled rate throughout the day. It has an osmotically active trilayer core surrounded by a semipermeable membrane that releases MPH gradually and an overcoating of rapidly available MPH producing an initial peak plasma concentration in approximately 1 to 2 hours. Plasma concentration then continues to gradually increase to an ultimate peak level in approximately 6 to 8 hours, following which levels gradually decline. Serum half-life is 3.5 ± 0.4 hours. Doses over 54 and 72 mg/day are not recommended for children and adolescents respectively; doses >2 mg/kg/day are not recommended for any age.

Contraindications for the Administration of Methylphenidate Hydrochloride

MPH is contraindicated in patients with marked anxiety, tension, and agitation as it may worsen these symptoms. It is contraindicated in patients with known hypersensitivity to the drug, glaucoma or motor tics or a family history or diagnosis of Tourette's disorder. It is also contraindicated during treatment with MAOIs or within 14 days of discontinuing such medication.

Adverse Effects and Adjustment of Methylphenidate Hydrochloride Dose Schedule

Children who develop significant behavioral or attention difficulties in the late afternoon or early evening may do so because of a return to baseline behavior as serum levels decline into subtherapeutic levels and/or because of a rebound effect as the drug wears off (Rapoport et al. 1978a). A third dose of medication given in the afternoon may be helpful for some such children. Johnston et al. (1988), however, suggested that psychostimulant rebound effects are not clinically significant for most children.

Insomnia may also occur. It is clinically important to distinguish those children whose insomnia is an untoward effect of the drug from those whose insomnia may be due to the recurrence of behavioral difficulties as the medication effect subsides and/or a rebound effect. For the first group of children, a reduction in milligram dosage of the last dose of the day may be necessary. For the latter group, an evening dose or a dose approximately 1 hour before bedtime may be helpful. Chatoor et al. (1983) prescribed late afternoon or evening dextroamphetamine sustained-release capsules to seven children who had strong rebound effects as their medication wore off and who developed marked behavioral problems and difficulty settling down and sleeping at bedtime. Parents reported significant behavioral improvement and markedly less bedtime oppositional behavior and increased ease in falling asleep. The authors compared sleep EEGs in seven children recorded during periods on dextroamphetamine sustained-release capsules and on placebo. Compared with placebo, dextroamphetamine tended to delay onset of sleep slightly, significantly increased rapid eye movement (REM) latency (time to first REM period), and significantly decreased REM time (by approximately 14%) and the number of REM periods. Length of stage 1 and stage 2 sleep was significantly increased, and sleep efficiency (amount of time asleep during recording) decreased. Reduction in sleep efficiency was only 5%, which seemed minor compared with the significant behavioral improvement that occurred (Chatoor et al. 1983).

There is some evidence that MPH may lower the convulsive threshold (manufacturer's package insert). McBride et al. (1986), however, found only a single case report in the literature in which a child who was previously seizure-free had a seizure soon after treatment with MPH. The authors treated 23 children and adolescents, aged 4 to 15 years and diagnosed with ADD who had seizure disorders of various types ($N = 20$) or epileptiform EEG abnormalities ($N = 3$), with MPH. Fifteen of the children with documented seizure disorder received concomitant antiepileptic drugs. Individual doses of 0.33 ± 0.13 mg/kg were administered with total daily doses of 0.63 ± 0.25 mg/kg) from 3 months to 4 years. The authors found no evidence of increased frequency of seizures following MPH treatment in 16 children with active seizure disorders or 4 children who had had active seizure disorders but who had been seizure-free and off antiepileptic drugs from 2 months to 2 years. The three children with epileptiform abnormalities also did not develop seizures during the period they received MPH. This evidence suggests that MPH may not lower the seizure threshold to a clinically significant degree at usual therapeutic doses and that the presence of a seizure disorder in a child or adolescent with ADHD is not an absolute contraindication for a trial of MPH (McBride et al. 1986). Crumrine et al. (1987) also reported that they had administered MPH 0.3 mg/kg twice daily to nine males 6.1 years to 10.1 years of age who had diagnoses of ADHD and seizure disorder. The boys had been previously stabilized on anticonvulsant medication and experienced no seizures or changes in EEG background patterns or epileptiform activity during 4-week, randomized, double-blind crossover trials of MPH or placebo. Subjects improved significantly on the hyperactivity, inattention, and hyperactivity index factors on the Conners Teacher Questionnaire (Crumrine et al. 1987).

These reports suggest that when clinically indicated, it is not unreasonable to undertake a trial of MPH in children and adolescents with coexisting seizure disorders and ADHD. Clearly, frequency of seizures should be carefully monitored, and if their frequency increases or seizures develop *de novo*, the clinician may discontinue MPH.

Swanson et al. (1986) reported on six children who developed behavioral and cognitive tolerance to their usual doses of MPH during long-term treatment. To maintain satisfactory clinical response, their pediatricians had to titrate the total daily doses to levels of 120 to 300 mg administered in as many as five individual doses of 40 to 60 mg. These children performed a cognitive task better at their usual high dose (average, 60 mg three times daily) than at a lower dose (average, 30 mg three times daily), confirming cognitive tolerance. Overall, these children had high serum levels compatible with the high doses, suggesting that neither metabolic tolerance nor differential absorption was responsible for the behavioral tolerance.

Garfinkel et al. (1983) compared efficacy of MPH with placebo, desipramine, and clomipramine in a double-blind crossover study of 12 males (mean age, 7.3 years; range, 5.9 to 11.6 years) diagnosed with ADD who required day hospital or inpatient hospitalization because of the severity of their impulsivity, inattention, and aggressiveness. MPH was significantly better in improving symptoms on the Conners Scale as rated by teachers ($P < .005$) and program child care workers ($P < .001$).

Indications for Methylphenidate Hydrochloride in Child and Adolescent Psychiatry

FDA approved for treating attention-deficit/hyperactivity disorder (ADHD) and narcolepsy in patients at least 6 years of age.

Immediate-Release Methylphenidate Dosage Schedule

- Children < 6 years of age: not approved for use.
- Children at least 6 years of age and adolescents up to 17 years of age: start with 5 mg once or twice daily (usually about 7:00 AM and noon) and raise dose gradually to 5 to 10 mg/week. Maximum recommended daily dosage is 60 mg. The usual optimal dose falls between 0.3 and 0.7 mg/kg administered two to three times daily (total daily dose range of 0.6 to 2.1 mg/kg) (Duncan, 1990).
- Adolescents at least 18 years of age and adults: start with an initial daily dose of 5 mg two or three times daily, usually before meals, and titrate based on clinical response. Average dose is 20 to 30 mg/day with a range of 10 to 60 mg/day.

Immediate-Release Methylphenidate Hydrochloride Dose Forms Available

Tablets: (Ritalin, Methylin): 5 mg, 10 mg (scored), and 20 mg (scored)
    Chewable tablets (Methylin chewable tablets): 2.5 mg, 5 mg, and 10 mg
    Oral solution (Methylin oral solution): 5 mg/5 mL, 10 mg/5 mL

Extended/Sustained-Release Methylphenidate Dosage Schedule

- Children < 6 years of age: not approved for use.
- Individuals at least 6 years of age.

Methylphenidate hydrochloride sustained-release tablets and extended-release capsules are administered once daily in the morning. Their duration of action is approximately 8 hours. Start with an initial dose of 10 to 20 mg once daily and increase by a maximum of 10 mg weekly to a maximum total daily dose of 60 mg. If a patient is already receiving immediate-release methylphenidate, an equivalent milligram dose of a sustained-release preparation may be substituted for the total dose of standard-release methylphenidate used during the same period. Extended-release tablets must be taken whole and not crushed or chewed; sustained-release capsules may be opened and sprinkled on applesauce.

Extended/Sustained-Release Methylphenidate Hydrochloride Dose Forms Available

- Sustained release tablets (Ritalin-SR 20 mg; Metadate ER 10 mg, 20 mg; Methylin ER 10 mg, 20 mg). Sustained-release tablets of equivalent strength may be substituted for the total dose of the immediate-release form given over 8 hours.
- Methylphenidate extended-release capsules: (Ritalin LA 10, 20, 30, and 40 mg; Metadate CD 10, 20, and 30 mg) The recommended initial dose is 20 mg once daily in the morning. Dosage may be titrated upward in 10 mg increments weekly. The maximum total daily dose recommended is 60 mg. The capsules may be opened and sprinkled on applesauce and consumed immediately without chewing, which

(continued)

Indications for Methylphenidate Hydrochloride in Child and Adolescent Psychiatry *(Continued)*

is advantageous for some younger children or if there is a question of compliance (swallowing the capsule).

OROS [Osmotic Release Oral System] methylphenidate hydrochloride tablets (Concerta, OROS: 18, 27, 36, and 54 mg) The maximum recommended once-daily dose is 54 mg in children and up to 72 mg/day (not to exceed 2 mg/kg/day) in adolescents. Concerta was designed to have clinical effects lasting approximately 12 hours. Swanson et al. (2000) have shown that OROS methylphenidate can be initiated once daily at 18 mg/day and titrated weekly to a maximum recommended dose of 54 mg/day in children; that is, without prior titration on standard (immediate-release) methylphenidate. Swanson et al. (2003) showed that OROS methylphenidate remains clinically effective for at least 12 hours and that its efficacy is comparable to that of immediate-release methylphenidate given three times daily.

Methylphenidate transdermal system (Daytrana, 10, 15, 20, and 30 mg patches).

Reports of Interest

OROS Methylphenidate Hydrochloride in the Treatment of Attention-Deficit/ Hyperactivity Disorder. Wilens et al. (2005) conducted a long-term open-label study of OROS MPH in the treatment of 407 children (age range 6 to 13 years, mean age 9.2 ± 1.8 years). Of those enrolled, 229 subjects continued treatment to the 21/24-month endpoint. Subjects were prescribed 18 to 54 mg daily; the mean daily dose at baseline was 35.2 mg and at endpoint was 44.2 mg. Using last observation carried forward (LOCF) analyses, 85% of parents/caregivers and 92% of investigators rated a good "2" or excellent "3" response on the Global Assessment of Effectiveness. Regarding Adverse Events (AEs), 282 (69.3%) reported at least one AE that investigators thought to be probably due to OROS MPH. The most frequent were headache (30.2%), insomnia (19.9%), decreased appetite (18.7%), abdominal pain (11.1%), and tics (0.8%). The authors concluded that OROS MPH was effective and tolerable in this population for up to 2 years.

Methylphenidate Hydrochloride in the Treatment of Attention-Deficit/ Hyperactivity Disorder in Preschoolers. In a double-blind, placebo-controlled comparison of two doses (0.3 and 0.5 mg/kg/day) of MPH and placebo, Musten et al. (1997) treated 31 preschoolers (26 males, 5 females, mean age 58.07 ± 6.51 months, range 48 to 70 months) diagnosed with ADHD by DSM-III-R (APA, 1987) criteria. Twenty-six (84%) of the subjects were also diagnosed with comorbid oppositional defiant disorder and six (19%) with conduct disorder. Bilingual children had a score of ≥ 72 and English-only-speaking children of ≥ 80 on the Peabody Picture Vocabulary Test. Efficacy was evaluated by ratings on the Gordon Diagnostic System Delay and Vigilance Tasks (for attention and impulsivity), and the Conners' Parent Rating Scale-Revised (CPRS-R). Subjects were randomly assigned to each of the three conditions for a period of 7 to 10 days.

MPH significantly improved impulsivity on the Gordon Delay Task. Subjects made more correct responses on MPH than on placebo ($P < .05$) and there was no difference between the two doses of MPH. On the Gordon Vigilance Task (assessing sustained attention and impulsivity under conditions of high arousal and low feedback), there was significantly better performance on MPH than on placebo ($P < .01$) and there were no significant differences between the two doses of MPH. Parents ratings on the three subscales of the CPRS-R (Learning, Conduct, and Hyperactivity Index) all showed MPH to be significantly better than placebo ($P = .001$). There was no difference in the two MPH doses for the Conduct or Hyperactivity Index, but MPH 0.5 mg/kg/day was significantly better than MPH 0.3 mg/kg/day on the learning subscale. There was no evidence of improvement with MPH in children's compliance with parental directives on three laboratory tasks; however, MPH significantly improved the children's ability to stay on task in the 0.5 mg/kg dose but not in the 0.3 mg/kg dose. Subjects' productivity in a "cancellation task" was significantly improved on the 0.5 mg/kg dose only. Compared with placebo, parents reported significantly more untoward effects of greater severity with MPH 0.5 mg/kg/day but not with MPH 0.3 mg/kg/day. The authors concluded that the treatment of their subjects with MPH resulted in improvement similar to that reported for older children. It significantly improved attention and parent-rated behaviors. Overall the results on using 0.5 mg/kg/day were superior to using the lower dose and supported using an initial dose of 0.5 mg/kg/day in this age-group. The authors also noted that their protocol had fixed doses and that optimal doses for some subjects may have been higher and resulted in further improvement (Musten et al. 1997).

In their review of stimulant medication, Wilens and Spencer (2000) reviewed seven earlier placebo-controlled studies of MPH in a total of 187 preschoolers, mean age 4.9 years, age range, 1.8 to 6 years. The studies were 3 to 9 weeks long; total mean MPH daily dose was 5 to 20 mg/day or 0.3 to 1.0 mg/kg/day. Overall there was mild to moderate improvement in ADHD symptomatology in all the studies. They noted that subjects' compliance increased with higher doses, which tended to improve the mother–child relationship.

Methylphenidate in the Treatment of Mentally Retarded Children Diagnosed with Attention-Deficit/Hyperactivity Disorder. Handen et al. (1999) reported a 3-week, double-blind, placebo-controlled study of methylphenidate (MPH) in treating 11 preschool children (9 males, 2 females; mean age, 58.9 ± 8.2 months; age range, 4.0 to 5.9 years), 9 were diagnosed with attention-deficit/hyperactivity disorder (ADHD) by DSM-III-R (APA, 1987) criteria and the other 2 had long-standing difficulty with inattention and overactivity. Two of the subjects with ADHD were diagnosed with comorbid oppositional defiant disorder. Most subjects had intelligence quotients (IQs) in the mentally retarded range (mean IQ, 60.0 ± 11.6; IQ range, 40 to 78). Receptive/expressive language functioning was consistent with IQ in most subjects, and no subjects had diagnoses in the pervasive developmental spectrum.

All subjects underwent an initial, week-long period of baseline studies and acclimation to the study/laboratory "classroom" setting. Following this, subjects were administered MPH in 0.3- and 0.6-mg/kg doses or placebo for 1 week each. The three conditions were randomly assigned, but because of concern of untoward effects, the 0.3 mg/kg dose always preceded the 0.6 mg/kg dose. Efficacy was measured on the Conners Teacher Rating Scale (CTRS), the Preschool Behavioral Questionnaire (PBQ), the Side Effects Checklist, and several measures of behavior in the laboratory classroom (waiting task, resistance-to-temptation task, an 8-minute play session, compliance task, and cleanup task). Data were analyzed for the ten children who completed the study as one child experienced significant increase in social withdrawal, irritability, tearfulness, whining, and anxiety on 0.3 mg/kg and further treatment with MPH was not recommended.

Overall, 8 (73%) of the 11 subjects responded positively to MPH with a minimum of 40% decrease on the Hyperactivity Index of the CTRS and/or the Hyperactive-Distractible subscale of the PBQ. Ratings on MPH, 0.6 mg/kg, compared with placebo on three of the CTRS indices (Hyperactivity [$P < .005$], Inattention-Passivity [$P < .05$], and Hyperactivity Index [$P < .05$]) and the PBQ Hyperactive-Distractible subscale ($P < .005$) all showed significant improvement. In the "laboratory classroom" play intensity and movement during free play decreased significantly, and during the compliance and cleanup tasks, vocalization and disruptive behavior decreased and compliance increased significantly on the omnibus test (but not the pairwise *post hoc* tests) while on MPH. Most children experienced a positive but not significant change on the MPH 0.3-mg/kg dose; the 0.6-mg/kg MPH dose was better for most of the variables, which showed significant improvement. Unfortunately, more clinically important untoward effects (e.g., social withdrawal and irritability) also occurred more frequently at the higher MPH dose. Overall, 45% of the 11 subjects developed untoward effects on MPH. The authors concluded that preschoolers with ADHD and mental retardation responded to MPH similarly to typically developing children with ADHD. They also noted that children with developmental disabilities (e.g., mental retardation) may be at greater risk for developing untoward effects on MPH, especially at higher doses, than children without such disabilities.

Pearson et al. (2003, 2004a, 2004b) reported on the behavioral adjustment, cognitive functioning, and individual variation in treatment response in a 5-week, within-subject, crossover, placebo-controlled, double-blind study of 24 children (18 males, 6 females; mean age 10.9 ± 2.4 years) diagnosed by DSM-III-R (APA, 1987) criteria with ADHD (22, combined type; 2, inattentive type) and mental retardation (17, mild mental retardation; 7, moderate mental retardation; estimated mean IQ of the 24 subjects using the Stanford Binet 4th edition, was 56.5 ± 10.24). Subjects were treated with placebo or methylphenidate (MPH) in doses of 0.15, 0.30, and 0.60 mg/kg administered twice daily, before breakfast and at lunch time. During the first week, all subjects received placebo; during the following 4 weeks they were randomly administered each of the four conditions for 1 week. None of the children had other comorbid psychiatric diagnoses.

Behavioral adjustment (Pearson et al. 2003) was assessed by rating scales completed by teachers and parents. Symptoms of inattention, hyperactivity, oppositional behavior, conduct problems, and asocial behavior declined steadily with increasing MPH doses. The most significant findings were reported by teachers for the 0.60 mg/kg dose as follows: attention ($P = .024$), hyperactivity ($P < .001$), and oppositional behavior ($P = .012$) compared with placebo on the ADD-H Comprehensive Teacher Rating Scale and hyperactivity ($P < .001$), conduct problem ($P < .001$), emotional overindulgence ($P = .006$), asocial ($P = .009$), daydream-attention ($P = .022$), and hyperactivity index ($P < .001$) on the Conners' Teacher Rating Scale. The only parent rating that showed significant improvement was Impulsive-Hyperactive ($P = .018$) on the Conners' Parent Rating Scale. The only adverse effects reaching significance were insomnia and loss of appetite, which were dose related. Parents reported that 16.7% (4/24) of the subjects experienced insomnia and that 29.2% (7/24) experienced significantly decreased appetite at the 0.60 mg/kg b.i.d. dose. Subjects did not experience significant increases in staring, social withdrawal, or anxiety. The authors noted that their findings of increasing improvement with increasing dose in the 0.15 to 0.60 mg range were consistent with the MTA study findings (MTA Cooperative Group, 1999a). The authors also noted that their results suggest that, whenever possible, dose regulation should be done when feedback from subjects' teachers is available.

In the same subjects, Pearson et al. (2004b) investigated the effects of MPH on cognitive functioning as assessed by their performance on tasks of sustained attention (using a modified version of the Continuous Performance Test [CPT]), visual sustained attention (using the Speeded Classification Task [SCT]), auditory selective attention (using the Selective Listening Task [SLT]), impulsivity/inhibition (using a Delay of Gratification Task [DGT] and the Matching Familiar Figure Test [MFFT]), and immediate memory (using the Delayed Match to Sample [DMTS]) task. Overall, higher MPH doses were associated with significantly greater gains in cognitive task performance on all the above measures except the DMTS, where no significant MPH effects were found. The 0.15 mg/kg b.i.d. dose was relatively ineffective compared with the 0.60 mg/kg b.i.d. dose. The authors noted that, for subjects who could not tolerate the 0.60 mg/kg b.i.d. dose because of untoward effects such as appetite suppression or insomnia, 0.30 mg/kg b.i.d. also produced significant, but lesser gains.

Pearson et al. (2004a) also looked at their 24 subjects' individual variations in cognitive and behavioral responses to MPH. The authors reported that 57% of subjects on 0.15 mg/kg b.i.d. 63% of subjects on 0.30 mg/kg b.i.d. and 71% of subjects on 0.60 mg/kg b.i.d. showed (any) gains in cognitive task performance. When "significant cognitive gains," defined as > 30% improvement relative to placebo on tasks where such a score was possible, were assessed, these percentages decreased to 31%, 37%, and 46% respectively. The authors also looked at deterioration in cognitive task performance. The authors reported that 35% of subjects on 0.15 mg/kg b.i.d. 29% of subjects on 0.30 mg/kg b.i.d. and 23% of subjects on 0.60 mg/kg b.i.d. showed some deterioration in cognitive task performance. When "significant cognitive deterioration," defined as > 30% deterioration relative to placebo, were assessed, these percentages decreased to 14%, 15%, and 9% respectively. The authors noted that these data suggest that MPH is not causing the deterioration, as fewer children exhibited cognitive deterioration as the MPH dose increased.

Regarding behavioral responses to MPH, Pearson et al. (2004a) reported that 45% of subjects on 0.15 mg/kg b.i.d. 58% of subjects on 0.30 mg/kg b.i.d. and 68% of subjects on 0.60 mg/kg b.i.d. showed (any) behavioral gains. When "significant behavioral gains," defined as > 30% improvement, were assessed, these percentages decreased to 25%, 38%, and 55% respectively. The authors also looked at deterioration in behavior. The authors reported that 38% of subjects on 0.15 mg/kg b.i.d. 24% of subjects on 0.30 mg/kg b.i.d. and 13% of subjects on 0.60 mg/kg b.i.d. showed some degree of deterioration in behavioral functioning. When "significant behavioral deterioration," defined as > 30% deterioration relative to placebo, were assessed, these percentages decreased to 22%, 16%, and 9% respectively.

Importantly, the authors noted that there was substantial independence between the effects of MPH on behavioral and cognitive changes and suggested that the clinician should monitor both responses when treating such children to determine the overall efficacy in a given child. The authors concluded that children with ADHD and MR show substantial improvement in cognitive and behavioral domains when treated with MPH and that the percentage of subjects who improve far outweighs subjects who substantially worsen, and that this favorable ratio improved as the study dose of MPH increased. They reported that at the 0.60 mg/kg b.i.d. dose, five times as many subjects showed substantial cognitive and behavioral gains compared with subjects who showed substantial declines in these domains. The authors concluded that treating children diagnosed with ADHD and mild to moderate MR with MPH results in improvement in both cognitive and behavioral domains and that, on average, higher doses are more effective. The authors also noted that the response rate of children with ADHD and mental retardation to MPH is not as favorable as in children with ADHD who are not retarded (Pearson et al. 2004a).

Methylphenidate in Conduct Disorder with and Without Attention Deficit Disorder. Klein et al. (1997) conducted a double-blind, placebo-controlled study in which 84 children (age range, 6 to 15 years; mean, 10.2 ± 2.3 years; 74 males, 10 females) who were diagnosed with conduct disorder by DSM-III criteria were randomly assigned to a 5-week trial of MPH ($N = 41$) or placebo ($N = 42$). One subject dropped out before beginning treatment. A comorbid diagnosis of ADHD consistent with DSM-IV criteria was made in 69% of the subjects. Medication was administered twice daily (morning and noon doses) and was gradually raised to a total of 60 mg/day unless untoward effects prevented this. Subjects received no psychosocial therapy, although their parents were given weekly supportive counseling.

Seventy-four subjects completed the study, four taking MPH and five receiving placebo withdrew. The average dose of MPH at the termination of the study was 41.3 mg/day or 1 mg/kg, with the morning and noon doses never varying more than 5 mg. Untoward effects were reported by 31 (84%) of the subjects receiving MPH; the most common were decreased appetite and delay of sleep, with only a few instances of the latter being severe. Seventeen (46%) of the subjects on placebo reported at least one untoward effect. The authors noted that 72 (97.6%) of the subjects completing the study had at least three symptoms of conduct disorder consistent with DSM-IV criteria and that 51 (69%) had comorbid ADHD.

Compared with subjects receiving placebo, those taking MPH were rated significantly better by teachers and parents on all ratings of ADHD symptoms and all ratings of conduct disorder except socialized aggression, which measures severe delinquent behavior, such as membership in a gang, which was rare in this population. Teachers' ratings specifically noted significant reductions in "obscene language, attacks others, destroys property and deliberately cruel," whereas parents' ratings on "cruel to others, bad companions, and steals outside the home" showed significant decreases. Global improvement ratings of improved or better versus slightly improved or worse were statistically significant ($P < .001$) for subjects on MPH compared with those on placebo (teachers, 59% vs .9%; mothers, 78% vs. 27%; and psychiatrists, 68% vs. 11%). Further analysis of the data showed that the significant improvements in symptoms of conduct disorder in subjects treated with MPH were not influenced significantly by the presence, absence, or severity of comorbid ADHD. The authors concluded that MPH had an independent positive influence on provocative, aggressive, mean behaviors and that MPH had a clinically significant effect in the treatment of conduct disorder that was independent of the presence or absence of ADHD.

Methylphenidate in the Treatment of Children Diagnosed with Autistic Disorder with Symptoms of Attention-Deficit/Hyperactivity Disorder. MPH has been investigated in the treatment of children diagnosed with autistic disorder who also have symptoms of ADHD. Although most of the earlier literature states that stimulants are contraindicated for autistic children and cause a worsening in behavior and/or stereotypies, several recent studies have reported that MPH is effective in treating some children with autistic disorder who also exhibit such symptoms as hyperactivity, impulsivity, short attention spans, and aggression. Strayhorn et al. (1988) reported on two autistic children, a 6-year-old autistic boy given MPH in a randomized trial with either placebo or MPH given each day, and a preschool child treated openly with MPH. The former child was reported to show improvement in attention and activity levels, less destructive behavior, and a decrease in stereotyped movements, but sadness and temper tantrums significantly worsened. The preschooler was said to have had similar results.

Birmaher et al. (1988) treated nine hyperactive autistic children aged 4 years to 16 years with 10 to 50 mg/day of MPH. Eight of the children improved on all rating scales; the oldest child improved on all scales except the one measuring behavior in school. In contrast, Realmuto et al. (1989), who treated two 9-year-old autistic boys with 10 mg of MPH administered twice daily, found that one became fearful and unable to separate from significant adults, had a worsening of his hyperactivity, and developed a rapid pulse. The second child's baseline behaviors did not change significantly, although he developed mild anorexia.

Quintana et al. (1995) reported a 6-week, double-blind, placebo-controlled crossover study of monotherapy with methylphenidate (MPH) in the treatment of 10 children (6 males, 4 females; mean age, 8.5 ± 1.3 years; age range, 7 to 11 years) who were diagnosed with autistic disorder by DSM-III-R (APA, 1987) criteria; subjects' mean developmental quotient was 64.3 ± 9.9. Efficacy was determined by ratings on the Childhood Autism Rating Scale (CARS; scores of ≤ 29 = nonautistic; 30 to 36.5 = mildly to moderately autistic; 37 to 60 = severely autistic) and the 10-item Conners Abbreviated Parent Questionnaire, the hyperactivity factor of the Conners Teacher Questionnaire (CTQ), the Aberrant Behavior Checklist (ABC; scores of 1 to 58 = slight behavioral problem; 59 to 116 = moderate problem; and 117 to 174 = severe problem) and three subscales of the ABC (I, irritability factor; III, stereotypies; and IV, hyperactivity factor). Untoward effects were rated on the Side Effects Checklist.

All subjects had previously been treated with neuroleptics but not with MPH; all were off medication for at least 1 month and completed a 2-week baseline rating period off medication. Subjects were then randomly assigned to 1 week of placebo or of MPH 10 mg twice daily (morning and noontime doses) dose range, 0.17 to 0.33 mg/kg/day, followed by a second week of placebo or MPH 20 mg twice daily or 0.34 to 0.68 mg/kg/day. Subjects then crossed over to receive the treatment they had not received for the final 2 weeks of the study.

Ratings over baseline improved significantly, more when subjects were taking MPH compared with placebo on the hyperactivity factor of the CTQ ($P = .02$), the ABC total score ($P = .04$), ABC irritability factor ($P = .01$), and the ABC hyperactivity factor ($P = .02$). However, all these ratings except the ABC irritability factor, also improved significantly over baseline when on placebo, but the improvements were significantly less than when receiving MPH. There were no statistically significant differences in improvement between the two doses of MPH or any correlation with age or developmental quotient. Untoward effects were few and not statistically different from placebo; there was no significant change in ratings on the Abnormal Involuntary Movement Scale (AIMS) or on stereotypy ratings on the ABC stereotypic movement subscale. The authors concluded that MPH produced modest but significant improvement in hyperactivity in these patients without clinically significant untoward effects. They also recommended that hyperactive children diagnosed with autistic disorder be given a trial of MPH before a neuroleptic is administered. In some cases this may result in sufficient improvement so that a neuroleptic is not required, and in some other cases, a lower dose of neuroleptic may be effective if combined with MPH (Quintana et al. 1995).

Handen et al. (2000) conducted a double-blind, placebo-controlled crossover study of methylphenidate (MPH) in the treatment of 13 children (10 males, 3 females; mean age, 7.4 years; age range, 5.6 to 11.2 years), 9 of whom were diagnosed by DSM-IV (APA, 1994) criteria with autistic disorder and 4 of whom were diagnosed with pervasive developmental disorder not otherwise specified. In addition, all had comorbid diagnoses of both ADHD and oppositional defiant disorder ((ODD; ($N = 5$), ADHD only ($N = 6$), or ODD only ($N = 2$). Intelligence quotients were in the following ranges: average ($N = 1$), mild mental retardation ($N = 4$), moderate mental retardation ($N = 5$), severe/profound mental retardation ($N = 3$). Seven children were in special education classes and six were inpatients or in an intensive day-treatment program. Subjects were administered MPH in 0.3- or 0.6-mg/kg doses or placebo for 1 week each. The three conditions were randomly assigned, but because of concern about untoward effects, the 0.3-mg/kg dose always preceded the 0.6-mg/kg dose. Doses were given to all subjects at breakfast and lunch times; 11 subjects were given an optional third dose at about 4:00 PM. Efficacy was assessed by ratings on the Conners Teacher Scale 10-item Hyperactivity Index (CTSHI), the IOWA Conners' Teacher Rating Scale, the Aberrant Behavior Checklist (ABC), the Child Autism Rating Scale (CARS), and the Side Effects Checklist. Responders were a priori defined as having a > 50% decrease on the CTSHI on MPH (either dose) versus placebo treatments.

Eight children (61.5%) were rated "responders"; seven of them showed improvement on both doses of MPH, and the eighth only on the higher (0.6 mg/kg dose). Significant improvements occurred on one or both doses of MPH on the CTSHI, the aggression subscale of the IOWA Conners' Teacher Rating Scale, and two (hyperactivity and inappropriate speech) of the five factors on the ABC. Significant change occurred on measures on the Stereotype and Inappropriate Speech subscales of the ABC, with the greatest improvements in "odd, bizarre behavior" and "repetitive speech." No significant changes in core features of autism were evident on the CARS, which is a global assessment of autistic symptoms. There were no significant differences in clinical response between the two doses of MPH and no correlation of response with age or IQ. The authors concluded that clinically significant behavioral gains were obtained on MPH at the lower 0.3 mg/kg dose and that children diagnosed with autism may be at greater risk for untoward effects, especially in the 0.6 mg/kg dose range. One child developed crying, tantrums, aggression, and skin picking on the 0.3 mg/kg dose and was dropped from the study without getting the 0.6 mg dose; two children on the 0.6 mg/kg dose were dropped during the week, one for severe staring spells and one for increased aggression in school. Other children developed increased levels or irritability and/or social withdrawal, especially at the higher dose. At the end of the study, eight children had benefited enough to continue to be prescribed MPH in doses of 0.2 to 0.6 mg/kg.

Dexmethylphenidate Hydrochloride (Focalin; Focalin-XR)

Note: There is a boxed warning concerning Drug Dependence that the FDA has directed manufacturers of methylphenidate products to include in the package insert: (name of methylphenidate product) should be given cautiously to patients with a history of drug dependence or alcoholism. Chronic, abusive use can lead to marked tolerance and psychological dependence with varying degrees of abnormal behavior. Frank psychotic episodes can occur, especially with parenteral abuse. Careful supervision is required during drug withdrawal from abusive use since severe depression may occur. Withdrawal following chronic therapeutic use may unmask symptoms of the underlying disorder that may require follow-up.

Pharmacokinetics of Dexmethylphenidate Hydrochloride

Dexmethylphenidate hydrochloride (d-MPH) is the d-threo-enantiomer, the more pharmacologically active enantiomer of racemic methylphenidate hydrochloride (d,l-MPH), which is a 50/50 mixture of the d-threo- and the l-threo-enantiomers. Dexmethylphenidate is thought to block the reuptake of norepinephrine and dopamine into the presynaptic neuron and increase the release of these monoamines into the extraneuronal space. The drug is well absorbed orally and it may be taken with or without food. Peak plasma concentrations are reached in approximately 1 to 1 1/2 hours after ingestion in the fasting state. When taken with a high fat breakfast, peak plasma levels are about the same but take about twice as long to be reached. The medication is administered twice daily with at least 4 hours between doses. There is evidence that the therapeutic effects of d-MPH are of somewhat longer duration compared to a dose of d,l-MPH containing an equivalent amount of the d-isomer (d-MPH) (Wigal et al. 2004).

Dexmethylphenidate is metabolised primarily to ritalinic acid, which has little or no pharmacologic activity and is excreted primarily by the kidneys. The mean plasma elimination half-life of dexmethylphenidate is approximately 2.2 hours.

Contraindications of Dexmethylphenidate Hydrochloride

Dexmethylphenidate is contraindicated in patients with marked anxiety, tension, and agitation as it may worsen such symptoms.

Dexmethylphenidate is contraindicated in patients with hypersensitivity to MPH or other components of the drug. It is contraindicated in patients with glaucoma. Patients with motor tics or with a family history or diagnosis or Tourette's disorder should not be prescribed dexmethylphenidate.

To avoid a potential hypertensive crisis, dexmethylphenidate should not be prescribed to patients who are taking monamine oxidase inhibitors or within a minimum of 14 days of discontinuation of such drugs.

Adverse Effects of Dexmethylphenidate Hydrochloride

In premarketing trials with a total of 684 children, age range 6 to 17 years, the most frequently reported untoward effects were: stomach pain, fever, decreased appetite, and nausea. Other, less frequent untoward effects included vomiting, dizziness, sleeplessness, nervousness, tics, allergic reactions, increased blood pressure, and psychosis (abnormal thinking or hallucinations). A total of 50 children (7.3%) experienced untoward effects that resulted in the drug's discontinuation. The untoward effects most frequently responsible for this were: twitching (described as motor or vocal tics), anorexia, insomnia, and tachycardia approximately 1% each.

Indications for Dexmethylphenidate Hydrochloride in Child and Adolescent Psychiatry

FDA approved for treating attention-deficit/hyperactivity disorder (ADHD).

Dexmethylphenidate Dosage Schedule:

Immediate-release dexmethylphenidate should be taken twice daily with at least a 4-hour interval between doses, and may be taken with or without food.

- **Children < 6 years of age:** not approved for use.
- **Children at least 6 years of age, adolescents, and adults who were not taking racemic methylphenidate or who were on other (nonmethylphenidate) stimulants:**

  Start with 2.5 mg twice daily. Titrate at approximately weekly intervals in increments of 2.5 to 5.0 mg to a maximum of 20 mg daily.

- **Children at least 6 years of age, adolescents, and adults who are currently taking racemic methylphenidate:**

  Start with one half the dose of racemic methylphenidate to a maximum of 20 mg daily (10 mg doses administered approximately 4 hours apart).

Dexmethylphenidate Hydrochloride Dose Forms Available

- Tablets: 2.5 mg, 5 mg, and 10 mg
- Extended-release capsules (Focalin-XR): 5 mg, 10 mg, and 20 mg. This preparation permits once-daily dosing and produces a bimodal plasma concentration-time profile of two distinct peaks—an initial immediate release and the second approximately 4 hours later.

Reports of Interest

Dexmethylphenidate Hydrochloride in the Treatment of Attention-Deficit/Hyperactivity Disorder

Wigal et al. (2004) compared dexmethylphenidate hydrochloride (d-MPH) and d, l-threo-methylphenidate (d,l-MPH) in a 5-week, multicenter, double-blind, placebo-controlled study of 132 subjects (age range, 6 to 17 years; mean 9.8 years; 116 male, 16 female), diagnosed by DSM-IV criteria (APA, 1994) with an Attention-deficit/Hyperactivity Disorder. Following a 1-week, single-blind placebo lead in, subjects received d-MPH ($N = 44$), d,l-MPH ($N = 46$), or placebo ($N = 42$) twice daily (between 7 and 8 AM and between 11:30 AM and 12:30 PM) for 4 weeks; dosage was adjusted on a weekly basis to a maximum of 10 mg twice daily for d-MPH (85% were titrated to the maximum dose) and 20 mg twice daily for d,l-MPH (69% were titrated to the maximum dose). At endpoint, the average daily dose for the d-MPH group was 18.25 mg and for the d,l-MPH group 32.14 mg.

Primary efficacy was rated on the Swanson, Nolan, and Pelham (SNAP) Rating Scale completed by the teacher (Teacher SNAP) twice weekly in the afternoon. Secondary efficacy measures included the Parent SNAP (Saturdays and Sundays at

3:00 PM and 6:00 PM), Clinical Global Impressions Scale-Improvement (CGI-I), and a math test; these ratings were obtained at 6:00 PM to test the hypothesis that the duration of action of d-MPH would be longer than that of d,l-MPH.

On the Teacher SNAP, both the d-MPH group ($P = .0004$) and the d,l-MPH group ($P = .0042$) had significantly greater improvement than the placebo group; the effect size was large (1) and equal for both drugs. Duration of significant efficacy was longer for the d-MPH group as measured by the Parent SNAP (d-MPH score significance at 3:00 PM $P < .0001$; at 6:00 PM $P = .0003$) than that for the d,l-MPH group (d,l-MPH score significance at 3:00 PM was 0.0073; at 6:00 PM $P = .0640$). On the CGI-I, 22% of subjects of placebo were rated "much" (16.2%) or "very much improved (5.4%). Compared with the placebo group, 67% of d-MPH subjects were rated "much" (35.7%) or "very much improved" (31%) with $P = .0010$; 49% of d,l-MPH subjects were rated "much" (26.8%) or "very much improved" (22.0%) with $P = .0130$. The d-MPH group improved significantly more from baseline to endpoint than the placebo group ($P = .0007$); the d,l-MPH group's improvement did not quite reach significance compared with the control group ($P = .0589$).

On the 6:00 PM math test, the d-MPH group scored significantly better that the placebo group; the placebo group worsened from baseline with an average of 3.9 fewer correct answers, whereas the d-MPH group got an average of 12.5 more problems correct ($P = .0236$). The d,l-MPH group scores on the 6:00 PM math test were not significantly different from those of the placebo group.

No patients experienced serious adverse effects (AEs). Headache, abdominal pain, nausea, diminished appetite were the most frequently reported AEs. Abdominal pain was reported more frequently in the d-MPH group compared to the d,l-MPH group ($P = .0252$). Clinically significant changes occurred in the vital signs of 13 subjects (3 d-MPH, 8 d,l-MPH and 2 placebo) respectively. Significant weight loss, ranging from 5% to 18% of baseline weight, was reported for four subjects in the d-MPH group, six subjects in the d,l-MPH group, and two subjects in the placebo group.

The authors concluded that d-MPH (mean, 18.25 mg) and d,l-MPH (mean, 32.14 mg) have similar efficacy and safety in treating ADHD, similar large effect sizes, and suggest that d-MPH has a longer duration of action that d,l-MPH after twice daily dosing (Wigal et al. 2004).

As part of a multicenter study, Arnold et al. (2004) administered dexmethylphenidate hydrochloride (d-MPH) to 89 subjects (72 males, 17 females; mean age 10.1 ± 2.9 years, age range 6 to 16 years) who were diagnosed with attention-deficit/hyperactivity disorder (ADHD); 71.9% were treatment naive. The first phase of the study was an open-label, dose-titration study of 6-weeks' duration; this was followed by a 2-week, double-blind, randomized, placebo-controlled withdrawal phase.

Efficacy was measured on the Clinical Global Impressions-Improvement (CGI-I) Scale, the Swanson, Nolan, and Pelham (SNAP)-ADHD Rating Scale, and a "Math Test," which was used as a measure of "duration-of-effect" of the medication. The CGI-Severity (CGI-S) Scale was used to assess the severity of the subject's illness.

Medication was begun at doses ranging from 2.5 to 10 mg twice daily (morning dose and a noontime dose) depending on subjects' prior medication histories. During the first 4 weeks, medication was titrated upward to a maximum total dose of 20 mg daily or until adverse effects prevented increase or a CGI-I score of 1 "very much improved" or 2 "much improved" was achieved. During weeks 5 and 6, the dose was held constant.

Of the 89 subjects, 76 completed the 6-week open-label phase. The 13 dropouts were due to therapeutic failure (4), adverse effects (4), lost to follow-up (3), withdrawn consent (1), and protocol violation (1). Seventy-three completers (82% of the subjects) were rated 1 or 2 on the CGI-I; 89.2% were rated "normal to mildly ill" on the CGI-S Scale versus only 1.1% at baseline ($P < .001$). A total of 77 patients (86.5%) experienced adverse effects. Four subjects were discontinued because of adverse effects (one with rambling speech and tremor, one with labile mood, one with moderate headaches, and one with sleep terrors with somnambulism). Eight subjects had reduction in dosage because of tremor and anergy, gastrointestinal distress (including nausea, emesis, and diarrhea), headache, insomnia, unusual sensory experience, and irritability; except for insomnia, these adverse effects remitted with dose reduction.

Seventy-five of the subjects entered the subsequent 2-week withdrawal phase; 35 were assigned to d-MPH and 40 to placebo; 1 dropped out from each group. At the time of assignment 88.6% of the subjects in the d-MPH group and 87.5% of those in the placebo group were rated as showing only mild to no ADHD symptoms. Similarly 70.6% of the d-MPH group and 80% of the placebo group were taking 10 mg of dexmethylphenidate twice daily. The placebo group showed significantly more treatment failures than the d-MPH group on the CGI-I: 61.5% had scores of 6 "much worse" or 7 "very much worse" versus 17.1% ($P = .001$), deterioration in the 3:00 PM Math Test ($P = .024$) and the 6 PM Math Test ($P < .0001$), Teacher SNAP-ADHD ($P = .028$) and the Parent SNAP-ADHD scores at 3:00 PM ($P = .0026$) and at 6:00 PM ($P = .0381$).

The authors also noted that adverse effects were similar to those of other stimulants and that scores on the Math Tests at 3 and 6 hours after the noon dose, confirmed the earlier reported duration of efficacy for dexmethylphenidate to be at least 6 hours after the second daily dose (Arnold et al. 2004).

Silva et al. (2006) reported a multicenter, 2-week, double-blind, placebo-controlled, crossover study in which 54 subjects, age range 6 to 12 years, mean age 9.4 ± 1.6 years who were diagnosed with Attention-deficit/Hyperactivity Disorder by DSM-IV criteria, were randomly assigned to treatment for a 7-day period, which consisted of a 20 mg dose of d-MPH-ER (extended release) for 5 days, a day off medication, then on the seventh day, ratings in the (period 1) classroom laboratory setting on d-MPH-ER followed by another 7-day period consisting of placebo for 5 days, a day off medication, and then on the seventh day ratings in the (period 2) classroom laboratory setting on placebo (sequence A) or the reverse order (sequence B). All subjects had been stabilized on a total daily dose of 20 to 40 mg of d,l-MPH for a minimum of 1 month before beginning the study. All subjects had four visits: an initial screening visit, a practice day in the classroom, and two evaluation classroom days.

The primary efficacy variable was the Swanson, Kotkin, Agler, M-Flynn, and Pelham (SKAMP)-Combined scores at time 1-hour postdose. Secondary efficacy variables over the 12-hour classroom session were SKAMP-Attention and SKAMP-Deportment scores and the written math test score; these ratings were done at postdose hours 1, 2, 4, 6, 8, 9, 10, 11, and 12. The adjusted mean change in the SKAMP-Combined score from predose to 1-hour postdose was -10.014 for subjects when on d-MPH-ER compared with 0.878 when on placebo ($P < .001$) and the scores on d-MPH-ER were consistently significantly superior to placebo for the 12-hour period of laboratory classroom measurements ($P < .001$). The authors estimated the duration of effect of d-MPH-ER to be from 1 to 12 hours postdose. Scores on the SKAMP-Attention and SKAMP-Deportment Scales were significantly better with d-MPH-ER than with placebo at all time points. Mean changes from pre-dose in the number of math problems attempted and the number of math problems correctly answered indicated that d-MPH-ER was significantly more effective than placebo (P < .001).

Because of imbalanced predose scores on the SKAMP-Combined and SKAMP–Attention; Math-Attempted and Math-Completed scores were significantly different between the two treatment weeks, a *post hoc* analysis was performed. In that analysis, for the SKAMP scores, the imbalance was mainly due to higher predose values in subjects given d-MPH-ER during the first week (period 1). The *post hoc* analysis of the 27 subjects who had d-MPH-ER during the first week was no longer significantly different from placebo at times 8, 10, 11, and 12 hours. Similarly, for both Math-Attempted and Math-Correct, scores at time 9, 10, 11, and 12 hours were not significantly different from placebo. The authors noted that this constraint may have contributed to the significant difference between drug and placebo during the later hours and recommended a larger sample without issues of imbalanced predose values to further clarify the duration of action of d-MPH-ER.

Adverse events (AEs) were obtained by observation in the laboratory classroom, spontaneous reporting by the subjects, and parental reports of the period preceding each assessment day. One subject, on placebo, dropped out of the study because of nausea. Reported AEs were mild or moderate; no clinically significant cardiovascular AEs or laboratory abnormalities occurred. AEs that occurred more frequently on d-MPH-ER than placebo and possibly related to the drug were: decreased appetite (9.4% vs. 0%), anorexia (7.5% vs. 0%) upper abdominal pain (5.7% vs. 1.9%), fatigue (3.8% vs. 0%), and insomnia (3.8% vs. 0%). The authors noted that because subjects had been stabilized on d,l-MPH prior to entering the study, the number and severity of adverse effects reported would tend to be less than would be the case if subjects were treatment naïve.

Overall, the authors concluded that in this group of subjects, d-MPH-ER was both safe and effective in treating ADHD. Its duration of action may last for up to 12 hours (Silva et al. 2006).

Amphetamine Sulfate: Dextroamphetamine Sulfate (Dexedrine); Mixed Amphetamine Salts (Adderall)

Pharmacokinetics of Dextroamphetamine Sulfate

Amphetamines are noncatecholamine sympathomimetic amines with central nervous system activity. Dextroamphetamine sulfate is the dextro isomer of racemic (dextro [d-] levo- [l-]) amphetamine sulfate (Benzedrine), which was historically the first stimulant used in child and adolescent psychopharmacology (Bradley, 1937). The d-isomer is biologically more active than the l-isomer. However, as noted in the preceding text, some individuals respond positively to the l-isomer and not to the d-isomer (Arnold et al. 1976). Maximal dextroamphetamine plasma concentrations occurs approximately 3 hours after oral ingestion. Average plasma half-life is approximately 12 hours.

Contraindications for the Administration of Dextroamphetamine Sulfate

The administration of dextroamphetamine sulfate is contraindicated in individuals with symptomatic cardiovascular disease, moderate to severe hypertension, hyperthyroidism, hypersensitivity to the sympathomimetic amines, or glaucoma. Sudden death has been reported in children with structural cardiac abnormalities who were treated with amphetamines at usual therapeutic doses.

Individuals who are in an agitated state or who have a history of drug abuse should also not be prescribed this drug.

Amphetamines should not be prescribed during or within 14 days of the administration of a monoamine oxidase inhibitor (MAOI) to avoid the risk of a hypertensive crisis.

Amphetamines should be used with caution in individuals who have motor or vocal tics, Tourette's disorder or a family history of such. This is discussed in more detail in the introductory part of this chapter.

Untoward Effects of Dextroamphetamine Sulfate

Dextroamphetamine sulfate elevates the systolic and diastolic blood pressure and has weak bronchodilator and respiratory stimulant action. Tachycardia may occur. The most frequent and troublesome immediate untoward effects include insomnia, anorexia, nausea, abdominal pain or cramps, vomiting, constipation or diarrhea, headache, dry mouth, thirst, lability of mood, irritability, sadness, weepiness, tachycardia, and blood pressure changes. Many of these symptoms diminish over a few weeks, although the cardiovascular changes may persist.

Clinical experience suggests that behavioral symptoms and thought disorder in psychotic children may be worsened by the administration of amphetamines. Amphetamines may cause short-term suppression of growth. Their long-term effects on growth inhibition are not certain and growth should be monitored during their administration. This is discussed in more detail in the introductory part of this chapter.

Indications for Amphetamine Preparations in Child and Adolescent Psychiatry

There is a "Black Box" warning for all amphetamine products:

Note: Amphetamines have a high potential for abuse. Administration of amphetamines for prolonged periods of time may lead to drug dependence. Particular attention should be paid to the possibility of subjects obtaining amphetamines for nontherapeutic use or distribution to others and the drugs should be prescribed or dispensed sparingly.
Misuse of amphetamine may cause sudden death and serious cardiovascular events.

Dextroamphetamine sulfate is FDA approved for treating attention deficit disorder with hyperactivity (ADDH), narcolepsy, and exogenous obesity. (ADDH is a DSM-III APA, 1980a diagnosis that, in large part, corresponds to the DSM-IV APA, 1994, 2000 diagnosis ADHD.)

Immediate-Release Amphetamine Sulfate Dosage Schedule for Treating ADHD

The serum half-life for standard-preparation dextroamphetamine sulfate is approximately 6 to 8 hours in children. This half-life makes it possible for some children to take the medication before leaving for school and maintain clinical effectiveness for

(continued)

Indications for Amphetamine Preparations in Child and Adolescent Psychiatry *(Continued)*

the duration of the school day without taking a noontime dose, which is required when the standard-preparation methylphenidate is used.

- Children < 3 years of age: not approved for use.
- Children 3 through 5 years of age: begin with 2.5 mg daily; raise by 2.5-mg increments once or twice weekly; titrate for optimal dose.
- Patients 6 years and older: begin with 5 mg daily; raise by 5-mg increments once or twice weekly; the usual maximum dose is 40 mg/day or less.

The usual optimal individual dose falls between 0.15 and 0.5 mg/kg for each dose (Duncan, 1990), administered two to three times daily (total daily dose range, 0.30 to 1.5 mg/kg/day).

Mixed amphetamine salts (Adderall), which is a combination of equal parts of dextroamphetamine saccharate, amphetamine aspartate, dextroamphetamine sulfate, and amphetamine sulfate, has been introduced for the treatment of attention deficit disorder with hyperactivity and narcolepsy. Peak plasma concentration occurs approximately 3 hours after ingestion. The manufacturer states that its plasma half-life is 7 to 8 hours, based on the amphetamine component. Usually the first dose is given soon after awakening or before leaving for school; this may be followed by an addition one or two doses at 4- to 6-hour intervals. Whether this combination has clinically significant benefits compared to standard- or extended-release dextroamphetamine sulfate is uncertain at present.

Immediate-Release Amphetamine Sulfate Dose Forms Available

- Tablets (Dexedrine): 5 mg
- Tablets (DextroStat): 5 mg, 10 mg

Immediate-Release Mixed Amphetamine Salts Preparations Available

- Tablets (Adderall): 5 mg, 7.5 mg, 10 mg, 12.5 mg, 15 mg, 20 mg, and 30 mg

Extended-Release Amphetamine Preparations Dosage Schedule and Available Dose Forms for Treating ADHD

Extended-Release Dextroamphetamine Sulfate (Dexedrine)

- Sustained-release capsules (Dexedrine spansules): 5 mg, 10 mg, 15 mg

The maximum dextroamphetamine plasma concentrations occurs approximately 8 hours after oral ingestion of the sustained-release capsule. The plasma half-life is approximately 12 hours, similar to that of the immediate release form. The manufacturer also noted that this "formulation has not been shown superior in effectiveness over the same dosage of the standard, noncontrolled-release formulation given in divided doses" (PDR, 2005, p 1465).

Extended-Release Mixed Amphetamine Salts (Adderall XR) and Dose Forms Available

- Extended-release capsules (Adderall XR): 5 mg, 10 mg, 15 mg, 20 mg, 25 mg, and 30 mg

The average time to maximum serum levels of Adderall XR is approximately 7 hours. Its duration of action is roughly equivalent to taking two doses of immediate release Adderall of the same total dose 4 hours apart. The capsule can be opened and sprinkled on applesauce without significantly changing its rate of absorption.

Dextroamphetamine in the Treatment of Attention Deficit Disorder with Hyperactivity/Attention-Deficit/Hyperactivity Disorder

Dextroamphetamine sulfate and Adderall, a preparation of four amphetamine salts, are the only amphetamines currently used with any frequency to treat ADHD in the United States and are the only stimulants currently in use that are approved by the FDA for administration to children as young as 3 years of age. Hence they are officially the standard treatment for children up to age 6 years; however, many clinicians do prescribe MPH for some patients < 6 years of age as there is considerable clinical experience and literature supporting this. Methamphetamine hydrochloride (Desoxyn) is approved for use in children above 6 years of age; however, as in the author's experience it is infrequently prescribed it is not discussed in this book. In addition, if MPH does not provide satisfactory benefit in controlling symptoms of ADHD, it is recommended that an amphetamine product be tried before moving on to another class of drugs.

Amphetamines may obtund the maximal electroshock seizure discharge and have been reported to prevent typical three-per-second spike-and-dome petit mal seizures and to abolish the abnormal EEG pattern in some children (Weiner, 1980). Amphetamine preparations may therefore be the stimulants of choice for individuals who have seizures or who are at risk for developing them, although, as noted earlier, MPH does not appear to increase the frequency of seizures or their development *de novo* when administered in usual therapeutic doses.

Reports of Interest

Amphetamine Sulfate in the Treatment of ADHD. Gillberg et al. (1997) reported a 12-month, randomized, double-blind, placebo-controlled study in which 62 subjects (52 males, 10 females; mean age, 9.0 ± 1.6 years; range, 6 to 11 years), diagnosed by DSM-III-R (APA, 1987) criteria with severe ADHD (26 [42%] of whom had various comorbid disorders) were treated with (racemic) amphetamine sulfate. For 72 subjects, the entire 18-month-long protocol was preceded by a 1-month baseline evaluation. During months 1 through 3, they were administered amphetamine sulfate in a single-blind fashion beginning with initial daily doses of 5 mg at breakfast and 5 mg at lunch times. Subsequent dose regulation permitted a maximum total daily dose of 60 mg. Ten subjects dropped out during this period because of untoward effects or lack of clinical response. The remaining 62 subjects all improved significantly. The 4th through 15th months consisted of the double-blind, placebo-controlled administration of amphetamine sulfate or placebo. The mean amphetamine sulfate dose of the 62 participating subjects at the beginning of this portion was 17 mg/day or 0.52 mg/kg/day, with a range of 5 to 35 mg/day or 0.20 to 1.10 mg/kg/day. During the double-blind portion, dosage was increased for 11 subjects and decreased for 8 subjects. Only 32 subjects (24 of 32 [75%] on active medication and 8 of 30 [27%] receiving placebo) completed the 12-month double-blind, placebo-controlled portion of the protocol. Most of the subjects assigned to the placebo group required switching to open treatment with amphetamine before the completion of the double-blind portion. Months 16 through 18 consisted of administration of single-blind placebo. Efficacy was assessed by ratings on Conners Parent and Teacher Scales and the Wechsler Intelligence Scale for Children—Revised (WISC-R).

During the 12-month placebo period, the group assigned to amphetamine retained the improvements achieved during the 3-month period on amphetamine, but the group assigned to placebo experienced reexacerbation of ADHD symptoms, as shown by comparison of ratings on the Conners Parent Scale, with mean scores declining from 43% to 47% ($P < .001$) and the Conners Teachers Scale with mean scores declining from 27% to 43% ($P < .01$). Comparing baseline WISC-R Scores to those at 15 months, the 35 subjects taking amphetamine for $\geq$ 9 months showed FSIQ a mean increase of 4.5 ± 4.7 points versus a mean increase of 0.7 ± 7.2 for the 8 subjects taking placebo for $\geq$ 6 months ($P < .05$). With the exception of decreased appetite for the amphetamine group, there were no significant differences in untoward effects for the placebo and amphetamine groups during the double-blind portion of the study. Four males developed hallucinations during the study; three were on active drug and one was on placebo. Upon stopping medication or with dose reduction, the hallucinations rapidly ceased. This study is one of the few long-term studies of amphetamines and suggests that the drug is safe and effective in treating children with ADHD for up to 15 months. Interestingly, when amphetamine was replaced with placebo during the 16th to 18th months of the study, there was no change in parent ratings and only a nonsignificant decline in teachers' ratings, suggesting that behavioral improvements were being maintained without the active drug.

Dextroamphetamine Sulfate in the Treatment of ADHD in Children Diagnosed with Pervasive Developmental Disorder. Geller et al. (1981) reported that dextroamphetamine administered to two children with pervasive developmental disorder and ADDH improved their attention spans with no significant worsening of behavior.

Adderall

Adderall (mixed amphetamine salts [MAS]) is composed of equal proportions of four amphetamine salts (D-amphetamine saccharate, D-amphetamine sulfate, d,l-amphetamine sulfate, and d,l-amphetamine aspartate), resulting in a 3:1 ratio of d-isomer to l-isomer.

Two double-blind placebo-controlled studies, the 4-week, multicenter study of Biederman et al. (2002) in naturalistic home and school settings with an N of 584 and the 6-week analog classroom study of McCracken et al. (2003) with an N of 51 reported that an extended-release formulation of MAS (Adderall XR) was effective and safe in treating children 6 to 12 years of age who were diagnosed with ADHD for at least 12 hours. In 2005, McGough et al. reported on the long-term tolerability and effectiveness of once-daily MAS XR in a 24-month, multicenter, open-label extension of these two studies. A total of 568 subjects who had completed one of the double-blind studies with no significant adverse effects (AEs) or had withdrawn for reasons other than AEs entered the long-term study. MAS XR was initiated in all subjects at a once-daily morning dose of 10 mg; 10-mg increases were permitted at weekly intervals during the first month to a maximum of 30 mg/day. The primary measure of effectiveness was the 10-item Conners Global Index Scale, Parent (CGIS-P) version. A total of 273 subjects (48%) completed the 24-month extension; the major reasons for discontinuing prematurely were: withdrew consent (87, 15.3%); AEs (84, 14.8%); and lost to follow-up (74, 13%). The mean once-daily dose for completers was 22.4 ± 6.9 mg. Improvement of $> 30\%$ in CGIS-P scores was maintained over the duration of the study ($P < .001$). Most AEs were of mild or moderate severity. The most frequent AEs responsible for withdrawal from the study were weight loss (27, 4.8%), anorexia/decreased appetite (22, 3.9%), insomnia (11, 1.9%), depression (7, 1.2%), and emotional lability (4, 0.7%). Mean systolic and diastolic blood pressure increased by 3.5 and 2.6 mm Hg respectively; heart rate increased by 3.4 beats/minute. There were no clinically significant changes in laboratory test values. The authors concluded that MAS XR in once-daily doses of between 10 to 30 mg was well tolerated and resulted in significant clinical benefits over the 24-month extention period in children diagnosed with ADHD (McGough et al. 2005).

Adderall Versus Methylphenidate

Several studies have compared Adderall and MPH in the treatment of children and adolescents diagnosed with attention-deficit/hyperactivity disorder.

Swanson et al. (1998) conducted a 7-week, double-blind, placebo-controlled, crossover study of placebo, methylphenidate (MPH), and Adderall in doses of 5, 10, 15, and 20 mg. All subjects had prior significant clinical responses to MPH (average total daily dose was 31.06 ± 13.59 mg divided into three doses), and each subject received an initial dose of MPH identical to that he or she had been taking (average dose was 12.5 mg) during the week on that condition. Each subject was on one of the six conditions for a week; during the seventh week one of the conditions was repeated randomly, or if one condition had been missed, the medication appropriate for that week was given.

Findings of particular clinical interest were as follows: peak clinical effects of MPH occurred at an average of 1.88 hours, more rapidly than Adderall at usual doses, where peak clinical effects occurred at 1.5, 2.6, 2.6 (sic), and 3 hours for the 5-, 10-, 15-, and 20-mg doses, respectively.

MPH had a shorter duration of action that ended rather abruptly at an average of 3.98 hours. The duration of action of Adderall was dose dependent, increasing with the dose; duration of action was 3.52, 4.83, 5.44, and 6.40 hours for the 5-, 10-, 15-, and 20-mg doses, respectively.

Adderall was efficacious in the treatment of ADHD and there were no unexpected or serious untoward effects; those that occurred were typical of stimulants.

Manos et al. (1999) compared the efficacy of methylphenidate (MPH) given twice daily (breakfast and lunch times) and a single breakfast-time dose of Adderall in a 4-week, double-blind titration, placebo-controlled study of 84 subjects (66 males, 18 females; mean age, 10.1 years; range, 5 to 17 years) diagnosed with attention-deficit/hyperactivity disorder by DSM-IV (APA, 1994) criteria. Each child's physician decided which active drug the child would be prescribed; parents and clinicians were aware of which active drug their child would receive but not of the dose titration or when placebo would be given. All subjects received 7 days of treatment with placebo, and 5-, 10-, and 15-mg doses of either MPH or Adderall. The four conditions were assigned randomly except that the week of the 10-mg dose had to precede the week of the 15-mg/day dose. Seven children on MPH and four on Adderall did not receive the 15-mg/day dose because their physician thought they were too young or weighed too little and had made an assessment that the optimal dose had already been achieved.

Efficacy was determined by the ADHD rating scale, the Conners Abbreviated Symptoms Questionnaire, Composite Ratings, School Situations Questionnaire—Revised, and the Side Effect Behavior Monitoring Scale. The average optimal dose of MPH was 19.5 mg/day and of Adderall was 10.6 mg/day, suggesting that Adderall is clinically about twice as potent as MPH. The optimal dose was significantly better than baseline or placebo conditions. There were no significant differences between parent and teacher ratings of subjects on MPH or Adderall. There were no clinically or statistically significant medication effects at any dose for pulse, blood pressure, or weight. The most commonly reported untoward effects at optimal dose for MPH were "anxious" (7/42, 16.7%), "perseveration" (5/42, 11.9%), "stares a lot" (4/42, 9.6%), "sad/unhappy" (9.6%), and "drowsiness" (3/42, 7.1%). For Adderall, the most common untoward effects at optimal dose were "insomnia" (5/42, 11.9%), "sad/unhappy" (11.9%), "prone to cry" (11.9%), and "irritability" (3/42, 7.1%). These children actually experienced more total untoward effects when not receiving medication, but the differences were not significant. The authors concluded that their data showed that the efficacy of a single morning dose of Adderall was comparable to that of morning and noon doses of MPH, and that therefore a single morning dose of Adderall can eliminate the need of a noontime dose in school and simplify the drug management of such children. Of additional clinical interest, all 15 of the Adderall subjects who had previously tried MPH without clinical benefit (7 were nonresponders and 8 had serious untoward effects) showed clinical improvement on Adderall. The only two subjects who showed no clinical improvement in the study were both receiving Adderall. No subjects receiving MPH had previous trials of MPH.

Pliszka et al. (2000) conducted a 3-week, double-blind, placebo-controlled, parallel-group study comparing placebo, Adderall, and MPH in the treatment of 58 children, mean age 8.2 ± 1.4 years diagnosed with attention-deficit/hyperactivity disorder. A flexible dosing algorithm was devised to permit blind titration of the dose at the end of the first and second weeks based on clinical response. At the end of the study, the mean dose of Adderall was 12.5 ± 4.1 mg/day and the mean dose of MPH was 25.2 ± 13.1 mg/day. The most important clinical findings of the study were that both drugs were superior to placebo. The positive effects of Adderall on behavior lasted longer than those of MPH. No subject receiving Adderall required a noon dose; however, 7 of the 13 MPH responders also did not require a noon dose. There was a greater tendency for the children on Adderall to have more stomachaches and to manifest a sad mood than for those receiving MPH.

Caffeine

Caffeine is included among the stimulants because there have been some suggestions that it may be useful in treating ADHD. Two reviews of the relevant literature concluded that caffeine is not a therapeutically useful drug in the treatment of ADHD (Klein, 1987; Klein et al. 1980).

Bernstein et al. (1994) investigated the effects of caffeine on learning, performance, and anxiety in 21 prepubescent normal children, 12 males and 9 females, 8 through 12 years old (mean age, 10.6 ± 1.3 years) who ingested a minimum of 20 mg/day of caffeine in their usual diets (average daily caffeine consumption by subjects was 50.9 ± 52.2 mg/day or 1.3 mg/kg/day). Children with significant medical conditions or those ever diagnosed with ADHD were excluded. Subjects were enrolled in a double-blind, placebo-controlled, crossover study in which they were seen for four 2-hour sessions spaced approximately 1 week apart. The four rated conditions were baseline, placebo, low-dose (2.5 mg/kg) caffeine, and high-dose (5 mg/kg) caffeine. Caffeine intake was restricted for 12 to 15 hours before the sessions. Children reported feeling less "sluggish" after receiving caffeine, and their performances improved significantly on two of four measures of attention and a test of manual dexterity for the dominant hand. Self-reported anxiety level showed a trend to increase.

Magnesium Pemoline (Cylert)

Between the second (1995) and third (2001) editions of this book, the situation regarding magnesium pemoline changed significantly. The manufacturer noted in the package insert that Cylert was associated with life-threatening hepatic failure and that 15 cases of acute hepatic failure had been reported to the FDA since it was first marketed in 1975. This was 4 to 17 times the rate expected in the general population. Twelve of the cases resulted in death or liver transplantation, usually within 4 weeks of onset of signs of liver failure.

Since the last edition was published, Pemoline has been withdrawn from the market (in 2005), after it was determined by the FDA that the overall risk of liver toxicity from pemoline magnesium outweighed its potential benefits. The interested reader may consult the prior edition if he/she requires further information.

CHAPTER 5

First Generation/Typical Antipsychotic Drugs

INTRODUCTION

Although antipsychotic drugs, also commonly known as *neuroleptics* or *major tranquilizers*, are used in adults primarily to treat psychoses, in children they have also been used to treat other common nonpsychotic psychiatric disorders. At present, antipsychotics are the drugs of first choice in childhood for schizophrenia and autistic disorder. There is, however, some evidence that antipsychotics are not as effective clinically in schizophrenia with childhood onset as in schizophrenia occurring in later adolescence and adulthood (Green et al. 1984). Meyers et al. (1980) noted that serum neuroleptic levels of 50 ng/mL of chlorpromazine equivalents correspond to the threshold for clinical response in adult patients with schizophrenia and suggest that similar therapeutic serum levels are necessary in children. Because children may metabolize and excrete antipsychotics more efficiently than adults, determination of serum neuroleptic levels, if they are available, is recommended before a trial of an antipsychotic is deemed a failure.

Shapiro and Shapiro (1989) concluded that antipsychotics were also the drugs of choice for treating chronic motor or vocal tic disorder and Tourette's disorder when psychosocial, educational, or occupational functioning was so impaired that medication was required.

Antipsychotic drugs are also clinically effective in children with severely aggressive conduct disorders, and some are approved for use in such children. Lithium is also effective in some such children, perhaps more so when an explosive affect is present, and lithium has fewer clinically significant untoward effects than neuroleptics. Because lithium is still not approved for use either in children younger than 12 years or for this indication, and because of the necessity of monitoring serum lithium levels, many clinicians prefer to use antipsychotic drugs.

The use of antipsychotics in the mentally retarded continues to be controversial, but they are prescribed frequently, especially for institutionalized patients. In optimal doses, antipsychotics are effective in decreasing irritability, sleep disturbances, hostility, agitation, and combativeness, and may improve concentration and social behavior in agitated, severely retarded individuals (American Medical Association, 1986). Aman and Singh (1988) cautioned that the influential studies of the mentally retarded by Breuning, which showed significant detrimental effects on cognition resulting from antipsychotic use, appear to have been fabricated.

ANTIPSYCHOTIC DRUGS IN THE TREATMENT OF ATTENTION-DEFICIT/HYPERACTIVITY DISORDERS

Some antipsychotic agents (e.g., haloperidol) have been approved for treating children with symptoms such as excessive motor activity, impulsivity, difficulty sustaining attention, and poor frustration tolerance, which would be found in most children diagnosed with attention- deficit/hyperactivity disorder (ADHD); however, the package insert for thioridazine was modified in 2000 to delete this indication. Double-blind, controlled studies have shown antipsychotic drugs to be effective in treating children who would meet the criteria for ADHD. However, studies comparing antipsychotic drugs with stimulants almost always show that, overall, stimulants are statistically more effective clinically than antipsychotics (Green, 1995; Gittelman-Klein et al. 1976). In addition, many clinicians are reluctant to use antipsychotics to treat patients with ADHD because of the risk that an irreversible tardive dyskinesia might develop and the worry that the sedative effects of antipsychotics may interfere significantly with cognition and learning. Because of such factors, antipsychotics should be thought of as third-rank drugs to be used primarily in the treatment of ADHD, which is severely disabling and which has not responded to stimulants and other drugs with untoward effects of more acceptable risk.

Although these caveats in using antipsychotics are not to be dismissed, some recent data moderating these dictums should be cited: (a) the influential studies of Breuning and his colleagues, which showed significant detrimental effects on cognition in mentally retarded patients treated with antipsychotic drugs, appear to have been fabricated (Aman and Singh, 1988); (b) later studies have reported minimal impairment of cognition in subjects diagnosed with ADHD who were treated with appropriate doses of antipsychotics (Klein, 1990/1991); (c) there is a suggestion that thioridazine may be superior to stimulants in treating subgroups of mentally deficient patients diagnosed with equivalents of ADHD (Alexandris and Lundell, 1968; Aman et al. 1991a, 1991b).

In a randomized, crossover, double-blind study, Weizman et al. (1984) reported that the combination of propericiazine, a neuroleptic agent prescribed by child psychiatrists in Israel, and a stimulant was statistically superior to placebo-stimulant treatment of 14 children diagnosed with attention deficit disorder with hyperactivity (ADDH) who had experienced some, but not satisfactory, improvement with stimulant medication only. The authors noted that the combination of a stimulant and neuroleptics may be useful in some children who do not respond adequately to stimulants alone. Clinically, this may be a potentially useful option for a small subgroup of children who do not respond adequately to stimulants or to other drugs alone. The combination of stimulant and neuroleptic would presumably achieve a satisfactory result that would either not be achieved by the neuroleptic alone or would require higher doses of neuroleptics, which would carry an increased risk of untoward effects, such as tardive dyskinesia and cognitive dulling.

PHARMACOKINETICS OF ANTIPSYCHOTIC DRUGS

Rivera-Calimlim et al. (1979) reported plasma chlorpromazine levels in a total of 24 children aged 8 to 16 years who were treated with chlorpromazine for psychiatric disorders, including various psychoses, mental retardation with aggression, hyperactivity, self-injurious behavior, and mood disorders with anxiety. The authors reported wide interpatient variations in chlorpromazine plasma levels for a given dose; for example, nine children receiving 0.8 to 2.9 mg/kg/day achieved mean plasma levels of 6.6 ng/mL, with a range from undetectable to 18 ng/mL. One child receiving 9.8 mg/kg/day showed only trace levels of plasma chlorpromazine. Children and adolescents had chlorpromazine plasma levels that were two to three-and-a-half times lower than those for adults, for a given dose per kilogram of body weight. Clinical improvement in these children usually began when plasma chlorpromazine concentration was at least 30 ng/mL, and optimal levels ranged between 40 ng/mL and 80 ng/mL; suggested optimal plasma levels for adults treated with chlorpromazine were higher, between 50 ng/mL and 300 ng/mL. A final clinically important observation was that plasma chlorpromazine levels declined over time in most patients who were on fixed doses (Rivera-Calimlim et al. 1979). It was suggested that one possible reason might be autoinduction of enzymes that metabolize chlorpromazine.

CONTRAINDICATIONS FOR THE ADMINISTRATION OF ANTIPSYCHOTIC DRUGS

Known hypersensitivity to the drug and toxic central nervous system depression or comatose states are absolute contraindications. If a severe adverse event develops (e.g., agranulocytosis, neuroleptic malignant syndrome tardive dyskinesia, or a withdrawal dyskinesia), children and adolescents should be managed without antipsychotics, if at all possible.

Neuroleptics may lower the seizure threshold; they should be used cautiously in patients with seizure disorders, and chlorpromazine probably should not be used in such patients.

INTERACTIONS OF ANTIPSYCHOTIC DRUGS WITH OTHER MEDICATIONS

The most frequent clinically important reactions are with other central nervous system depressants such as alcohol, sedatives and hypnotics, benzodiazepines, antihistamines, opiates, and barbiturates, in which an additive central nervous system depressive effect occurs.

Antipsychotic drugs also have varying degrees of anticholinergic effects. When combined with another anticholinergic (antiparkinsonian) agent, such as when one is used prophylactically to prevent acute dyskinesia, pseudoparkinsonism, or akathisia, central nervous system symptoms of cholinergic blockade may result. These symptoms may include confusion, disorientation, delirium, hallucinations, and worsening of preexisting psychotic symptoms. Of clinical importance, this picture may be mistaken for inadequate treatment or worsening of the psychosis, rather than an untoward effect.

The combination of antipsychotic drugs and lithium carbonate, particularly if high doses are used, may lead to an increased incidence of central nervous system toxicity, including neuroleptic malignant syndrome.

Combined use of antipsychotic drugs with tricyclic antidepressants or monoamine oxidase inhibitors may increase plasma levels of antidepressants.

Neuroleptics may also have noteworthy interactions with many other medications.

UNTOWARD EFFECTS OF ANTIPSYCHOTIC DRUGS

Although antipsychotic drugs may have numerous serious untoward effects, those of greatest concern in children and adolescents are the effects of sedation on cognition and the extrapyramidal syndromes, in particular the possible development of irreversible tardive dyskinesia with the standard antipsychotics.

Agranulocytosis

Agranulocytosis is a major concern in patients treated with clozapine; it is discussed in more detail later. Agranulocytosis has also been reported with other antipsychotics. It usually occurs relatively early in treatment (e.g., for chlorpromazine, usually between the 4th and 10th weeks). Parents and older patients should be warned to report indications of sudden infections, such as fever and sore throat, to the physician. White blood cell count should be determined immediately, and if it is significantly depressed, medication should be stopped and therapy instituted.

Untoward Cognitive Effects

Both high-potency and low-potency antipsychotic agents are effective when given in equivalent doses, but they differ in the frequency and severity of their untoward effects. Usually, the higher-potency antipsychotic drugs cause less sedation, fewer autonomic side effects, and more extrapyramidal untoward effects; the lower-potency antipsychotic drugs cause greater sedation, more autonomic side effects, and fewer extrapyramidal effects (Baldessarini, 1990). Because of the great importance of minimizing any cognitive dulling in schoolchildren and in the mentally retarded, whose cognition is already compromised, high-potency, less-sedative antipsychotic drugs are often preferred. Over a period of days to weeks, however, considerable tolerance often develops to the sedative effects of high-dose, low-potency antipsychotic drugs, and thus they are still useful when untoward effects are carefully monitored (Green, 1989).

Extrapyramidal Syndromes

Significant numbers of children and adolescents receiving antipsychotic medication develop extrapyramidal syndromes. Baldessarini (1990) has enumerated six types of extrapyramidal syndromes associated with the use of antipsychotic drugs. The risk of extrapyramidal syndromes with clozapine and other atypical antipsychotics appears to be considerably reduced compared with that of standard antipsychotics.

Effects Usually Appearing During Drug Administration

Acute Dystonic Reactions

The period of maximum risk is within hours to 5 days of initiation of neuroleptic therapy. There may also be increased risk following increments in dose. High-potency, low-dose antipsychotic drugs are more likely to precipitate an acute dystonic reaction than are low-potency, high-dose antipsychotic drugs, and young males, both children and adolescents, may be at increased risk (APA, 1980b). Untreated acute dystonic reactions may last from a few minutes to several hours, and they may recur. Symptoms, which may be painful and frightening, particularly if the patient does not understand what is happening, include muscular hypertonicity; tonic contractions (spasms) of the neck (torticollis), mouth, and tongue, which may make speaking difficult; oculogyric crisis (eyes rolling upward and remaining in that position); and opisthotonos (spasm in which the spine and extremities are bent with an anterior convexity). Acute dystonic reactions respond rapidly to anticholinergic and antiparkinsonian drugs, such as 25 to 50 mg diphenhydramine (Benadryl) orally or intramuscularly, or 1 to 2 mg benztropine (Cogentin) intramuscularly. (The manufacturer of benztropine cautions that, because of its atropine-like untoward effects, its use is contraindicated in children younger than 3 years and that it should be used with caution in older children (PDR, 1995).) If the dystonia is very severe, administering either 25 mg of diphenhydramine or 1 to 2 mg of benztropine intramuscularly will reverse the dystonia within a few minutes. The prophylactic use of anticholinergic and antiparkinsonian agents to prevent acute dystonic reactions is discussed following the section on "Akathisia."

Parkinsonism (Pseudoparkinsonism)

Symptoms of parkinsonism include tremor, cogwheel rigidity, drooling, and decrease in facial expressive movements (mask-like or expressionless facies), and akinesia (slowness in initiating movements). These symptoms respond to antiparkinsonian medications; for example, benztropine (Cogentin), 1 to 2 mg given two or three times daily, usually provides relief within a day or two. Antiparkinsonian medication may be withdrawn gradually after 1 or 2 weeks to see if it is still necessary for symptomatic relief.

The period of maximum risk for developing parkinsonism is 5 to 30 days after initiation of neuroleptic therapy. The risk for development of parkinsonism appears to be greater for females and to increase with age. It is rarely seen in preschool children treated with therapeutic doses of neuroleptics; it occurs commonly in school-aged children and adolescents (Campbell et al. 1985). Richardson et al. (1991) reported that 21 (34%) of 61 hospitalized children and adolescents, of whom only 7 were diagnosed with psychotic or affective disorders, who were taking neuroleptics at the time of evaluation exhibited symptoms of parkinsonism when rated on several movement disorder scales. Three (14.3%) of the 21 children were rated as having parkinsonism despite the fact that they were concurrently receiving antiparkinsonian drugs. Development of parkinsonism was significantly ($P = .05$) associated with a longer duration on medication at the time of evaluation (mean of 117 days for patients with parkinsonism and mean of 34 days for patients without parkinsonism).

Akinesia, perhaps the most severe form of parkinsonism, is defined by Rifkin et al. (1975) as a "behavioral state of diminished spontaneity characterized by few gestures, unspontaneous speech and, particularly, apathy and difficulty with initiating usual activities" (p. 672). It may be particularly difficult to differentiate from the negative symptoms of schizophrenia, such as apathy and blunting. Van Putten and Marder (1987) suggested that akinesia might be the most toxic behavioral side effect of antipsychotic drugs. The authors noted that a subjective sense of sedation or drowsiness, excessive sleeping, and a lack of any leg-crossing during an interview of approximately 20 minutes correlated with the presence of akinesia. Akinesia also interferes with social adjustment, and the patient may appear to have a "postpsychotic depression." Patients with akinesia are often less concerned with any psychotic symptoms and report that everything is fine; they may experience an absence of emotion and appear emotionally dead (Van Putten and Marder, 1987). Although antiparkinsonian drugs may be helpful, in some cases they do not adequately control symptoms of akinesia. There is some evidence that antiparkinsonian drugs become less effective at higher daily dosages of antipsychotics (Van Putten and Marder, 1987).

The prophylactic use of anticholinergic and antiparkinsonian agents to prevent pseudoparkinsonism is discussed following the section on "Akathisia."

Akathisia (Motor Restlessness)

The period of maximum risk for developing this condition is 5 to 60 days after initiation of neuroleptic therapy, but it has been reported to occur in as few as 6 hours after an oral dose of a neuroleptic (Van Putten et al. 1984). Symptoms include constant uncomfortable restlessness, a feeling of tension in the lower extremities often accompanied by a strong or irresistible urge to move them, inability to sit still, and foot-tapping or pacing. Clinically, blunted affect, emotional withdrawal, and motor retardation may also be observed (Van Putten and Marder, 1987).

Akathisia may or may not respond to antiparkinsonian drugs such as trihexyphenidyl (Artane). Van Putten and Marder (1987) noted the dual nature of akathisia: a subjective experience of restlessness and observable motor restlessness. In their clinical experience, all patients with moderate or severe akathisia exhibited either rocking from foot to foot or walking on the spot. Akathisia was also strongly associated with depression, dysphoria, and, at times in severe and treatment-resistant cases, exacerbation of psychotic symptoms and homicidal and suicidal ideation and behavior (Van Putten and Marder, 1987). Of particular clinical importance, patients who have unpleasant untoward effects, especially akathisia, with antipsychotics, are more likely to be noncompliant and to unilaterally discontinue medication early in treatment (Van Putten and Marder, 1987).

Fleischhacker et al. (1989) have published a rating scale for akathisia that includes two subjective items: "a sensation of inner restlessness" and "the urge to move," and three items that characterize the frequency and magnitude of observed akathisia phenomena.

Propranolol may be helpful in ameliorating akathisia (Adler et al. 1986); benzodiazepines and clonidine have also been reported to be effective in some cases.

Clonazepam was administered to 10 first-onset psychotic adolescents (eight of whom were diagnosed with schizophrenia, paranoid subtype) between 16 and 19 years of age who experienced distressing akathisia following treatment with antipsychotics (Kutcher et al. 1987). Nine of the patients had also been receiving benztropine concomitantly with their antipsychotic medication. All patients reported subjective improvement, and scores on an akathisia subscale decreased significantly after 1 week's treatment with 0.5 mg/day of clonazepam.

In some cases, reduction in dose of the antipsychotic may be necessary. Neppe and Ward (1989) recommend that if only akathisia develops (i.e., without accompanying parkinsonism), a beta-blocker be used rather than an anticholinergic agent.

Prophylactic Use of Antiparkinsonian Agents for Acute Dystonic Reaction, Parkinsonism, and Akathisia

The use of antiparkinsonian (anticholinergic) agents prophylactically to minimize the likelihood of the patient's developing an acute dystonic reaction, parkinsonism, or akathisia from antipsychotic drug use is controversial. Some of the reasons relate to the effects caused by the anticholinergic agents themselves. Anticholinergic agents may adversely affect cognition and may aggravate psychotic symptomatology. In addition, there is some suggestion that at least part of the effectiveness of these agents is that they may lower the serum concentration of the antipsychotic drug (Rivera-Calimlim et al. 1976). Because of their reluctance to give an additional medication that itself may have untoward effects, many clinicians choose to minimize the risk of these extrapyramidal effects by beginning with a low dose and titrating the medication slowly. If an acute dystonic reaction should occur, it may be treated with diphenhydramine and the dosage of antipsychotic lowered temporarily if necessary. Conversely, some clinicians routinely prescribe an agent such as benztropine for approximately 1 month to 6 weeks, covering the period of maximal risk for the development of both acute dystonic reactions and parkinsonian untoward effects. Another option for outpatients is to prescribe a small amount of an anticholinergic (e.g., diphenhydramine) with an explanation of how it is to be administered should a dystonic reaction occur (e.g., to take one capsule should such a reaction begin, to take another dose in 20 to 30 minutes if there is no improvement, and to go to an emergency room if the reaction is severe and alert the physician to the medication being taken).

In their review of the management of acute extrapyramidal syndromes induced by neuroleptics, Neppe and Ward (1989) note that anticholinergics can significantly reduce the rate of acute dystonias especially in the highest-risk group, males younger than 30 years of age treated with high-potency antipsychotic agents. However, as acute dystonic reactions tend to be transient, prophylactic treatment for more than 2 weeks is not usually indicated. These authors recommend no prophylaxis for parkinsonism and akathisia, because they rarely present as dramatically emergent a picture as acute dystonia. The parents and/or patient, as appropriate, may be carefully informed about the possibility of these conditions arising, to aid in their early detection. The clinician can then decide how best to treat the particular symptom in the particular patient (Neppe and Ward, 1989).

Van Putten and Marder (1987) point out that prophylactic use of antiparkinsonian drugs may not fully prevent symptoms of akinesia from developing, and that some schizophrenic patients who have been stabilized using antiparkinsonian medication may experience increased anxiety, depression, general dysphoria, and suffering when the anticholinergics are withdrawn.

The clinician should decide on a case-by-case basis which of the preceding possibilities is best for a given patient. This decision will be based on such factors as whether a high- or low-potency neuroleptic is given, how rapidly the dose is increased, previous experience of the patient, whether it is administered to an outpatient or an inpatient (who has ready access to clinical staff), how such a reaction might affect the relationship with the patient and/or the parents and subsequent compliance, and the patient's environment. For example, it can be particularly difficult for a patient and family if the patient develops an acute dystonic reaction while attending school.

Neuroleptic Malignant Syndrome

Neuroleptic malignant syndrome is life-threatening and can occur after a single dose, but occurs most frequently within 2 weeks of initiation of neuroleptic therapy or an increase in dosage; males and younger individuals appear to be most often affected (for review see Kaufmann and Wyatt, 1987). Symptoms include severe muscular rigidity, altered consciousness, stupor, catatonia, hyperpyrexia, labile pulse and blood pressure, and occasionally myoglobinemia. Most patients have elevated creatine phosphokinase (CPK) levels. Neuroleptic malignant syndrome can persist for up to 2 weeks or longer after medication is discontinued and can be fatal. Treatment consists of immediate cessation of medication and hospitalization with supportive treatment. Dopaminergic agonists (e.g., bromocriptine and amantadine) and/or dantrolene have also been reported to reduce the mortality rate significantly (Sakkas et al. 1991). Antiparkinsonian drugs are not useful.

Latz and McCracken (1992) conducted an extensive literature search and reported a total of 49 cases of neuroleptic malignant syndrome (NMS) in patients 18 years or younger. The youngest reported case was that of an 11-month-old. Five (83%) of the six preschoolers developed NMS after a single dose of neuroleptic that either was an accidental overdose or was prescribed for a nonpsychiatric illness. Overall lethality for all cases reviewed was 16.3% (8 of 49). However, the death rate for patients 12 years of age or younger was 27% (3 of 11), more than twice the death rate of 13% (5 of 38) for adolescents 13 to 18 years old.

Steingard et al. (1992) also published a review with detailed summaries of 35 cases of neuroleptic malignant syndrome in patients younger than 19 years of age. Fever, rigidity, altered mental status, and tachycardia were present in > 70% of the cases. Five (14%) of the patients died; however, only one of these died within the past two decades, and that was a 2-year-old who had ingested chlorpromazine accidentally.

Late-Appearing Syndromes (After Months or Years of Treatment)

Tardive Dyskinesia

Definitions and descriptions of tardive dyskinesia (TD) and related dyskinesias (withdrawal, masked dyskinesias) vary. Perhaps the most influential definition at present is the research diagnostic criteria proposed in 1982 by Schooler and Kane. They note that, if possible, the absence of abnormal involuntary movements before beginning pharmacotherapy should be documented. Schooler and Kane's (1982) research diagnostic criteria for tardive dyskinesia proposed three prerequisites for making the diagnosis:

1. Exposure to neuroleptic drugs for a minimum total cumulative exposure of 3 months.
2. The presence of at least "moderate" abnormal involuntary movements in one or more body areas (face, lips, jaw, tongue, upper extremities, lower extremities, trunk) or at least "mild" movements in two or more body areas.
3. Absence of other conditions that might produce abnormal movements.
   Once these prerequisites have been met by a patient, Schooler and Kane (1982) proposed six diagnostic categories of tardive dyskinesia:
   a. (i) Probable tardive dyskinesia "concurrent neuroleptics" if the patient is currently receiving neuroleptic therapy, or (ii) probable tardive dyskinesia "neuroleptic-free" if no longer receiving neuroleptic medication. (Only one of these two diagnoses would be possible the first time the patient is examined.)
   b. Masked probable tardive dyskinesia: within 2 weeks of an increase in dose in a patient diagnosed with 1a or resumption of neuroleptic drug treatment in a patient diagnosed with 1b, prerequisite 2 is no longer met.

   c. Transient tardive dyskinesia: within 3 months of a patient being diagnosed with 1a and with no increase in dose of neuroleptic (a dose reduction is permissible), prerequisite 2 is no longer met; or, within 3 months of a patient being diagnosed with 1b, prerequisite 2 is no longer met, and the patient has remained neuroleptic-free.
   d. Withdrawal tardive dyskinesia: while receiving neuroleptics the patient does not meet prerequisite 2, but within 2 weeks of cessation of neuroleptics with usual serum half-lives or 5 weeks after stopping a long-acting neuroleptic (e.g., a depot dosage form), the patient develops abnormal movements consistent with prerequisite 2. If the movements cease or no longer satisfy prerequisite 2 within 3 months, this diagnosis stands.
   e. (i) Persistent tardive dyskinesia "concurrent neuroleptics" if the patient was diagnosed with 1a and has continuously received neuroleptics over the subsequent 3 months and continues to satisfy prerequisite 2. (ii) Persistent tardive dyskinesia "neuroleptic-free" if the patient was diagnosed with 1a (and neuroleptic drug was immediately stopped), with 1b, or with 4 (withdrawal TD) and no neuroleptic was administered during the subsequent 3 months and the patient continues to fulfill prerequisite 2. (iii) Persistent tardive dyskinesia "unspecified" if the patient was diagnosed 1a, 1b, or 4, and the patient received neuroleptics for part of the subsequent 3-month period and still meets prerequisite 2.
   f. Masked persistent tardive dyskinesia if a patient diagnosed with 5a or 5c no longer meets prerequisite 2 within 3 weeks of an increase in dosage of the neuroleptic agent or if a patient diagnosed with 5b no longer meets prerequisite 2 within 3 weeks of resumption of a neuroleptic.

Four additional diagnostic criteria were suggested by the American Psychiatric Association Task Force on Tardive Dyskinesia (American Psychiatric Association, 1992):

1. The abnormal movements are exacerbated or may be provoked by a decrease or withdrawal of an antipsychotic drug. Increasing the dose of antipsychotic will suppress (or dampen) the movements at least temporarily.
2. Anticholinergic medication does not ameliorate and may worsen the movements.
3. Emotional stress may worsen the movements.
4. The movements decrease or disappear during sleep.

Tardive dyskinesia develops while actively receiving a neuroleptic drug, as opposed to a withdrawal dyskinesia that occurs when a neuroleptic is withdrawn or its dose is decreased. Tardive dyskinesia, which may be both severely disabling and irreversible, is the most clinically significant common long-term untoward effect of antipsychotic use. Baldessarini (1990) notes that in some cases, especially in younger patients, tardive dyskinesia will disappear over the course of weeks to as much as 3 years. It is believed that the risk of developing irreversible tardive dyskinesia increases with both total cumulative dose and duration of treatment. Older females appear to be at increased risk. It has been reported that fine, worm-like (vermicular) movements of the tongue may be an early sign of tardive dyskinesia and that discontinuation of the medication when this occurs may prevent further development of the syndrome (PDR, 1995). Symptoms of tardive dyskinesia most typically include involuntary choreoathetotic movements that affect the face; tongue; perioral, buccal, and masticatory musculature; and neck but may also involve the torso and extremities.

Atypical and less common forms of tardive dyskinesia, such as tardive akathisia, a persisting restlessness, and tardive dystonia, also occur. Burke et al. (1982) reported 42 cases of tardive dystonia that they diagnosed by the following criteria:

1. The presence of chronic dystonia.
2. History of antipsychotic drug treatment preceding or concurrent with the onset of dystonia.
3. Exclusion of known causes of secondary dystonia by appropriate clinical and laboratory evaluation.
4. A negative family history for dystonia.

Symptoms of tardive dystonia began after as few as 3 days and up to 11 years after initiation of antipsychotic medication. The incidence of tardive dystonia was more frequent in younger male patients than in older patients; was characterized by sustained abnormal postures accompanied by torticollis, torsion of the trunk and extremities, blepharospasm, and grimacing; and was incapacitating in severe cases. Spontaneous remission occurred in a few patients, but dystonia persisted for years in most. Of the many medications used to ameliorate the tardive dystonia, the most helpful were tetrabenzine, which improved symptoms in 68% of patients, and anticholinergics, which were helpful in 39% of patients (Burke et al. 1982).

In tardive dyskinesia and other choreoathetotic syndromes, emotional stress typically causes worsening of the movements, drowsiness or sedation causes them to diminish, and sleep causes them to disappear (APA, 1980b). There is no adequate treatment; antiparkinsonian drugs may worsen the condition (for review see APA, 1980b). There is evidence, however, that the atypical antipsychotic drug clozapine not only produces little or no tardive dyskinesia when it is the only neuroleptic ever used, but also significantly decreases or eliminates existing symptoms of tardive dyskinesia during the period it is prescribed (Small et al. 1987; Birmaher et al. 1992; and Mozes et al. 1994). Upon its discontinuation, however, the dyskinetic movements that were suppressed by clozapine rapidly returned in 18 of 19 patients (Small et al. 1987).

Vitamin E and Tardive Dyskinesia

Vitamin E has also been reported to be helpful in treating tardive dyskinesia in adults. Adler et al. (1993) treated 28 adult patients diagnosed with tardive dyskinesia in a double-blind parallel-group comparison study of 8 to 12 weeks' duration. The 16 patients who received 1,600 IU of vitamin E daily showed significantly greater improvement on their scores on the AIMS than the 12 patients who received placebo. The authors noted that their data also supported earlier findings that patients whose onset of tardive dyskinesia was within the preceding 5 years were more likely to respond to vitamin E therapy than patients with more long-standing tardive dyskinesia.

Adler et al. (1999) note that although several short-term, controlled studies found vitamin E to be helpful, they were from a single site, had relatively small numbers, and treatment duration was short. To further investigate the effectiveness of vitamin E, the authors conducted a prospective, randomized, nine-site, double-blind, placebo-controlled study that compared up to 2 years of treatment with d-vitamin E (1,600 IU/day) and placebo in 158 subjects diagnosed with tardive dyskinesia who were taking typical neuroleptics or risperidone. Seventy-three subjects were assigned to vitamin E treatment and 85 to placebo; 107 subjects completed at least 1 year of the study. Efficacy was rated on the Abnormal Involuntary Movements Scale (AIMS), the Barnes Akathisia Scale, and the Modified Simpson-Angus Scale; electromechanical assessments of dyskinesia were also recorded. Psychiatric status was assessed with the Brief Psychiatric Rating Scale (BPRS) and the Global Assessment of Functioning (GAF). The authors reported no significant differences between vitamin E and placebo on any of the rating scales at the end of the study and concluded that vitamin E is not effective in treating tardive dyskinesia in patients who are actively being treated with neuroleptics. The authors also noted that changing prescribing practices may have resulted in their subjects being more treatment resistant than subjects in earlier studies.

In addition, a withdrawal dyskinesia may emerge when neuroleptic medication is withdrawn or the dose is reduced. Withdrawal-emergent dyskinesias can occur for two different reasons. First, antidopaminergic drugs, including antipsychotics, can suppress tardive dyskinesia; thus, decreasing their serum levels can "unmask" ongoing tardive dyskinesia. Second, Baldessarini (1990) points out that a "disuse supersensitivity" to dopamine agonists may also occur following withdrawal of antidopaminergic drugs; he suggests that this phenomenon may explain withdrawal dyskinesias that resolve within a few weeks.

The reported prevalence of neuroleptic-induced tardive dyskinesia and withdrawal tardive dyskinesia in children and adolescents has ranged from 0% to 51% (Wolf and Wagner, 1993). It is thought that the risk of developing tardive dyskinesia that will become irreversible increases with both total cumulative dose and duration of treatment. No cases of irreversible tardive dyskinesia developing in children or adolescents have been reported; the longest neuroleptic-free persistent tardive dyskinesia was reported to last 4.5 years. Usually, withdrawal dyskinesias resolve within a few weeks to a few months of discontinuation of the neuroleptic (Wolf and Wagner, 1993).

Richardson et al. (1991) reported that 5 (12%) of 41 hospitalized children and adolescents (mean age, 15.5 years), of whom only 10 were diagnosed with psychotic or affective disorders, who had taken neuroleptics for at least one period of 90 continuous days before the time of evaluation exhibited symptoms of treatment-emergent tardive dyskinesia (occurring while receiving neuroleptics) when rated on the Simpson Abbreviated Dyskinesia Scale. The five patients who developed tardive dyskinesia were significantly more likely to have had a history of assaultive behavior ($P = .003$) and a first-degree relative who had been hospitalized for a psychiatric disorder ($P = .009$) than patients who did not develop tardive dyskinesia. Using the more stringent research criteria of Schooler and Kane (1982), three (7%) were diagnosed with tardive dyskinesia.

If tardive dyskinesia develops, every effort should be made to discontinue or at least reduce the dose of antipsychotic drug as much as possible. The dyskinesia should be monitored with serial ratings on the AIMS. If the severity of the psychiatric disorder precludes discontinuation of antipsychotic medication (e.g., in a patient diagnosed with autistic disorder who exhibits severe self-injurious behavior (SIB) and aggressiveness and who has not responded adequately to other medications such as lithium or propranolol), the clinician must carefully document the rationale for reinstituting antipsychotic medication and verify that the legal guardians (and patient when appropriate) have given their informed consent. Reinstating or increasing the dose of antipsychotic may suppress or mask tardive dyskinesia.

Because of such risks, antipsychotic agents should be given only to children and adolescents for whom no other potentially less harmful treatment is available; for example, although effective in some children diagnosed with ADHD, antipsychotic drugs should not be used unless stimulant medications and other nonstimulant drugs with safer untoward-effect profiles have been treatment failures (Green, 1995).

Although antipsychotics are the only drugs that result in persistent tardive dyskinesia in a significant proportion of patients, a number of different drugs may cause dyskinesias after short- or long-term treatment. Jeste and Wyatt (1982) note that the dyskinesia produced by L-dopa most closely resembles the tardive dyskinesia resulting from antipsychotics and that, typically, the dyskinesias caused by most other drugs are usually acute, sometimes toxic, effects and almost always remit when the drug is discontinued. Among the drugs used in child and adolescent psychopharmacotherapy for which dyskinesias have been reported are amphetamines, methylphenidate, monoamine oxidase inhibitors, tricyclic antidepressants, lithium, antihistamines, benzodiazepines, and antiepileptic drugs (Jeste and Wyatt, 1982).

Rabbit Syndrome (Perioral Tremor)

Rabbit syndrome (perioral tremor), which may be a late-onset variant of parkinsonism, is uncommon. Its name derives from the fact that patients so afflicted make rapid chewing movements similar to those of rabbits (Villeneuve, 1972). It may respond to antiparkinsonian medication.

Other Untoward Effects of Antipsychotic Drugs

Table 5.1 is a compilation of most of the reported untoward effects of chlorpromazine, the prototype antipsychotic drug. Most of these untoward effects have also been reported to occur to a greater or lesser degree with other antipsychotic drugs.

REPRESENTATIVE FIRST GENERATION/TYPICAL ANTIPSYCHOTIC DRUGS

Table 5.2 summarizes representative first-generation/typical antipsychotic drugs commonly used in child and adolescent psychiatry, as well as clozapine. It compares their relative potencies and expected potential sedative, autonomic, and extrapyramidal untoward effects with chlorpromazine, the prototype of the antipsychotics. FDA age limitations and recommended dosages for approved use in children and adolescents are also given when available.

(text continues on page 104)

TABLE 5.1 ● **Untoward Effects of Chlorpromazine**

Allergic
  Mild urticaria
  Photosensitivity, exfoliative dermatitis
  Asthma
  Anaphylactoid reactions
  Laryngeal edema
  Angioneurotic edema
Autonomic nervous system
  Antiadrenergic effects
    Orthostatic hypotension
    Ejaculatory disturbances
  Anticholinergic effects
    Decreased secretion, resulting in dry mouth, dry eyes, nasal congestion
    Blurred vision, mydriasis
    Glaucoma attack in patients with narrow-angle closure
    Constipation, paralytic ileus
    Urinary retention
    Impotence
Cardiovascular
  Postural (orthostatic) hypotension
  Tachycardia
  ECG changes
  Sudden death due to cardiac arrest
Central nervous system
  Neuromuscular effects
    Dystonias
    Akasthisia (motor restlessness)
    Pseudoparkinsonism
    Tardive dyskinesia
  Seizures, lowering of seizure threshold
  Drowsiness, sedation
  Behavioral effects
    Increased psychotic symptoms
    Catatonic-like states
Dermatological
  Photosensitivity
    Skin pigmentation changes in exposed areas
    Rashes
Endocrinological
  Elevated prolactin levels
  Gynecomastia
  Amenorrhea
  Hyperglycemia, glycosuria, and hypoglycemia

(continued)

TABLE 5.1 ● *(Continued)*

Hematological
  Agranulocytosis
  Eosinophilia
  Leukopenia
  Hemolytic anemia
  Aplastic anemia
  Thrombocytopenic purpura
  Pancytopenia
Hepatological
  Jaundice
Metabolic
  Weight gain, increased appetite
Ophthalmologic
  Blurred vision
  Precipitation of acute glaucoma attack in persons with narrow-angle glaucoma
  Deposition of pigmented material and star-shaped opacities in lens
  Deposition of pigmented material in cornea
  Pigmentary retinopathy
  Epithelial Keratopathy
Teratogenic effects possible (seen in animal studies)
Other
  Neuroleptic malignant syndrome
  Sudden death, which may be related to cardiac failure or suppression of cough reflex

Considerations About Dosage

The antipsychotic effects of neuroleptic agents evolve gradually. The depolarization inactivation of dopaminergic neurons, which is necessary for antipsychotic efficacy, takes approximately 3 to 6 weeks to develop. Hence it is important to have a trial of adequate duration of an antipsychotic drug at usual therapeutic doses rather than rapidly increasing the dose, which can lead to the erroneous clinical impression that a much higher dose than necessary was responsible for the patient's clinical improvement. Studies have also suggested that there is a therapeutic window of approximately 300 to 1,000 mg of chlorpromazine or its equivalent for most psychotic adult patients. Patients receiving < 300 mg tend to improve less, and those receiving > 1,000 mg of chlorpromazine or its equivalent show no increased benefit (for review see Levy, 1993). It is usually recommended that antipsychotic agents initially be administered in divided doses, most frequently three or four times daily. Once the optimal dose is established, however, their relatively long serum half-lives usually permit either once-daily dosage (e.g., before bedtime) or twice-daily dosage (in the morning and before bedtime).

TABLE 5.2 ● **Representative First Generation/Typical Antipsychotic Drugs and Clozapine**

Antipsychotic Drug /Trade Name	Chemical Classification	Therapeutically Equivalent Oral Dose in Mgs	Effects			Approved Age for Use	Usual Optimal Dose/Maintenance Dose Range
			Sedation	Autonomic[a]	Extrapyramidal Reaction[b]		
Chlorpromazine/ Thorazine	Phenothiazine: aliphatic compound	100	+ + +	+ + +	+ +	Over 6 months	See text
Thioridazine/Mellaril	Phenothiazine: piperidine compound	100	+ + +	+ + +	+	2 years	See text
Clozapine/Clozaril	Dibenzodiazepine	75	+ + +	+ + +	0?	16 years	As per adults; see text
Mesoridazine/Serentil	Phenothiazine: piperidine compound	50	+ + +	+ +	+	12 years	No specific doses for children
Loxapine/Loxitane	Dibenzoxazepine	15	+ +	+/ + +	+ + / + + +	16 years	As per adults
Molindone/Moban	Dihydroindolone	10	+ +	+	+	12 years	No specific doses for children
Perphenazine/Trilafon	Phenothiazine: piperazine compound	10	+ +	+	+ + / + + +	12 years	No specific doses for children

(continued)

TABLE 5.2 ● *(Continued)*

Antipsychotic Drug/Trade Name	Chemical Classification	Therapeutically Equivalent Oral Dose in Mgs	Effects Sedation	Effects Autonomic[a]	Effects Extrapyramidal Reaction[b]	Approved Age For Use	Usual Optimal Dose/Maintenance Dose Range
Trifluoperazine/ Stelazine	Phenothiazine: piperazine compound	5	+ +	+	+ + +	6 years	See text
Thiothixene/Navane	Thioxanthene	5	+	+	+ + +	12 years	No specific doses for children
Fluphenazine/Permitil, Prolixin	Phenothiazine: piperazine compound	2	+	+	+ + +	16 years	See text
Haloperidol/Haldol	Butyrophenone	2	+	+	+ + +	3 years	See text
Pimozide[c]/Orap	Diphenyl- butylpiperidine	10	+	+	+ + +	Over 12 years	0.2 mg/kg/day or maximum, 10 mg/day

Adapted from American Medical Association. Drug Evaluations Annual, 1994. Chicago: American Medical Association, 1994.

[a] α-antiadrenergic and anticholinergic effects.

[b] excluding tardive dyskinesia, which appears to be produced to the same degree and frequency by all agents except clozapine with equieffective antipsychotic doses. Clozapine has produced agranulocytosis; therefore, recommendations for its use are limited (see text).

[c] only indicated for tourette's disorder that has not responded to other standard treatments; not approved for use in psychoses.

FIRST GENERATION/TYPICAL ANTIPSYCHOTIC DRUGS
Chlorpromazine Hydrochloride (Thorazine)

Indications for Chlorpromazine Hydrochloride in Child and Adolescent Psychiatry

In addition to being approved for uses similar to those for adults, including psychotic disorders, chlorpromazine is approved for the treatment of severe behavioral problems in children, marked by combativeness and/or explosive hyperexcitable behavior. It is also noted that dosages > 500 mg/day are unlikely to further enhance behavioral improvement in severely disturbed mentally retarded patients.

Chlorpromazine may lower the threshold to seizures; another antipsychotic should be chosen for seizure-prone individuals.

Chlorpromazine Dosage Schedule for Children and Adolescents

- Infants younger than 6 months of age: not recommended.
- Children aged 6 months to 12 years with severe behavioral problems or psychotic conditions:

  Oral: 0.25 mg/kg every 4 to 6 hours as needed. Titrate upward gradually. In severe cases, daily doses of 200 mg or higher may be required.
  Rectal: 1 mg/kg every 6 to 8 hours as needed.
  Intramuscular: 0.5 mg/kg every 6 to 8 hours as needed. Maximum daily intramuscular dose for a child younger than 5 years or under 22 kg is 40 mg; for a child 5 to 12 years of age or 22 kg to 45 kg, maximum daily dose is 75 mg.
- Adolescents: depending on severity of symptoms, begin with 10 mg three times to 25 mg four times daily. Titrate upward with increases of 20 mg to 50 mg twice weekly. For severely agitated patients, 25 mg may be given intramuscularly and repeated if necessary in 1 hour. Any subsequent intramuscular medication should be at 4- to 6-hour intervals.

Chlorpromazine Hydrochloride Dose Forms Available

- Tablets: 10 mg, 25 mg, 50 mg, 100 mg, 200 mg
- Spansules (extended release, not recommended for children) 30 mg, 75 mg, 150 mg
- Syrup: 10 mg/5 mL
- Oral Concentrate 30 mg/mL, 100 mg/mL
- Suppositories: 25 mg, 100 mg
- Injection (intramuscular): 25 mg/mL

Reports of Interest
Chlorpromazine in the Treatment of Children and Adolescents Diagnosed with Attention-Deficit/Hyperactivity Disorder

Werry et al. (1966) reported that chlorpromazine was significantly superior to placebo ($P = .005$) in reducing hyperactivity in a double-blind, placebo-controlled, 8-week study of 39 hyperactive children (mean age, 8.5 years; IQ, 85 or greater), a large number of whom had additional symptoms of distractibility, irritability, and specific cognitive defects. Intellectual functioning and symptoms of distractibility, aggressivity, and excitability did not appear significantly affected by the drug. The authors concluded that chlorpromazine could be used for behavioral symptoms in therapeutic doses (mean dose was 106 mg/day with a maximum daily dose of

5 mg/kg or 150 to 200 mg) without fear of significantly impairing learning. The most frequent untoward effects were mild sedation and mild photosensitization of the skin (Werry et al. 1966).

Weiss and her colleagues (1975) reported that 5 years after initial diagnosis, there were no differences on measures of emotional adjustment, antisocial behavior, and academic performance among a group of hyperactive children treated with chlorpromazine for 1.5 to 5 years, a similar group treated for 3 to 5 years with methylphenidate, and a group whose medication was discontinued after 4 months because of poor response.

Thioridazine Hydrochloride (Mellaril)

In July of 2000, Novartis, the manufacturer of Mellaril (thioridazine hydrochloride), issued major changes in their labeling. This included a **boxed warning** indicating that thioridazine has been shown to prolong the QT_c interval in a dose-related manner and that drugs with this potential, including thioridazine, have been associated with torsade de pointes and sudden death.

At present, thioridazine is indicated only for the treatment of schizophrenic patients who have failed to respond adequately to trials with appropriate doses and duration of at least two antipsychotics because of the lack of clinical efficacy or intolerable untoward effects.

The use of thioridazine in the treatment of significant behavioral problems, including combativeness, explosive hyperexcitable behavior, ADHD with marked conduct problems, aggressivity, mood lability, poor frustration tolerance, and impulsivity, is no longer approved by the FDA or the package insert. Any such use would not only be "off-label" but would be ignoring the new recommendations and warnings, and cannot be recommended.

Contraindications for the Administration of Thioridazine Hydrochloride

Thioridazine is contraindicated with fluvoxamine, propranolol, and pindolol, which appear to appreciably inhibit its metabolism, drugs that inhibit cytochrome P450 2D6 isozyme (e.g., fluoxetine and paroxetine) and drugs known to prolong the QT_c interval. Thioridazine is also contraindicated in patients known to have genetically related reduced levels of p450 2D6 activity, which occur in approximately 7% of the general population, and patients with congenital long QT syndrome, a baseline QTc > 450 msec, or a history of cardiac arrhythmia.

Indications for Thioridazine Hydrochloride in Child and Adolescent Psychiatry

In July 2000, the FDA issued a warning about the use of Thioridazine, restricting its use. The current Black Box Warning (PDR, 2006) states: **Thioridazine has been shown to prolong the QTc interval in a dose-related manner, and drugs with this potential, including thioridazine, have been associated with torsade de pointes-type arrhythmias and sudden death. Because of its potential for significant, possibly life-threatening proarrhythmic effects, thioridazine should be reserved for use in the treatment of schizophrenic patients who fail to show an acceptable response to**

(continued)

Indications for Thioridazine Hydrochloride in Child and Adolescent Psychiatry (Continued)

adequate courses of treatment with other antipsychotic drugs, either because of insufficient effectiveness or the inability to achieve an effective dose due to intolerable adverse effects from those drugs.

Currently, thioridazine no longer has FDA approval for treating severe behavioral problems marked by combativeness and/or explosive hyperexcitable behavior, or for the short-term treatment of hyperactive children who show excessive motor activity with accompanying conduct disorders consisting of some or all of the following symptoms: impulsivity, difficulty sustaining attention, aggressivity, mood lability, and poor frustration tolerance.

Thioridazine Dosage Schedule

- Children younger than 2 years of age: not recommended.
- Children 2 to 12 years of age: usual dosage ranges from 0.5 mg/kg/day to a maximum of 3 mg/kg/day. Start with a low dose and titrate upward for optimal therapeutic effect. More severely disturbed children may initially require 25 mg once or twice daily.
- Adolescents and adults: a maximum of 800 mg/day is permitted to minimize the likelihood that pigmentary retinopathy will develop. The initial dose depends on the severity of the disorder; frequently, 25 to 50 mg two or three times daily is an appropriate starting dosage.

Thioridazine Hydrochloride Dose Forms Available

- Tablets: 10 mg, 15 mg, 25 mg, 50 mg, 100 mg, 150 mg, 200 mg
- Oral Concentrate: 30 mg/mL, 100 mg/mL
- Oral Suspension: 25 mg/5 mL, 100 mg/5 mL

Reports of Interest

The following studies were conducted prior to the changes in labeling and are no longer FDA-approved uses of thioridazine.

Thioridazine in the Treatment of Children and Adolescents Diagnosed with ADHD. Klein (1990/1991) analyzed data collected in a 4-week, double-blind, placebo-controlled study of thioridazine in treating 77 children (ages 6 to 12 years) who would meet DSM-III-R (APA, 1987) diagnostic criteria for ADHD. Subjects were administered a large number of tests to measure general and specific cognitive functions. The mean daily doses of thioridazine at 4 and 12 weeks were 193 mg and 160 mg, respectively. At both 4 and 12 weeks, only a single psychometric test was significantly worse for patients on thioridazine than for those on placebo. Although significant decrements in cognitive test performance were expected on these relatively high doses of thioridazine, they did not occur. Klein concluded that thioridazine does not have a general deleterious effect of cognitive performance on children diagnosed with ADHD and treated for up to 12 weeks with therapeutic doses of thioridazine. It was suggested that thioridazine be administered in one nighttime dose to minimize the sedative effects, which are most acute following ingestion. Interestingly, Klein noted that more than half of the subjects were rated as having at least mild-to-moderate daytime drowsiness; however, on testing, there was minimal effect on cognitive performance.

Thioridazine in Patients Diagnosed with ADHD and Mental Retardation. Aman et al. (1991b) studied the effects on cognitive-motor performance in 27 children with a mean IQ of 54 (range, 30 to 90) who also had a DSM-III diagnosis of attention deficit disorder (ADD) and/or a conduct disorder in a double-blind, placebo-controlled, crossover study of methylphenidate (0.4 mg/kg/day) and thioridazine (1.75 mg/kg/day). Thioridazine had no adverse effect on the performance of any of the cognitive-motor performance tests and had no deleterious effect on IQ when correct answers of the subjects were reinforced. Aman et al. (1991a) noted that more severely retarded children with IQs of 45 or less or a mental age below 4.5 years, whose functioning is characterized by a narrow attentional focus, tended to respond poorly to stimulants, in contrast to less retarded individuals who responded more positively to stimulants. No such relationship was apparent between IQ and response to thioridazine. At the doses employed, thioridazine had relatively minor behavioral effects, although it was superior to placebo on teachers' ratings of conduct problems, hyperactivity, and overall improvement. The authors suggested that higher doses of thioridazine, up to 2.5 mg/kg, might be more effective in treating severe behavioral disorders and hyperactivity in more retarded individuals; they also noted that some such individuals might benefit from stimulants (Aman et al. 1991a, 1991b).

In an earlier study, Alexandris and Lundell (1968) compared the effects of thioridazine, amphetamine, and placebo in 21 mentally deficient (IQ range, 55 to 85) children (ages 7 to 12 years) diagnosed with hyperkinetic syndrome. Thioridazine was significantly superior to amphetamine on scores related to concentration, aggressiveness, sociability, interpersonal relationship, comprehension, work interest, and work capacity. In no case was amphetamine or placebo significantly superior to thioridazine. The average dose of thioridazine after 6 months was 95 mg/day; dose range was 30 to 150 mg/day.

Trifluoperazine Hydrochloride (Stelazine, Vesprin)

Indications for Trifluoperazine Hydrochloride in Child and Adolescent Psychiatry

One manufacturer has a specific disclaimer that trifluoperazine has not been proved effective in the management of behavioral complications in patients with mental retardation, and recommends it only for the treatment of psychotic individuals and for the short-term treatment of nonpsychotic anxiety in individuals with generalized anxiety disorder who have not responded to other medications.

Trifluoperazine Dosage Schedule

- Children younger than 6 years of age: not recommended.
- Children aged 6 to 12 years of age: a starting dose of 1 mg once or twice daily with gradual upward titration is recommended. Dosages in excess of 15 mg/day are usually required only by older children with severe symptoms.
- Adolescents: 1 to 5 mg twice daily. Usually the optimal dose will be 15 to 20 mg/day or less; occasionally, up to 40 mg/day will be required. Titration to optimal dose can usually be accomplished within 2 to 3 weeks.

(continued)

Indications for Trifluoperazine Hydrochloride in Child and Adolescent Psychiatry *(Continued)*

Trifluoperazine Hydrochloride Dose Forms Available

- Tablets: 1 mg, 2 mg, 5 mg, 10 mg
- Oral Concentrate: 10 mg/mL
- Injection, Intramuscular: 2 mg/mL. (One manufacturer notes that there is little experience using intramuscular trifluoperazine with children and recommends 1 mg intramuscularly once, or maximally twice, daily if necessary for rapid control of severe symptoms.)

Haloperidol (Haldol)

Pharmacokinetics of Haloperidol

Morselli et al. (1983) noted that steady-state haloperidol plasma levels in children may vary up to 15-fold at a given mg/kg daily dosage, but for a given individual the relationship between dosage and plasma level is fairly consistent. Most children had haloperidol plasma half-lives that were shorter than those of adolescents and adults. However, the authors also emphasized that despite their more rapid metabolism of haloperidol, children did not require proportionally higher daily doses, because they also appear to be more sensitive to both the therapeutic and the untoward effects of haloperidol at lower plasma concentrations than were older adolescents and adults (Morselli et al. 1983).

Indications for Haloperidol in Child and Adolescent Psychiatry

Haloperidol is indicated for the treatment of acute and chronic psychotic disorders and for the control of tics and vocal utterances in Tourette's disorder. Only after the failure of treatment with psychotherapy and nonantipsychotic medications has haloperidol been approved for treating children with severe behavioral disorders (e.g., "combative, explosive hyperexcitability [which cannot be accounted for by immediate provocation]" [package insert]) and for the short-term treatment of hyperactive children with coexisting conduct disorders, who exhibit such symptoms as "impulsivity, difficulty sustaining attention, aggressivity, mood liability, and poor frustration tolerance."

Haloperidol Dosage Schedule for Children and Adolescents with Psychotic Disorders, Tourette's Disorder, or Severe Nonpsychotic Behavioral Disorders

- Children younger than 3 years of age: not recommended.
- Children 3 to 12 years of age (weight: 15 to 40 kg): begin with 0.5 mg daily; titrate upward by 0.5-mg increments at 5- to 7-day intervals. Therapeutic dose ranges are usually from 0.05 to 0.075 mg/kg/day for nonpsychotic behavioral disorders and Tourette's disorder; for psychotic children the upper range is usually 0.15 mg/kg/day, but may be higher in severe cases. Morselli et al. (1983) reported good therapeutic results in children with tics and Tourette's disorder associated with haloperidol plasma levels in the range of 1 to 3 ng/mL. Higher haloperidol

(continued)

Indications for Haloperidol in Child and Adolescent Psychiatry (Continued)

plasma levels, usually between 6 and 10 ng/mL, were necessary for significant improvement in psychotic conditions.

- Adolescents: depending on severity, 0.5 to 5 mg two or three times daily. Higher doses may be necessary for more rapid control in some severe cases.

Haloperidol Dose Forms Available

- Tablets: 0.5 mg, 1 mg, 2 mg, 5 mg, 10 mg, 20 mg
- Oral Concentrate: 2 mg/mL
- Injectable immediate release, (intramuscular): Haloperidol lactate (Haldol IR injection): 5.0 mg/mL. Safety has not been established for children and younger adolescents. If necessary, in acutely agitated older adolescents an initial dose of 2 to 5 mg may be given intramuscularly. Additional medication may be given every 1 to 8 hours as determined by ongoing evaluation of the patient.
- Injection, long-acting, (intramuscular) Haloperidol Decanoate: 50 mg, 100 mg Haldol Decanoate Injection 50 and Haldol Decanoate Injection 100 contain 50 mg and 100 mg of haloperidol (present as 70.52 mg and 141.04 mg of haloperidol decanoate), respectively. The safety and efficacy of haloperidol decanoate has not been established for children and younger adolescents, and it is currently used primarily for treating adults diagnosed with chronic schizophrenia. However, in some severely disturbed adolescents, particularly when compliance is a major therapeutic issue, haloperidol decanoate may be indicated. Peak plasma concentration is reached approximately 6 days after injection and plasma half-life is approximately 3 weeks. The usual interval between doses is 4 weeks, but this may need to be adjusted for some patients.

Reports of Interest

Haloperidol in the Treatment of Schizophrenia with Childhood Onset. Green et al. (1992) administered haloperidol on an open basis to 15 hospitalized children younger than 12 years of age diagnosed with schizophrenia. They reported the optimal dose to range between 1 and 6 mg/day. Acute dystonic reactions occurred in approximately 25% of the children despite low initial doses and gradual increments of the drug.

Spencer et al. (1992) administered haloperidol to 12 patients (9 males, 3 females; ages 5.5 to 11.75 years) in an ongoing, double-blind, placebo-controlled study of hospitalized children diagnosed with schizophrenia. Optimal haloperidol dose ranged from 0.5 to 3.5 mg/day (range, 0.02 to 0.12 mg/kg/day; mean, 2.02 mg/day). Haloperidol was significantly better than placebo on staff Global Clinical Judgments ($P = .003$), and on four of the eight Children's Psychiatric Rating Scale (CPRS) items selected for their pertinence to schizophrenia: ideas of reference ($P = .04$); persecutory ($P = .01$), other thinking disorders ($P = .04$), and hallucinations ($P = .04$). Two children (16.7%) experienced acute dystonic reactions. All 12 improved on haloperidol and were discharged on that medication.

In a double-blind, head-to-head comparison of haloperidol and clozapine, Kumra et al. (1996) reported that clozapine was significantly superior to haloperidol in treating treatment-resistant adolescents with childhood-onset schizophrenia.

Because of its severe untoward-effect profile, however, clozapine is not a first-line therapeutic drug for schizophrenia. This study is reviewed in detail later under clozapine.

Haloperidol in the Treatment of Tourette's Disorder. Shapiro and Shapiro (1989) concluded that the most effective neuroleptics in the treatment of tics and Tourette's disorder were pimozide (Orap), haloperidol, fluphenazine (Prolixin, Permitil), and penfluridol (Semap, an investigational drug). Studies by Shapiro and Shapiro (1984); Shapiro et al. (1983); and Sallee et al. (1997) comparing haloperidol and pimozide found pimozide to be more efficacious and to have significantly less severe untoward effects in treating Tourette's disorder. These studies are reviewed later under pimozide.

Haloperidol in the Treatment of Autistic Disorder and Atypical Pervasive Developmental Disorders. Haloperidol is the most well-studied first generation antipsychotic used in the treatment of autistic disorder. In a study of 40 autistic children 2.33 to 6.92 years of age, haloperidol in optimal doses of 0.5 to 3 mg/day yielded global clinical improvement and significantly decreased the symptoms of withdrawal, stereotypies, abnormal object relationships, hyperactivity, fidgetiness, negativism, and angry and labile affect (Anderson et al. 1984). However, a high rate of dyskinesias remains a problem. Significant numbers of autistic children (22%, or 8 of 36) developed tardive dyskinesia or withdrawal dyskinesia in a prospective study in which 0.5 to 3 mg/day of haloperidol was administered for periods ranging from 3.5 to 42.5 months; thus close monitoring is necessary (Perry et al. 1985).

In autistic disorder, stereotypies existing at baseline may be suppressed by administration of haloperidol. When the drug is withdrawn, there is potential for confusion between the reappearance of stereotypies and a withdrawal dyskinesia; this is of special concern if a physician unfamiliar with the child at baseline assumes treatment responsibilities for the child while he or she is on maintenance medication.

Joshi et al. (1988) administered fluphenazine or haloperidol to 12 children aged 7 to 11 years who were hospitalized and diagnosed with childhood onset or atypical pervasive developmental disorders (PDDs) (i.e., approximately equivalent to the DSM-III-R [APA, 1987] diagnoses of autistic disorder with childhood onset and PDD not otherwise specified [PDDNOS]). The children responded with remarkable improvement in peer interactions and reality testing and decreases in autistic-like behavior, aggressiveness, impulsivity, and hyperactivity. Seven of the 12 children were able to return home rather than be admitted for residential treatment as had been planned. Haloperidol was begun at a dose of 0.02 mg/kg/day and titrated based on behavioral response, with increases at 3- to 5-day intervals. Mean optimal dose of haloperidol was 0.04 ± 0.01 mg/kg/day. Untoward effects were remarkably infrequent. Drowsiness occurred initially in some children, but it was transient and did not interfere with their later cognitive performance. Two children receiving haloperidol developed some rigidity and cogwheeling that responded to oral diphenhydramine during the first few days of treatment; the extrapyramidal symptoms did not recur when the diphenhydramine was discontinued.

Haloperidol in the Treatment of Aggressive Conduct Disorder. In a double-blind, placebo-controlled study of 61 treatment-resistant hospitalized children, aged 5.2 to 12.9 years, with undersocialized aggressive conduct disorder, both haloperidol and lithium were found to be superior to placebo in ameliorating behavioral symptoms (Campbell et al. 1984b). Optimal doses of haloperidol ranged from 1 to 6 mg/day. The authors reported that, at optimal doses, the untoward effects of haloperidol appeared to interfere more significantly with the children's daily routines than did those of lithium.

Haloperidol in the Treatment of ADHD. Werry and Aman (1975) investigated the effects of methylphenidate and haloperidol on attention, memory, and activity in 24 children (ages 4.11 to 12.4 years), more than half of whom were diagnosed with hyperkinetic reaction and the remainder with unsocialized aggressive reaction. Each child received one of four drug conditions—placebo, methylphenidate (0.3 mg/kg), low-dose haloperidol (0.025 mg/kg), or high-dose haloperidol (0.05 mg/kg)—in a double-blind, placebo-controlled, crossover (within subject) design. For all statistically significant measures of cognitive functions of vigilance and short-term memory, the rank order of the means was methylphenidate, haloperidol (low dose), placebo, and haloperidol (high dose). The data suggested that methylphenidate and low-dose haloperidol, although to a lesser degree, improved these cognitive functions, whereas high-dose haloperidol appeared to cause them to deteriorate (Werry and Aman, 1975). The clinical importance of observing this biphasic effect is that it is the dose of haloperidol, not the drug itself, that may cause cognitive impairment. Based on this study, most children and adolescents treated for ADHD with haloperidol should receive doses between 0.5 and 2.0 mg/day (i.e., 0.025 mg/kg for a weight range of 20 to 80 kg).

Thiothixene (Navane)

Indications for Thiothixene in Child and Adolescent Psychiatry

Thiothixene is an antipsychotic drug of the thioxanthene series. It is indicated in the management of symptoms of psychotic disorders. It has not been evaluated in the management of behavioral disturbances in the mentally retarded nor is its use recommended in children younger than 12 years of age, because safe conditions for its use in that age-group have not been established (PDR, 2000).

Thiothixene Dosage Schedule

- Children younger than 12 years of age: not recommended.
- Adolescents aged at least 12 years of age and adults: for milder conditions an initial dose of 2 mg three times daily with titration to 5 mg three times daily if needed is usually effective. For more severe conditions, use an initial dose of 5 mg twice daily. The usual optimal dose is 20 to 30 mg/day; occasionally, up to 60 mg/day are required. Daily doses of > 60 mg rarely increase the beneficial response (PDR, 2000).

Thiothixene Dose Forms Available

- Capsules: 1 mg, 2 mg, 5 mg, 10 mg, 20 mg
- Concentrate: 5 mg/mL
- Intramuscular injectable preparation: 2 mg/mL, 5 mg/mL

Report of Interest
Thiothixene in the Treatment of Adolescents Diagnosed with Schizophrenia

Realmuto and his colleagues (1984) assigned 21 adolescent inpatients (mean age, 15.1 years; range, 11.75 to 18.33 years) diagnosed with chronic schizophrenia, to either thiothixene or thioridazine. Optimal dose was individually titrated over a period of approximately 2 weeks. For the 13 patients who received thiothixene, the mean optimal dose was 16.2 mg/day (range, 4.8 to 42.6 mg/day) or 0.30 mg/kg/day for 4 to 6 weeks. Hallucinations, anxiety, tension, and excitement decreased the most during the first week. Cognitive disorganization improved more slowly. There were no significant differences between the two drugs in rapidity of symptom improvement or extent of improvement at the end of the study. Approximately 50% of patients improved, regardless of the medication. There was a suggestion, however, that untoward effects, particularly drowsiness, were less severe with thiothixene than with thioridazine and that because of this, high-potency antipsychotics may be preferable to the more sedating low-potency antipsychotics in treating adolescents with schizophrenia (Realmuto et al. 1984).

Loxapine Succinate (Loxitane)

Indications for Loxapine Succinate in Child and Adolescent Psychiatry

Loxapine is a dibenzoxazepine compound with antipsychotic properties used in treating psychotic disorders. The manufacturer does not recommend its use in persons younger than 16 years of age.

Loxapine Dosage Schedule

- Children and adolescents younger than 16 years of age: not recommended.
- Adolescents at least 16 years of age and adults: an initial dose of 10 mg twice daily is recommended and is titrated according to clinical response. The usual therapeutic and maintenance dose ranges from 60 to 100 mg daily. A maximum of 250 mg/day is recommended.

Loxapine Succinate Dose Forms Available

- Capsules: 5 mg, 10 mg, 25 mg, 50 mg
- Oral Concentrate: 25 mg/mL
- Injectable preparation (intramuscular): 50 mg/mL

Report of Interest

Loxapine Succinate in the Treatment of Adolescents Diagnosed with Schizophrenia

Pool and colleagues (1976) conducted a 4-week, double-blind study comparing the efficacies of loxapine, haloperidol, and placebo in 75 adolescents, 13 to 18 years of age, diagnosed with acute schizophrenia or chronic schizophrenia with an acute exacerbation. Loxapine was begun at a dose of 10 mg daily and titrated to a maximum of 200 mg daily (average daily dose, 87.5 mg). Extrapyramidal reactions, most commonly parkinsonian muscular rigidity, were the most frequent untoward effects of loxapine and occurred in 19 of 26 subjects. The second most frequent untoward effect, sedation, occurred in 21 of the 26 subjects. Both loxapine and haloperidol were significantly superior to placebo in diminishing schizophrenic symptoms. The authors concluded that loxapine was relatively safe and efficacious in the treatment of adolescent schizophrenia.

Molindone Hydrochloride (Moban)

Molindone hydrochloride is a dihydroindolone compound with antipsychotic properties; it is structurally unrelated to the phenothiazine, butyrophenone, and thioxanthene antipsychotics. Its clinical action resembles that of the piperazine phenothiazines (e.g., perphenazine [Trilafon]) (Drug Facts and Comparisons, 1995). Moban is rapidly absorbed from the gastrointestinal tract, and peak blood levels of unmetabolized drug are achieved approximately 1.5 hours after ingestion. Moban has many metabolites, and pharmacologic effects from a single dose may last up to 36 hours (PDR, 2000). Although molindone has been associated with sinus tachycardia, it is one of the few antipsychotics that has no warning of increased QT_c intervals in the package insert (Gutgesell et al. 1999).

Indications for Molindone Hydrochloride in Child and Adolescent Psychiatry

Molindone hydrochloride is approved for the treatment of psychotic disorders. Its use in children younger than 12 years of age is not recommended as its efficacy and safety have not been established for use in that age-group (PDR, 2000).

Molindone Dosage Schedule

- Children younger than 12 years of age: not recommended.
- Adolescents and adults: the usual starting dose for treatment of psychotic symptoms is 50 to 75 mg/day, with an increase to 100 mg/day in 3 to 4 days. The medication should be titrated according to symptom response; up to 225 mg/day may be required in severely disturbed patients.

Molindone Hydrochloride Dose Forms Available

- Tablets: 5 mg, 10 mg, 25 mg, 50 mg, 100 mg
- Oral Concentrate: 20 mg/mL

Report of Interest

Molindone Hydrochloride in the Treatment of Children Diagnosed with Conduct Disorder

Greenhill et al. (1985) compared molindone and thioridazine in treating 31 hospitalized boys, ages 6 to 11 years, who were diagnosed with undersocialized conduct disorder, aggressive type. Children were assigned randomly to either medication in an 8-week, double-blind, parallel-design study. Subjects were drug-free for the baseline week and were on placebo the second week of the study. During week 3, medication was raised until it produced sedation; this was followed by a fixed dose of drug during weeks 4 through 6. The final 2 weeks of the study were again placebo. The mean dose of thioridazine over the 4-week treatment period was 169.9 mg/day (4.64 mg/kg/day), and the mean dose of molindone was 26.8 mg/day (1.3 mg/kg/day).

The groups were similar on baseline ratings, which showed them to be severely aggressive. In fact, the initial or terminal placebo periods had to be shortened for

11 subjects and drug begun because of their severe symptomatology. Symptoms improved significantly during the 4 weeks on either drug compared to the placebo periods. On Clinical Global Impressions (CGI), nurses rated the severity of illness at the end of the study as less in the molindone group ($P < .08$) and the degree of improvement as significantly greater ($P < .035$). Untoward effects differed, although not significantly, between the drugs; acute dystonic reactions occurred more frequently in the molindone group (23.5% vs. 6.1%), whereas sedation and gastrointestinal symptoms were more frequent among subjects treated with thioridazine. The authors concluded that molindone is relatively safe for inpatient children and adolescents and thought its efficacy in this population was similar to the more commonly used neuroleptics.

Fluphenazine Hydrochloride (Prolixin, Permitil)

Indications for Fluphenazine Hydrochloride in Child and Adolescent Psychiatry

Fluphenazine hydrochloride is approved for the treatment of psychotic disorders. It is not approved for administration to children younger than 12 years of age, however, because of lack of studies proving its efficacy and safety in this age-group. A manufacturer notes that it has not been shown to be effective in treating behaviorally disturbed patients who are mentally retarded.

Fluphenazine Dosage Schedule

- Children younger than 12 years of age: safety and efficacy have not been established; however, USPDI (2005) recommends 0.25 to 0.75 mg one to four times daily for psychotic disorders in children.
- Adolescents and adults: the manufacturer recommends an initial daily total dose of 2.5 to 10 mg for adults, divided and administered every 6 to 8 hours. One should be at least this conservative in adolescents (see also Joshi et al. [1988]).

Fluphenazine Hydrochloride Dose Forms Available

- Tablets: 1 mg, 2.5 mg, 5 mg, 10 mg
- Elixir: 0.5 mg/mL (2.5 mg/5 mL)
- Oral Concentrate: 5 mg/1 mL
- Injectable preparation (intramuscular): 2.5 mg/mL
- Long-acting preparations for parenteral administration: fluphenazine enanthate, 25 mg/mL, and fluphenazine decanoate, 25 mg/mL, are available. (They are used primarily in treating adults diagnosed with chronic schizophrenia. However, USPDI (2005) suggests an intramuscular or subcutaneous dose of between 3.125 mg and 12.5 mg every 1 to 3 weeks as needed and tolerated in children aged 5 to 11 years. In children aged 12 years and older, an initial dose of 6.25 to 18.75 mg is suggested with a subsequent increase to12.5 to 25 mg, with injections every 1 to 3 weeks.)

Report of Interest

Fluphenazine Hydrochloride in the Treatment of Children Diagnosed with Pervasive Developmental Disorders

As discussed earlier for haloperidol, Joshi et al. (1988) found fluphenazine to be efficacious in treating children diagnosed with childhood-onset PDD or atypical

PDD. Fluphenazine was begun at 0.02 mg/kg/day and increased at 3- to 5-day intervals based on behavioral responses. Mean optimal dose of fluphenazine was 1.3 ± 0.7 mg/day. Untoward effects of fluphenazine were remarkably infrequent. Initial drowsiness occurred in some children, but it was transient.

Pimozide (Orap)

Pimozide is an antipsychotic of the diphenyl-butylpiperidine series. It is indicated for the suppression of motor and phonic tics in patients with Tourette's disorder who have failed to respond to standard treatment (e.g., haloperidol). It is not intended as a treatment of first choice. A "Dear Health Care Provider" letter dated September 1999, from the manufacturer warned that sudden, unexpected deaths have occurred in patients taking pimozide at doses > 10 mg/day.

Pharmacokinetics of Pimozide

Peak serum levels usually occur 6 to 8 hours after ingestion of pimozide. Pimozide is metabolized primarily in the liver; the drug and its metabolites are excreted primarily through the kidneys. There are wide interindividual variations in half-life and in peak serum levels for equivalent doses. Mean serum half-life in patients with schizophrenia is approximately 55 hours. There are few correlations between plasma levels and clinical findings (package insert). The cytochrome P4503A4 enzyme system (CYP 3A) is important in the metabolism of pimozide and it should not be taken simultaneously with drugs that may inhibit CYP 3A. Likewise, patients taking pimozide should avoid drinking grapefruit juice, which may inhibit the metabolism of pimozide by CYP 3A. As CYP 1A2 may also be involved in the metabolism of pimozide, clinicians should be alert to the potential for drug interactions with CYP 1A2 inhibitors.

Untoward Effects of Pimozide

Pimozide prolongs the QT interval of the ECG. An ECG should be done at baseline and monthly during the period of dose titration. Increase of the QT interval beyond an absolute limit of 0.47 second in children or 0.52 second in adults or > 25% above the patient's original baseline should be considered a mandate for no further increase in dose and possibly for lowering it. Because hypokalemia is associated with ventricular arrhythmias, potassium levels should be monitored during therapy.

Contraindications for Pimozide Administration

In addition to considerations for antipsychotics in general, pimozide is contraindicated in the treatment of simple tics or tics other than those associated with Tourette's disorder. Pimozide should not be given together with other drugs (e.g., stimulants) that may cause tics. An ECG should be performed before initiating treatment with pimozide, which should not be given to patients with congenital long QT intervals or a history of cardiac arrhythmias, or to those who are taking drugs that prolong the QT interval. Pimozide is contraindicated in patients receiving drugs that inhibit cytochrome P450 3A (CYP 3A) enzyme system, which may impede pimozide metabolism, including macrolide antibiotics, azole antifungal agents, protease inhibitors, nefazodone, and zileuton. Two sudden deaths have occurred when pimozide and the antibiotic clarithromycin, a P450 inhibitor, were administered simultaneously (PDR, 2000).

Indications for Pimozide in Child and Adolescent Psychiatry

Pimozide is indicated only in the treatment of patients diagnosed with Tourette's disorder whose development and/or daily life function is severely compromised by the presence of motor and phonic tics and who have not responded satisfactorily to or cannot tolerate standard treatments, such as haloperidol. Pimozide should not be considered a drug of first choice.

Unexplained deaths, perhaps cardiac related, and grand mal seizures have occurred in patients taking high doses of pimozide (> 20 mg/day) (PDR, 1995). More recently (September, 1999), the manufacturer reported that sudden, unexplained deaths had occurred with doses > 10 mg/day.

Pimozide Dosage Schedule

- Children younger than 2 years: not recommended. Safety and efficacy have not been determined for this age-group.
- Children aged 2 years and older and adolescents up to 17 years of age: because very limited information is available on the use of pimozide in children younger than 12 years of age, it should be introduced at a very low dose and gradually adjusted upward; it is suggested that treatment be initiated with 0.05 mg/kg/day taken at bedtime and gradually increased by increments of 0.5 mg every third day to a maximum of 0.2 mg/kg/day, not exceeding 10 mg/day.
- Adolescents 18 years of age and older and adults: recommended initial dose is 1 to 2 mg/day given in divided doses and titrated upward every other day. Most patients are maintained at < 0.2 mg/kg/day or 10 mg/day. Doses > 0.2 mg/kg/day or 10 mg/day are not recommended (PDR, 2006).

Pimozide Dose Forms Available

- Scored tablets: 1 mg, 2 mg

Reports of Interest

Use of Pimozide in Children and Adolescents with Tourette's Disorder. Shapiro et al. (1983) treated 31 patients aged 10 to 50 years (mean age, 19.6 ± 9.2 years) diagnosed with Tourette's syndrome with pimozide in an open study. All had previously received haloperidol and either had unsatisfactory symptom control, an unacceptable level of untoward effects, or a desire to try pimozide. Pimozide was titrated in 1-mg increments every 4 to 7 days until optimal dose was achieved. The mean optimal dose of pimozide was 12.9 ± 12.5 mg/day (median dose, 8 mg/day; range, 1 to 64 mg/day). In this subgroup of patients, the therapeutic efficacy of pimozide was superior to that of haloperidol. Significantly, more patients treated with pimozide (74.4%) achieved > 70% symptomatic improvement than with haloperidol (45.4%). The mean score for untoward effects was significantly less for pimozide than for haloperidol. The authors hypothesized that the superiority of pimozide was related to its relative lack of norepinephrine antagonism compared with haloperidol, which decreases norepinephrine levels and more readily induces untoward effects such as sedation, depression, impaired motivation, cognitive dulling, irritability, phobias, and dysphoria, limiting the use of higher doses of haloperidol (Shapiro et al. 1983).

Shapiro and Shapiro (1984) performed a double-blind placebo-controlled study of pimozide in 20 patients (mean age, 24.6 ± 2.7 years; range, 11 to 53 years) diagnosed with Tourette's syndrome. Six patients had a concomitant diagnosis of ADDH. The study was for a duration of 14 weeks—2 drug-free weeks followed by 6 weeks' study of one condition and then 6 weeks of the other. Initial dose of pimozide was 1 mg/day at bedtime, and dosage was flexibly adjusted every 2 to 3 days over 6 weeks to a maximum of 10 mg/day (approximately 0.2 mg/kg/day) for children and 20 mg/day for adults. Average optimal dose for pimozide was 6.88 ± 1.26 mg/day. The authors noted that the effective dosage was relatively independent of age and that younger patients often required higher dosages than adults. Benztropine was used in 18 patients at some time during treatment to counteract extrapyramidal and akinesic effects. Pimozide was significantly more clinically effective (most measures at the $P = .0001$ level) than placebo on multiple dependent measures. The untoward effects of pimozide were similar to those of other high-potency antipsychotic drugs but were mostly of only slight to moderate intensity, an advantage over haloperidol (Shapiro and Shapiro, 1984).

Sallee et al. (1997) reported that pimozide was significantly superior to equivalent doses of haloperidol in treating children and adolescents with a primary diagnosis of Tourette's disorder using DSM-III criteria (APA, 1980a). The authors treated 22 outpatients (age range, 7 to 16 years; mean, 10.2 years; 5 females and 17 males) in a double-blind, placebo-controlled double-crossover study comparing haloperidol and pimozide. Following a 2-week placebo baseline period, haloperidol, pimozide, and placebo were administered randomly for 6 weeks each, with a 2-week washout between each condition. Medication was begun at 1 mg/day and titrated upward at a maximum of 2 mg/week for 4 weeks and then maintained for the final 2 weeks with a goal of reducing the tic symptoms present at baseline by 70%. With the exception of diphenhydramine for nasal congestion, the subjects received only the study medications. Total scores on the Tourette Syndrome Global Scale were reduced by the targeted 70% in five subjects (23%) during placebo administration and in 14 subjects (64%) while on either active medication. Optimal doses of pimozide, 3.4 ± 1.6 mg/day (range, 1 to 6 mg/day), and of haloperidol, 3.5 ± 2.2 mg/day (range, 1 to 8 mg/day), were equivalent. Detailed evaluations of the subjects using the "total" and "tic subscale" scores of the Tourette Syndrome Global Scale and the "tic subscale" score of the Tourette's Syndrome Symptom List were performed at the end of baseline and the end of each 6-week medication trial. Pimozide, but not haloperidol, was superior to placebo on each of the three scores. On the Children's Global Assessment Scale Tic Severity Scale both pimozide and haloperidol were rated superior to placebo ($P = .01$). The differences in the untoward-effect profile of the two medications were strikingly in favor of pimozide. Treatment limiting untoward effects occurred three times more frequently during treatment with haloperidol (nine subjects [41%]) than with pimozide (three subjects [13.6%]). General untoward effects such as headache, stomachache, and irritability did not differ among the three conditions. Most of haloperidol's untoward effects were extrapyramidal, including akathisia ($N = 2$) and akinesia ($N = 2$). In addition, three subjects developed treatment-emergent depression or anxiety and two experienced academic failure while receiving haloperidol. Of particular interest, because of pimozide's known effects on cardiac function, the authors reported that electrocardiovascular effects on heart rate, rhythm, and waveform had no discernible differences from either placebo or haloperidol. The authors concluded that, overall, pimozide is superior to haloperidol in the treatment of Tourette's disorder in this age-group, although there may be occasional individuals who are helped more by haloperidol.

Use of Pimozide in Children and Adolescents with Other Psychiatric Disorders. Pangalila-Ratulangi (1973) reported a pilot study in which eight boys and two girls aged 9 to 14 years, eight of whom were diagnosed with schizophrenia or schizophrenia-like symptoms and two of whom had symptoms suggestive of epilepsy and blunted affect, improved clinically on doses of 1 to 2 mg/day of pimozide.

Naruse and colleagues (1982) assigned 87 children and adolescents, aged 3 to 16 years, randomly to haloperidol, pimozide, or placebo in a crossover double-blind study. The subjects were diagnosed with various behavioral disorders, and 34 were autistic. Global ratings found pimozide to be clinically as effective as haloperidol, and both to be superior to placebo. Pimozide, however, was more clinically efficacious than haloperidol on behavioral rating scales. Sleepiness was the most common untoward effect and occurred in 24% (20) of the subjects receiving pimozide and 23% (19) of those receiving haloperidol versus only 4% (3) receiving placebo. Insomnia was the next most common side effect, occurring in 4% (3) of subjects on pimozide, 5% (4) of subjects on haloperidol, and 11% (9) of subjects on placebo.

CHAPTER 6

Second Generation/ Atypical and Other Antipsychotic Drugs

"ATYPICAL" ANTIPSYCHOTIC DRUGS

The FDA has directed manufacturers of atypical antipsychotic drugs to add a black box warning that elderly patients with dementia-related psychosis treated with atypical antipsychotic drugs are at increased risk of death of 1.6 to 1.7 times that seen in placebo-treated patients. Atypical antipsychotic drugs are not approved for treatment of patients with dementia-related psychoses.

Atypical antipsychotic drugs, including clozapine, risperidone, olanzapine, quetiapine, ariprazole, and ziprasidone differ from the traditional antipsychotic drugs in that in addition to being dopamine receptor (D_2) blockers, they are significant serotonin receptor (S_2) blockers. The simultaneous blocking of D_2 and S_2 receptors in the brain is thought to account for the increased efficacy of these drugs in improving "negative" symptoms of schizophrenia as well as the decreased incidence of extrapyramidal untoward effects that occur with the atypical antipsychotic drugs compared with standard antipsychotic drugs (Borison et al. 1992; PDR, 2000). These drugs may also have a positive therapeutic effect when administered to some patients with preexisting tardive dyskinesia TD (Chouinard et al. 1993; Birmaher et al. 1992; Mozes et al. 1994).

Because prepubertal children diagnosed with schizophrenia differ from adolescents and adults diagnosed with schizophrenia on some significant parameters and frequently respond less satisfactorily to treatment with standard antipsychotics, specific investigations of the various atypical antipsychotics will be necessary to determine their efficacy in this age-group (Green and Deutsch, 1990).

Clozapine (Clozaril)

The FDA has directed manufacturers of atypical antipsychotic drugs to add a black box warning that elderly patients with dementia-related psychosis treated with atypical antipsychotic drugs are at increased risk of death of 1.6 to 1.7 times that seen in placebo-treated patients. Clozapine is not approved for treatment of patients with dementia-related psychosis.

Clozapine, a dibenzodiazepine, was approved by the FDA for marketing in the United States in late 1989. It differs from typical antipsychotic drugs in its dopaminergic effects. It functions as a dopamine blocker at both D_1 and D_2 receptors but does not induce catalepsy or inhibit apomorphine-induced stereotypy. Clozapine also appears to block limbic dopamine receptors more than striatal dopamine receptors. This may account for the fact that no confirmed cases of tardive dyskinesia have been reported in more than 20 years of worldwide experience in patients who have received only clozapine (PDR, 2000).

Volavka (1999) suggested that clozapine's antiaggressive effect in patients diagnosed with schizophrenia may result from its unique pharmacologic properties of preferentially blocking the D1-mediated function and its serotonergic actions.

Clozapine has significantly greater efficacy in treating the "negative" symptoms of schizophrenia and a lower incidence of extrapyramidal symptoms than traditional antipsychotics. There is also evidence that clozapine has a positive therapeutic effect on some patients with preexisting tardive dyskinesia. Like traditional antipsychotic drugs, clozapine initially suppresses the involuntary movements, but, unlike traditional antipsychotics, the abnormal movements do not worsen over time with clozapine, sometimes even with dose reduction. There is a suggestion that, although it may not be curative, clozapine may alleviate tardive dyskinesia over time in some patients (Jann, 1991).

Because of the increased risk for serious and potentially life-threatening untoward effects that has been reported in patients receiving clozapine, its administration is appropriate only for severely dysfunctional patients with schizophrenia who have not responded satisfactorily to adequate trials of at least two other antipsychotic drugs or who cannot tolerate the untoward effects present at therapeutic dose levels.

In their comparison of clozapine and olanzapine in the treatment of treatment-resistant schizophrenia with childhood onset, Kumra et al. (1998) reported that clozapine was superior to olanzapine and remains the "gold standard" treatment for schizophrenia. They also concluded that all children and adolescents with treatment-refractory schizophrenia should be given a trial of clozapine despite the increased risk of serious untoward effects (agranulocytosis/neutropenia and seizures) and the inconvenience of mandatory and necessary monitoring.

Pharmacokinetics of Clozapine

Peak plasma concentrations during steady-state maintenance at 100 mg twice daily occurred on an average of 2.5 hours (range, 1 to 6 hours) after dosing; mean peak plasma concentration was 319 ng/mL (range, 102 to 771 ng/mL). Clozapine is almost completely metabolized to demethylated, hydroxylated, and N-oxide derivatives, of which approximately 50% are secreted in the urine and 30% in the feces. Serum half-life after a single 75-mg dose averages 8 hours (range, 4 to 12 hours); at steady state on 100 mg twice daily, serum half-life averaged 12 hours (range, 4 to 66 hours). Food does not affect the absorption/bioavailability of clozapine; it may be taken with or without food.

Contraindications for Clozapine Administration

Hypersensitivity to clozapine is a contraindication. Also, patients with myeloproliferative disorders, uncontrolled epilepsy, or a history of clozapine-induced agranulocytosis or severe granulocytopenia should not take clozapine. Clozapine should not be administered together with another drug known to cause agranulo-cytosis or to suppress bone marrow function.

Adverse Effects of Clozapine

Agranulocytosis is reported to occur in association with administration of clozapine in 1% to 2% of patients. Because of this, weekly monitoring of white blood cell (WBC) counts is mandatory, with discontinuation of treatment if the WBC decreases significantly. It has been recommended that if the WBC falls below 3,500, monitoring should be increased to twice weekly, and if the WBC falls below 3,000, clozapine should be discontinued. Alvir et al. (1993) reported that 73 of 11,555 patients who received clozapine during a 15-month period developed agranulocytosis; of these, 2 died from complications of infection. The cumulative incidence of agranulocytosis was 0.80% after 1 year and 0.91% after 18 months. Agranulocytosis occurred during the first 3 months of treatment in the large majority of cases (61 [83.6%] of 73). In general, older patients and females appear to be at higher risk for developing agranulocytosis. However, an exception appeared to be that patients younger than 21 years of age were at somewhat higher risk than patients between 21 and 40 years of age. The authors also noted that subsequent to the period of their study, an additional five patients between 40 and 72 years of age died from complications resulting from agranulocytosis within 3 months of taking clozapine (Alvir et al. 1993). The manufacturer reports that more than 68,000 patients in the United States had been prescribed clozapine as of January 1, 1994. Of these, 317 developed agranulocytosis; despite weekly monitoring, 11 cases were fatal (PDR, 1995). As of August 21, 1997, the number of patients who were prescribed clozapine had increased to 150,409, with 585 cases of agranulocytosis and 19 fatalities (PDR, 2000).

Kumra et al. (1996) reported that five (24%) of 21 adolescent patients enrolled for up to 30 ± 15 months in their study had mild to moderate neutropenia, compared with an estimated cumulative risk of 1.5% to 2.0% in adults. They suggested that this might occur because, in metabolizing clozapine, children produce relatively higher concentrations of N-desmethyl-clozapine, which is associated with hematopoietic toxicity, than do adults.

Administration of clozapine is also associated with an increased incidence of seizures that is apparently dose dependent. At doses below 300 mg/day, approximately 1% to 2% of patients develop seizures; at moderate doses of 300 to 599 mg/day, approximately 3% to 4% develop seizures; at high doses of 600 to 900 mg/day, approximately 5% of patients develop seizures. Baseline EEG and periodic monitoring should be mandatory for children and adolescents receiving clozapine.

Gerbino-Rosen et al. (2005) reported a retrospective chart review of the hematologic adverse events (HAE) in 172 children and adolescents admitted over a 12-year period to a long-term chronic care facility for treatment-resistant disorders, defined as having failed treatment (i.e., continued need for hospitalization secondary to potential for self-harm, harm to others, or inability to care for self) with at least two antipsychotics in at least two chemical classes in clinically appropriate doses; the large majority of patients were diagnosed with schizophrenia spectrum disorders ($N = 139$) or bipolar disorder ($N = 25$). Patients, none of whom had previously received clozapine, were administered clozapine (mean age at clozapine initiation was 15.03 ± 2.13 years) on an open-label basis following a standard drug-monitoring program, with weekly assessments of white blood cell counts (WBC) counts with differential, including absolute neutrophil counts (ANCs). The median observation period was 8 months. Neutropenia (an ANC $< 1500/mm^3$) occurred in 29 (16.9%) patients; 5 of these patients continued clozapine as a repeated blood sample had a safe ANC and were not included among the patients who developed clozapine-induced HAE ($N = 24$). One of the 24 (0.6%) developed agranulocytosis (ANC $< 500/mm^3$). The cumulative probability of developing an HAE over a 1-year period was 16.1%, (95% CI, 9.7% to 22.5%); for developing agranulocytosis the cumulative probability over a 1-year period was 0.99% (95% CI, 0.98% to 1.0%). Twenty of the 24 patients with an HAE were rechallenged with clozapine; of these 11 did not develop another episode of HAE and remained on clozapine. The nine patients who developed a second episode were administered a third trial of clozapine, with five being successfully maintained on clozapine without subsequent HAE and four patients eventually stopping because of HAEs. Overall only eight (5%) patients stopped clozapine because of HAEs. The authors noted that the risk for agranulocytosis in children and adolescents treated with clozapine is similar to that reported for adults and that with careful monitoring and prompt discontinuation of clozapine at the first sign of an HAE, there were no long-term negative sequelae in these patients (Gerbino-Rosen et al. 2005).

BOXED WARNING [Summary]: Because of significant risk of developing potentially fatal agranulocytosis, only severely ill patients who have failed to respond adequately to (or could not tolerate) at least two other antipsychotics should be considered for treatment with clozapine. If given, mandatory monitoring protocols must be followed. READ PACKAGE INSERT COMPLETELY BEFORE PRESCRIBING.

Indications for Clozapine in Child and Adolescent Psychiatry

Clozapine is indicated for the management of severely ill, treatment-resistant, schizophrenic patients, and to reduce the risk of recurrent suicidal behavior in patients with schizophrenia or schizoaffective disorder who are judged to be at risk of re-experiencing suicidal behavior. The manufacturer noted that safety and efficacy of clozapine have not been established in children younger than 16 years of age.

Clozapine Dosage Schedule

- Children and adolescents 15 years of age and less: not recommended.
- Adolescents 16 years of age and adults: initially, a dose of 12.5 mg once or twice daily is recommended. The dose can be increased daily by 25 to 50 mg, if tolerated, to reach a target dose of 300 to 450 mg by 2 weeks' time. Subsequent dose increases of a maximum of 100 mg may be made once or twice weekly. Total daily dosage should not exceed 900 mg.

Clozapine Dose Forms Available

- Scored tablets: 25 mg, 100 mg

(continued)

BOXED WARNING [Summary]: Because of significant risk of developing potentially fatal agranulocytosis, only severely ill patients who have failed to respond adequately to (or could not tolerate) at least two other antipsychotics should be considered for treatment with clozapine. If given, mandatory monitoring protocols must be followed. READ PACKAGE INSERT COMPLETELY BEFORE PRESCRIBING. (Continued)

Mandatory Monitoring

Baseline white blood cell (WBC) count must be $\geq 3,500/mm^3$, with the differential having an absolute neutrophile count (ANC) of $\geq 1,500/mm^3$. Weekly monitoring of these parameters is required, with WBC counts $\geq 3,000/mm^3$ and ANCs $\geq 1,500/mm^3$ necessary to continue on medication. If lower counts occur, clozapine must be interrupted and the patient monitored daily. If both counts for the first 6 months are always within the acceptable range, biweekly monitoring may be initiated after 6 months. Read the complete monitoring instructions in package insert or PDR before prescribing.

Other untoward effects include adverse cardiovascular effects such as orthostatic hypotension, tachycardia, and ECG changes.

Reports of Interest

Clozapine in the Treatment of Children and Adolescents Diagnosed with Schizophrenia

Siefen and Remschmidt (1986) administered clozapine to 21 inpatients, 12 of whom were younger than 18 years (average age, 18.1 years). Their patients had an average of 2.4 inpatient hospitalizations and had been tried on an average of 2.8 different antipsychotics without adequate therapeutic response or with severe extrapyramidal effects. In addition, the authors considered it a risk that their patients' psychotic symptoms would become chronic if clozapine was not administered.

Clozapine was administered over an average of 133 days. The average maximum dose was 415 mg/day (range, 225 to 800 mg/day) and the average maintenance dose was 363 mg/day (range, 150 to 800 mg/day). In addition, 11 of the 21 subjects were administered one or more other unidentified drugs for about half of the time they were receiving clozapine.

Approximately 67% of symptoms that had been relatively resistant to previous treatment with antipsychotics disappeared or improved markedly in 11 (52%) of the patients, and an additional six (29%) patients showed at least slight improvement in the same number of symptoms. Four patients, however, had no changes or worsening of more than half of their psychopathologic symptoms during clozapine therapy. Positive symptoms of schizophrenia improved more than negative symptoms. Specifically, improvements in incoherent/dissociative thinking, aggressiveness, hallucinations, agitation, ideas of reference, anxiety, inability to make decisions, psychomotor agitation, motivation toward achievement, impoverished and restricted thinking, and ambivalent behavior were reported. Symptoms such as lack of self-confidence, fear of failure, psychomotor retardation, irritability, slowed thinking, blunted affect, and unhappiness showed no improvement or deteriorated during treatment with clozapine (Siefen and Remschmidt, 1986).

The most frequent untoward effects observed early in treatment with clozapine were daytime sedation, dizziness, tachycardia, orthostatic hypotension, sleepiness, and increased salivation. No patients developed agranulocytosis, and the hematologic changes that occurred in approximately 25% of patients were clinically insignificant and normalized during continued maintenance on clozapine (Siefen and Remschmidt, 1986).

Schmidt et al. (1990) reported a total of 57 cases of children and adolescents (age range, 9.8 to 21.3 years; mean, 16.8 years; 30 males and 27 females) who were treated with clozapine. Forty-eight patients were diagnosed with a schizophrenic disorder, five with schizoaffective disorder, two with monopolar manic disorder, and two with pervasive developmental disorders (PDDs). These patients had a mean duration of illness of 19.4 months (range, 0 to 74 months) before this hospitalization, which was the first for 16 patients, the second for 16 patients, and the third or more for the remaining 25 patients. Clozapine was begun on an average approximately 3 months after hospitalization following treatment failures with other antipsychotic drugs and concern about chronicity, intolerable untoward effects, or uncontrolled excitation. Average dose during the length of hospitalization was 318 mg/day (range, 50 to 800 mg/day); average dose at discharge was somewhat lower, 290 mg/day (range, 75 to 800 mg/day). Thirty-five patients received only clozapine. In 22 cases, one or more additional other neuroleptics, primarily phenothiazines, were administered simultaneously, but in about one half of these cases the additional drugs were tapered off and discontinued so that eventually 80% of the patients were on clozapine only. Mean duration on clozapine during hospitalization was 78 days (range, 7 to 355 days), and 17 (31%) patients were discharged on clozapine.

Clozapine was discontinued in 15 (28%) of the patients between the 8th and 132nd days of treatment (average, 50th day) when they were taking a mean dose of 143 mg/day (range, 25 to 350 mg/day) for the following reasons: insufficient antipsychotic effect in seven cases; poor compliance and a change to depot medication in five cases; and severe untoward effects in three cases (cholinergic delirium, seizure, and questionable clinically significant decrease of erythrocytes to 2.3 million).

The authors reported that two-thirds of the patients significantly improved in the whole range of symptoms. Paranoid-hallucinatory symptoms and excitation responded best, followed by a reduction in aggressivity. Clozapine was less effective in decreasing agitation and improving negative symptoms, and these symptoms sometimes worsened. Untoward effects were noted in all subjects. These included increased heart rates (during the first 8 weeks only) from 94 to 109 beats per minute in 37 (65%) patients, daytime sedation in 29 (51%) patients, hypersalivation in 20 (35%) patients, orthostatic hypotension in 20 (35%) patients, and an unspecified rise in temperature in 15 (26%) patients. Abnormal movements were observed in nine patients, including tremor (six cases), akathisia (one case), and unspecified extrapyramidal symptoms in two cases. During the first 16 weeks of clozapine therapy, a significant decrease of various hematologic parameters, including number of erythrocytes, was observed, but did not reach pathologic values; a relative shift from lymphocytes to neutrophils was seen in the differential during the first 2 weeks. There was a reversible increase in liver enzymes, which peaked during the third and fourth weeks. On EEGs, there was evidence that clozapine induced increased neuronal disinhibition (e.g., spike discharges) and a shift in background activity to lower frequencies. Pathologic EEG changes were present in 30 (55%) patients on clozapine compared with 17 (30%) patients before its administration ($P < .01$). One patient developed a seizure (Schmidt et al. 1990). The authors later noted that they considered EEG monitoring before and during treatment with clozapine to be mandatory (Blanz and Schmidt, 1993).

Birmaher et al. (1992) treated three inpatient adolescents (an 18-year-old female and two 17-year-old males) with clozapine; they were diagnosed with schizophrenia that was chronic and resistant to treatment with standard antipsychotics. Clozapine was titrated upward, resulting in markedly better symptom control than was achieved in previous drug trials. Doses at discharge were 100 mg/day for the female and 300 mg/day for the two males. The female patient experienced a reexacerbation of symptoms after approximately 1 year despite good compliance, and rehospitalization was required. She was discharged in 2 weeks, but it was necessary to increase clozapine to 400 mg/day; her functioning was described as satisfactory, but some auditory hallucinations remained.

The only untoward effects that these three patients complained about were sedation and increased salivation, and these gradually remitted. The buccolingual dyskinesia, which one of the males had developed during treatment with standard antipsychotics, disappeared while on clozapine (Birmaher et al. 1992).

Mandoki (1993) administered clozapine to two hospitalized males, of age 14 and 16 years, diagnosed with schizophrenia who had unsatisfactory responses to trials of many medications, including antipsychotics. The younger patient had predominantly severe negative symptoms and the older one predominantly severe positive symptoms. Clozapine in doses of 300 to 400 mg/day resulted in significant improvements. The 14-year-old was discharged on 300 mg/day of clozapine 11 weeks after clozapine treatment began. At follow-up he was attending school. Clozapine had been increased to 200 mg every morning and 400 mg at bedtime. Untoward effects were significant weight gain, mild hypersalivation, and severe drowsiness. The 16-year-old was discharged on 300 mg/day of clozapine 2 months after beginning clozapine. Dose was increased to 400 mg/day after 2 months because inappropriate touching behaviors recurred. No untoward effects were reported. At follow-up, both adolescents were continuing to experience gradual clinical improvement.

Remschmidt et al. (1994) reported a retrospective study of 36 adolescent inpatients, age range of 14 to 22 years, diagnosed with schizophrenia who were treated on an open basis with clozapine following treatment failures with at least two other antipsychotic drugs. Doses ranged from 50 to 800 mg/day (mean, 330 mg/day), and the mean duration of clozapine administration was 154 ± 93 days. Twenty-seven patients (75%) had clinically significant improvement; four (11%) had complete remissions. Three patients (8%) showed no improvement. Six (17%) developed untoward effects necessitating the discontinuation of clozapine: leukopenia without agranulocytosis (two patients); hypertension, tachycardia, and ECG abnormalities (two); elevations in liver transaminases to 10 times normal values without other signs of hepatitis (one); and worsening of symptoms and development of stupor when given in combination with carbamazepine 400 mg/day (one). Five patients developed extrapyramidal symptoms over a period of several months: four (11%) developed akathisia and one developed a course tremor. Overall, positive symptoms improved significantly more than negative symptoms. For example, delusions, hallucinations, and excitation improved in approximately 65% of patients. Some negative symptoms (e.g., flat affect and autistic behavior) showed little improvement, but other negative symptoms (e.g., anergy, muteness, bizarre behavior, and thought blocking) showed improvement in 11% to 22% of the patients. Nine (90%) of 10 patients who had predominantly negative symptoms did not improve clinically.

Levkovitch et al. (1994) treated 13 adolescents (seven males and six females; mean age, 16.6 years; range, 14 to 17 years) who were diagnosed with adolescent-onset schizophrenia with clozapine. All had experienced treatment failures, with an average of three traditional antipsychotics. Patients received an average daily dose of 240 mg of clozapine for a mean of 245 days. After 2 months, 10 patients (76.9%) showed significant improvement of at least a 50% decrease in scores on the Brief Psychiatric Rating Scale (BPRS); two patients showed more modest improvements. Clozapine was discontinued after 2 days in one patient because of significant orthostatic hypotension. Other untoward effects were tiredness in four (30.8%) patients, hypersalivation in one (7.7%), and temperature elevation in one (7.7%). No leukopenia occurred during weekly monitoring.

Frazier et al. (1994) treated 11 hospitalized adolescents (age range, 12 to 17 years; mean, 14.0 ± 1.5 years) diagnosed with childhood-onset schizophrenia with a 6-week open trial of clozapine. Subjects were chronically and severely ill and had received at least two previous neuroleptic medications without significant clinical benefit or experienced intolerable untoward effects. Following a 4-week washout/observation period, clozapine was begun at 12.5 mg/day or 25 mg/day. Dose was titrated individually based on symptom response versus untoward effects and increased by one to two times the initial dose every 4 days to a potential maximum of 900 mg/day. The main untoward effects responsible for limiting dose increases were tachycardia (three patients) and sedation (seven patients). Other untoward effects reported included hypersalivation (eight patients), weight gain (seven), enuresis (four), constipation (four), orthostatic hypotension (two), nausea (one), and dizziness (one).

Extrapyramidal untoward effects also occurred: four adolescents developed akathisia after several months and one developed a coarse tremor. The mean dose of clozapine at the end of the 6-week period was 370.5 mg/day (range, 125 to 825 mg/day). Six (55%) of the patients improved over 30% on the Brief Psychiatric Rating Scale (BPRS) on optimal dose of clozapine, compared with admission ratings when nine of the patients were receiving other drugs; nine (82%) of the patients improved on clozapine over 30% on the BPRS compared with ratings during the washout period. Nine of the 11 patients also received 6-week courses of haloperidol following 4-week washout/observation periods during their hospitalizations; of these, five (56%) showed more than a 30% improvement on the BPRS while on clozapine, compared with earlier ratings while on haloperidol. Both positive and negative symptoms of schizophrenia improved (Frazier et al. 1994).

Mozes et al. (1994) treated four children with clozapine; the three males and one female, 10 to 12 years of age, were diagnosed with schizophrenia and had not responded satisfactorily to other neuroleptics. Clozapine was begun in doses of 25 to 100 mg/day and titrated upward. Three patients had significantly reduced symptomatology in < 2 weeks. Further decreases in both positive and negative symptoms occurred during the next 10 to 15 weeks of treatment. All four children improved significantly on the BPRS, with a mean reduction of 41 within 15 weeks. At the time of the report, patients had been in treatment between 23 and 70 weeks, and maintenance dosage ranged from 150 to 300 mg/day. The most frequent untoward effect was drooling, which spontaneously decreased over time; drowsiness, experienced by three patients, peaked during the first week and then gradually faded away. Excitatory EEG changes occurred in three patients, and dosage was not increased to decrease the likelihood of seizures. Of note, two cases of tardive dyskinesia caused by previous neuroleptic drugs disappeared on clozapine.

Kumra et al. (1996) reported a double-blind study comparing clozapine and haloperidol in 21 hospitalized patients (11 males, 10 females; mean age, 14.0 ± 2.3 years) who had been diagnosed with schizophrenia by DSM-III-R (APA, 1987) criteria by age 12 and who were treatment refractory. All patients had failed to respond to at least two standard neuroleptics, often at high doses, and augmented with mood stabilizers or antidepressants; most patients also had failed to respond to risperidone. Medications were discontinued over a 2-week period, which was followed by a 4-week washout before active medication whenever this could be tolerated. Patients were randomly assigned to a 6-week parallel treatment with clozapine ($N = 10$) or haloperidol ($N = 11$); the two groups did not differ significantly on any demographic variables. To maintain the blind and to minimize any extrapyramidal effects secondary to haloperidol, all patients receiving that drug were prescribed up to 6 mg/day of benztropine, whereas subjects on clozapine received identical placebo tablets. Initial doses were based on patients' weights and ranged from 6.25 to 25 mg/day for clozapine and from 0.25 to 1.0 mg/day for haloperidol. Increases in the dose by one or two times the initial dose were permitted every 3 to 4 days if clinically indicated. Three patients receiving clozapine and one patient on haloperidol were unable to complete the 6-week trial because of severe untoward effects and were dropped during the fourth and fifth weeks, and the ratings of the final week were carried forward in data analysis. The mean dose of haloperidol during the last treatment week was 16.0 ± 8 mg/day (range, 7 to 27 mg/day) or 0.29 ± 0.19 mg/kg/day (range, 0.08 to 0.69 mg/kg/day). The mean dose of clozapine during the last treatment week was 176 ± 149 mg/day (range, 25 to 525 mg/day) or 3.07 ± 2.59 mg/kg/day (range, 0.34 to 7.53 mg/kg/day); the mean dose of clozapine for the seven subjects who completed the entire 6-week trial was higher: 239 ± 134 mg/day. Clozapine was statistically superior to haloperidol on ratings at the 6-week endpoint on the Brief Psychiatric Rating Scale ($P = .04$), the Bunney-Hamburg Psychosis Rating Scale ($P = .02$), the Scale for the Assessment of Positive Symptoms ($P = .01$), and the Scale for the Assessment of Negative Symptoms ($P = .002$). Clozapine was also superior to haloperidol on the depression ($P = .02$), thinking disturbance ($P = .05$), withdrawal ($P = .03$), and total ($P = .03$) rating scores on the Brief Psychiatric Rating Scale. After the double-blind study was completed, the 11 patients who received haloperidol were administered clozapine openly for 6 weeks. The combined sample of 21 subjects was rated on the Clinical Global Impressions Scale (CGI) as follows: very much improved, two (9.5%); much improved, 11 (52.4%); minimally improved, seven (33%); and worsened, one (4.8%). The authors also noted that for some patients, clinical improvement continued and peaked only after 6 to 9 months of treatment, as has been reported for adults.

Despite the superiority of clozapine over haloperidol, Kumra et al. (1996) noted serious untoward effects secondary to clozapine. Five of the 10 patients in the double-blind portion developed toxic hematopoietic effects with an absolute neutrophil count of < 1,500. In three patients, the WBC normalized spontaneously and they were successfully restarted on clozapine; the other two patients, however, had recurrences of neutropenia when rechallenged with clozapine and were dropped from the study. One patient developed myoclonus and had a tonic-clonic seizure the next day; epileptiform spikes continued on the EEG despite lowering the dose of clozapine and antiepileptic medication, and clozapine was discontinued. Another patient who had bifrontal and posterior delta wave slowing during the study had tonic-clonic seizures as an outpatient on 275 mg/day of clozapine and continued to have petit mal seizures despite a reduction in dosage and treatment with valproate sodium, necessitating discontinuation of clozapine. Three of the 11 patients treated openly with clozapine also developed significant EEG changes associated with worsening behavior, such as increased aggression, psychosis, or irritability. Two of these individuals improved with a reduction of the dose of clozapine and addition of valproate sodium; however, the third experienced further clinical deterioration and facial myoclonus with associated EEG spikes, which required the discontinuation of clozapine. Children and adolescents appear to be at greater risk than adults to develop clinically significant EEG changes. One patient on clozapine had clinically significant increases in liver enzymes and two had tachycardias of more than 100 beats/minute. The authors also felt that excessive weight gain occurred secondary to clozapine; the two best responders during the double-blind protocol gained the most weight. Only one patient was dropped from the haloperidol group, and that was for signs of incipient neuromalignant syndrome; the discontinuing of haloperidol and initiation of supportive measures resulted in normalization of laboratory abnormalities and vital signs within a few days. The extrapyramidal tract untoward effects expected from haloperidol were minimized by the prophylactic benztropine. This study provides significant support for the importance of clozapine in treatment-resistant schizophrenia in children and adolescents but underscores the importance of monitoring the WBC for untoward effects, such as neutropenia/agranulocytosis, and to monitor EEGs for epileptiform changes, to observe for myoclonic movements that may progress to tonic-clonic seizures, and for seizures as the pediatric age-group may be at greater risk for all of these than adults.

In a naturalistic treatment study, Kranzler et al. (2005) administered open-label clozapine, using a flexible titration schedule, to 20 treatment-refractory adolescents (14 males, 6 females; median age 14.19 years; age range 8.5–18 years) diagnosed with schizophrenia and hospitalized in a long-term treatment facility (Bronx Children's Psychiatric Center) to evaluate its effectiveness in the treatment of aggression. Subjects were judged to be acutely ill and required a change of medication because of the severity of their psychosis and aggression when clozapine was introduced. The current medication regime was continued and there was a slow cross taper with clozapine. Using a mirror-image study design, effectiveness was measured by comparing the number of emergency oral and injected medications and frequency of seclusion or restraint events in the 12 weeks immediately preceding the trial of clozapine and during a similar period (from week 12 through week 24 of clozapine treatment) when optimal clozapine levels had been reached. The mean dose at week 24 was 476 ± 119 mg/day, and 11 of the 20 subjects were on clozapine monotherapy. Comparison of pre-clozapine and optimal clozapine measures implemented for aggressive behavior showed significant decreases in emergency oral medication ($P = .000$), injectable medication ($P = .007$) and seclusion events ($P = .003$). Another significant finding was that patients who had been hospitalized for a shorter length of time when started on clozapine showed a significantly greater reduction in seclusion events than subjects who had been hospitalized for longer periods when the switch to clozapine was made ($P = .033$). These data suggested that, in such a patient population, clozapine reduces the incidence and severity of violence and aggression and may hasten discharge to a less restrictive setting. The authors think that clozapine treatment may be underutilized because of concerns about its untoward effects and the necessary frequent monitoring with blood tests.

Risperidone (Risperdal)

The FDA has directed manufacturers of atypical antipsychotic drugs to add a black box warning that elderly patients with dementia-related psychosis treated with atypical antipsychotic drugs are at increased risk of death of 1.6 to 1.7 times that seen in placebo-treated patients. Risperidone is not approved for treatment of patients with dementia-related psychosis.

Risperidone belongs to the new chemical class of benzisoxazole derivatives. It was approved by the FDA for marketing in the United States in 1993. The manufacturer suggests that its antipsychotic properties may be mediated through its antagonism of dopamine type 2 (D_2) and serotonin type 2 ($5HT_2$) receptors; it also has a high affinity for alpha-1 and alpha-2 adrenergic and H_1 histaminergic receptors (package insert).

Risperidone appears to have significantly greater efficacy in improving "negative" symptoms of schizophrenia than the traditional antipsychotics (Chouinard et al. 1993).

Risperidone has significantly fewer extrapyramidal symptoms than typical antipsychotics. At the usual recommended dose of 6 mg/day and at doses up to 10 mg/day, the incidence of extrapyramidal symptoms in patients treated with risperidone is not significantly different from the incidence of such symptoms in patients treated with placebo. However, the appearance of extrapyramidal symptoms is dose related and becomes increasingly greater than that for placebo with further increases in dosage.

Although the manufacturer notes that there have been isolated reports of tardive dyskinesia associated with risperidone, it is likely that the incidence of tardive dyskinesia occurring with risperidone only will be significantly less than that with typical antipsychotic agents.

Pharmacokinetics of Risperidone

Food does not affect the rate or extent of the absorption of risperidone. Peak serum levels of risperidone occur at a mean of 1 hour after ingestion. Risperidone is metabolized in the liver by cytochrome $P_{450}IID_6$ to 9-hydroxyrisperidone, its major metabolite, which is similar to risperidone in its receptor binding activity. Because of genetic polymorphism, approximately 7% of Caucasians and a very low percentage of Asians are slow metabolizers. Peak 9-hydroxyrisperidone levels occur in approximately 3 hours in extensive metabolizers and 17 hours in poor metabolizers. Half-life ($T_{1/2}$) of risperidone is approximately 3 hours in extensive metabolizers and 20 hours in poor metabolizers; $T_{1/2}$ of 9-hydroxyrisperidone is approximately 21 hours in extensive metabolizers and 30 hours in poor metabolizers.

Contraindications for Risperidone Administration

Risperidone is contraindicated in patients with a known hypersensitivity to it.

Risperidone should be administered with caution to patients with hepatic impairment, which may increase free risperidone by up to 35%, and/or renal impairment, which may decrease clearance of risperidone and its active metabolite by up to 60%.

Interactions of Risperidone with Other Drugs

Carbamazepine: plasma concentrations of risperidone and 9-hydroxyrisperidone were decreased by approximately 50% with coadministration of carbamazepine over a 3-week period. Plasma levels of carbamazepine did not appear to be affected.

Valproate: oral doses (4 mg/day) of risperidone did not affect the pre-dose or average plasma concentrations and exposure area under the curve (AUC) of valproate (a total of 1000 mg administered in three divided doses), but there was a 20% increase in valproate peak plasma concentration after concomitant administration of risperidone.

Lithium: risperidone (6 mg day in two divided doses) did not affect the exposure (AUC) or lithium's peak plasma concentration.

Fluoxetine: fluoxetine in doses of 20 mg/day increased risperidone's plasma concentration from 2.5 to 2.8 times, but did not affect the plasma concentration of 9-hydroxyrisperidone.

Paroxetine: paroxetine in doses of 20 mg twice daily increased risperidone's plasma concentration by 3 to 9 times and lowered the concentration of 9-hydroxyrisperidone by approximately 13%.

Adverse Effects of Risperidone

Black Box Warning. There is a "Black Box Warning" that there is increased mortality in elderly patients with dementia-related psychosis who are treated with atypical antipsychotic drugs including risperidone.

Extrapyramidal Symptoms. The incidence of extrapyramidal symptoms in patients treated with risperidone appears to be dose related; however, for patients receiving up to 10 mg daily, it is not significantly different from that in patients receiving placebo.

Hepatotoxicity. Kumra et al. (1997) reviewed the medical records of the 13 children and adolescents (3 males and 10 females) diagnosed with schizophrenia who were admitted to the NIMH over a period of 28 months and treated with risperidone. Two of the 3 males, but none of the females, showed evidence of steatohepatitis with obesity, elevated liver enzyme values, and evidence of fatty liver on ultrasound, which was confirmed by biopsy in one case. Following discontinuation of risperidone, liver function tests returned to normal within 2 weeks to 3 months. The authors noted that two additional males who were subsequently admitted developed hepatotoxicity during long-term treatment with risperidone. The authors strongly recommended determining baseline liver function tests, obtaining liver aminotransferases, cholesterol, and triglycerides every 3 months, and monitoring weight frequently in pediatric patients who are being maintained on risperidol. Males in this age range may be particularly at risk for hepatotoxicity.

Szigethy et al. (1999) retrospectively reviewed the charts of 38 children and adolescents (32 males, six females; mean age, 10.6 ± 3.7; age range, 4 to 17 years) who had been treated with a mean dose of 2.5 mg/day (range, 0.5 to 10.0 mg/day) or 0.05 mg/kg/day (range, 0.01 to 0.11 mg/kg/day) of risperidone for a mean of 15.2 ± 10.0 months (range, 1 to 35 months) to assess hepatic function during risperidone treatment and to identify any clinical factors associated with hepatic dysfunction. Diagnoses of the subjects were autistic disorder (N = 12), other pervasive developmental disorders (N = 8), mood disorders (N = 6), disruptive behavior disorders (DBDs) ($N = 7$) and psychotic disorders ($N = 5$). Thirty-seven (97.4%) of the subjects had normal values for aspartate aminotransferase (AST), alanine aminotransferase (ALT), and total bilirubin after treatment with risperidone for a mean duration of 12.2 ± 9.8 months (range, 1 to 30 months). The thirty-eighth subject, who had received 24 months of risperidone and a peak dose of 4 mg/day, had an ALT of 46 U/L, 7 U/L above the upper limit of normal, which was not considered clinically significant. Baseline liver function tests were available for 14 subjects; comparison of these values with those obtained after an average of 5.47 ± 4.9 months (range, 1 to 19 months) showed no clinically meaningful increases. All subjects for whom baseline weights were available gained weight during treatment (see following text). The authors noted that obesity itself is associated with both steatohepatitis and elevated transaminases, and that weight gain alone may have caused the elevated ATL in their patients. Overall, the authors concluded from their review that the risk for risperidone-induced hepatotoxicity is probably low in relatively short-term therapy in this age-group.

Weight Gain. Weight gain is often a problem in patients treated with risperidone, usually secondary to a marked increase in appetite. Horrigan and Barnhill (1997) noted a positive correlation between the degree of clinical improvement, increased appetite, and weight gain. They noted that serotonin plays a role in signaling satiety and that, by blocking $5HT_2$ receptors, risperidone may cause dysregulation of the "satiety switch."

In their chart review of 38 patients who received risperidone, Szigethy et al. (1999) reported that weight gain occurred in all 23 subjects for whom baseline weights were available; mean baseline weight was 37.92 ± 16.0 kg (range, 15.0 to 73.6 kg), and mean end-of-study weight was 48.28 ± 18.97 kg (range, 19.10 to 82.95 kg). The mean weight gain was 1.01 ± 0.73 kg/month (range, 0.18 to 3.1 kg/month). The mean duration of risperidone therapy for all 38 subjects was 15.2 ± 10.0 months (range, 1 to 35 months), demonstrating that risk of weight gain with risperidone therapy is an important therapeutic issue.

Martin et al. (2000) conducted a retrospective chart review comparing 37 child and adolescent inpatients treated for a minimum of 6 continuous months with risperidone, with 33 inpatients having no exposure to atypical antipsychotics with regard to baseline weight, standardized z scores of weight for age and gender, and percentage of subjects whose weight increased $\geq$ 7% (chosen a priori as the standard cutoff for extreme weight gain in clinical trials). After 6 months of risperidone, significantly more subjects on risperidone (78%) versus 24% of controls gained $\geq$ 7% of their baseline weight ($P = .001$). A significant difference was evident within 2 months of treatment ($P = .001$). Risperidone-treated subjects gained an average of 1.2 kg/month over the 6-month study, and their weight gain showed no tendency to plateau during that period. There was no correlation between dose of risperidone and demographic or clinical characteristics such as discharge diagnosis or concomitant medication. Weight gain is an important consideration in the treatment of children and adolescents with risperidone and must be considered in the risks and benefits discussed as part of the informed consent process.

Hyperprolactinemia. Risperidone may cause elevations of prolactin that are significantly above normal values and may persist during chronic administration.

This is discussed in detail and relevant literature reviewed under the section on "Prolactin Levels" in Chapter 2.

Hyperglycemia and Type 2 Diabetes. Epidemiologic studies suggest an increased risk of treatment emergent hyperglycemia-related adverse events (AEs) in patients treated with atypical antipsychotic drugs, including risperidone (PDR, 2006).

Other Untoward Effects. Orthostatic hypotension, dizziness, tachycardia, increase of QT_C interval on ECG to > 450 msec, insomnia or somnolence, constipation, rhinitis, and many other untoward effects have been reported.

Indications for Risperidone in Child and Adolescent Psychiatry

Risperidone is indicated for the management of the manifestations of schizophrenia and the short-term (3-week) treatment of bipolar mania of acute manic or mixed episodes associated with Bipolar I disorder.

Risperidone Dosage Schedule

- Children and adolescents 15 years of age or less: not recommended. The safety and effectiveness of risperidone in the pediatric age-group have not been established.
- Adolescents at least 16 years of age and adults: an initial dose of 1 mg bid is recommended, with an increase to 2 mg twice daily on the second day and a further increase to 3 mg twice daily on the third day. It is recommended that any subsequent adjustments of dosage be made at weekly intervals to allow adequate time for steady-state serum levels to be achieved. If adjustments are necessary, small (e.g., 0.5 mg or 1 mg twice daily) increments or decrements are suggested. Doses above 6 mg/day have not been demonstrated to have any increased clinical efficacy and are associated with more untoward effects, including extrapyramidal symptoms. The safety of doses over 16 mg/day has not been evaluated in clinical trials.

Risperidone Dose Forms Available

- Tablets: 0.25 mg, 0.5 mg, 1 mg, 2 mg, 3 mg, and 4 mg
- Orally Disintegrating Tablets (Risperdal M-TAB) 0.5 mg, 1 mg, and 2 mg
- Oral solution: 1 mg/mL
- Long-acting injection (Risperal Consta) 25 mg, 37.5 mg and 50 mg vials. This dosage form is indicated for the treatment of schizophrenia and is designed to provide 2 weeks of medication coverage. Its use is not recommended in patients younger than 18 years of age as its safety and efficacy has not been studied in this age-group.

Reports of Interest

Risperidone in the Treatment of Children and Adolescents Diagnosed with Schizophrenia. Cozza and Edison (1994) treated two 15-year-old adolescents, one male and one female, with risperidone; they were diagnosed with schizophrenia and had not responded satisfactorily to usual antipsychotics. Risperidone was begun at 1 mg daily and rapidly titrated to 6 mg/day. Both adolescents developed significant extrapyramidal side effects, suggesting that adolescents may be more sensitive to these effects than adults. Risperidone was decreased to 1 mg twice daily and the untoward effects improved. Both patients showed significant improvement in positive and negative symptoms within 1 week. However, both patients also reported an upwelling of such uncomfortable emotions that they were ambivalent about continuing on risperidone, and the female eventually became noncompliant.

In their 1995 publication, Simeon et al. reported that three males, ages 11, 15, and 17, who were diagnosed with schizophrenia and had not improved during previous trials of standard medications improved markedly when treated openly with risperidone. Onset of the schizophrenia was at 5 years of age in the first two patients and at 15 years of age in the third. Optimal daily doses were 2.5 mg (0.051 mg/kg), 2 mg (0.022 mg/kg), and 4 mg (0.048 mg/kg), respectively. The authors noted that paranoid ideation, delusions, depressed mood, aggressiveness, and negative symptoms such as withdrawal improved markedly within 3 weeks. None of the patients experienced significant untoward effects.

Armenteros et al. (1997) administered risperidone for 6 weeks on an open basis to 10 adolescents (seven males and three females; age range, 11 to 17 years) who were diagnosed with schizophrenia by DSM-IV criteria. Two subjects were inpatients; the others were in a research day hospital. Seven subjects were considered nonresponders to standard neuroleptics, either because of intolerable untoward effects or inadequate clinical improvement; three adolescents had never received a neuroleptic.

Following a 2-week washout period, during which those subjects on psychoactive medication had it tapered and discontinued, risperidone was begun at a dose of 2.0 mg/day given in divided doses at 9:00 AM and 1:00 PM. Dose was individually titrated over 3 weeks with 1-mg increments every 2 days to a maximum of 10 mg/day, unless untoward effects prevented further increase. Maximum therapeutic doses of risperidone ranged from 4.0 mg/day to 10.0 mg/day (mean, 6.6 mg/day) or from 0.05 mg/kg/day to 0.17 mg/kg/day (mean, 0.09 mg/kg/day). These doses were maintained for the remaining 3 weeks of the study. Outcome as measured by the Positive and Negative Syndrome Scale for Schizophrenia (PANSS) at time 6 weeks showed a decrease ranging from 4.6% to 47.7% ($P = .000$), with six (60%) subjects meeting the criterion for improvement, which was at least a 20% reduction. As a group there was also a significant improvement on the Brief Psychiatric Rating Scale (BPRS) ($P = .001$). On the Clinical Global Impressions (CGI) there was again significant improvement ($P = .007$); however, as on the PANSS, four subjects did not show noteworthy improvement; three were rated as minimally improved, and one was rated as unimproved.

Untoward effects included mild somnolence that subsided within 2 weeks of the dose increase ($N = 8$); weight gain ($N = 8$, with a mean gain of 4.85 kg before nutritional counseling was begun); acute dystonic reaction ($N = 2$); parkinsonian syndrome that required ongoing treatment with benztropine ($N = 3$); mild orofacial dyskinesia that remitted when the dose was decreased ($N = 1$); blurred vision ($N = 1$); and impaired concentration ($N = 1$). Electrolytes, CBC, ECG, and liver enzymes were normal throughout the study (Armenteros et al. 1997).

Risperidone in the Treatment of Children and Adolescents with Pervasive Developmental Disorders. Simeon et al. (1995) reported significant improvement in two adolescent males, ages 13 and 14 years, who were diagnosed with pervasive developmental disorders and ADHD. In addition, it was suspected that the 13-year-old might have negative symptoms secondary to schizophrenia, and the 14-year-old was diagnosed with a conduct disorder. Both had significant social withdrawal, aggression, and violent behavior. Optimal daily doses were 1 mg (0.018 mg/kg) and 1 mg (0.016 mg/kg), respectively. Both patients improved markedly, and no significant untoward effects were reported.

Simeon et al. (1995) also treated a 13-year-old female diagnosed with borderline mental retardation, developmental delays, and a somatic delusional disorder, who also had aggressive behavior, temper tantrums, social inappropriateness, inattentiveness, and enuresis. Risperidone, 2 mg/day (0.047 mg/kg/day), was effective in controlling delusional thinking and in reducing aggressive outbursts. It was necessary to coadminister a stimulant (d-amphetamine, 5 mg twice daily) to improve her attention span and concentration.

Fisman and Steele (1996) treated 14 patients (10 males, four females; age range, 9 to 17 years; mean, 12.7 ± 4.0 years) diagnosed as having pervasive developmental disorders with risperidone in an open study, nine with Asperger's disorder, four with autistic disorder, and one with pervasive developmental disorder not otherwise specified (PDDNOS). Five patients had comorbid disorders; none was retarded. Three patients received clomipramine, and one patient, diagnosed with comorbid bipolar disorder, received lithium carbonate and carbamazepine in addition to risperidone during the study. Twelve patients had previously been treated with psychoactive medication. Five of the eight patients who had been previously treated with clomipramine experienced worsening agitation and behavioral deterioration that necessitated discontinuing the drug.

Risperidone was usually initiated with a dose of 0.25 mg twice daily and increased by 0.25 mg every 5 to 7 days. Optimal doses ranged from 0.75 to 1.5 mg/day in divided doses. Improved functioning was rated on the Children's Global Assessment Scale in 13 (93%) of the 14 subjects; 10 (71%) showed a marked decrease in agitation and anxiety. Disruptive behaviors such as hyperactivity, aggression, and temper outbursts decreased notably following administration of risperidone. Inattention and obsessional behaviors were markedly improved on risperidone in 13 patients and the obsessions that worsened in 1 patient improved significantly when clomipramine 50 mg twice daily was added to the risperidone. Social awareness showed marked improvement in 10 subjects, moderate improvement in 3 subjects, and slight improvement in 1 subject. Improvement occurred most rapidly during the first 2 months but continued during follow-ups from 2 to 7 months' duration (mean, 7.4 months). No patient on risperidone had a major relapse during the follow-up period. Untoward effects were minimal and no extrapyramidal effects or agitation were observed. Initial drowsiness, the most frequent untoward effect, occurred in five (36%) of the patients and was managed by reduction in dose. The authors felt that, with these positive clinical findings, risperidone merits further systematic study as a potentially useful agent in treating children and adolescents with pervasive developmental disorders (Fisman and Steele, 1996).

McDougle et al. (1997) administered risperidone to 18 subjects (15 males and 3 females; age range, 5 to 18 years, mean, 10.2 ± 3.7) diagnosed with pervasive developmental disorders in a 12-week, open-label trial. Diagnoses included autistic disorder ($N = 11$), Asperger's disorder ($N = 3$), childhood disintegrative disorder ($N = 1$), and pervasive developmental disorders not otherwise specified ($N = 3$). Mental retardation was also present in 14 subjects: profound ($N = 1$), severe ($N = 11$), and moderate ($N = 2$). All the subjects had been treated previously with psychoactive drugs.

After a minimum of 4 drug-free weeks and baseline behavioral ratings, risperidone was initiated at a dose of 0.5 mg at bedtime and was individually titrated by weekly increases of 0.5 mg given in divided morning and bedtime doses. The optimal dose of risperidone ranged from 1 mg/day to 4 mg/day (mean, 1.8 mg/day ±1.0 mg/day). Twelve (67%) of the subjects were considered responders based on ratings of "much improved" or "very much improved" on the Clinical Global Impressions (CGI) Scale. Three subjects diagnosed with autistic disorders were rated minimally worse, and one was rated "unchanged." One subject with PDDNOS was rated "minimally worse" and one was rated "unchanged." Based on significant improvement on several rating scales, the authors concluded that risperidone may be useful in some children and adolescents diagnosed with PDDs, with significant improvements in reducing repetitive, ritualistic behaviors and in reducing impulsive aggression and maladaptive behaviors, including some impairments in social relatedness (McDougle et al. 1997). Untoward effects included weight gain, ranging from 10 to 35 pounds, with a mean of 17.8 ± 7.5 pounds ($N = 12$), sedation ($N = 6$), nocturnal enuresis ($N = 1$), sialorrhea ($N = 1$), blunted affect ($N = 1$), agitation ($N = 1$), and gross motor incoordination ($N = 1$). No clinically significant cardiovascular changes were noted, and no acute extrapyramidal untoward effects occurred.

Horrigan and Barnhill (1997) reported treating 11 males with risperidone (mean age, 18.3 years; age range, 6 to 34 years); 10 of these subjects were diagnosed with autistic disorder with comorbid moderate to severe mental retardation. All 11 exhibited explosive aggressive behavior, including self-injurious behavior of such a magnitude that their present caretakers were considering placing them elsewhere; 8 of them had poor sleep patterns, which additionally aggravated the situation. On average, the 11 patients had prior trials on 5.45 psychotropic drugs with no, or only partial, improvement. After appropriate washout, five subjects were begun on risperidone only, and six had risperidone added to partially efficacious medications, which were continued. Risperidone was initiated with a bedtime dose of 0.5 mg daily and titrated upward in 0.25 to 0.5 mg increments every 5 to 7 days. All patients improved, with the most significant clinical gains apparent within 24 hours. Aggression, self-injury, explosivity, overactivity, and poor sleep patterns improved the most, and caregivers reported that many of the patients tolerated frustration and transitions better, and appeared more calm and focused. Optimal daily dose after 4 weeks ranged from 0.5 mg to 2.0 mg, with a modal dose of 0.5 mg b.i.d. ($N = 10$); after 4 months, the modal dose remained unchanged for the eight patients who continued on the study. Untoward effects reported included three patients with initial mild sedation that ceased by the third week. One patient developed possible chemical hepatitis, with gammaglutamyltranspeptidase (GGT) increasing from a baseline of 32 to 295 at week 10, necessitating discontinuation. Possible precipitation of a new complex partial seizure disorder and a weight loss of 3.5 kg occurred in one patient, and significant weight gain was reported in eight patients, with gains of 1.6 to 3.6 kg within 4 weeks. None of the patients developed any extrapyramidal tract symptoms or significant changes in blood pressure or heart rate.

Perry et al. (1997) treated six subjects with risperidone (five males, one female; mean age, 10.7 ± 3.3 years; range, 7 to 14 years) in an open-label trial. Five subjects were diagnosed with autistic disorder and one with pervasive developmental disorder not otherwise specified (PDDNOS), and five of the six with mental retardation (one moderate, three severe, and one profound) by DSM-III-R criteria. Two patients were hospitalized and four were treated as outpatients. Target symptoms were severe behavioral symptoms, including aggression toward others and temper tantrums. Efficacy was evaluated by ratings on the Clinical Global Impressions Scale-Improvement (CGI-I), the CGI-Severity (CGI-S) Scale, and selected items from the Children's Psychiatric Rating Scale (CPRS), which included "hyperactivity," "withdrawal," "negative/uncooperative," "angry affect/erupts easily," "lability of affect," and "rhythmic motions" (stereotypy). Risperidone was initiated at a dose of 0.5 mg once or twice daily and titrated in 0.5 mg increments every few days based on clinical response. Four subjects received risperidone only, one also took carbamazepine, and one received medication for sleep. The mean optimal dose was 2.7 ± 2.2 mg/day, with a range of 1 to 6 mg/day. Mean duration on risperidone was 5.2 ± 2.3 months (range, 1 to 8 months). The CGI and CPRS ratings used for analysis were data collected after 1 to 2 months on medication for inpatients and after 3 to 5 months for the outpatients.

There was significant improvement on the CGI-I Scale ($P < .001$), although there was only a slight, insignificant improvement of the CGI-S Scale, which meant that the subjects remained seriously impaired. On the CPRS items, there was a significant decrease in "angry affect/erupts easily" ($P = .04$) and "lability of affect" ($P = .03$). The other four items did not show significant improvement. There were no serious untoward effects, but five subjects gained a mean of 5.4 kg over a period of 7 weeks on medication. There were no extrapyramidal symptoms. Therapeutic gains were maintained for more than 2 years in three patients who continued to take risperidone (Perry et al. 1997).

Nicolson et al. (1998) treated 10 outpatient males (mean age, 7.2 ± 2.2 years, range, 4.5 to 10.8 years) diagnosed with autistic disorder by DSM-IV (APA, 1994) criteria with a 12-week, open trial of risperidone. Eight subjects were functioning intellectually in the mild to severely retarded range based on the academic scale of the Developmental Profile II. Only three of the subjects had received previous psychopharmacotherapy. Target symptoms included hyperactivity, stereotypies, tantrums, withdrawal, self-injurious behavior, and aggression. Efficacy was assessed by ratings on the Clinical Global Impressions-Severity (CGI-S) and CGI—Improvement (CGI-I) Scales, the Children's Psychiatric Ratings Scale (CPRS), Childhood Autism Rating Scale (CARS), and the Conners Parent-Teacher Questionnaire (PTQ). Risperidone was initiated at a dose of 0.5 mg/day and titrated upward with a maximum weekly increase of 0.5 mg/day to optimal dose; a maximum of 6 mg/day or 0.1 mg/kg/day or till untoward effects prevented further increase. The mean optimal dose was 1.3 ± 0.5 mg/day (range, 1 to 2.5 mg/day) or 0.05 ± 0.02 mg/kg/day. Based on a CGI-I rating of "very much improved" or "improved," eight (80%) of the subjects improved. The two oldest males did not improve, and both had had treatment failures with typical antipsychotics, SSRIs and clonidine. Significant improvement was shown in the ratings on the CGI-S ($P = .001$), 14-item CPRS ($P < .001$), the CPRS Autism factor ($P = .001$), the CPRS Hyperactivity factor ($P = .02$), CARS ($P < .001$) and the PTQ ($P < .001$). Parents noted a 50% reduction in "temper outbursts" (explosive and unpredictable behavior) on the PTQ ($P = .004$), and teachers noted improvement in aggression behavior. Clinically significant improvements in social interaction were noted in several males. Weight gain occurred commonly, with a mean increase of 3.5 kg over the 12 weeks. Transient sedation, usually after the initial dose or an increase in dose, was seen in three subjects. Other untoward effects were generally few and mild. There was no evidence of extrapyramidal symptoms and no significant changes in heart rate or blood pressure.

Zuddas et al. (2000) conducted an open-label, 12-month prospective study administering risperidone to 11 outpatients (eight males, three females; mean age, 12.3 ± 3.8 years) diagnosed with autistic disorder ($N = 9$) or pervasive developmental disorder not otherwise specified (PDDNOS; $N = 2$) by DSM-IV (APA, 1994) criteria. All had comorbid mental retardation (mild, $N = 2$; moderate, $N = 6$; or severe, $N = 3$). All subjects had shown no significant improvement on prior trials of standard neuroleptics. Efficacy was assessed by ratings in the Childhood Autism Rating Scale (CARS), the Child Psychiatric Rating Scale (CPRS), the Clinical Global Impressions-Improvement Scale (CGI-I), and the Child-Global Assessment Scale (C-GAS). Risperidone was initiated at a dose of 0.5 mg/day and titrated individually based on clinical response in increments of 0.5 mg every 5 days to a maximum of 6 mg/day or 0.1 mg/kg/day, whichever was less. Patients who showed no improvement on the CGI-I after 2 months were considered nonresponders and risperidone was discontinued. Responders were treated for 6 months and given the choice to continue on risperidone with final assessments to be done after 12 months of treatment. One male developed worsening compulsory behavior and fidgetiness after 4 weeks and was dropped from the study. The 10 responders, rated "much" or "very much improved" on the CGI-I, had a mean risperidone dose at 6 months of 2.7 ± 2 mg/day. Mean ratings on the CPRS-14, the CARS, and the C-GAS were all significantly improved at 6 months ($P < .001$ for all three scales). Seven patients continued on risperidone for the additional 12 months; gains were maintained, and there was no significant difference between the 6- and 12-month ratings. The three patients who discontinued treatment after 6 months did so for facial dystonia in one case, amenorrhea in the second case, and parental choice of a nonmedical treatment in the third. The 12-month ratings of these three patients showed progressive deterioration and had returned to baseline in two cases and were minimally worse than baseline in the third. Overall behavioral symptoms such as fidgetiness, hyperactivity, stereotypies, and liability of affect improved more than the core symptoms of autism, such as speech deviance, distorted sensory response, and unspontaneous relationship to the examiner. Weight gain was a common untoward effect, with a mean increase of approximately 5 kg at 6 months. All subjects experienced mild transient sedation early in the treatment. Although no extrapyramidal symptoms were reported during the first 6 months, two patients subsequently developed facial dystonias, which remitted after dose reduction in one case and discontinuation of risperidone in the other. The authors concluded that risperidone is effective as a first-line drug in the long-term management of behavioral disorders in children and adolescents with pervasive developmental disorders.

Members of the Research Units on Pediatric Psychopharmacology (RUPP) Autism Network conducted an 8-week, multi-site, randomized, double-blind, placebo-controlled study comparing the safety and efficacy of risperidone and placebo in the treatment of severe tantrums, aggression, and/or self injurious behavior (SIB) in 101 children (82 males, 19 females; age range 5–17 years, mean age 8.8 + 2.7 years) who were diagnosed with autistic disorder by DSM-IV (APA, 1994) criteria (McCracken et al. 2002). The primary outcome measures were the Irritability subscale of the Aberrant Behavior Checklist (ABC) and the Clinical Global Impressions-Improvement (CGI-I) Scale; a positive response required a minimum 25% reduction on the Irritability score and a rating of 1 or 2 (much improved or very much improved) on the CGI-I Scale at time 8 weeks. Forty-nine subjects were assigned to risperidone and 52 to placebo.

Initial dose of risperidone was determined by subjects' weights: children weighing < 20 kg received 0.25 mg daily; those weighing 20–45 kg received 0.5 mg daily at bedtime for the first 3 days and then increased to 0.5 mg twice daily on day 4 followed by titration in 0.5 mg increments to a maximum of 1 mg in the morning and 1.5 mg at bedtime by day 29. Children weighing > 45 kg were prescribed medication at a somewhat accelerated rate to achieve a maximum permitted dose of 1.5 mg in the morning and 2.0 mg at bedtime. The final mean dose of risperidone was $1.8 + 0.7$ mg/day, with a range of 0.5 to 3.5 mg.

At time 8-weeks, subjects on risperidone had a 56.9% decrease on the Irritability subscale of the ABC versus 14.1% decrease for subjects receiving placebo ($P < .001$). On the CBI-I Scale, 75.5% of subjects on risperidone were rated 1 or 2 (very much improved or much improved) versus only 11.5% of subjects on placebo. Positive responders included 69% of the risperidone group versus only 12% of the group on placebo ($P < .001$). The authors also noted that, compared to the group receiving placebo, the risperidone group improved significantly on the Stereotypy and Hyperactivity Scales, but there were no significant differences on the Social Withdrawal and Inappropriate Speech Scales of the ABC. The authors also noted that 23 of the 34 subjects who were "responders" continued to show benefit after 6 months on medication.

No child dropped out of the study because of adverse events (AEs); no serious AEs occurred in the risperidone group and most were mild and self-limited (e.g., fatigue/drowsiness subsided in most subjects within 4 to 6 weeks). Increased appetite ("mild" 49% vs. 25%, $P = .03$; "moderate" 24% vs. 4%, $P = .01$), fatigue 59% versus 27%, drowsiness 49% versus 12% ($P < .001$), dizziness, 16% versus 4% ($P = .05$), and drooling 27% versus 6% ($P = .02$) were each significantly more frequent in the risperidone group than in the placebo group. Over the 8-week study, subjects on risperidone gained significantly more weight—an average of $2.7 + 2.9$ kg versus $0.8 + 2.2$ kg for subjects in the placebo group ($P < .001$). Three (6%) of the subjects in the risperidone group withdrew from the study because of lack of clinical efficacy versus 18 (35%) of the subjects in the placebo group, of whom 12 withdrew because of lack of clinical efficacy ($P = .001$).

The authors concluded that risperidone was safe and effective with a favorable risk-benefit ratio in the short-term treatment of children diagnosed with autistic disorder. Significant improvements were noted in tantrums, aggression, self-injurious behavior, stereotypic behavior, and hyperactivity.

Aman et al. (2005) reported further on the long-term safety and efficacy of risperidone for up to 6 months in the subjects in an 8-week double-blind, placebo-controlled trial reported by McCracken et al. (2002). Upon completion of this 8-week study, 37 placebo nonresponders were treated with risperidone on an open basis for an additional 8 weeks; of these subjects, 30 who responded to risperidone then entered a 16-week open extension phase of treatment with risperidone (Scahill et al. 2001). Of the 34 risperidone responders in the initial 8-week double-blind, placebo-controlled trial, 30 entered the 16-week open extension phase of treatment with risperidone. An additional 3 subjects who were in the risperidone group during the initial 8-week placebo-controlled double-blind study but did not meet all criteria to be "responders" were also enrolled in the 16-week extension phase for a total of 63 subjects; the authors noted that including these 3 subjects in the analyses did not alter clinical results for any outcome. Finally, upon completing the 16-week open extension, 32 of the 63 subjects were rerandomized in an additional 8-week, double-blind phase to either continue therapy with risperidone ($N = 16$) or to enter a placebo substitution phase ($N = 16$) during the first 4 weeks of which risperidone was reduced by 25% of the dose each week with only placebo being given for the last 4 weeks. The authors noted that only 32 subjects participated in this final phase as interim analysis showed that significantly more subjects relapsed on placebo compared to those maintained on risperidone (62.5% vs. 12.5%, $P = .01$), and they then stopped this portion of the study.

Regarding adverse events (AEs), subjects on risperidone experienced the following significantly more frequently than those on placebo: daytime tiredness (94% vs. 54% "at all" and 37% vs. 12% moderate/severe; $P < .0001$), difficulty waking ($P = .05$); excessive saliva/drooling (29% vs. 16%; $P = .04$); and dizziness/loss of balance (22% vs. 8%; $P = .04$). On the other hand, difficulty falling asleep (65% vs. 47%; $P = .02$) and anxiety (48% vs. 32%; $P = .05$) were significantly more frequent in the placebo group than in the risperidone group. Excessive appetite was reported in 82% of the risperidone group versus 38% in the placebo group. There was significantly greater weight gain in the risperidone group; however, the authors noted that weight gain decelerated over time with ongoing risperidone treatment. There were no significant changes in height. As noted in the preceding text, only three (6.1%) of the subjects who were treated with risperidone dropped out of the study during the initial 8-week period (McCracken et al. 2002). During the 16-week extension, six (9.5%) of the subjects treated with risperidone dropped out because of AEs and two of these were because of seizures, which did not appear to be related to risperidone (Aman et al. 2005). The authors concluded that safety and tolerability remained favorable in treating these subjects. They cautioned that the number of patients in the study was too small to identify infrequent/rare adverse events and likewise too short in duration to determine rates of tardive dyskinesia, obesity, and diabetes.

Risperidone in the Treatment of Children and Adolescents Diagnosed with Bipolar Disorder. Frazier et al. (1999) conducted a retrospective chart review of outpatients at a university center who were diagnosed by DSM-IV criteria (APA, 1994) with bipolar disorder and treated with risperidone. Twenty-eight such subjects, mean age 10.4 ± 3.8 (range, 4 to 17 years; 27 males, one female), were identified. Twenty-five subjects were diagnosed with bipolar I disorder, most recent episode mixed, and three with bipolar I disorder, most recent episode hypomanic. In addition, there was an average of 2.6 ± 0.8 comorbid diagnoses, including ADHD in 25 (89%) and PDD in 8 (29%), and 13 subjects had psychotic symptoms. Subjects had been previously medicated with an average of 3.6 ± 1.7 drugs. Outcome was measured using the NIMH Clinical Global Impressions (CGI) Scale, including CGI-S (illness severity) and CGI-I (global improvement).

Risperidone was begun at a low dose and titrated to reach the lowest dose, achieving acceptable clinical improvement. Mean optimal daily dose of risperidone was 1.7 ± 1.3 mg. Mean length of treatment was 6.1 ± 8.5 months (range, 1 week to 34 months). A mean of 1.8 ± 1.1 drugs was administered concurrently to 27 (96%) of the subjects. Optimal clinical response to risperidone was 1.9 ± 1.0 months; 16 (57%) responded within the first month. CGI-S scores stratified for syndromes of mania, psychosis, and aggression all showed significant improvement, with decreases from marked severity to within the mild severity range. Such scores for ADHD declined significantly but still remained in the moderately severe range. Using a CGI-I rating of 2 or less ("much" or "very much improved") to define robust improvement, 82% of subjects improved for mania, 82% for aggression, 69% for psychosis, and 8% for ADHD. No serious untoward effects were reported; common untoward effects were weight gain (18%), mild sedation (18%), and drooling (7%). There were no cases of extrapyramidal side effects. Prolactin levels were available for 11 subjects; mean prolactin level was 32.8 ± 12.05 ng/mL (normal range, 0 to 15 ng/mL) and was above normal in nine (82%) of these subjects.

The authors concluded that risperidone treatment resulted in rapid and sustained improvement of manic, psychotic, and aggressive symptoms in these 28 children diagnosed with bipolar I disorder, all but one of whom had been previously medicated with limited success. They noted that the efficacy of risperidone was in contrast to similar subjects treated with mood stabilizers, which, although efficacious, took many months to reach maximum clinical improvement and were associated with a high percentage of relapse.

Biederman et al. (2005) conducted an 8-week, open-label, prospective study of risperidone monotherapy in 30 subjects, mean age 10.1 ± 2.5 years, 22 (73%) males, 8 (27%) females, diagnosed by DSM-IV criteria with Bipolar I or Bipolar disorder NOS. All subjects had clinically significant mania and a Young Mania Rating Scale (YMRS) score > 15; at entry the overall mean YMRS score was 27.9 ± 9.1, which is in the severe range. Risperidone was begun at a daily dose of 0.25 mg for subjects 12 years of age or younger and 0.50 mg/day for subjects 13 years of age or older. Based on clinical response, dose was titrated at weekly intervals to a maximum of 2.0 mg/day in the younger subjects and a maximum of 4.0 mg/day in the older group. Subjects taking stimulants as treatment of comorbid ADHD were permitted to continue if the dose had remained constant for a minimum of 30 days prior to the study.

Subjects were rated on the YMRS, the Children's Depression Rating Scale-Revised (CDRS-R), the Brief Psychiatric Rating Scale (BPRS), and the Clinical Global Impressions-Severity (CGI-S) and Improvement (CGI-I) Scales. A positive response was defined as a $\geq 30\%$ reduction in YMRS or a score of ≤ 2 (much or very much improved) on the CGI-I Scale. Euthymia was defined as a score of < 10 on the YMRS and a CDRS-R score of ≤ 28.

Twenty-two (22) subjects completed the entire 8-week study. Analyses were intention to treat (ITT) with the last observation carried forward (LOCF) for non-completers. At endpoint, there was significant improvement in manic symptoms ($P < .0001$) on the YMRS (baseline 27.9 ± 9.2 vs. endpoint 13.5 ± 9.7) although subjects remained with residual manic symptoms; 21 (70%) of subjects had at least a 30% reduction in baseline YMRS scores and 15 (50%) had reductions of at least 50%. The reduction in depressive symptoms as measured on the CDRS-R (baseline rating of 40.9 ± 11.5 vs. endpoint rating of 30.7 ± 11.0) was also significant ($P = .0001$), but indicated that symptoms of depression continued. Overall, euthymia was achieved in 7 (23%) subjects and remitted mania with residual depression in 5 (16%) subjects. Of note, 5 (55%) of subjects with a codiagnosis of conduct disorder, 10 (46%) of the subjects with a codiagnoses of depression, and 9 (35%) of the subjects with a codiagnosis of ADHD, were rated ≤ 2 (much or very much improved) on the CGI-I.

Regarding adverse events, the most commonly reported were gastrointestinal complaints (20%), increased appetite (16%), and sedation (13%). Prolactin levels increased significantly from a baseline of 7.9 ± 5.3 ng/dL to 34.4 ± 21.9 ng/dL at endpoint ($P < .001$). Subjects also had a significant increase in weight, 2.1 ± 2.0 kg ($P < .001$), and pulse rate from a baseline of 90.6 ± 13.3 bpm to 98.0 ± 14.0 bpm ($P = .006$) (Biederman et al. 2005).

Risperidone in the Treatment of Children and Adolescents Diagnosed with Conduct Disorder (and Various Intelligence Quotients). Findling et al. (1999) conducted a randomized, 10-week, double-blind, placebo-controlled study of risperidone in the treatment of 20 outpatients (age range, 6 to 14 years; mean age, 9.2 ± 2.9 years; 19 males and one female) who were diagnosed by DSM-IV criteria with conduct disorder and had prominent aggressive behavior. Ten subjects were assigned to each group. Risperidone was begun with a single morning dose of 0.25 mg/day for subjects weighing < 50 kg and 0.50 mg/day for subjects weighing ≥ 50 kg and titrated upward weekly by an amount equal to that received on day 1 for the first 6 weeks of the study, to a maximum of 1.5 mg/day for the subjects initially weighing < 50 kg, and a maximum of 3.0 mg/day for the heavier subjects.

The Rating of Aggression Against People and/or Property (RAAPP) Scale was used as the primary outcome measure, and the NIMH Clinical Global Impressions Scale assessing illness severity (CGI-S), and global improvement (CGI-I) was used as a secondary outcome measure. The average estimated end-of-study dose of risperidone was 0.028 ± 0.004 mg/kg/day, with a range of 0.75 to 1.5 mg/day. Six subjects assigned to risperidone completed the study, with three being withdrawn for lack of clinical improvement, and the other because of a rash developed during week 4 of the study. Three subjects assigned to placebo completed the study and four were withdrawn for lack of clinical improvement, two were discharged for failing to follow study protocol, and one was lost to follow-up (Findling et al. 1999).

Over the 10-week study, there was a significant $(P = .01)$ difference in the RAAPP scores in the group by time interaction with the means model, indicating that the mean RAAPP score differences between the subjects on placebo and those on risperidone increased with time, with the scores of subjects on risperidone decreasing more, which was indicative of greater improvement. During weeks 7 to 10 of the study, RAAPP scores of the subjects receiving risperidone were significantly $(P = .008)$ lower than those of the subjects receiving placebo. During the same period of the study, CGI-S scores of the subjects receiving risperidone were significantly $(P = .01)$ lower, indicating less aggression, than scores of the subjects receiving placebo.

Over the 10-week study, there was also a significant $(P = .01)$ difference in the CGI-I scores in the group by time interaction with the means model, indicating that the mean CGI-I score differences between the subjects on placebo and those on risperidone increased with time, with the scores of the subjects on risperidone decreasing more, which was indicative of greater improvement. During weeks 7 to 10 of the study, average CGI-I scores for the risperidone group were significantly less $(P = .0006)$ than those of the placebo group. In general, untoward effects were mild and transient. Increased appetite was noted in three of the subjects on risperidone, and the predicted end-of-study weight gain for the risperidone group was 4.2 ± 0.7 kg versus 0.74 ± 0.9 kg for the placebo group $(P = .003)$.

Findling et al. (1999) noted that, despite the small sample size, clinical improvement on almost all measures of aggressive behavior were highly significant in patients receiving risperidone compared with those on placebo. Risperidone, in low daily doses, appears to be a promising short-term treatment for at least some youngsters diagnosed with conduct disorder and exhibiting prominent aggressive behavior.

Aman et al. (2000) conducted a 6-week, randomized, double-blind, placebo-controlled study of risperidone in the treatment of 118 children (age range, 5 to

12 years) exhibiting severe conduct problems and who had intelligence quotients ranging from 35 (moderate retardation) to 84 (borderline intelligence). Efficacy was determined by ratings on the Nisonger Child Behavior Rating Form (N-CBRF), the Aberrant Behavior Checklist (ABC), the Behavior Problems Inventory, and the Clinical Global Impressions Scale. Risperidone dosage was titrated to be within a range of 0.02 to 0.06 mg/kg/day. The mean treatment dose was 1.23 mg/day. Patients on risperidone improved significantly more on the N-CBRF than patients on placebo, beginning within the first week and continuing for the duration of the study. At endpoint, risperidone was also significantly better than placebo, as evidenced by ratings on the other scales. No serious untoward effects were reported.

Croonenberghs et al. (2005) conducted an international multi-site (16 European, 11 North American, and 5 South African) 1-year open-label trial of risperidone with 504 patients (419 males, 85 females; mean age 9.7 ± 2.5 years, range 4 to 14 years; 375 [74.4%] were older than 12 years of age and 425 [84.3%] were White) diagnosed with disruptive behavior disorders and subaverage intelligence to determine risperidone's long-term safety and effectiveness in the treatment of such disorders. Subjects had DSM-IV Axis Diagnoses of conduct disorder (23.8%), conduct disorder and Attention-Deficit/Hyperactivity Disorder (ADHD, 20.8%), oppositional defiant disorder (ODD, 17.9%), ODD and ADHD (18.8%), disruptive behavior disorder (DBD) NOS (6.5%), DBDNOS and ADHD (10.1%), and ADHD only (2.0%) and Axis II diagnoses of borderline intelligence (37.6%), or mild (43.1%) or moderate (19.3%) mental retardation (mean IQ was 64.2 ± 13.4; range 36–84).

The primary rating scales employed in measuring results were the Nisonger Child Behavior Rating Form (N-CBRF) Conduct Problem Subscale and the Vineland Adaptive Behavior Scale for conduct problems; a modified children's version of the California Verbal Learning Test (MCVLT-CV) and the Continuous Performance Task for cognitive functioning; and the Extrapyramidal Symptom Rating Scale and Adverse Effects "Query" were also recorded. The Aberrant Behavior Checklist and the Clinical Global Impressions (CGI) Scale were used to assess overall effectiveness. After an initial 3-day screening, eligible subjects were treated with a weeklong, single-blind, placebo period. At the end of this period, they were administered the N-CBRF Conduct Problem Subscale and the Vineland Adaptive Behavior Scale; those scoring < 24 on the former or > 84 on the latter were excluded. Subjects were administered 0.01 mg/kg of an oral risperidone solution once daily for the first two days of the study; this was increased to 0.02 mg/kg beginning the third day. Thereafter, doses could be adjusted at weekly intervals, but increases could not be > 0.02 mg/kg/day and the maximum permitted dose was 0.06 mg/kg/day.

Of the 504 subjects, 367 (73%) completed the 1-year study. The primary reasons for noncompletion were adverse effects (43; 8.5%), lost to follow-up (26; 5.2%), withdrawal of consent (18; 3.6%), and noncompliance (17; 3.4%). The most frequent reason for discontinuing was weight gain (9 subjects). The median dose was 1.5 mg/day (range, 0.1–4.3 mg/day).

Subjects' scores improved significantly on both measures of cognitive functioning ($P < .001$). On the conduct problem subscale of the N-CBRF, the mean score decreased from 32.9 ± 7.5 at baseline to 17.0 ± 11.0 at endpoint, a 48% decrease ($P < .001$). On the positive social behavior subscale of the N-CBRF compliant/calm and adaptive/social behavior, both improved significantly ($P < .001$) from baseline, and on the problem behavior subscale, insecure/anxious, hyperactive, self-injury/stereotypic, self-isolated/ritualistic and overly sensitive behaviors decreased significantly ($P < .001$). On the CGI Scale, at baseline 72% were rated as having marked to extremely severe symptoms; at the end of the study only 12% were so rated and 66% had mild symptoms or were rated as not ill. Scores on the ABC decreased from 64.3 ± 25.0 at baseline to 37.4 ± 27.4 at endpoint ($P < .001$).

At least one adverse effect was reported by 462 (91.7%) of the subjects and most were mild or moderate in intensity. The most common adverse effects that appeared to be related to the medication were somnolence (149, 29.6%), weight gain (87, 17.3%), fatigue (69; 13.7%), hyperprolactinemia (56, 11.1%), and increased appetite (53, 10.5%). There was a low baseline incidence of extrapyramidal symptoms (EPS) and ratings decreased over time throughout the study. However, five subjects required antiparkinsonian medication during the study and six patients discontinued the study because of EPS. Two subjects developed tardive dyskinesia, which remitted after medication was discontinued and one subject possibly experienced a withdrawal dyskinesia within 12 hours of discontinuing risperidone.

The authors concluded that risperidone is generally safe and well tolerated by children and adolescents over a period of up to one year.

Snyder et al. (2002) conducted a double-blind, placebo-controlled 6-week study of 110 children (age range, 5 to 12 years) with subaverage IQs (15 were moderately retarded [IQ = 35–49], 42 were mildly retarded [IQ = 50–69] and 53 had borderline IQs [IQs = 70–85]) to determine the efficacy of risperidone in reducing the severe disruptive behaviors they exhibited, including aggression, destruction of property, impulsivity, and defiance of authority. The children were diagnosed with Conduct Disorder, Oppositional Defiant Disorder, or Disruptive Behavior Disorder NOS; 80% of subjects were also diagnosed with ADHD and 45 of these continued treatment with the stimulant medication they were already receiving at time of entry to this study. Subjects had to have a score of 24 or greater on Conduct Problem subtest of the Nisonger Child Behavior Rating Form (N-CBRF) at baseline and at the end of a weeklong single-blind placebo run-in period that preceded the 6-week study to enter the double-blind phase. Of the 133 children beginning the study, 23 (17.3%) were placebo responders who dropped out of the study before the double-blind phase.

Subjects were randomly assigned to placebo ($N = 57$) or risperidone ($N = 53$). Twenty-five subjects dropped out of the double-blind portion; the most common reason being insufficient response. All 19 dropouts from the placebo group were for insufficient response whereas only 2 of the 6 dropouts from the risperidone group were for this reason ($P < .001$).

Risperidone or placebo was administered as an oral solution, beginning at 0.01 mg/kg/day and titrated upward with a maximum permitted weekly increase of 0.02 mg/kg to a total maximum dose of 0.06 mg/kg/day. The mean dose of risperidone at the endpoint was 0.98 ± 0.06 mg/day (range 0.40–3.80 mg/day) or 0.033 ± 0.001 mg/kg/day. The risperidone group showed a significantly greater reduction in ratings on the primary outcome variable, the N-CBRF Conduct Problem subtest, than the placebo group (47.3% reduction vs. 20.9% reduction, $P < .001$). In addition, significant improvements for subjects on risperidone were reported on several other subscales of the N-CBRF (conduct problem scale) and on various subscales of the Behavior Problems Inventory (aggressive behavior), the Aberrant Behavior Checklist (irritability), and the Visual Analogue Scale (VAS) (symptom) compared to the placebo group. Ratings on the Clinical Global Impressions Scale-Improvement (CGI-I) for subjects who completed the 6-week double-blind phase were significantly better for the risperidone group ($N = 42$), which improved significantly more than the placebo group ($N = 37$). No clinically significant ECG changes occurred. There were no significant cognitive changes on the Continuous Performance Task (CPT) or on the modified California Verbal Learning Test for Children (MCVLT-CV).

The most common adverse effects reported in the risperidone group were somnolence (41.5%), headache (17%), appetite increase (15.1%), and dyspepsia (15.1%). At endpoint, the risperidone group gained significantly more weight than the placebo group, 2.2 kg versus 0.2 kg ($P < .001$). Prolactin levels increased significantly in both males (from 6.96 at baseline to 27.08 at endpoint) and females (from 11.30 at baseline to 30.38 and endpoint) taking risperidone; the authors attributed this increase in the group to a minority of subjects whose increased prolactin levels fell within the 35 to 105 ng/mL range (normal range is 2 to 18 ng/mL for males and 3 to 30 ng/mL for females.

The authors concluded that risperidone was effective in reducing aggression, hyperactivity, and self-injury associated with disruptive behavior disorders and that it was adequately tolerated.

Risperidone in the Treatment of an Adolescent Diagnosed with Obsessive-Compulsive Disorder. Simeon et al. (1995) reported that a 16-year-old male diagnosed with severe obsessive-compulsive disorder, symptoms of anxiety, and aggressive and oppositional behavior and who had failed prior trials of clomipramine alone and in combination with standard neuroleptics and fluvoxamine showed minimal improvement and remained severely dysfunctional when risperidone was used in combination with clomipramine and fluvoxamine.

Risperidone in the Treatment of Children and Adolescents Diagnosed with Tic Disorders. Gilbert el al. (2004) conducted a randomized, double-blind crossover trial comparing risperidone and pimozide in 19 children and adolescents (15 males, 4 females; age range, 7–17 years, mean 11 ± 2.5 years) who were diagnosed with Tourette's disorder ($N = 16$) or chronic motor tic disorder ($N = 3$). Subjects were randomized to active treatment for a 4-week period; this was followed by a 2-week washout and administration of the other drug for 4 additional weeks. All subjects received placebo for an initial 2-week period, at the completion of which baseline tic severity was determined. The active drugs were titrated for the first two weeks and then held constant for the final two weeks of each period. Doses were increased if there was minimal or no improvement and held constant if untoward effects developed. Both treatments were administered twice daily; however, the morning dose of pimozide was a placebo. Pimozide was begun at a dose of 1 mg at bedtime and could be titrated up to a maximum of 4 mg/daily. Risperidone was begun at a dose of 0.5 mg twice daily (morning and bedtime) and could be titrated up to a maximum of 2 mg twice daily. Two subjects taking risperidone and one subject taking pimozide discontinued the study because of worsening tics. Thirteen (13) subjects completed the study. The final daily doses of risperidone ranged from 1 to 4 mg (mean 2.5 mg/day); final daily doses of pimozide ranged from 1 to 4 mg (mean 2.4 mg/day). Changes in tic severity were rated on the Yale Global Tic Severity Scale (YGTSS; baseline rating $= 43.3 \pm 17.5$). For the first 4-week period, subjects on risperidone had significantly lower tic severity scores on the YGTSS than subjects on pimozide (25.2 ± 13.6 vs. 34.2 ± 14.2; $P = .05$). The mean 18 point (42%) decrease on the YGTSS in the subjects receiving risperidone is clinically meaningful. Subjects on both drugs experienced weight gain; during the 4-week treatment periods, subjects on risperidone gained a mean of 1.9 kg while those on pimozide gained about half as much, 1.0 kg. Untoward effects were rated as mild. The authors conclude that their study supports the idea that risperidone and other atypical dopamine blocking agents are effective in treating Tourette's disorder, but caution that excessive weight gain and high drop out rates in this and other studies suggest that, when such drugs are used as monotherapy, the efficacy to adverse-effect ratio is unfavorable for some patients.

Olanzapine (Zyprexa)

The FDA has directed manufacturers of atypical antipsychotic drugs to add a black box warning that elderly patients with dementia-related psychosis treated with atypical antipsychotic drugs are at increased risk of death of 1.6 to 1.7 times that seen in placebo-treated patients. Olanzapine is not approved for treatment of patients with dementia-related psychosis.

Olanzapine belongs to the thienobenzodiazepine class. It was approved by the FDA for marketing in the United States in 1997. The manufacturer suggests that its antipsychotic properties may be mediated through a combination of dopamine and serotonin type 2 ($5HT_2$) antagonism. Olanzapine also antagonizes muscarinic M_{1-5} receptors, which may explain its anticholinergic effects; histamine H_1 receptors, which may explain the somnolence that may occur; and adrenergic alpha-1 receptors, which may explain the orthostatic hypotension sometimes observed.

Pharmacokinetics of Olanzapine

Food does not affect the rate or extent of absorption of olanzapine. Peak serum concentrations occur approximately 6 hours after oral administration. The half-life of olanzapine ranges from 21 to 54 hours in 90% of the population, with a mean half-life of 30 hours. With once-daily dosing, steady-state serum concentrations occur in approximately 7 days.

Olanzapine is metabolized primarily by direct glucuronidation and cytochrome P450 (CYP)- mediated oxidation. The major circulating metabolites during steady state, 10-N-glucuronide and 4'-N-desmethyl olanzapine, are clinically inactive at usual doses. The drug is highly metabolized, with only approximately 7% being recovered unchanged in the urine. Approximately 60% of the drug is excreted through the kidneys and approximately 30% is recovered in the feces.

Tobacco smoking induces cytochrome CYP1A2, a principal enzyme mediating the metabolism of olanzapine; hence adult smokers have lower plasma olanzapine levels than nonsmokers.

It is noted that olanzapine clearance is approximately 30% greater in males than in females and approximately 40% greater in smokers than in nonsmokers; however, dosage modifications are not usually necessary.

Olanzapine Pharmacokinetics In Child and Adolescent Inpatients Diagnosed with Schizophrenia

Grothe et al. (2000) studied the pharmacokinetics of olanzapine in an 8-week, open-label treatment of eight inpatients (four males, four females; age range, 10 to 18 years) diagnosed with schizophrenia who were subjects in the NIMH study investigating the efficacy and safety of atypical antipsychotic drugs in treatment-refractory schizophrenia with childhood onset. As all eight were nonsmokers, their olanzapine pharmacokinetics were compared with those reported for adult nonsmokers. Olanzapine was begun at a dose of 2.5 mg/day, with an increase to 5.0 mg/day on day 3. Subsequently, olanzapine was titrated upward in 2.5- to 5.0-mg increments every 5 to 9 days based on clinical response up to a maximum of 20 mg/day. Blood samples were drawn weekly; at the end of treatment, plasma level determinations were made for 0, 1, 2, 4, 8, 12, 24, and 36 hours after the final dose. At the end of the 8-week study, seven subjects were receiving olanzapine 20 mg/day and one was receiving 15 mg/day. Plasma olanzapine levels increased linearly in this dose range, making dose adjustments relatively predictable. At a fixed dose, steady-state levels developed in approximately 7 days, with olanzapine's concentration approximately doubling over that period. The seven subjects receiving 20 mg/day had an average steady-state plasma olanzapine concentration of 92.6 ± 27.0 ng/mL; average trough concentration (measured 24 hours after the last dose) was 75.6 ± 27.2 ng/mL. The seven subjects' mean maximum plasma concentration (C_{max}) was 115.6 ± 26.7 ng/mL, which occurred at a mean time (T_{max}) of 4.7 ± 3.7 hours after the dose was given. Mean elimination half-life ($T_{1/2}$) was 37.2 ± 5.1 hours. Olanzapine plasma levels of these seven mostly adolescent subjects were comparable to those reported for adult nonsmokers.

Interactions Of Olanzapine with Other Drugs

Of particular note, carbamazepine, a potent inducer of CYP1A2 activity, in doses of 200 mg b.i.d. causes an increase of approximately 50% in the clearance of olanzapine; higher doses may cause an even greater increase, necessitating upward adjustment of the dose of olanzapine.

Contraindications for Olanzapine Administration

Olanzapine is contraindicated in patients with known hypersensitivity to the drug.

Adverse Effects of Olanzapine

Extrapyramidal Symptoms. At doses up to 15 ± 2.5 mg, there were no statistically significant differences in treatment-emergent extrapyramidal symptoms assessed by rating scales between placebo and olanzapine. This was also true for adverse effects spontaneously reported by patients, except that akathisia was reported significantly more frequently at doses of 10 ± 2.5 mg or more for olanzapine than for placebo.

Other Adverse Effects. Orthostatic hypotension, tachycardia, weight gain, liver transaminase elevations, somnolence, insomnia, constipation, dizziness, agitation, and dry mouth have been reported to occur in patients treated with olanzapine.

Indications for Olanzapine in Child and Adolescent Psychiatry

Olanzapine is indicated for the management of the treatment of schizophrenia, the treatment of acute mixed or manic episodes associated with Bipolar I Disorder, maintenance monotherapy of Bipolar Disorder, and the treatment of agitation associated with Schizophrenia and Bipolar I Mania.

Olanzapine Dosage Schedule

(continued)

Indications for Olanzapine in Child and Adolescent Psychiatry (Continued)

- Children and adolescents 17 years of age and less: not recommended. The safety and effectiveness of olanzapine have not been established for pediatric populations.

Treatment of Schizophrenia

Adolescents 18 years of age and adults: an initial dose of 5 to 10 mg is recommended, with titration to 10 mg/day within several days. Further titrations should occur at weekly intervals to allow steady-state levels to develop. Doses above 10 mg/day have not been demonstrated to increase efficacy, and the safety of doses over 20 mg/day has not been evaluated in clinical trials.

Treatment of Acute Mixed or Manic Episodes Associated with Bipolar I Disorder

Adolescents 18 years of age and adults: an initial daily dose of 10 to 15 mg is recommended. Adjustments of 5 mg/day may be made at recommended intervals of not < 24 hours. Antimanic efficacy has been demonstrated at daily doses of 5 to 20 mg/day; safety of doses greater than 20 mg/day has not been evaluated in clinical trials.

Olanzapine Dose Forms Available

- Tablets: 2.5 mg, 5 mg, 7.5 mg, 10 mg, 15 mg, 20 mg
- Orally Disintegrating Tablets (Zyprexa Zydis): 5 mg, 10 mg, 15 mg, 20 mg
- Injection, Intramuscular: 10 mg vial

Reports of Interest

Olanzapine in the Treatment of Children and Adolescents Diagnosed with Schizophrenia. Sholevar et al. (2000) treated with olanzapine 15 hospitalized subjects (9 males, 6 females; age range, 6 to 13 years; mean age, 9.4 ± 1.99 years) who were diagnosed with childhood-onset acute schizophrenia by DSM-IV criteria before age 12. Medication was begun between 24 and 48 hours after admission. Because the first 3 subjects experienced morning sedation and lethargy on initial doses of 5 mg of olanzapine daily, the subsequent 12 patients were begun on 2.5 mg daily. Medication was increased to 5 mg daily after 5 days if no untoward effects were apparent. Average hospitalization during which this study took place was 11.3 days. At the end of hospitalization, 14 (93%) of the subjects were maintained on 5 mg olanzapine daily. Psychiatric improvement was rated on a four-point scale: 0 = no improvement, 1 = slight improvement, 2 = moderate improvement, and 3 = great improvement. Five subjects (33.3%) were greatly improved, five (33.3%) were moderately improved, three (20%) were slightly improved, and two (13.3%) showed no improvement. Sedation was the most common untoward effect and lasted from 0 to 4 days. There were no clinically significant changes in laboratory values or vital signs. The authors reported that longer duration of initial sedation was significantly positively correlated with increased clinical improvement ($P = .004$). Younger age was significantly correlated with increased clinical improvement ($P < .05$). The 11 subjects who were being treated for the first time with an antipsychotic showed greater clinical improvement than the 4 subjects who had failed prior treatments with antipsychotics.

Kumra et al. (1998) compared the efficacy of olanzapine in an 8-week, open-label trial in 8 patients (mean age, 15.3 ± 2.3 years) with that of clozapine in a 6-week, open-label trial in 15 patients (mean age, 13.6 ± 1.5 years) in the treatment of subjects diagnosed with schizophrenia by DSM-III-R (APA, 1987) criteria. Subjects receiving olanzapine in this study had treatment-resistant schizophrenia (all had failed prior treatment with at least two other neuroleptics) with childhood onset, which comprises an even rarer subgroup than schizophrenia with childhood onset. In addition, four of the subjects on olanzapine had experienced good clinical response to clozapine but developed significant untoward effects requiring its discontinuation. In addition, most clinicians would now administer a trial of an atypical antipsychotic rather than a standard neuroleptic as a first-line medication.

Mean dose of olanzapine at the sixth week of treatment was 17.5 ± 2.3 mg/day (range, 12.5 to 20 mg/day) or 0.27 ± 0.11 mg/kg/day (range, 0.15 to 0.41 mg/kg/day). The mean dose of clozapine at the sixth week of treatment was 317 ± 147 mg/day (range, 100 to 600 mg/day) or 5.42 ± 2.84 mg/kg/day (range, 1.28 to 8.88 mg/kg/day). Efficacy was rated using scores of the Brief Psychiatric Rating Scale (BPRS) and the Clinical Global Impressions Scale (CGI).

The most clinically important findings of this study were that eight (53%) of the 15 subjects on clozapine and none of the 8 subjects on olanzapine met "responder" criteria by week 6. At week 8, two (25%) of the subjects receiving olanzapine met "responder" criteria and one (12.5%) was a partial responder. Clinical improvement of subjects on clozapine at 6 weeks was rated better than that of subjects on olanzapine at 8 weeks for all clinical ratings. Even the four subjects who could not tolerate clozapine because of untoward effects had shown greater clinical improvement on clozapine than on olanzapine. Of the eight patients on olanzapine, three were rated "much improved"; two, "minimally improved"; one, "no change"; one, "minimally worse"; one, "much worse." Four subjects, who improved on olanzapine at 8 weeks and continued to take the drug, showed further clinical improvement. Untoward effects of olanzapine were moderate but frequent; the most common were insomnia (seven, 87.5%), transient liver transaminase elevation (seven, 87.5%), increased appetite (six, 75%), nausea/vomiting (six, 75%), headache (six, 75%), sustained tachycardia (six, 75%), increased agitation (six, 75%), difficulty concentrating (five, 62.5%), and constipation (five, 62.5%). During the 8-week trial, seven (87.5%) of the patients on olanzapine were treated with lorazepam, 2 to 8 mg/day, for agitation or insomnia. No patient on olanzapine required prophylactic anticonvulsant treatment for developing an abnormal EEG or convulsions, but four of the patients on clozapine required such medication (Kumra et al. 1998). The authors concluded that clozapine remains the "gold standard" for the treatment of schizophrenia but that, because of olanzapine's much more favorable untoward-effect profile and indication of therapeutic efficacy in some of their subjects, it is a good first-line choice for treating schizophrenia with childhood onset.

Olanzapine in the Treatment of Children and Adolescents Diagnosed with Pervasive Developmental Disorders. Potenza et al. (1999) reported a 12-week, open-label, pilot study in which olanzapine monotherapy was prescribed to eight patients (mean age, 20.9 ± 11.7 years; range, 5 to 42 years), of whom four were children or adolescents, diagnosed by DSM-IV (APA, 1994) criteria with autistic disorder ($N = 5$) or with pervasive developmental disorder not otherwise specified (PDDNOS) of at least moderate severity. Four subjects had full-scale intelligence quotients (FSIQs) in the mildly retarded range, and three subjects had FSIQs in the moderately retarded range. Seven of the subjects had prior drug trials, including at least one typical antipsychotic that was clinically ineffective or produced unacceptable untoward effects. Efficacy was assessed using the Yale-Brown Obsessive-Compulsive Scale Compulsion subscale (Y-BOCS-CS), the Self-Injurious Behavior Questionnaire (SIB-Q), the Vineland Adaptive Behavior Scale Maladaptive Behavior subscales (VMBS), the Ritvo-Freeman Real-Life Rating Scale (RFRLRS), the Clinical Global Impressions-Improvement Scale (CGI-I), and the Clinician-Rated Visual Analog Scale(VAS).

All subjects had a 4-week, drug-free period before beginning the 12-week protocol. An initial daily dose of 2.5 mg of olanzapine was prescribed for the first 2 weeks. Olanzapine was then titrated upward in 2.5- to 5.0-mg increments to a maximum of 20 mg/day, usually given at bedtime. Seven subjects completed the study and the eighth dropped out after 9 weeks because of failure to improve, the last observation of that case was carried forward, intent-to-treat methodology was used in the data analysis. The mean dose of olanzapine at week 12 was 7.8 ± 4.7 mg/day (range, 5 to 20 mg/day). Six patients were considered responders, and the response was not correlated with dose, age, IQ, SIB or repetitive behaviors, or baseline severity of illness. By the end of week 4, subjects showed a significant mean improvement over baseline on the CGI-I ($P = .015$) with further improvement at the end of the 8th and 12th weeks ($P < .001$). There was also significant improvement on items of the VAS, such as temper tantrums, impulsivity, anxiety, social withdrawal, rocking, destruction of property, and inappropriate sexual behavior; the RFRLRS behavioral constellations for sensory motor behaviors, social relationship to people, affectual reactions, sensory responses, and language use and response; and the SIB-Q showed a significant reduction in aggressive behavior over time. Repetitive behaviors rated on the Y-BOCS-CS showed no significant improvement. The most clinically significant untoward effects were sedation in three subjects and significant weight gain in six subjects. The group mean weight at the end of the 12-week period was 70.88 ± 25.06 kg, compared with 62.50 ± 25.37 kg at baseline ($P = .008$). The guardians of two children who were responders discontinued their olanzapine 2 and 8 weeks after the initial period because they felt the clinical benefit was not sufficient to tolerate the significant weight gain.

Olanzapine in the Treatment of Children and Adolescents Diagnosed with Bipolar Disorder. Frazier et al. (2000) treated 23 subjects (age range, 5 to 14 years), diagnosed with bipolar disorder and currently manic or mixed, with olanzapine on an open-label basis for up to 8 weeks. The dose ranged from 2.5 to 20 mg/day. Efficacy was evaluated by ratings on the Young Mania Rating Scale (YMRS) with responders defined a priori as having $\geq 30\%$ improvement in total score from baseline to endpoint and by ratings of ≤ 3 ("very much improved," "much improved," or "improved") on the Clinical Global Impressions-Bipolar Mania (CGI-BP) Improvement Scale. Twenty-two (95.7%) completed the study, the twenty-third developed depressive symptoms and dropped out. Mean ratings on the YMRS decreased by 19.04 ± 9.21 ($P < .001$), and 60.9% were rated as responders. No significant extrapyramidal symptoms were noted; however, subjects' weights increased significantly (4.98 ± 2.32 kg over the course of the treatment).

Quetiapine Fumarate (Seroquel)

The FDA has directed manufacturers of atypical antipsychotic drugs to add a black box warning that elderly patients with dementia-related psychosis treated with atypical antipsychotic drugs are at increased risk of death of 1.6 to 1.7 times that seen in placebo-treated patients. Quetiapine fumarate is not approved for treatment of patients with dementia-related psychosis.

Quetiapine fumarate (Seroquel) belongs to a new chemical class, the dibenzothiazepine derivatives. The drug antagonizes $5HT_{1A}$, $5HT_3$, dopamine D_1, dopamine D_2, histamine H_1, adrenergic alpha-1, and adrenergic alpha-2 neurotransmitter receptors in the brain. It has no appreciable affinity at cholinergic muscarinic and benzodiazepine receptors. It is suggested that its antipsychotic properties may be mediated through its antagonism of dopamine type 2 (D_2) and serotonin type 2 ($5HT_2$) receptors. Quetiapine's antagonism of H_1 and adrenergic alpha-1 receptors may explain the sedation and hypotension, respectively, sometimes observed with the drug. It was approved by the FDA in 1997.

Pharmacokinetics of Quetiapine Fumarate

Food affects the bioavailability of quetiapine fumarate only marginally. Peak serum levels occur at a mean of 1.5 hours after ingestion. Quetiapine fumarate is extensively metabolized, primarily in the liver, by sulfoxidation by cytochrome P450 3A4 isoenzyme, to its major, sulfoxide metabolite, and by oxidation; both metabolites are pharmacologically inactive.

Steady-state serum concentrations occur after approximately 2 days on a given dose regimen. Terminal serum half-life is approximately 6 hours.

Gender, race, and smoking have no clinically significant effects on the metabolism of quetiapine fumarate.

Contraindications for Quetiapine Fumarate Administration

Quetiapine fumarate is contraindicated in patients with a known hypersensitivity to it.

Quetiapine fumarate should be administered with caution to patients with hepatic impairment, which may increase plasma levels.

Advantages of Quetiapine Fumarate

Quetiapine fumarate does not cause statistically significant changes in the QT, QT_C, and PR intervals of the ECG.

Adverse Effects of Quetiapine Fumarate

Extrapyramidal Symptoms. The incidence of treatment-emergent extrapyramidal symptoms in patients treated with quetiapine fumarate is not significantly different from that in patients treated with placebo over a daily dose range of 75 to 750 mg.

Other Adverse Effects. Orthostatic hypotension, dizziness, tachycardia, weight gain, somnolence, constipation, dry mouth, dyspepsia, and many other untoward effects have been reported in patients taking quetiapine.

Indications for Quetiapine Fumarate in Child and Adolescent Psychiatry

Quetiapine is indicated for the management of the manifestations of schizophrenia and Acute Manic Episodes associated with Bipolar I Disorder.

Quetiapine Dosage Schedule

- Children and adolescents 17 years of age and less: not recommended. The manufacturer notes that the safety and effectiveness of quetiapine fumarate in the pediatric age-group have not been established.

Treatment of Schizophrenia

- Adolescents 18 years of age and adults: an initial dose of 25 mg bid is recommended, with increases in increments of 25 to 50 mg bid or tid on the second and third days, as tolerated, to a target daily total dose of 300 to 400 mg given bid or tid by the fourth day. It is recommended that any subsequent adjustments of dosage be made at intervals of at least 2 days to allow adequate time for steady-state serum levels to be achieved. If further adjustments are necessary, increments or decrements of 25 to 50 mg bid are suggested. Efficacy has been demonstrated for a dose range of 150 to 750 mg/day in clinical trials. However, doses above 300/day were not more effective than 300 mg/day in a dose response study. The safety of doses > 800 mg/day has not been evaluated in clinical trials.

Treatment of Acute Manic Episodes associated with Bipolar I Disorder.

Quetiapine should be administered twice daily. A starting dose of 50 mg bid is recommended on the first day. This should be increased by increments of up to 100 mg daily to reach a total of 400 mg/day (200 mg bid) on day 4. Titration may continue to a maximum of 800 mg/day with increments no > 200 mg/day. The safety of doses > 800 mg/day has not been evaluated in clinical trials.

Quetiapine Fumarate Dose Forms Available

- Tablets: 25 mg, 100 mg, 200 mg, and 300 mg

Report of Interest

Quetiapine Fumarate in the Treatment of Children and Adolescents Diagnosed with Autistic Disorder

Martin et al. (1999) treated six male outpatients (mean age, 10.9 ± 3.3 years; age range, 6.2 to 15.3 years) diagnosed with autistic disorder by DSM-IV (APA, 1994) criteria with quetiapine in a 16-week, open-label study. All were mentally retarded (two mild, three moderate, one severe). Target symptoms for five patients were aggression, self-injury, and poor impulse control, and for the sixth interfering stereotypies and repetitive behaviors. Quetiapine was begun with a nighttime dose of 25 mg and titrated on the basis of clinical response, with increases up to 100 mg/week permitted. Efficacy was assessed by ratings on the Aberrant Behavior Checklist (ABC), the Clinical Global Impressions-Improvement Scale (CGI-I), with subjects rated "much improved" or "very much improved" considered responders, the Ritvo-Freeman Real Life Rating Scale (RFRLRS), and the Children's Yale-Brown Obsessive-Compulsive Scale (CY-BOCS). Only two subjects completed the

16-week study. Three (50%) dropped out (two after 4 weeks and one after 8 weeks) because sedation and the lack of clinical improvement were so problematic that the dose of quetiapine could not be increased (one of the three also had an apparent seizure), and the fourth dropped out after 4 weeks because of behavioral activation and apparent akathisia. Mean dose of quetiapine at endpoint or at dropout was 225 ± 108 mg/day (range, 100 to 350 mg/day). Based on the CGI-I, only the two subjects who completed the 16 weeks were responders, one "very much improved" and the other "much improved'; of the four nonresponders, one was "much worse," two were "minimally worse," and one was "no change." Four subjects experienced increased appetite and a mean weight gain of 2.9 ± 3.6 kg. Overall, quetiapine was poorly tolerated and/or ineffective for two-thirds of the subjects, and only one of the two responders continued to benefit from long-term treatment with quetiapine.

Findling et al. (2004) reported a 12-week, open-label study in nine subjects (age range 12.0 to 17.3 years; eight males, one female) diagnosed with autistic disorder and having a score of > 30 on the Childhood Autism Rating Scale (CARS), and a rating on the Clinical Global Impressions-Severity (CGI-S) of at least moderately ill. Target symptoms included aggression, self-injurious behavior, tantrums, irritability, overactivity, and social withdrawal. Quetiapine was begun at 25 mg twice daily for 3 days and then increased to 50 mg twice daily for the next 11 days. At the beginning of week 3, the dose was increased by 50 mg twice daily every other week to reach a target dose of 150 mg twice daily (300 mg/day). Following this, the dose could be increased by a total of 25–75 mg/week, based on tolerability and clinical response, to a maximum of 750 mg/day.

Mean total quetiapine daily dose was 291.7, dose range 100 mg to 450 mg. Responders were defined as having ratings of 1 (very much improved) or 2 (much improved) on the CGI-Improvement (CGI-I) rating at endpoint. Six patients completed the study; one dropped out because of increased aggression/agitation and one dropped out because of drowsiness, while the final patient was lost to follow-up after one week. Only two of the eight patients (25%) who received medication were responders. The most frequent side effects reported by parents were sedation ($N = 7$), weight gain ($N = 5$), agitation ($N = 4$), and aggression ($N = 2$). The authors noted that quetiapine was not particularly effective clinically in these treatment-resistant adolescents with autistic disorder (Findling et al. 2004).

Aripiprazole (Abilify)

The FDA has directed manufacturers of atypical antipsychotic drugs to add a black box warning that elderly patients with dementia-related psychosis treated with atypical antipsychotic drugs are at increased risk of death of 1.6 to 1.7 times that seen in placebo-treated patients. Aripiprazole is not approved for treatment of patients with dementia-related psychosis.

Aripiprazole belongs to the chemical class of quinolinone derivatives. It was approved by the FDA for marketing in the United States in 2002. The manufacturer suggests that its antipsychotic properties may be mediated through its partial agonism of dopamine type 2 (D_2) and serotonin type 1 ($5HT_{1A}$) receptors and antagonism of serotonin type 2 ($5HT_{2A}$) receptors.

Pharmacokinetics of Aripiprazole

Taken orally, aripiprazole is well absorbed and peak plasma concentrations occur within 3 to 5 hours. Taking it with food does not significantly alter peak plasma concentrations; however, it may delay them for several hours. Activity is due to aripiprazole (approximately 60%) and its major metabolite dehydro-aripiprazole (approximately 40%) at steady-state plasma levels, which are achieved for both within 14 days. Mean elimination half-lives are approximately 75 hours for aripiprazole and approximately 94 hours for dehydro-aripiprazole. The major metabolism is through the hepatic P450 isomers CYP2D6 and CYP3A4. Most of the metabolites and some unchanged drug are excreted in the feces; a lesser but significant amount is excreted by the kidneys.

Approximately 8% of Caucasians are poor metabolizers of aripiprazole because they have decreased ability to metabolize CYP2D6 substrates. Such individuals have a net increase of approximately 60% on exposure to the drug, compared to extensive (normal) metabolizers of the drug. The elimination half-life of aripiprazole for poor metabolizers is approximately 146 hours, nearly twice that of extensive metabolizers.

Interactions of Aripiprazole with Other Drugs

Drugs such as quinine, which inhibit CYP2D6, can result in more than a doubling of plasma levels and require downward adjustment of the dose of aripiprazole. If fluoxetine or paroxetine, both potential CYP2D6 inhibitors, is given concomitantly, the aripiprazole dose should be reduced by at least one-half of the usual dose.

Contraindications for Aripiprazole Administration

Aripiprazole is contraindicated in patients with known hypersensitivity to the drug.

Adverse Effects of Aripiprazole

ECG changes: No significant ECG differences were found between subjects administered placebo and aripiprazole in the pooled data of the premarketing trials; within the dose range of 10 to 30 mg, aripiprazole tended to slightly shorten the QT_C interval. There was a median increase in heart rate of 4 beats per minute in subjects treated with aripiprazole.

Weight: In premarketing studies of 4 to 6 weeks duration, subjects receiving aripiprazole gained a mean of 0.7 kg compared with subjects on placebo who lost a mean of 0.05 kg. In a 52-week study, weight gain or loss was related to initial BMI. Subjects with a BMI of < 23 gained a mean of 2.6 kg and 30% had an increase in weight of > 7% over baseline measures. The data for subjects with baseline BMIs of 23 to 27 were a mean weight gain of 1.4 kg with 19% experiencing a weight gain of > 7%. Subjects with a BMI > 27 lost a mean weight of 1.2 kg, but 8% of them still gained > 7% of their baseline body weight.

Indications for Aripiprazole in Child and Adolescent Psychiatry

Aripiprazole is indicated for the treatment of schizophrenia, acute manic episodes and acute mixed episodes of Bipolar I Disorder, and for the maintenance therapy of these disorders.

(continued)

Indications for Aripiprazole in Child and Adolescent Psychiatry *(Continued)*

Aripiprazole Dosage Schedule

- Children and Adolescents 17 years of age and less: not recommended. The safety and efficacy of aripiprazole have not been established for pediatric populations.
- Adolescents 18 years of age and older and adults: a single initial and target dose of 10 to 15 mg daily is recommended. Doses > 15 mg/day resulted in no increased efficacy in premarketing trials. As it takes up to 2 weeks for steady-state kinetics to be achieved, any increases in dose should be made after that period.

Aripiprazole Dose Forms Available

- Tablets: 5 mg, 10 mg, 15 mg, 20 mg, and 30 mg
- Oral solution: 1 mg/mL

Ziprasidone Hydrochloride (Geodon)

The FDA has directed manufacturers of atypical antipsychotic drugs to add a black box warning that elderly patients with dementia-related psychosis treated with atypical antipsychotic drugs are at increased risk of death of 1.6 to 1.7 times that seen in placebo-treated patients. Ziprasidone hydrochloride is not approved for treatment of patients with dementia-related psychosis.

The manufacturer suggests that ziprasidone's antipsychotic properties may be mediated through its antagonism of dopamine type 2 (D_2) and serotonin type 2 ($5HT_{2A}$) receptors.

It was approved by the FDA for marketing in the United States in 2001.

Pharmacokinetics of Ziprasidone Hydrochloride

Taken orally, ziprasidone is well absorbed and peak plasma concentrations occur within 6 to 8 hours. Absorption is increased up to twofold when taken with food. Elimination is mainly through hepatic metabolism; about one-third of the excretory metabolites are oxidized by P450 CYP3A4 and about two-thirds result from reduction by aldehyde oxidase. Approximately 20% is excreted in the urine and 66% in the feces. Mean terminal half-life is approximately 7 hours for doses in the recommended clinical range. Steady-state plasma levels are achieved within 1 to 3 days at a constant dose.

Interactions of Ziprasidone with Other Drugs

Carbamazepine, an inducer of CYP3A4, resulted in a decrease of approximately 35% in ziprasidone AUC ([area under the curve], "the total amount of drug absorbed into the systemic circulation and available for distribution to the target organ and site of action" [Ayd, 2000]).

Contraindications for Ziprasidone Administration

Ziprasidone is contraindicated in patients with known hypersensitivity to the drug, or patients who have familial long QT syndrome or a history of cardiac arrhythmias or other significant cardiovascular illnesses.

Ziprasidone should not be prescribed concomitantly with other drugs that are known to prolong the QTc interval.

Adverse Effects of Ziprasidone

ECG changes: Ziprasidone is associated with increases in the QTc interval. In placebo-controlled trials, ziprasidone increased the QTc interval by approximately 10 msec at a dose of 160 mg/day compared to placebo. In direct comparisons with five other antipsychotic medications, the mean increase in QTc over baseline in subjects receiving ziprasidone ranged from 9 to 14 msec greater than for subjects receiving risperidone, olanzapine, quetiapine, and haloperidol but was approximately 14 msec less than for subjects receiving thioridazine.

Indications for Ziprasidone Hydrochloride in Child and Adolescent Psychiatry

Ziprasidone is indicated for the treatment of schizophrenia and the treatment of acute mania episodes or mixed episodes associated with Bipolar Disorder. Ziprasidone intramuscular is indicated for the treatment of acute agitation in patients with schizophrenia and patients who need intramuscular antipsychotic medication for rapid control of the agitation.

Because of ziprasidone's greater capacity to increase the QT/QTc interval compared to several other antipsychotics, careful clinical consideration should be given to prescribing one or more trials of such alternative antipsychotics before undertaking a trial with ziprasidone.

Ziprasidone Dosage Schedule

- Children and Adolescents 17 years of age and less: not recommended. The safety and efficacy of ziprasidone have not been established for pediatric populations.
- Adolescents 18 years of age and older and adults: an initial dose of 20 mg twice daily is recommended. Maximum total daily doses over 160 mg are not usually recommended. As it takes 1 to 3 days to achieve steady-state plasma levels, adjustments in dose should not be made at intervals of < 2 days. In long-term studies (52 weeks) of subjects maintained on ziprasidone doses ranging from 20 to 80 mg bid, no clinical advantage was demonstrated for doses over 20 mg bid.

Ziprasidone Hydrochloride Dose Forms Available

- Capsules: 20 mg, 40 mg, 60 mg, and 80 mg
- Injection: (ziprasidone mesylate) single use vials 20 mg/mL for intramuscular injection. Doses are different from the oral doses; read package insert before use.

Reports of Interest

Ziprasidone in the Treatment of Children and Adolescents Diagnosed with Autistic Disorder. McDougle et al. (2002) conducted an open-label trial to evaluate the safety and effectiveness of ziprasidone in treating 12 subjects (mean age 11.62 ± 4.38 years; age range 8 to 20 years) who were diagnosed with autistic disorder ($N = 9$) or pervasive developmental disorder not otherwise specified (PDDNOS); ($N = 3$) by DSM-IV criteria; 11 subjects had codiagnoses of mental retardation (mild = 4, moderate = 6, and severe = 1). Target symptoms were aggression, self-injury, property destruction, agitation, irritability, and mood instability. Most subjects were treatment resistant and 11 were previously treated with one or more other atypical antipsychotic drugs, with significant weight gain often causing their discontinuation. At the beginning of the study 5 subjects were receiving an atypical antipsychotic, which was discontinued over a 4-week taper. Four subjects were permitted to continue on their usual dose of other medications during the study.

The initial dose of Ziprasidone was 20 mg at bedtime and titrated upward according to clinical response and adverse events (AEs), in increments of 10 to 20 mg/week, and divided into 2 daily doses. All subjects completed a minimum of 6 weeks of the study; mean duration was 14.15 ± 8.29 weeks, range 6 to 30 weeks. The final mean ziprasidone dose was 59.23 ± 34.76 mg/day, dose range 20 to 120 mg/day. Responders were defined as subjects with a Clinical Global Impressions-Improvement (CGI-I) rating of 1 (very much improved) or 2 (much improved). Six (50%) subjects were responders; two subjects with comorbid bipolar disorder were rated much worse. Adverse events (AEs) were evaluated using a checklist used by the RUPP Autism Network. Four subjects reported no AEs. Sedation ($N = 5$), usually transient, was the most frequent AE, three experienced increased appetite and two had insomnia. Both the subjects with comorbid bipolar disorder experienced agitation and insomnia. One subject who had a history of tardive dyskinesia of the hands developed an oral dyskinesia that resolved when ziprasidone was discontinued. The mean weight change was -5.83 ± 12.52 pounds, range -35 to $+6$ pounds. No cardiovascular AEs were reported; however, only a baseline ECG was performed. The authors suggested that ziprasidone is a potentially useful treatment for aggression, agitation, and irritability in children, adolescents, and young adults diagnosed with autistic disorder or PDDNOS, and that further studies should be undertaken (McDougle et al. 2002).

Ziprasidone [Intramuscular] in the Treatment of Children and Adolescents Exhibiting Acute Agitation, Aggression or Anxiety. Staller (2004) conducted a retrospective chart review of 49 children and adolescents (17 males, 32 females; age range 8 to 16 years) who were administered intramuscular ziprasidone for acute agitation and agitation/anxiety/threat ($N = 47$) or psychosis ($N = 2$) during hospitalization in an acute care private psychiatric hospital in central upstate New York. Most subjects (87%) were administered 20 mg injections; however, six subjects (two males and four females), all 13 years of age or younger, received 10 mg injections. Nursing notes indicated that only two patients continued to exhibit agitation and aggression during the subsequent shift and only one of these was given a repeat 20 mg dose. There were no adverse reactions reported.

CHAPTER 7

Antidepressant Drugs

Note: The FDA directed, in October 2004, manufacturers of antidepressant medications to add the following Black Box Warning to their labeling. "Warning: Suicidality in Children and Adolescents—Antidepressants increased the risk of suicidal thinking and behavior (suicidality) in short-term studies in children and adolescents with major depressive disorder (MDD) and other psychiatric disorders. Anyone considering the use of [drug name] or any other antidepressant in a child or adolescent must balance this risk with the clinical needs. Patients who are started on therapy should be observed closely for clinical worsening, suicidality, or unusual changes in behavior. Families and caregivers should be advised of the need for close observation and communication with the prescriber. [Drug name] is not approved for use in pediatric patients except for patients with [Any approved pediatric claims here]. (See Warnings and Precautions:Pediatric Use.)

Pooled analyses of short-term (4 to 16 weeks) placebo-controlled trials of nine antidepressant drugs (SSRIs and others) in children and adolescents with MDD, obsessive-compulsive-disorder (OCD), or other psychiatric disorders (a total of 24 trials involving over 4,400 patients have revealed a greater risk of adverse events representing suicidal thinking or behavior (suicidality) during the first few months of treatment in those receiving antidepressants. The average risk of such events on drug was 4%, twice the placebo risk of 2%. No suicides occurred in these trials."

Furthermore, in the labeling under "Warnings" the following is indicated: "All pediatric patients being treated with antidepressants for any indication should be observed closely for clinical worsening, suicidality, and unusual changes in behavior, especially during the initial few months of a course of drug therapy, or at times of dose changes, either increases or decreases. Ideally, such observation would include at least weekly face-to-face contact with patients or their family members or caregivers during the first 4 weeks of treatment, then biweekly visits for the next 4 weeks, then at 12 weeks, and as clinically indicated beyond 12 weeks. Additional contact by telephone may be appropriate between face-to-face visits.

Adults with MDD or comorbid depression in the setting of other psychiatric illness taking antidepressants should also be observed for clinical worsening and suicidality, especially during the first few months of treatment, or at times of dose increases or decreases."

INTRODUCTION

The selective serotonin reuptake inhibitor (SSRI) antidepressants are now the most frequently prescribed antidepressants for children and adolescents, and continue to be prescribed with increasing frequency because of their significantly safer untoward-effects profile, in particular, the reduced risks of cardiotoxicity and lethality of overdose compared with the risks associated with tricyclic antidepressants. For these reasons, Ambrosini et al. (1993) recommended prescribing SSRIs and not tricyclics to depressed patients with suicidal and/or impulsive tendencies. The SSRIs have also been approved for the treatment of several other psychiatric disorders and are used off-label for several additional ones. In 2005, the FDA, directed manufacturers of all antidepressants, including SSRIs, to label their package inserts with a warning of increased suicidal thoughts and behavior in children and adolescents, noting that a pooled analysis of short-term studies in subjects less than 18 years old showed an increase from 2% in subjects receiving a placebo to 4% in subjects receiving an antidepressant.

SUICIDAL RISK AND ANTIDEPRESSANTS

Simon et al. (2006) provided an excellent and succinct review of the events leading up to the FDA's issuing a warning about increased suicidal risk in children and adolescents being treated with newer antidepressants and the FDA's advisory requiring a "black box" warning for all antidepressants as of October 2004 as an introduction to their important study on suicidal risk during antidepressant treatment.

The authors identified 65,103 patients with 82,285 episodes of antidepressant treatment over a period of $12\frac{1}{2}$ years ending June 30, 2003. The subjects were members of the Group Health Cooperative (GHC), a mixed-model prepaid health plan with about 500,000 members in the states of Washington and Idaho. An "episode" was defined as an outpatient antidepressant prescription filled (the index prescription) during the study period with no prior antidepressant prescription filed in the preceding 180 days and a ICD-9 diagnosis of unipolar major depressive disorder, dysthymia, or depressive disorder NOS made during a treatment visit within 30 days before or after the index prescription. Data were obtained from four computerized record systems, including GHC pharmacies where about 95% of members fill their prescriptions, outpatient visit registration records, hospital discharge data, and mortality records (Simon et al. 2006). A total of 11,436 patients had 2 or more treatment episodes and 5,107 (6.2%) of the episodes occurred in patients < 17 years. Females comprised 69.5% of the sample.

The authors evaluated the risks of death by suicide and serious suicide attempts (defined as leading to hospitalization), whether these risks increased during the month after starting an antidepressant, and whether the ten newer antidepressants (bupropion, citalopram, fluoxetine, fluvoxamine, mirtazapine, nefazodone, paroxetine, sertraline, escitalopram, and venlafaxine) initially identified by the FDA warnings were associated with higher risks of serious suicidal attempts or death by suicide compared to older antidepressants.

During the 3 months before the index prescription, a total of 73 serious suicide attempts were identified. During the 6-month follow-up period after the index prescription was filled, there were 76 (93/100,000) serious suicide attempts and 31 (40/100,000) completed suicides. The probability of death by suicide was much higher in males (odds ratio [OR] = 6.6; 95% confidence interval [CI] = 2.9 to 14.7) but did not vary significantly with age. The probability of serious suicide attempts was not significantly different between males and females; however, it strongly correlated with younger age ($Z = 3.18$, $P < .001$) with an absolute rate of 314/100,000 (95% CI = 160 to 468) in children and adolescents and of 78/100,000 in adults (95% CI = 58 to 98).

The highest risk of serious suicide attempts was during the month before the index prescription and was primarily because of the increased risk in the 7 days preceding the index prescription; the authors attributed this to the fact that such an attempt may result in beginning treatment with antidepressants. Compared to the month before treatment, there was a decrease in serious suicide attempts during the first month after the index prescription; however, the number of attempts during the first month was greater than in any of the following 5 months, over which a continuing gradual decline occurred. This risk of suicide death during the first month after the index prescription was not significantly higher than in the subsequent 5 months (OR = 1.2; 95% CI = 0.5 to 2.9). During the 6-month follow-up there was a total of 3 suicide deaths in adolescents. The pattern of serious suicide attempts in adolescents over the 6-month period ($N = 17$) was similar to that in adults with the highest risk in the month before the index prescription, a sharp decline immediately after starting treatment and continuing to gradually decline over the next 5 months.

The authors found differences in the risks between the ten newer antidepressants and older antidepressants (primarily tricyclics and trazodone). The risk of suicidal death over the 6-month follow-up period was 34/100,000 for the ten newer antidepressants and 51/100,000 for the older antidepressants. The risk of serious suicidal attempts was 76/100,000 for the 10 newer antidepressants and 129/100,000 for the older antidepressants. Patients treated with the ten newer antidepressants had the highest risk of serious suicidal behavior in the month before starting antidepressants and the risk in the first months after the index prescription was not significantly different from that in months 2 through 5 (OR = 1.6; 95% CI = 0.9 to 3.1). Patients treated with the older antidepressants had the highest risk in the first month of treatment, which was significantly higher than in months 2 through 6 (OR = 3.6; 95% CI = 1.8 to 6.9).

The authors concluded that their data did not support the contention of increased risk of suicide deaths or serious suicidal attempts during the first month of antidepressant therapy; however, the risk of serious suicidal attempts was higher during the first week of therapy. The risk of suicide deaths appeared to be relatively constant during the first six months of therapy. The authors found no evidence that the newer antidepressants increased the risk of suicidal deaths or serious suicidal attempts compared to the risks of older antidepressants (Simon et al. 2006).

TRICYCLIC ANTIDEPRESSANTS

Indications for Tricyclic Antidepressants in Child and Adolescent Psychiatry

The tricyclic antidepressants have FDA approval for the treatment of depression only in those children at least 12 years of age, although it is well established that prepubertal children can be diagnosed with major depressive disorder (MDD) using research diagnostic criteria (RDC) (Spitzer et al. 1978) or Diagnostic and

Statistical Manual of Mental Disorders, Third Edition DSM-III (APA, 1980a) criteria (Puig-Antich, 1987).

A review of the literature on the use of tricyclic antidepressants in children and adolescents with major depression found them to be clinically effective in several open studies, but no double-blind placebo-controlled study has reported that tricyclics were superior to placebo (Ambrosini et al. 1993). However, the placebo-controlled double-blind study of Preskorn et al. (1987) found that desipramine (DMI) was superior to placebo when plasma levels were controlled (reviewed later). Geller et al. (1993) caution that the use of tricyclic antidepressants in depressed 6- to 12-year-olds may precipitate switching to mania and hasten the onset of bipolarity and perhaps increase later rapid cycling.

Imipramine (IMI) is also approved for the treatment of enuresis in those at least 6 years of age. There is, however, a considerable body of literature suggesting that IMI is effective in the treatment of attention-deficit/hyperactivity disorder (ADHD), school phobia (separation anxiety disorder), disorders of sleep (sleep terror disorder and sleepwalking disorder), and MDD in some children treated on an open basis.

Clomipramine, another tricyclic antidepressant, has been approved for the treatment of childhood obsessive-compulsive disorder.

Currently, there are no formal criteria for the prophylactic use of tricyclic antidepressants in children and adolescents. The risks versus the benefits of long-term use for prevention of recurrences of mood disorders in this age group have not yet been established, and such use must be based on the physician's clinical judgment (National Institute of Mental Health/National Institutes of Health Consensus Development Panel, 1985).

Tricyclic Antidepressants in the Treatment of Children and Adolescents Diagnosed with ADHD

Although the treatment of ADHD is not an approved indication, tricyclic antidepressants were among the second-line drugs most frequently prescribed in treating patients diagnosed with ADHD who have not responded to stimulant medication; they were used as the drug of first choice by some clinicians when comorbid diagnoses such as depression or anxiety disorder are present (Green, 1995). The use of tricyclic antidepressants (TCAs) has significantly decreased since the reports of sudden death with their use and the introduction of the SSRI antidepressants. Of the TCAs, imipramine hydrochloride (IMI) and desipramine hydrochloride (DMI) are the best studied and were the most frequently used, although nortriptyline hydrochloride, amitriptyline hydrochloride, and the antiobsessional drug, clomipramine hydrochloride, have also been found to be effective. Overall, desipramine hydrochloride appears to have a lower risk of untoward effects than IMI, amitriptyline, and clomipramine (Biederman et al. 1989a); however, cardiotoxicity is a major concern (see following text). There are few studies on long-term safety and efficacy of the tricyclic antidepressants in treating ADHD (Green, 1995).

The mechanism of action of tricyclic antidepressants in ADHD is different from that in depression. Optimal doses are usually considerably lower, and the onset of clinical response is rapid (Donnelly et al. 1986; Linnoila et al. 1979), although one study required 3 to 4 weeks for subjects treated with DMI to show significant clinical improvement compared with subjects receiving placebo (Biederman et al. 1989b). When used to treat ADHD, tricyclics improve mood and decrease hyperactivity but usually are sedating and do not appear to improve concentration (Wender, 1988). Tricyclic antidepressants have also been reported to cause small but significant declines in motor performance, which are usually of limited clinical significance (Gualtieri et al. 1991).

The preponderance of published studies strongly suggests that tricyclic antidepressants are effective in the treatment of ADHD. In fact, in the early 1970s, some authors considered IMI to be the drug of choice in treating ADHD (Huessy and Wright, 1970; Waizer et al. 1974). Most double-blind studies comparing tricyclic antidepressants with a stimulant, a placebo, or both have found that both drugs are superior to placebo; however, the stimulant drug is usually equal or superior to the tricyclic on most of the clinically significant measures of improvement and, overall, the literature suggests that stimulants are superior (Campbell et al. 1985; Klein et al. 1980; Pliszka, 1987; and Rapoport and Mikkelsen, 1978b).

Parallel to the situation with stimulants, there is evidence that patients diagnosed with ADHD may not respond to one tricyclic antidepressant but may have a markedly positive response to another. For example, Wilens et al. (1993b) found that 31 (70%) of 44 subjects who had had unsatisfactory responses to desipramine subsequently had positive responses to nortriptyline.

One difference noted in several studies relates to the longer serum half-lives of the tricyclic antidepressants compared with those of methylphenidate and dextroamphetamine; the therapeutic effects last longer with the tricyclics, and behavior after school and in the evenings of subjects receiving tricyclics is typically rated better by parents and others than behavior of subjects on the stimulants. The latter is true because when the last dose of the stimulant is given at lunchtime, it loses its clinical efficacy by late afternoon (Green, 1995; Yepes et al. 1977).

Pharmacokinetics of Tricyclic Antidepressants

About 7% of the general population has a genetic variation that results in decreased activity of the drug-metabolizing enzyme cytochrome P450 2D6 (PDR, 1995). Such individuals metabolize tricyclic antidepressants more slowly than usual and may develop toxic serum levels at therapeutic doses of < 5 mg/kg. Individuals taking the same oral dose of desipramine have been reported to have up to a 36-fold variation in plasma levels (PDR, 1995, p. 1417).

There may be large interindividual variations in steady-state plasma levels of tricyclics and their metabolites, although intraindividual levels are usually reproducible and correlate linearly with dose. Preskorn et al. (1989a) reported that steady-state IMI plus DMI levels varied 22-fold (from 25 to 553 ng/mL) among 68 hospitalized children, aged 6 to 14 years, who were prescribed a fixed daily dose of 75 mg of IMI to treat major depression ($N = 48$) or enuresis ($N = 20$); likewise, Biederman et al. (1989b) found that DMI serum levels varied up to 16.5-fold when fixed doses of DMI were administered.

Potter et al. (1982) found that about 5% of 47 subjects, including 32 enuretic males aged 7 to 13 years, were deficient DMI hydroxylators and that such subjects had 2 to 4 times the steady-state concentrations of either IMI or DMI per unit dose as the general population. Preskorn et al. (1989b) warned that persons who metabolize tricyclics slowly may develop central nervous system toxicity, which may be confused with worsening of depression, or severe cardiotoxicity when taking conventional doses of tricyclics and that deaths have occurred. Because of these variables, it is necessary to obtain plasma levels to avoid treatment failures for subtherapeutic levels or possible toxic effects from excessive levels.

Dugas et al. (1980) have recommended administering tricyclic antidepressants to children in two or three divided doses daily if more than 1 mg/kg/day is given to avoid or minimize untoward effects related to peak serum levels. Long-acting preparations (e.g., imipramine pamoate capsules) are designed for once-daily dosing; their use is not recommended in children and younger adolescents because of their high unit potency and the greater sensitivity of this age group to cardiotoxic effects.

Table 7.1 summarizes the development of symptoms of central nervous system toxicity. Preskorn et al. (1989b) have urged that therapeutic drug monitoring of tricyclic antidepressants be considered a routine standard of care for patients receiving these drugs.

Tricyclic Antidepressant Discontinuation/Withdrawal Syndrome

Some children experience a flu-like withdrawal syndrome, with gastrointestinal symptoms including nausea, abdominal discomfort and pain, vomiting, headache, and fatigue. These symptoms result from cholinergic rebound and may be considered a cholinergic overdrive phenomenon. Ryan (1990) noted that because of their rapid metabolism of tricyclics, some prepubertal children and younger adolescents may show daily withdrawal effects if they receive their entire daily tricyclic medication in one dose; hence, it may be necessary to divide the medication into two or three doses.

When maintenance medication is discontinued, tapering the medication down over 10 days to 2 weeks rather than abruptly withdrawing the medication will usually avoid the development of a clinically significant withdrawal syndrome. The clinician is cautioned that in patients with poor compliance, who in essence may undergo periodic self-induced acute withdrawals, the resulting withdrawal syndrome may be confused with untoward effects of the medication, inadequate treatment, or worsening of the underlying condition.

TABLE 7.1 ● **Evolution of Central Nervous System Tricyclic Antidepressant Toxicity**

Affective Symptoms	Motor Symptoms	Psychotic Symptoms	Organic Symptoms
Mood	Tremor	Thought disorder	Disorientation
↓Concentration	Ataxia	Hallucinations	↓Memory
Lethargy	Seizures[a]	Delusions	Agitation
Social withdrawal			Confusion

[a]Seizures typically occur late but can occur earlier in the evolution.
From Preskorn SH, Jerkovich GS, Beber JH, et al. Therapeutic drug monitoring of tricyclic antidepressants: a standard of care issue. *Psychopharmacol Bull* 1989;25:281–284.

Contraindications for Tricyclic Antidepressant Administration

Known hypersensitivity to tricyclic antidepressants is an absolute contraindication.

Tricyclic antidepressants are contraindicated for children and adolescents with cardiac conduction abnormalities.

Tricyclic antidepressants should not be administered concomitantly with a monoamine oxidase inhibitor (MAOI). At least 14 days must pass after discontinuing a MAOI before administering a tricyclic antidepressant.

Tricyclics may lower the seizure threshold and should be used with caution in individuals with seizure disorder.

Tricyclic antidepressants may activate psychotic processes in schizophrenic patients.

Interactions of Tricyclic Antidepressants with Other Drugs

Hyperpyretic crises or severe convulsive seizures may occur in patients receiving MAOIs and tricyclic antidepressants simultaneously.

Anticholinergic effects of tricyclic antidepressants may be additive with those of antipsychotics and result in central nervous system anticholinergic toxicity.

The central nervous system depressive effects of tricyclic antidepressants may be additive with those of alcohol, benzodiazepines, barbiturates, and antipsychotics.

Tricyclic antidepressants may diminish or reverse the efficacy of antihypertensive agents.

Cigarette smoking may decrease the efficacy of tricyclic antidepressants.

Many other interactions with various drugs have also been reported.

Untoward Effects of Tricyclic Antidepressants

Tricyclic Antidepressants and Cardiotoxicity

Reports of Sudden Death

At least eight sudden deaths have been reported in children taking tricyclic antidepressants. Although these deaths have not been proven to be cardiac related, cardiac arrhythmias, particularly tachyarrhythmias and torsade de pointes, are suspected.

Certain circumstances may increase the risk of the occurrence of torsade de pointes and/or sudden death in association with the use of drugs that prolong the QTc interval, including (i) bradycardia; (ii) hypokalemia or hypomagnesemia; (iii) concomitant use of other drugs that prolong the QTc interval; and (iv) presence of congenital prolongation of the QT interval (PDR 2005, p. 2611).

Six of the sudden deaths occurred in children taking DMI and two occurred in children taking IMI (one IMI only and one IMI and thioridazine). Four of the sudden deaths occurred after strenuous exercise (three on DMI and one on a combination of IMI and thioridazine); however, whether strenuous exertion might have been a precipitating or contributing cause was not addressed for several subjects. Six of the children who died were 9 years old or younger, one was 12 years, and one was 16 years.

A 6-year-old girl taking IMI for chronic school phobia and separation anxiety died 3 days after the dose had been raised to 300 mg (14.7 mg/kg) at bedtime (Saraf et al. 1974).

Sudden deaths were reported in three boys treated with DMI ("sudden death," June 1, 1990). These were two 8-year-old boys diagnosed with ADD (one received DMI for 2 years at an unknown dose and one received the same drug for 6 months at 50 mg/day) and a 9-year-old boy whose diagnosis, dose, and duration of DMI administration were not reported. All three of the boys had plasma levels in the therapeutic or subtherapeutic ranges (Sudden Death, 1990). A fifth child, a 12-year-old girl who had been prescribed a single daily 125-mg dose of DMI for the treatment of ADD, died a few days after the dose was increased to 50 mg three times daily; she was found unconscious after playing tennis and retiring for a nap and was not successfully revived (Riddle et al. 1993). The sixth sudden death, reported by Popper and Zimnitzky (1995), was a 14.7-year-old male who was prescribed 300 mg/day of DMI. His serum level on 225 mg/day was 132 ng/mL. He was in a residential treatment facility and collapsed and died a short time after swimming in the pool. In 1997, Varley and McClellan reported yet two more (the seventh and eighth) sudden deaths: one a 9-year-old male with multiple psychiatric problems who was started on DMI for treatment of depression during an inpatient hospitalization. He died suddenly 29 days after discharge after a total of 5 weeks of treatment with DMI. At the time of his death, he was taking 50 mg twice daily (3.3 mg/kg). The other child was a 7-year-old male with disruptive behavior and multiple psychiatric diagnoses, including adjustment disorder with mixed disturbance of emotion and conduct, oppositional defiant disorder, possible posttraumatic stress disorder (PTSD), and possible MDD. Two months before his death, IMI was increased to 150 mg at bedtime, and thioridazine, 25 mg, was added for extreme agitation, to be given if needed (p.r.n), every 2 hours. At the time of death, thioridazine was reportedly given as "25 to 75 mg at night p.r.n. for agitation;" it was not known when the last thioridazine was administered. After running several blocks home from school, the boy collapsed, went into cardiac arrest, and could not be resuscitated.

Several publications, reports, editorials, and commentaries rapidly followed the reports of these deaths. It became clear how little was known about the cardiac effects of tricyclics in prepubertal and even older subjects. Basically, the response was to be even more cautious when administering tricyclics not only to children but also to adolescents (Geller, 1991). In particular, it was recommended that a rhythm strip be obtained at baseline, during titration of medication, and at maintenance levels emphasizing measurement of the QTc to aid in identifying potentially vulnerable children (Riddle et al. 1991). Elliot and Popper (1990/1991) recommended obtaining electrocardiograms (ECGs) at baseline, at a dose of about 3 mg/kg/day, and at a final dose of not > 5 mg/kg/day. They also suggested using the following parameters as guidelines for cardiovascular monitoring in children and adolescents receiving tricyclic antidepressants.

PR interval: < 210 msec

QRS interval: widening to no more than 30% over baseline

QT_c interval: < 450 msec

Heart rate: maximum of 130 beats/min

Systolic blood pressure: maximum of 130 mm Hg

Diastolic blood pressure: maximum of 85 mm Hg

Although a more conservative viewpoint would be to obtain an ECG after each dose increase, Elliot and Popper (1990/1991) have pointed out that simply increasing the frequency of ECG monitoring does not necessarily reduce the risk of sudden death.

Cardiovascular toxicity of tricyclic antidepressants is of concern in all age groups, but especially in children and younger adolescents. Of particular concern is the slowing of cardiac conduction as reflected on the ECG by increases in PR and QRS intervals, cardiac arrhythmias, tachycardia, and heart block.

Schroeder et al. (1989) reported that the cardiovascular effects of DMI in 20 children, aged 7 to 12 years, who were treated with an average dose of 4.25 mg/kg/day (maximum of 5 mg/kg/day) were a 21% increase in cardiac rate and a 2.5% increase in the QT interval. Arrhythmias and clinically meaningful blood pressure changes did not occur. The authors concluded, concerning potential cardiotoxicity, that DMI was safe in children without heart disease, although ECG monitoring was essential (Schroeder et al. 1989). Baldessarini (1990) noted that children are more sensitive to cardiotoxic effects of tricyclic antidepressants than adolescents and adults; he suggested that this increased vulnerability may be related to the relative efficiency with which they convert tricyclic antidepressants to potentially cardiotoxic 2-OH metabolites. However, Wilens et al. (1992) studied steady-state serum concentrations of DMI and 2-OH-DMI (OHDMI) in 40 child, 36 adolescent, and 27 adult psychiatric patients. Serum levels of DMI per weight-corrected (mg/kg) dose rose from 50 ng/mL in children (age range, 6 to 12 years), to 56 ng/mL in adolescents (age range, 13 to 18 years), and to 91 ng/mL in adults (age range, 19 to 67 years). Contrary to expectations, 2-OH-DMI levels also increased with age from 17 ng/mL in children to 20 ng/mL in adolescents, and to 26 ng/mL in adults. The results did not support the hypothesis that children would develop relatively higher levels of OHDMI than adolescents and adults because of more efficient hepatic oxidative metabolism of DMI. Children either were more efficient in clearing both DMI and OHDMI than adults or absorbed DMI relatively inefficiently. In fact, the data supported the clinical impression that children and adolescents usually require higher mg/kg doses of DMI than adults to reach similar serum DMI and OHDMI concentrations (Wilens et al. 1992).

In a subsequent study, Wilens et al. (1993a) analyzed the effects of serum levels of DMI and 2-OH-DMI on ECGs in 50 children, 39 adolescents, and 30 adult psychiatric patients treated with DMI. With these expanded numbers of subjects, children and adolescents continued to have lower serum levels of DMI and OHDMI for weight-corrected doses compared to adults. Children and adolescents showed no significant associations between serum drug and metabolite levels and heart rate or conduction (PR and QRS) intervals, although there was a weak relationship between sinus tachycardia and higher total DMI plus OHDMI levels. When data from all the 119 subjects were combined, there was a modest correlation among DMI, OHDMI, and DMI plus OHDMI serum levels and PR and QRS intervals; however, the authors concluded that these were not likely to be clinically significant in any age group. About 10% of the subjects had combined DMI plus OHDMI serum levels of 250 ng/mL or greater, which may increase risk of cardiovascular toxicity. They recommended monitoring serum levels, and obtaining a baseline ECG and ECGs with increases in daily dose of > 3 mg/kg (Wilens et al. 1993a).

Because routine ECGs may not record infrequent cardiac arrhythmias, Biederman et al. (1993) examined 24-hour ECG recordings and echocardiographic findings in 35 children and 36 adolescents receiving long-term (1.5 ± 1.2 years) DMI therapy for psychiatric disorders. Compared with untreated healthy children, subjects' ECGs had significantly higher rates of single or paired premature atrial contractions and runs of supraventricular tachycardia and a decreased rate of sinus pauses and junctional rhythm. DMI levels correlated significantly only with paired premature atrial contractions. All echocardiographic findings but one were normal; the abnormal one was thought to be caused by a pericardial effusion of viral origin and not drug related. Overall, the data supported earlier impressions that treatment with DMI is associated with minor and benign cardiac effects (Biederman et al. 1993).

Walsh et al. (1994) reported on the effects of DMI on the autonomic control of the heart in 13 children, adolescents, and young adults (mean age, 17.5 ± 6.4 years; age range, 7 to 29 years). They noted that parasympathetic input to the heart decreases substantially with age and suggested that, because of the tricyclics' anti-cholinergic effects and their blockading the more active parasympathetic nervous systems of this age group, they increase supine blood pressure and pulse notably more in children and adolescents than in middle-aged and older adults. Their study documented that DMI reduces parasympathetic input to the heart and suggested that DMI may increase the ratio of sympathetic to parasympathetic cardiac input more in younger patients because of their relatively higher pretreatment levels of autonomic activity. This may explain the findings that DMI increased the ratio of low-frequency to high-frequency variability in heart rate and overall substantial decrease in heart period variability found in their study. Because reductions in heart period variability are associated with increased vulnerability to serious arrhythmias, treatment with tricyclic antidepressants may increase the risk of arrhythmias in children and adolescents. The authors emphasized that their data were preliminary and that further studies were needed before clinical recommendations could be made.

In a subsequent study designed to further evaluate the cardiac effects of DMI on autonomic input to the heart, Walsh et al. (1999) obtained 24-hour ECGs from 42 subjects; 12 subjects were 7 to 18 years of age and 30 subjects were between 19 and 66 years old. Ten of the subjects < 19 years old were diagnosed with ADHD that had not responded to stimulants, and one with MDD that had not responded to an SSRI. The authors assessed cardiac autonomic input using spectral analysis of the RR interval variability to determine heart rate variability. Pretreatment (off-medication) ECGs were done before administration of DMI in 41 cases. The ECG on DMI was done at optimal clinical dose, but 5 mg/kg/day could not be exceeded. Average duration on DMI was 33.1 ± 18.4 days for all ages. The mean dose of DMI was lower and the mean dose in mg/kg/day was higher in subjects < 19 years old than in older subjects (148 ± 99 mg/day vs. 195 ± 57 mg/day and 3.30 ± 0.77 mg/kg/day vs. 2.80 ± 0.87 mg/kg/day, respectively).

The authors reported that DMI treatment was associated with a significant increase in heart rate and significant decreases in RR interval variability at all frequencies. DMI had no selective effect on the ratio of high-frequency bands, which are thought to reflect parasympathetic input, to low-frequency bands, which are thought to reflect sympathetic input. Hence DMI had no impact on cardiac sympathetic/vagal (parasympathetic) balance. Although the RR interval variability was greater in the younger age group both with DMI and off medication, the magnitude of the effect of DMI on RR interval variability was similar in children, adolescents, and adults. The authors noted that the decrease in cardiac vagal modulation with DMI theoretically should increase the risk of arrhythmia, because parasympathetic input to the heart generally protects against the development of arrhythmias. However, they did not resolve the issue as to whether DMI treatment would significantly increase the risk of developing a life-threatening arrhythmia.

The preceding studies appear to conclude that tricyclic antidepressants in the usual clinical dose range (< 5 mg/kg/day) and at the usual serum drug and metabolite levels (250 to 300 ng/mL or less of DMI plus OHDMI) are usually associated with minor and clinically benign effects on cardiac function in all age ranges. They further suggest that children and adolescents are not at significantly greater risk for developing such effects compared to adults. The Ad Hoc Committee on Desipramine and Sudden Death of the American Academy of Child and Adolescent Psychiatry, established to investigate these concerns, reported at a members' forum at the 1992 Annual Convention that the risk of sudden death for children 5 to 14 years old who are treated with DMI in therapeutic doses is approximately the same as the risk of sudden death for similarly aged children in the general population, between 1.5 and 4.2/million/year ($P > .23$) (AACAP, 1992, p. 8). The matter remains controversial, however. Werry (1994), in a letter to the editor of the *Journal of the American Academy of Child and Adolescent Psychiatry* proposed severe restrictions on the use of DMI, whereas Riddle et al. (1994) rebutted his suggestion, noting "based on the available data, there is as yet no established cause of the deaths nor any scientific evidence that they were related to the DMI. As the number of sudden deaths is so small, the causal mechanism(s) are unknown and no specific cardiac finding has any known predictive value, clinically it should be considered mandatory to monitor both ECG changes and serum drug and metabolite levels and to keep them within recommended parameters whenever tricyclic antidepressants are prescribed."

Amitai and Frischer (2006) used the large database of the American Association of Poison Control Centers (AAPCC) Toxic Exposure Surveillance System (TESS) for the 20-year period, 1983 to 2002, to determine the relative risk of death that was associated with the ingestion of desipramine compared to other tricyclic antidepressants (amitriptyline (AMI), imipramine, nortriptyline, and doxepin) in younger children (< 6 years old) and older children and adolescents (6 to 17 for years 1983 to 1992 and 6 to 19 for years 1993–2002). (The case fatality rate [CFR] was defined as the ratio of the number of deaths divided by the number of exposures, an exposure being a report to the AAPCC-TESS concerning an individual ingestion of a drug or toxin.) The authors reported that there was a total of 24 deaths in the younger group and 144 deaths in the older group during these 20 years; most ingestions in the younger group were thought to be accidental while those in the older group were usually intentional or "suicide." The authors noted that poisoning fatalities are vastly underreported to poison control centers and that the actual number of fatalities is much higher. The CFR for desipramine was significantly higher than that of the other 4 drugs in both groups ($P = <.001$). Specifically, the CFR for desipramine exceeds that for amitriptyline by 7- to 8-fold, for doxepine by 4-fold; for imipramine by 6- to 12-fold; and for nortriptyline by 7- to 10-fold. The authors concluded that the reports on sudden death in children treated with desipramine coupled with its increased lethality compared to other tricyclic antidepressants when ingested accidently or in a suicide attempt, indicate that restrictions should be place on the use of desipramine in children and adolescents (Amitai and Frischer, 2006).

Other Untoward Effects of Tricyclic Antidepressants

Untoward effects to the central nervous system may include drowsiness, EEG changes, seizures, incoordination, anxiety, insomnia and nightmares, confusion secondary to anticholinergic toxicity, delusions, and worsening of psychosis.

Tricyclic antidepressants may cause blood dyscrasias; if patients develop fever and sore throats during treatment with tricyclics; a complete blood count should be taken.

Anticholinergic untoward effects may include dry mouth, blurred vision, and constipation.

Changes in libido, both increases and decreases, have been reported; gynecomastia and impotence have also been reported.

Preskorn et al. (1988) reported that cognitive toxicity was associated with supratherapeutic plasma levels of tricyclics.

Tricyclic antidepressants, including clomipramine, may cause acute psychotic episodes if inadvertently administered to some individuals with schizophrenia who have been incorrectly diagnosed.

TRICYCLIC ANTIDEPRESSANTS IN CHILD AND ADOLESCENT PSYCHIATRY

Imipramine Hydrochloride (Tofranil), Imipramine Pamoate (Tofranil-PM)

Because imipramine hydrochloride has been the most widely used clinically and has been more thoroughly studied in children and adolescents than the other tricyclics, it will serve as the prototype.

Untoward Effects of Imipramine

Imipramine has many untoward effects, some of which are potentially life threatening. Cardiovascular effects, including arrhythmias, tachycardia, blood pressure changes, impaired conduction and heart block, and a decreased seizure threshold, are particularly worrisome. See also the preceding section "Untoward Effects of Tricyclic Antidepressants."

Imipramine in the Treatment of Enuresis

Although the pharmacological treatment of enuresis has been shown to be effective (Poussaint and Ditman, 1965; Rapoport et al. 1980b), it should not be employed until possible organic etiologies have been ruled out by appropriate physical examination and tests. It should be emphasized that behavioral therapies (e.g., conditioning with an alarm and pad apparatus) are the treatments of choice for functional enuresis. There is a tendency for some children to become tolerant of IMI's antienuretic effects, and many children relapse after medication withdrawal. Desmopressin acetate (DDAVP, a synthetic analog of the natural hormone, arginine vasopressin) nasal spray or tablets may be effective in some cases of enuresis that do not respond satisfactorily to other treatments.

Imipramine's antienuretic effect occurs rapidly and appears to be unrelated to its antidepressant effects; it may directly inhibit bladder musculature and increase outlet resistance (American Medical Association, 1986). It also appears that the IMI plus DMI plasma level required for the effective treatment of enuresis is lower than that required for treating MDD. DeGatta et al. (1984) treated 90 enuretic patients, aged 5 to 14 years, with IMI and reported that the minimum efficient serum concentration of IMI plus DMI in most cases was 80 ng/mL. However, about 20% of the subjects did not respond satisfactorily to IMI even with adequate serum levels.

Fritz et al. (1994) reviewed prior studies of plasma levels of IMI and DMI, its metabolite, in enuretic children treated with IMI and reported on levels in 18 additional patients. The therapeutic efficacy of IMI was moderately but significantly related to increasing levels of mg/kg dosage. Intersubject plasma combined IMI and DMI levels varied at least sevenfold at every dosage. The combined IMI and DMI levels at 2.5 mg/kg averaged 136.0 ng/mL (range, 35 to 170 ng/mL) for complete responders, 116 ng/mL (range, 37 to 236 ng/mL) for partial responders, and 96.0 ng/mL (range, 60 to 157 ng/mL) for nonresponders. The authors noted that despite the lack of a clear therapeutic window, serum-level monitoring is useful in identifying subjects with low serum levels and suboptimal responses. In such cases, the dose of IMI may be raised before concluding that the medication is ineffective. Knowledge of the serum level is essential, however, to avoid the danger of further dose increases resulting in toxic serum levels in nonresponsive subjects who have relatively high serum levels.

A trial of IMI may occasionally be indicated when safer and more efficacious methods have failed and the symptom is psychologically a handicap or distressing to the patient, or perhaps when rapid control is essential to permit a child to go to summer camp or to travel.

The most frequent untoward effects reported in the treatment of enuretic children with IMI are nervousness, sleep disorders, tiredness, and mild gastrointestinal disturbances (PDR, 1995). DeGatta et al. (1984) reported that 40% of their 90 enuretic subjects had at least one side effect; 42% had loss of appetite, 16% had light sleep, 11% had abdominal pains, 8% had dry mouth, and 8% had headaches.

In clinical practice, initial ECGs often have not been done for the treatment of enuresis, because the final total daily dosage of IMI usually remains below 2.5 mg/kg and the risk of cardiotoxicity is low. In the light of the several sudden deaths reported in children receiving tricyclic antidepressants, even in usual doses, the author recommends a baseline ECG to screen for cardiac abnormalities that may increase the risk of conduction disorders secondary to tricyclic administration. It is suggested that bedwetters who void soon after falling asleep benefit if IMI is given earlier and in divided doses (e.g., 25 mg in midafternoon and 25 mg before bed) (PDR, 1995). A maximum dose of 2.5 mg/kg should not be exceeded because of the possibility of developing ECG abnormalities. Doses of more than 75 mg/day do not increase efficacy and do increase untoward effects (PDR, 1995).

Indications for Imipramine Hydrochloride Child and Adolescent Psychiatry

Note: Review the Black Box Warning at beginning of chapter or in package insert before prescribing.

Imipramine is approved for use in treating symptoms of depression in adolescents and adults. Its use in children is restricted to the treatment of enuresis in children who are at least 6-years old. Manufacturers state that a maximum dose of 2.5 mg/kg should not be exceeded in children (PDR, 1995).

Imipramine Dosage Schedule

● Children ≤ 11 years of age:

   Treatment of depression: Not recommended (however, see the relevant reviews later of the use of IMI in this age group).

(continued)

Indications for Imipramine Hydrochloride Child and Adolescent Psychiatry *(Continued)*

Treatment of enuresis: Not recommended for children < 6 years.

For children 6 years through 11 years of age, begin with 25 mg 1 hour before bedtime. If not effective within 1 week, increase to a maximum dose of 50 mg.

Treatment of attention-deficit/hyperactivity disorder: No official recommendations for age or dose exist. Based on the literature and experimental protocols, the following is suggested for children > 6 years of age: monitoring prerequisites for IMI should be followed. Begin with a low dose, either 25 mg/day or 0.5 mg/kg/day, and slowly titrate upward with increases of 25 mg once or twice weekly.

● Adolescents ≥ 12 years of age and adults:

Treatment of depression: An initial dosage of 30 to 40 mg with gradual titration upward is suggested. It is generally not necessary to exceed 100 mg/day (manufacturer's package insert) (however, see the discussion in the following text on treating adolescents and the importance of determining serum levels.)

Treatment of enuresis: Begin with 25 mg 1 hour before bedtime. If not effective within 1 week, increase to 50 mg with a maximum recommended dose of 75 mg.

Treatment of attention-deficit/hyperactivity disorder: No official recommendations for age or dose exist. Based on the literature and experimental protocols, the following is suggested: Begin with a low dose, either 25 mg/day or 0.5 mg/kg/day, and slowly titrate upward with increases of 25 mg once or twice weekly. Monitoring prerequisites for IMI should be followed.

Imipramine Hydrochloride Dose Forms Available

● Tablets (imipramine hydrochloride): 10, 25, and 50 mg
● Capsules (imipramine pamoate): 75, 100, 125, and 150 mg. These capsules are designed for once-daily dosing. Because of their high unit potency and the greater sensitivity of children to the cardiotoxic effects of IMI, their use is not recommended in children and younger adolescents.

Reports of Interest

Imipramine in the Treatment of Childhood (Prepubertal) Major Depressive Disorder. Imipramine and nortriptyline were the only tricyclics approved by the FDA for investigational use in the treatment of MDD in children 12 years of age and younger. FDA guidelines for ECG changes during treatment with either drug were as follows:

1. The PR interval should not exceed 0.21 second.
2. Resting heart rate should be < 130 beats per minute.
3. The QRS interval should not exceed 0.02 second more than the baseline interval.

The blood pressure of children receiving IMI, which can both elevate the blood pressure and produce orthostatic hypotension, should not be permitted to exceed 145/95 mm Hg (Geller and Carr, 1988). IMI levels above 5 mg/kg are not usually permitted in investigational protocols (Hayes et al. 1975).

Baseline studies that should be completed before initiating treatment with a tricyclic antidepressant include sitting and supine blood pressure, complete blood count with differential, electrolytes, thyroid function tests, blood urea nitrogen (BUN), serum creatinine, urinalysis with osmolality, liver function tests, and an ECG.

Several investigators have noted that in clinical practice an absolute upper-dose maximum for tricyclic antidepressants is not very useful because of the marked intersubject variability in pharmacokinetics (e.g., metabolism and elimination) and the fact that, although children as a group tend to metabolize and/or eliminate tricyclic antidepressants more rapidly than older adolescents and adults, some children, perhaps genetically slow hydroxylators, may reach very high serum levels on doses well below the recommended maximum (Biederman et al. 1989b). Hence, careful clinical monitoring, including serum levels, is essential.

Puig-Antich et al. (1987) investigated the use of IMI in prepubescent children diagnosed with MDD. In a double-blind placebo-controlled study of 38 subjects, there was no significant difference between response to IMI (56%; 9 of 16 subjects) and response to placebo (68%; 15 of 22 subjects).

These authors also studied total maintenance plasma levels (IMI plus DMI) in 30 prepubescent children and found a positive correlation between plasma level and clinical response. Responders had significantly higher ($P < .007$) mean maintenance total plasma levels (284 ± 225 ng/mL) than nonresponders (145 ± 80 ng/mL). The authors reported that a maintenance total plasma level of 150 ng/mL was the most important differentiating point between responders and nonresponders. Eighty-five percent (17) of 20 subjects whose values were above 150 ng/mL had positive responses, but only 30% (three) of 10 children with lower values responded positively. The authors also found nothing, including dosage, that predicted plasma levels (Puig-Antich et al. 1987). This is consonant with the finding that combined IMI and DMI steady-state plasma levels varied sixfold (from 56 to 324 ng/mL) in 11 boys receiving 75 mg/day of IMI (Weller et al. 1982).

Other important findings of Puig-Antich et al. (1987) were: (a) the more severe the pretreatment depressive symptoms on the Kiddie-Schedule for Affective Disorders and Schizophrenia (K-SADS) nine-item depressive score, the less likely was a favorable response to IMI ($P < .008$); (b) prepubescent children with the RDC psychotic subtype of MDD were much less likely to have a favorable response to IMI than nonpsychotic depressed children ($P < .05$); and (c) some children would require dosages of more than 5 mg/kg/day to reach plasma levels in the range associated with positive response.

These authors also reported that the following untoward effects were found in more than 30% of the children treated with IMI: excitement, irritability, nightmares, insomnia, headache, muscle pain, increased appetite, abdominal cramps, constipation, vomiting, hiccups, dry mouth, bad taste in the mouth, sweating, flushed face, drowsiness, dizziness, tiredness, and restlessness. Similar untoward effects were present in the placebo group, although at lower frequencies. The untoward effects were severe enough in 17 of the 30 children to prevent upward titration to 5 mg/kg/day; cardiac side effects were responsible in 10 of these cases. Nine children had increases in the PR interval to the maximum, and one child's resting heart rate reached 130 beats per minute. No child on placebo showed ECG changes from baseline, whereas nearly every child receiving IMI had at least minor changes (Puig-Antich et al. 1987).

Preskorn et al. (1987) reported a double-blind, randomly assigned, placebo-controlled study of 22 hospitalized, prepubertal depressed children aged 6 to 12 years; IMI was found to be statistically better than placebo ($P < .05$) by 3 weeks, when IMI plus DMI plasma levels were used by laboratory workers to adjust dosage of IMI to reach a therapeutic range of 125 to 250 ng/mL. Doses of IMI could range between 25 and 150 mg/day. The authors also noted that dexamethasone suppression test (DST) nonsuppressors showed greater improvement than DST suppressors. Total plasma levels below 125 ng/mL yielded a response rate only somewhat better than placebo, and levels above 250 ng/mL were associated with a lower response rate and an increased incidence of toxic untoward effects. The latter included prolongation of intracardiac conduction, increased blood pressure and heart rate, and mental confusion. The authors noted that, in a prior study in which clinicians were unaware of plasma levels and further increased dosages resulting in some children developing total IMI plus DMI plasma levels > 450 ng/mL, the antidepressant response was poor and several children developed toxic confusion that was incorrectly interpreted as a worsening of the depressive condition. This underscored the importance of monitoring plasma drug levels because a reduction in dosage, not an increase, would be indicated.

Based on their own data and those of Puig-Antich et al. Preskorn et al. (1989a) concluded that plasma IMI plus DMI levels ranging from 125 to 250 ng/mL were both efficacious and safe in treating MDD in children. These authors suggested using an initial oral dose of 75 mg IMI daily and then determining the combined plasma concentration of IMI plus DMI 7 to 10 days later, when steady-state levels would be expected. Based on their experience, 78% of children initially had plasma levels outside of the therapeutic range; 66% were below 125 ng/mL and 12% were above 250 ng/mL. Because intraindividual plasma levels were reproducible and linearly correlated with dose, the authors used the following formula to adjust the dosage :

$$\text{new dose} = (\text{initial dose/initial level}) \times \text{desired level}$$

The desired level was 185 ng/mL, the midpoint of the optimal range. Using this strategy, 84% of their patients achieved levels within the therapeutic range. The remaining 16% had subtherapeutic levels, possibly requiring additional adjustments (Preskorn et al. 1989a).

Imipramine in the Treatment of Comorbid Prepubertal Major Depressive Disorder and Conduct Disorder. Puig-Antich (1982) reported that 16 of 43 prepubertal males accepted for treatment of MDD had a codiagnosis of conduct disorder. These subjects did not differ on significant demographic and clinical variables from subjects diagnosed with MDD only. Approximately one-third of each group had auditory hallucinations consistent with RDC criteria for psychotic subtype major depression. A history of major depression was found to precede the onset of conduct disorder in 14 (87%) of the 16 cases. Thirteen of the 16 patients who completed the study had a full antidepressant response between 5 and 18 weeks after beginning medication. Although this was a double-blind study, only one patient had a full response during the 5-week double-blind period; the others received either IMI openly or were switched to DMI and titrated upward. Dosage of 5 mg/kg/day was the desired dosage, but doses above and below this were administered; exact dosage was not reported for these patients. Of particular interest, however, was the fact that 11 of the 13 boys who definitely recovered from the major depression also experienced total remission of their conduct disorders. In a majority of cases, conduct disorders reappeared following recurrence of another major depressive episode. In six of these patients, who were treated with the same drug and dosage associated with remission, conduct disorders persisted in two (33%) following remission of the depressive symptoms. Puig-Antich (1982) emphasized the potential importance of treating these comorbid disorders and avoiding the recurrence of the depression during childhood and adolescence in significantly improving the prognosis of this subgroup of conduct disorders, which appear to develop following the onset of major depression.

Imipramine in the Treatment of Adolescent MDD. Thirty-four adolescents with MDD treated with IMI in an open study with monitoring of plasma IMI levels showed some differences from prepubescent children (Ryan et al. 1986). Imipramine was titrated to a dose of 5 mg/kg/day; the adolescents had an overall positive response rate of 44% (15) of 34, but there was no relationship between positive response and higher plasma IMI levels. Another difference between the adolescents and prepubertal children with MDD was that, as a group, nonpsychotic subjects did not respond more favorably than the psychotic subtype. The authors hypothesized that adolescents with MDD were less responsive to IMI because of an antagonistic effect of sex hormones, levels of which increase during adolescence (Ryan et al. 1986).

Strober et al. (1990) treated 35 adolescents (mean age, 15.4 years; age range, 3 to 18 years) openly with IMI; they had been hospitalized and diagnosed by RDC criteria with MDD with at least probable certainty. Ten of the adolescents also met criteria for delusional subtype. After failing to improve after 1 week's hospitalization, subjects were treated for 6 weeks with IMI. Six (17.7%) of the 34 subjects who completed the study were unable to achieve the target dose of 5 mg/kg/day, because of untoward effects. Average daily dose was 222 ± 49 mg/day, and steady-state IMI plus DMI levels varied 11-fold (mean, 237 ± 168 ng/mL; range, 79 to 888 ng/mL). Eight (33%) of the 24 nondelusional subjects and one (10%) of the 10 delusional subjects were considered responders, suggesting greater refractoriness in patients with psychotic features. None of the responders had a plasma IMI plus DMI level below 180 ng/mL, but the difference between responders and nonresponders was not significant. Overall, only 10 (29.4%) patients were rated very much improved or much improved on the Clinical Global Impressions-Improvement Scale.

Lithium Augmentation in Adolescents Diagnosed with Major Depressive Disorder Who Were Treatment Resistant to Imipramine. Ryan et al. (1988a) reported in a retrospective chart review their treatment of 14 adolescents, aged 14 to 19 years (mean, 16.9 years), who were diagnosed by Research Diagnostic Criteria (RDC) with nonbipolar MDD; these patients had not responded to treatment with various tricyclic antidepressants (for a period of at least 6 weeks in 12 cases and for 4 weeks in two cases) by lithium augmentation while continuing treatment with amitriptyline, DMI, or nortriptyline. Lithium carbonate was titrated to achieve therapeutic serum levels. Six patients (43%) were responders and improved to the extent that they had, at most, mild symptoms of depression and were no longer being functionally impaired by their depression. Most responders improved gradually over the first month after the addition of lithium treatment. Their serum lithium level was 0.65 ± 0.06 mEq/L and was not significantly different from that of the nonresponders. The authors suggested that the addition of lithium carbonate could be a useful adjunct to the treatment of some adolescents with major depression who do not respond satisfactorily to treatment with tricyclic antidepressants (Ryan et al. 1988a).

Strober et al. (1992) treated 24 adolescents diagnosed with MDD who had not responded to 6 weeks of treatment with IMI by augmentation with lithium. The dosage of IMI at the end of the sixth week was held constant, and lithium was added on an open basis for a 3-week period beginning with doses of 300 mg three times a day that were then titrated upward based on clinical response to a final mean serum lithium level of 0.89 mEq/L. As a comparison group, the authors used 10 patients diagnosed with MDD in an earlier study who did not respond to IMI during the first 6 weeks and who continued receiving IMI only for the subsequent 3 weeks. Both groups improved significantly during the final 3 weeks of treatment as measured on the Hamilton Rating Scale for Depression (Ham-D). Although the group receiving lithium showed greater improvement, the difference between the two groups was not significant. Two patients (8.3%) in the lithium-augmented group were rated as "marked responders," as evidenced by a decrease of at least 50% in the Ham-D and a final score of < 10, between 2 and 7 days after addition of lithium. Eight additional patients (33.3%) showed partial improvement over a period of 14 to 21 days following lithium administration. The authors noted that lithium's efficacy as an adjunct in adolescents with tricyclic-resistant major depression appears to be much less compared to that in adults, in whom up to 70% respond favorably. They also suggested that a small subgroup of adolescents may show an initial robust positive effect and that other adolescents may show gradual but less improvement over time. A trial of longer than 3 weeks may be necessary to determine if additional adolescents might benefit and whether further clinical gains would occur in adolescents who showed some improvement. The authors noted that Thase et al. (1989) reported on a subgroup of adults who showed improvement only after 4 to 6 weeks of lithium augmentation.

Imipramine in the Treatment of Attention-deficit/Hyperactivity Disorder. A considerable body of literature attests to the clinical efficacy of IMI in the treatment of ADHD, although most studies find stimulants superior (for review see Campbell et al. 1985; Rapoport et al. 1978c; and Rapoport et al. 1974). Although IMI does not have FDA approval for use in the treatment of ADHD, some clinicians consider IMI or DMI the next drug of choice if a patient does not respond to stimulants. Wender (1988), however, notes that when used to treat ADHD, tricyclics improve mood and decrease hyperactivity but usually are sedating and do not appear to improve concentration.

The mechanism of action of IMI in ADHD is different from that in depression; it is rapidly effective, and lower doses are often required. Mean dosages reported in the literature have ranged from 20 to 173.7 mg/day. The development of tolerance by some children to the therapeutic effects of IMI within about 6 weeks presents difficulties.

Rapoport et al. (1974) compared IMI and methylphenidate in a double-blind placebo-controlled study of 76 hyperactive boys. Mean daily dose of IMI was 80 ± 21 mg (maximum, 150 mg), and mean daily dose of methylphenidate was 20 mg (maximum, 30 mg). Although both drugs were significantly better than placebo, most measures favored the stimulant drug. Some tolerance to the therapeutic effects of IMI appeared to develop after about 10 weeks of treatment.

In a double-blind, placebo-controlled, crossover-design study of 30 hyperactive children, Werry et al. (1980) found IMI to be statistically more effective than methylphenidate in its overall therapeutic effect. Untoward effects of IMI, however, were greater and more troublesome than those of methylphenidate. Methylphenidate was given in doses of 0.40 mg/kg; IMI was given in doses of

1 and 2 mg/kg/day. The authors found few significant differences between the two IMI doses but thought that the lower dose resulted in a slightly better clinical response and milder side effects (Werry et al. 1980).

A 1-year follow-up study of 76 hyperactive boys treated with IMI or methylphenidate found that significantly more subjects on IMI discontinued the medication because of lack of benefit or untoward effects, but that subjects in both treatment groups who continued on either drug improved equally (Quinn and Rapoport, 1975). The large dropout rate is a considerable clinical disadvantage in using IMI. It appears that tolerance to IMI may develop, resulting in deterioration after an initial improvement (Gross, 1973; Klein et al. 1980; Quinn and Rapoport, 1975; and Waizer et al. 1974).

Imipramine in the Treatment of Separation Anxiety Disorder (School Phobia/ School Refusal). Gittelman-Klein and Klein (1971) reported a double-blind, placebo-controlled study using IMI to treat 35 children diagnosed with school phobia (separation anxiety). Of the 45 children between 6 and 14 years of age who entered the study, 35 (19 females and 16 males; mean age, 10.8 years) completed the 6-week protocol. Dosage was administered in the morning and evening for a total of 75 mg/day for the first 2 weeks and then adjusted weekly. At the completion of the study, doses ranged from 100 to 200 mg/day (mean, 152 mg/day). Also, all subjects were treated simultaneously with a multidisciplinary treatment program.

Dry mouth was much more frequent in the active drug group, occurring in 50% of the subjects ($P < .003$). One child developed orthostatic hypotension requiring reduction of dosage, but all other side effects reportedly disappeared without dosage adjustment. The authors noted that doses of IMI < 75 mg/day were indistinguishable from placebo in this study.

Using 'return to school regularly within 6 weeks' as the criterion, there was no statistical difference between IMI and placebo at the 3-week mark, but by 6 weeks, IMI was significantly ($P < .05$) better than placebo (Gittelman-Klein and Klein, 1971).

Klein et al. (1980) emphasize that IMI is effective in reducing separation anxiety but that anticipatory anxiety may continue to be problematic. Imipramine doses of between 75 and 200 mg/day were effective for school-phobic children between 6 and 14 years of age; however, children with severe separation anxiety without school phobia sometimes responded to doses as low as 25 to 50 mg/day. School-phobic children who responded to IMI were found to show at least some improvement when doses reached 125 mg/day; once improvement began, further dose increases usually produced additional benefit. Response was usually maximal within 6 to 8 weeks. It was suggested that maintenance be continued for a minimum of 8 weeks following remission of symptoms and then tapered and discontinued (Klein et al. 1980).

Klein et al. (1992) compared the efficacy of IMI and placebo in a double-blind, randomized study of 21 children (14 males and 7 females; age range, 6 to 15 years; mean, 9.5 ± 0.8 years) diagnosed with separation anxiety disorder by DSM-III criteria. Nine subjects (43%) were diagnosed with comorbid DSM-III anxiety disorders, overanxious disorder being the most frequent. The 21 subjects comprised the nonresponders of a larger group ($N = 45$) who were treated for the month preceding entry into the study with vigorous behavioral therapy. Behavioral treatment continued throughout the 6-week treatment period, during which 11 patients received IMI and 10 patients received placebo.

Imipramine was begun at 25 mg/day for 3 days, increased to 50 mg for the next 4 days, and then titrated to a maximum dose of 5 mg/kg/day. Baseline ECGs were obtained, with subsequent ECGs recorded after every dose increase above 50 mg/day. Daily doses of IMI ranged from 75 to 275 mg/day (mean, 153 mg/day or 4.67 mg/kg) at the completion of the study. Children treated with IMI had significantly more untoward effects than those who received placebo. Irritability or angry outbursts occurred in five (45%), dry mouth in five (45%), and drowsiness in two (18%) of the children receiving IMI. ECG changes occurred, but no dosage reductions were required, because they did not exceed the recommended maximum values or changes from baseline (Klein et al. 1992).

There were no significant differences between the IMI and placebo groups on any measure; both groups showed about 50% overall improvement. These results are strikingly different from those in the earlier study (Gittelman-Klein and Klein, 1971). The authors note that although IMI may still be useful in treating separation anxiety disorder, its efficacy appears to be considerably less than previously thought (Klein et al. 1992).

Bernstein et al. (2000) conducted a double-blind, placebo-controlled study of 63 adolescents (mean age, 13.9 ± 3.6 years; 38 females, 25 males) with school refusal and comorbid anxiety and MDDs, who were treated randomly for 8 weeks with either IMI or placebo; in addition, all subjects received concurrent, manual-based, monitored cognitive-behavioral therapy (CBT). Adolescents with conduct disorder were excluded from the study. The study period was preceded by a 1-week single-blind placebo washout; no subjects were eliminated because of improvement during this period. Efficacy was assessed by clinicians using the Anxiety Rating for Children's-Revised (ARC-R) and Children's Depression Rating Scale-Revised (CDRS-R). Imipramine was administered twice daily and gradually increased every 3 to 5 days to reach a target dose of 3 mg/kg/day by the end of the second week. A nonblind psychiatrist monitored serum blood levels at week 3 and recommended increases or decreases in dose if levels were outside the therapeutic range of 150 to 300 μg/L; to maintain the blind, a similar number of patients receiving placebo were instructed to increase or decrease the dosage. The mean IMI dose after 3 weeks was 184.6 ± 33.3 mg/day and the mean IMI plus DMI blood level was 246.6 ± 227.6 μg/L. Eight subjects had levels < 150 μg/L and seven subjects had levels > 300 μg/L. At completion of the study, mean IMI dose was 182.3 ± 50.3 mg and the mean IMI plus DMI blood level was 151.2 ± 90.2 μg/L; nine subjects had levels < 150 μg/L, including three with no detectable drug or metabolite; the mean IMI plus DMI level was 58.0 ± 51.4 μg/L. Subjects receiving IMI with concomitant CBT improved significantly more than subjects on placebo and CBT in weekly hours of school attendance (70.1 ± 30.6 hours vs. 27.6 ± 36.1 hours; $P = .017$) and in decreased depression as rated on the CDRS-R (34.6 ± 8.9 vs. 45.7 ± 16.5; $P = .037$). There were no significant differences between the groups on the ARC-R and two self-report measures. The authors noted that although recent studies had shown CBT to be efficacious in school refusal without medication, the present study suggests that a multimodal approach (i.e., CBT plus pharmacotherapy) results in a superior response. The authors also noted that many subjects remained with significant symptoms at the end of the 8-week study despite their improvement. Only a little more than half of the subjects receiving IMI plus CBT were attending school 75% of the time. Follow-up to see if further improvement occurred, gains were maintained, or school attendance worsened was being pursued but the results are not yet available (Bernstein et al. 2000).

Three children with panic disorder who also had severe separation anxiety and agoraphobia responded well to a combination of IMI and alprazolam, a benzodiazepine (Ballenger et al. 1989).

Imipramine in the Treatment of Somnambulism and Night Terrors. Four children with night terrors, two children with somnambulism, and one child with both disorders were treated with IMI (10 to 50 mg at bedtime). The sleep disorders remitted completely in all children (Pesikoff and Davis, 1971).

Nortriptyline Hydrochloride (Pamelor)

Untoward effects of nortriptyline and other tricyclic antidepressants are discussed earlier in the introduction to the tricyclic antidepressants. Untoward effects of nortriptyline are also discussed later in the summaries of its use in children and adolescents.

Indications for Nortriptyline Hydrochloride in Child and Adolescent Psychiatry

Note: Review the Black Box Warning at beginning of chapter or in package insert before prescribing.

Nortriptyline is approved by the FDA for the treatment of symptoms of depression in adolescents and adults. The drug is not recommended for use in the pediatric age group because its safety and effectiveness have not been established in children.

Nortriptyline Dosage Schedule

- Children and adolescents ≤ 17 years of age: Not recommended. Safety and efficacy have not been determined for this age group.
- Adolescents at least 18 years of age and adults: Manufacturer recommends giving a total of 30 to 50 mg/day. One should start at a low dose and titrate upward based on clinical response (however, see recommendations of Geller et al. in the subsequent text, on the usefulness of serum levels.)

Nortriptyline Hydrochloride Dose Forms Available

- Capsules: 10 mg, 25 mg, 50 mg, and 75 mg

Nortriptyline Dosage Schedule for Children and Adolescents

Pharmacokinetic studies of tricyclic antidepressants in adults have shown that their elimination half-lives are sufficiently long to permit the frequent practice of giving a single bedtime dose once titration is completed (Rudorfer and Potter, 1987). Geller et al. (1987b), however, noted that 41 children, aged 5 to 12 years, had a significantly shorter mean nortriptyline plasma half-life (20.8 ± 7.2 hours; range, 11.2 to 42.5 hours) than 32 adolescents aged 13 to 16 years (31.1 ± 19.8 hours; range, 14.2 to 76.6 hours). Geller et al. (1985) also found that correlations between the mg/kg dose of nortriptyline and steady-state plasma levels were not significant in 33 children and adolescents aged 5 to 16 years. The clinical significance of these data, including the interindividual variation of half-life by as much as six- or sevenfold, prompted Geller et al. (1987b) to advise that nortriptyline should be administered twice daily for all patients up to 16 years of age and that plasma level monitoring is essential to ensure achieving therapeutic plasma nortriptyline levels.

Geller et al. (1985) have used a single test dose of nortriptyline to predict steady-state plasma levels and to determine the initial dose of nortriptyline and presented tables suggesting daily doses to reach therapeutic nortriptyline plasma levels (Table 7.2).

To use this method, the clinician must have access to a laboratory that can reliably assay nortriptyline levels of < 20 ng/mL. To use this table clinically Geller et al. (1985) and Geller and Carr (1988) suggested the following:

1. At 9:00 AM administer a single dose of 25 mg to patients aged 5 to 9 years, or 50 mg to patients aged 10 to 16 years.
2. Twenty-four hours later (9:00 AM the next day) draw blood to determine the plasma nortriptyline level.
3. Use the table to determine the suggested medication dose for the patient's nortriptyline level and age.
4. Seven days later determine plasma nortriptyline level 9 to 11 hours after a dose. If the level is not in the therapeutic range (60 to 100 ng/mL), adjust the dosage using the following equation (Geller and Carr, 1988):

TABLE 7.2 ● **Suggested Nortriptyline Hydrochloride Dose Schedules for Children and Adolescents**

Predicted doses from 24-h plasma levels after a single dose of 25 mg administered to 5- to 9-y-olds.[a]

24-h Plasma Level (ng/mL)	Suggested Total Daily Dose (mg)
6–10	50–75
11–14	35–40
15–20	25–30
21–25	20

Predicted doses from 24-h nortriptyline plasma levels after a single dose of 50 mg administered to 10- to 16-y-olds.[a]

24-h Plasma Level (ng/mL)	Suggested Total Daily Dose (mg)
10–14	75–100
15–19	50–75
20–24	40–50
25–29	35
30–34	30
35–40	25
> 40	20

[a] Total daily dose should be divided and given twice daily because of relatively short half-life.
Adapted from Geller B, Cooper TB, Chestnut EC, et al. Child and adolescent nortriptyline single dose kinetics predict steady state plasma levels and suggested dose: preliminary data. *J Clin Psychopharmacol* 1985;5:154–158.

Day 7 plasma levels/current dose = 80 ng/mL/adjusted dose

Geller et al. (1987b) have recommended that nortriptyline be withdrawn gradually over approximately 10 days to 2 weeks to avoid withdrawal symptoms. Only 6 of 30 children and adolescents 6 to 16 years old developed withdrawal symptoms when this was done. In all cases symptoms were mild, and in five subjects they were limited to the gastrointestinal system and consisted of stomachache, nausea, and/or emesis.

Reports of Interest

Nortriptyline in the Treatment of Major Depressive Disorder in Children and Adolescents. Geller et al. have studied pharmacokinetic parameters of nortriptyline and its use in treating children and adolescents diagnosed with MDD (Geller et al. 1985, 1986, 1987a, 1987b, 1989, 1990, 1992). There are no double-blind, placebo-controlled studies establishing nortriptyline's superiority over placebo in treating MDD in children or adolescents.

In an open study, Geller et al. (1986) found that therapeutic efficacy correlated with nortriptyline plasma levels. Twenty-two children, aged 6 to 12 years, diagnosed with MDD were treated on an outpatient basis with fixed doses of either 10 mg twice daily or 25 mg twice daily for 8 weeks. Initial dose was based on individual subjects' rate of metabolism of nortriptyline, as determined by baseline single-dose kinetics, with the slower metabolizers receiving the lower fixed dose. Fourteen subjects (63.6%) responded favorably to nortriptyline. Responders were not significantly different from nonresponders in terms of age, sex, weight, social class, duration of illness, or baseline or 2-week Children's Depression Rating Scale scores. Responders, however, had significantly higher mean mg/kg daily doses (1.02 ± 0.21 mg/kg; range, 0.64 to 1.57 mg/kg) than nonresponders (0.82 ± 0.51 mg/kg; range, 0.40 to 2.01 mg/kg). The mean nortriptyline steady-state plasma level was also higher in responders (60.31 ± 20.90 ng/mL; range, 18.8 to 111.5 ng/mL) than in nonresponders (30.86 ± 17.64 ng/mL; range, 12 to 54.3 ng/mL). Twelve of the 13 subjects who received at least 0.89 mg/kg/day responded. All subjects with steady-state nortriptyline plasma levels of at least 60 ng/mL responded, as did 4 of 7 children with levels ranging from 40 to 59 ng/mL. At the end of the 8-week protocol, 7 of the 8 nonresponders recovered when the dose was increased to achieve steady-state nortriptyline plasma levels of 60 to 100 ng/mL. Overall, 21 of the 22 subjects had good clinical response with minimal and transient side effects, and all ECGs remained within recommended parameters for prepubertal children. The authors thought that because children's plasma nortriptyline levels are stable over time, ECGs need to be performed only at baseline and once at steady-state plasma levels if they remain within recommended parameters (Geller et al. 1986).

Geller et al. (1989, 1992) enrolled 72 prepubescent children, aged 6 to 12 years, who were diagnosed with MDD, nondelusional type, by RDC (Spitzer et al. 1978) and DSM-III (1980) criteria in a double-blind, placebo-controlled study of the efficacy of nortriptyline. The study design was a 2-week, single-blind, placebo washout phase followed by an 8-week random assignment, double-blind, placebo-controlled phase. All subjects were outpatients, and most had coexisting separation anxiety. The children were chronically depressed: 96% had been ill for at least 2 years, and 50% had MDD for 5 or more years before entering the study. Of the 72 subjects entering the study, 12 (16.7%) responded during the placebo phase,

10 were discontinued for various reasons during the active treatment phase, and 50 (24 on placebo and 26 on nortriptyline) completed the study.

Using Table 7.2, the initial dose necessary to achieve a steady-state nortriptyline level of 80 ± 20 ng/mL was determined from 24-hour plasma levels. Any necessary adjustments to obtain mean steady-state plasma levels of nortriptyline and of total, trans-10-hydroxynortriptyline, and cis-10-hydroxynortriptyline (10-OH-NT) were made during the first 4 weeks of the double-blind phase.

Both the nortriptyline and the placebo groups had a low rate of positive response (30.8% on nortriptyline and 16.7% on placebo), and there was no significant difference between them. There was no significant correlation between mean nortriptyline plasma level and response, or between mean nortriptyline plus mean total, cis-10-OH-NT, or trans-10-OH-NT plasma levels and response. Because of the poor response rate and the unlikelihood of finding a statistical difference between the placebo and active groups if the protocol were completed, Geller et al. (1989, 1992) stopped their study at this point.

Geller et al. (1990) enrolled 52 postpubertal adolescents, aged 12 to 17 years and diagnosed with MDD by RDC (Spitzer et al. 1978) and DSM-III (1980a) criteria, in a random assignment, double-blind, placebo-controlled study of nortriptyline. Adolescents with delusional symptoms were not enrolled. Subjects had scores on the Children's Depression Rating Scale (CDRS) and the Kiddie Global Assessment Scale (KGAS) placing them in the severe range of pathology. Of the 31 subjects completing the study, 27 (87.1%) had a duration of symptoms of at least 2 years (10 [32.3%] between 2 and 5 years and 17 [54.8%] more than 5 years). The study comprised a 2-week, single-blind, placebo washout phase and an 8-week, double-blind, placebo-controlled phase. Using Table 7.2, the initial dose necessary to achieve a steady-state nortriptyline level of 80 ± 20 ng/mL was determined from 24-hour plasma levels. Mean nortriptyline plasma level was 91.1 ± 18.3 ng/mL.

Of the 52 subjects enrolled, 17 (32.7%) responded to placebo by the end of week 2, and four additional subjects dropped out for other reasons. Of the 31 completing the study, 12 were assigned to nortriptyline and 19 to placebo. The results of the study showed such a low rate of response to nortriptyline that the study was terminated early. Only 1 (8.3%) of 12 subjects receiving nortriptyline responded, whereas 4 (21.1%) of the 19 subjects on placebo responded. (The one responder to nortriptyline went on to have a bipolar course.) Subjects with higher nortriptyline levels achieved significantly worse scores on the CDRS ($P = .002$). There were, however, no significant differences between the two groups on final CDRS or KGAS scores.

It is most interesting that 17, or about one-third, of enrolled patients with chronic and severe depression responded to placebo within 2 weeks. However, 13 of the 17 placebo responders relapsed, 9 of them within 1 to 4 weeks (Geller et al. 1990).

Nortriptyline in the Treatment of Children and Adolescents Diagnosed with ADHD. Saul (1985) treated 60 patients diagnosed with ADD (age range, 9 to 20 years) with nortriptyline. The first group of 30 subjects was diagnosed with ADD and scored more than nine points on the Kovacs Children's Depression Inventory (KCDI). The second group of 30 subjects had ADD but scored 9 or less on the KCDI. They were initially prescribed stimulant medication but responded poorly and were switched to nortriptyline. Nortriptyline for both groups was begun at 10 mg nightly for 2 weeks. Because no patients experienced difficulty at this dose level, the dose was then increased to 25 mg twice daily. Fifty-four (90%) of the

60 subjects had positive responses. Satisfactory clinical response usually occurred at 50 mg daily; 75 mg/day was the maximum dose given. Within 5 to 6 weeks, typically there was a marked change in attitude followed by an increase in attention span and a decrease in impulsivity. The most clinically significant untoward effects at the initial dose were dizziness and sleepiness; their inconvenience was minimized by administering the drug near bedtime.

Wilens et al. (1993b) conducted a retrospective chart review of 58 patients (mean, 12.1 ± 2.9 years; age range, 7 to 18 years) who were diagnosed with ADHD and received nortriptyline. All but nine subjects had comorbid diagnoses, including 34 with mood disorder, 18 with oppositional defiant disorder, and five with conduct disorder. These were treatment-resistant patients who had not responded satisfactorily to an average of four prior medication trials. About half of the subjects were also receiving one or two other medications concomitantly. Nortriptyline was administered for a mean of 11.9 ± 14.0 months (range, 0.4 to 57.9 months) in mean daily doses of 73.6 ± 33.1 mg (range, 20 to 200 mg/day) or a mean weight-corrected daily dose of 1.94 ± 0.99 mg/kg (range, 0.4 to 4.5 mg/kg). Overall, 28 patients (48%) were rated as marked responders and 16 (28%) as moderate responders. Subjects with and without comorbidity responded equally well; all five subjects with comorbid conduct disorder responded favorably.

There were no significant differences between responders and nonresponders in mean daily dose (74.8 ± 31.9 vs. 70.0 ± 38.0 mg), in weight-corrected mean daily dose (1.9 ± 0.9 vs. 2.1 ± 1.2 mg/kg), or serum nortriptyline levels (96.3 ± 51.6 vs. 83.4 ± 43.1. ng/mL). Significantly more ($P < .03$) of the "markedly improved" subjects had serum nortriptyline levels between 50 and 150 ng/mL. Untoward effects were usually mild and necessitated stopping nortriptyline in only one child who became agitated. No clinically significant conduction abnormalities were noted on ECG follow-up assessment.

Prince et al. (2000) conducted a two-phase, 9-week, controlled study of 35 subjects (28 males, 7 females; mean age, 9.8 ± 2.6 years) diagnosed with ADHD by DSM-IV (APA, 1994) criteria. Nineteen (59%) had lifetime comorbid oppositional defiant disorder (ODD) and four (13%) had lifetime comorbid conduct disorder. During the first 6-week, open-label phase, subjects were administered nortriptyline in divided doses (before school and after dinner) that were individually titrated up to a maximum of 2 mg/kg/day over the first 2 weeks (unless clinical efficacy was achieved at a lower dose or untoward effects prevented further increase) and then maintained for the subsequent 4 weeks. Responders were determined *a priori* by ratings on the Clinical Global Impressions ADHD Improvement Scale of 1 "very much improved" or 2 "much improved" or by a reduction of $> 30\%$ on the DuPaul ADHD DSM-IV symptom checklist. Oppositional defiant disorder symptoms were rated on a DSM-IV checklist of ODD symptoms.

Mean nortriptyline dose at the end of week 4 was 79 ± 36 mg/day or 1.9 mg/kg/day, with a mean serum nortriptyline concentration of 81 ± 66 ng/mL (range, 10 to 316 ng/mL). At the end of 6 weeks, the mean nortriptyline dose was 77 ± 35 mg/day or 1.8 mg/kg/day. Thirty-two subjects completed the first phase; two subjects had dropped out because of untoward effects and one because of nonresponse. By the end of week 6, there was an overall mean reduction in the ADHD symptom checklist of 53% ($P < .001$); 29 subjects (84%) had reductions of $> 30\%$ of their baseline ratings. Opposition defiant symptoms also significantly decreased by 48% ($P < .001$) during the 6-week open phase, with 25 subjects (71%) having a $> 30\%$ reduction compared to baseline ratings. There was no significant correlation between dose or serum level of nortriptyline and improvement in ADHD or opposition symptoms.

Twenty-five of the 29 responders elected to participate in the 3-week double-blind discontinuation phase; of the 23 subjects who completed this phase, 12 had been randomized to nortriptyline and 11 to placebo. The subjects who continued to receive nortriptyline had significantly lower scores on the DSM-IV ADHD checklist compared to subjects receiving placebo ($P < .04$). Overall, subjects randomized to nortriptyline maintained their clinical improvements in ADHD and ODD symptoms, whereas those randomized to placebo had a significant reexacerbation of these symptoms and their week-9 ratings were not significantly different from baseline. During the study, heart rate increased by 18% ($P < .05$) but there were no clinically significant changes in blood pressure, in PR, QRS, QTc, or any new ECG abnormality. The data suggest that nortriptyline is efficacious in treating both ADHD and oppositional symptoms in ADHD and ADHD with comorbidity (Prince et al. 2000).

Nortriptyline in Comorbid Attention-deficit/Hyperactivity Disorder and Chronic Motor Tic Disorder or Tourette's Syndrome. In a retrospective study of 12 children and adolescents (age range, 5 to 16 years; mean, 10.9 ± 1.0 years) diagnosed with ADHD and comorbid chronic motor tic disorder ($N = 2$) or Tourette's syndrome ($N = 10$), Spencer et al. (1993c) reported that 8 (67%) subjects were rated as being markedly or very much improved ($P = .01$) in their movement disorders, and 11 (92%) were rated much or very much improved ($P = .0001$) in their ADHD symptoms. The average dose of nortriptyline was 105 ± 11.7 mg/day or 2.8 ± 0.3 mg/kg/day. Mean serum nortriptyline level was 122.7 ± 12.1 ng/mg for the 10 patients for whom such values had been determined. There were few untoward effects. The only cardiac symptom was a mild tachycardia in one patient; no clinically significant changes occurred in EEGs.

Amitriptyline Hydrochloride (Elavil, Endep)

Amitriptyline hydrochloride is a tertiary amine tricyclic antidepressant. Although the tricyclic antidepressants block reuptake of both norepinephrine and serotonin, evidence suggests that the tertiary amine tricyclics block the reuptake of serotonin more than the reuptake of norepinephrine, whereas the secondary amine tricyclics may block norepinephrine uptake more than serotonin uptake.

Pharmacokinetics of Amitriptyline Hydrochloride

Untoward effects of amitriptyline are discussed earlier in "Untoward Effects of Tricyclic Antidepressants" as well as in the summaries of its use in children and adolescents later.

Indications for Amitriptyline Hydrochloride in Child and Adolescent Psychiatry

Note: Review the Black Box Warning at the beginning of the chapter or in the package insert before prescribing.

(continued)

Indications for Amitriptyline Hydrochloride in Child and Adolescent Psychiatry *(Continued)*

Amitriptyline is approved to treat symptoms of depression. It is noted that endogenous depression is more likely to be alleviated than other depressive states.

Amitriptyline Dosage Schedule

- Children ≤ 11 years of age: Not recommended because of limited experience with treating this age group.
- Adolescents at least 12 years of age and adults: An initial dose of 25 mg/day titrated upward in 25-mg increments is suggested. Ten milligrams 3 times daily and 20 mg at bedtime may be adequate for adolescents who do not tolerate higher doses. Adequate therapeutic response may take up to 30 days to develop. Usual maintenance is 50 to 100 mg/day.

Amitriptyline Hydrochloride Dose Forms Available

- Tablets: 10 mg, 25 mg, 50 mg, 75 mg, 100 mg, and 150 mg
- Injectable: 10 mg/mL

Reports of Interest

Amitriptyline Hydrochloride in the Treatment of Children and Adolescents Diagnosed with Attention-deficit/Hyperactivity Disorder. Yepes et al. (1977) administered amitriptyline, methylphenidate, or placebo to 50 children diagnosed with hyperkinetic reaction of childhood for randomly determined 2-week periods during which each drug was titrated. The initial dose of amitriptyline was 25 mg 3 times daily; dose was titrated to achieve optimal clinical response. Dose range was 50 to 150 mg/day; the mean was 92.1 mg/day. Amitriptyline was, with few exceptions, comparable to methylphenidate in effectiveness in reducing hyperactivity and aggression in both the home and school environments. The authors noted, however, that amitriptyline was more sedating than IMI and that, frequently, doses of amitriptyline sufficiently high to control symptoms could not be tolerated. Sedation remained a problem throughout the 2-week period on amitriptyline. In an earlier study (Krakowski, 1965), however, 50 children with various diagnoses with hyperkinesis received maintenance doses of 20 to 75 mg/day (i.e., about one-half that used in the preceding study) for up to 9 months with positive results, and only one instance of severe sedation occurred. (The other subjects developed tolerance or the sedative effect disappeared with reduction of dosage.)

Amitriptyline Hydrochloride in Children Diagnosed with Major Depressive Disorder. Kashani et al. (1984) performed a double-blind, crossover study comparing amitriptyline and placebo in nine prepubertal children diagnosed with MDD. Dosage ranged from 45 to 110 mg/day. Six (66.7%) of the subjects improved on amitriptyline, a finding that was not significant ($P < .09$).

Amitriptyline Hydrochloride in Adolescents Diagnosed with Major Depressive Disorder. Kramer and Feiguine (1981) compared the efficacy of amitriptyline and placebo in treating 20 adolescents diagnosed with depression. Age range was

13 to 17 years. Amitriptyline was initially given in 25-mg doses 4 times daily and increased within 3 days to a maximum of 200 mg/day in divided doses. The length of the study was 6 weeks. Both placebo and active medication groups improved over the 6-week period, and there was no significant difference between the two groups. Although this pilot study suggests that amitriptyline is no more effective than placebo in treating adolescent depression, more studies and larger numbers are necessary before coming to this conclusion definitively.

Amitriptyline Hydrochloride in Adolescents with "Treatment-Resistant" Major Depression. Birmaher et al. (1998) conducted a 10-week, randomized, double-blind, placebo-controlled, flexible-dose study of amitriptyline (AMI) in 27 hospitalized adolescents (19 females, 8 males; mean age, 16.2 ± 1.4 years,) diagnosed by DSM-III-R (APA, 1987) criteria with nonpsychotic MDD. All subjects were taking antidepressants, and seven were also taking lithium at the time of hospitalization. They underwent a 4-week period of withdrawal and still met MDD criteria before beginning the study protocol. Amitriptyline was begun at 50 mg/day in divided doses and titrated, based on clinical response, upward by 50 mg/week to a maximum of 5 mg/kg/day, a total of 300 mg/day, or AMI plus nortriptyline (NTP) serum levels of 300 ng/mL. The average dose of amitriptyline at the end of the study was 173.1 ± 56.3 mg/day or 2.8 ± 1.0 mg/kg/day and the average total AMI plus NTP blood levels were 226.2 ± 80.8 ng/mL. Both the placebo and the AMI groups had clinically significant reductions in scores on the Hamilton Depression Rating Scale, the Beck Depression Inventory, and the National Institute of Mental Health Clinical Global Impressions-Improvement (CGI-I) and Clinical Global Impressions-Severity of Illness (CGI-S) Scales, but there was no significant difference between the two groups. Overall, about 70% to 80% of these chronically depressed patients who were admitted to a state hospital as treatment failures showed similar significant symptomatic improvement on both placebo and AMI. Approximately 30% of the subjects continued to meet criteria for MDD, and 60% had subsyndromal symptoms of MDD. The dose of AMI or blood level of AMI plus NTP was not related to clinical outcome or untoward effects. The only untoward effect reported significantly more frequently with AMI was dry mouth. Patients in the AMI group had significantly higher resting and orthostatic heart rates at the end of the study.

Desipramine Hydrochloride (Norpramin, Pertofrane)

Desipramine is a secondary amine tricyclic antidepressant. Although the tricyclic antidepressants block reuptake of both norepinephrine and serotonin, evidence suggests that the secondary amine tricyclics block the reuptake of norepinephrine more than the reuptake of serotonin, whereas tertiary amine tricyclics may block serotonin uptake more than norepinephrine uptake.

Pharmacokinetics and Adverse Effects of Desipramine Hydrochloride
Pharmacokinetics and adverse effects of DMI, including sudden death, are discussed earlier under "Pharmacokinetics of Tricyclic Antidepressants" and "Untoward Effects of Tricyclic Antidepressants" and later under the "Reports of Interest" for DMI that follow.

Indications for Desipramine Hydrochloride in Child and Adolescent Psychiatry

Note: Review the Black Box Warning at the beginning of the chapter or in the package insert before prescribing.

Desipramine is indicated in the treatment of symptoms in various depressive syndromes, especially endogenous depression.

Desipramine Dosage Schedule

- Children and adolescents < 18 years of age: Not recommended. Its efficacy and safety have not been established in the pediatric age group.
- Adolescents at least 18 years of age and adults: Usual dose is between 25 and 100 mg/day. One should start at a lower dose and titrate according to clinical response. A dose of 150 mg/day should not be exceeded. Adequate treatment response may take 2 to 3 weeks to develop. Therapeutic total plasma levels of IMI plus DMI are usually considered to range between 100 and 300 ng/mL.

Desipramine Hydrochloride Dose Forms Available

- Tablets: 10 mg, 25 mg, 50 mg, 75 mg, 100 mg, and 150 mg

Reports of Interest

Desipramine Hydrochloride in the Treatment of Adolescent Major Depressive Disorder. From 113 adolescents referred for depression, Boulos et al. (1991) identified a group of 52 who were diagnosed with nonpsychotic MDD by DSM-III criteria and who did not have an eating disorder, had not been treated with psychiatric medication, and had ratings of at least 17 on the Hamilton Rating Scale for Depression (Ham-D) and of at least 16 on the Beck Depression Inventory. These subjects were enrolled in single-blind placebo washout for 1 week. The 43 subjects whose rating scores continued to fulfill the preceding criteria then entered a 6-week double-blind protocol in which they received either placebo or DMI in identical capsules. Desipramine was initiated at a dose of 100 mg at bedtime. Additional doses of 50 mg were added the next two mornings to achieve a daily dose of 200 mg (100 mg twice daily), which was maintained for the duration of the study. Thirty patients completed the study; 12 received DMI and 18 received placebo. Seven patients dropped out for "personal reasons" and six because of untoward effects. A positive treatment response was reported if there was a reduction of at least 50% in the pretreatment score on the Ham-D. There was no significant difference ($P < .59$) between the placebo group (6 [33%] of 18) and the DMI group (6 [50%] of 12). No significant differences between the groups in subjective untoward effects were reported. However, major adverse effects that necessitated discontinuing medication in six patients occurred only in the DMI group ($P < .05$) and included an allergic-type pruritic maculopapular rash (three patients), vomiting and laryngospasm (one), and orthostatic hypotension (two). ECG abnormalities, including tachycardia, sinus arrhythmia, and nonspecific T-wave changes, occurred only in the DMI group but were clinically nonsymptomatic and did not require withdrawal from the study. Serum metabolite levels were not reported.

Kutcher et al. (1994) enrolled 70 adolescents who were diagnosed with MDD in a fixed-dose, placebo-controlled DMI protocol. During the initial single-blind, 1-week placebo period, 10 subjects were judged to be placebo responders and were dropped. The remaining 60 subjects (42 females, 18 males; age range, 15 to 20 years; mean age, 17.8 years) were assigned randomly to 6 weeks of placebo ($N = 30$) or DMI ($N = 30$). Desipramine was begun with a 100-mg 8:00 PM dose, and 50 mg was added at 8:00 AM the second day and increased to 100 mg on the third day. Desipramine was continued at 100 mg twice daily throughout the remaining 6 weeks.

Eighteen subjects dropped out. Significantly, more of these were on active medication (13 [72%] of 18), and 10 of them did not complete the study because of untoward effects. Nine (90%) of the 10 were receiving DMI; five subjects had allergic-type reactions (four had maculopapular rashes and one had mild laryngospasm), two patients had clinically significant orthostatic hypotension, and two had significant gastrointestinal complaints. The patient receiving placebo dropped out because of severe agitation. At the completion of the protocol, two of the 26 items on the Side Effects Scale were rated significantly higher among subjects in the DMI group: trouble sleeping ($P = .03$) and delay in urinating ($P = .007$). Although heart rate significantly increased in the DMI group, there were no significant differences in systolic blood pressure while seated or standing, diastolic blood pressure while seated, or PR and QRS intervals on the ECG between the DMI and placebo groups.

Forty-two subjects completed the protocol; the ratings of 15 subjects (36%) decreased by at least 50% from baseline on the Hamilton Depression Rating Scale at the end of week 6. There was no significant difference ($P = .53$) between improved subjects receiving IMI ($N = 8$ [47%] of 17) and placebo ($N = 7$ [28%] of 25).

Mean combined DMI level (205.06 ng/mL) plus 2-OH-DMI level (70.01 ng/mL) was 275.07 ng/mL. There was no significant correlation between DMI, 2-OH-DMI, or combined serum levels and the outcome of treatment. In fact, the 17 subjects receiving DMI who did not improve had higher mean values of DMI, 2-OH-DMI, and combined serum levels than the eight subjects who improved. The authors concluded that their data were consonant with other studies of tricyclic medication in depressed adolescents, which did not show the significant treatment benefit seen in adults but did show a relatively high rate of significant and unpleasant untoward effects (Kutcher et al. 1994).

Desipramine Hydrochloride in the Treatment of Enuresis. Rapoport et al. (1980b) found that 75 mg of DMI at bedtime had a short-term antienuretic effect that was not statistically different from that of IMI.

Desipramine Hydrochloride in the Treatment of Attention-deficit/Hyperactivity Disorder. Garfinkel et al. (1983) studied 12 males (mean age, 7.3 years; range, 5.9 to 11.6 years) who were diagnosed with attention deficit disorder and required day hospital or inpatient treatment for the severity of their symptoms of impulsiveness, inattention, and aggression. The subjects received placebo, methylphenidate, DMI, and clomipramine in a double-blind, crossover experiment. The mean dose of DMI was 85 mg/day and did not exceed 100 mg/day or 3.5 mg/kg/day for any subject. Methylphenidate was significantly better than the other three conditions in improving overall classroom functioning as rated on the Conners Scale by teachers ($P < .005$) and program child care workers ($P < .001$).

In an open study, Gastfriend et al. (1984) treated 12 adolescents (age range, 12 to 17 years) who were diagnosed with ADD with DMI for 6 to 52 weeks.

Eleven of them had previously responded poorly to stimulants or had intolerable untoward effects. Although these were outpatients, their symptoms were so severe that residential schooling or hospitalization had been considered for many of them. Desipramine was initiated with a dose of 10 or 25 mg/day and increased weekly to a maximum of 5 mg/kg or until an optimal clinical result was obtained or untoward effects prevented further increase. The mean daily dose after 4 weeks was 1.57 mg/kg (range, 0.58 to 2.63 mg/kg); 11 of the 12 patients improved, and five were rated "much" or "very much" improved on the Clinical Global Impressions Scale. Ten patients were followed for 21 to 52 weeks; their optimal daily doses ranged from 0.93 to 5.95 mg/kg. Nine of the 10 patients sustained their improvement for more than 6 months, and 8 of these were rated "much" or "very much" improved. Plasma levels for a given dose varied as much as 10-fold. Untoward effects were most troublesome during the first month; six patients (50%) experienced drowsiness; three (25%), postural dizziness; three (25%), weight loss and/or decreased appetite; two (16%), headache; one (8%), insomnia; and one (8%), racing thoughts. The untoward effects lessened in all cases following reduction in dosage.

Subsequently, in another open study, Biederman et al. (1986) treated 18 children diagnosed with ADD with DMI for 4 to 52 weeks. Initial dose was 10 or 25 mg of DMI, and the dose was titrated weekly. Dose at 4 weeks ranged from 0.7 to 4 mg/kg/day (mean, 2.0 ± 0.9 mg/kg/day); on later follow-up, doses were significantly higher, ranging from 1.3 to 6.3 mg/kg/day. Improvement at follow-up time (mean time at follow-up, 22.9 ± 15.9 weeks) was also significantly greater than at 4 weeks. Although there was sufficient time for tolerance to medication to have developed, it was not observed.

Biederman et al. (1989a, 1989b) reviewed earlier work in this area and studied the efficacy of DMI in treating 42 children and 20 adolescents diagnosed with attention deficit disorder with hyperactivity ($N = 60$) or without hyperactivity ($N = 2$). Sixty-nine percent of their subjects had responded poorly to earlier treatment with stimulants. The subjects were randomly assigned to a 6-week, double-blind, parallel-groups, placebo-controlled protocol. Desipramine was titrated upward to an average daily dose of 4.6 ± 0.2 mg/kg, a relatively high dose. This high dose was selected because of inconsistent findings in studies using lower doses of DMI in subjects with ADD (Biederman et al. 1989a). Patients treated with DMI had statistically significant improvement in symptoms rated on the Conners Abbreviated Parent and Teacher Questionnaires, compared to subjects receiving placebo ($P = .0001$). The patterns of improvement were similar in adolescents and children. There was no significant relationship between serum DMI levels and clinical response, making the designation of an optimal level inappropriate. Some subjects who improved had serum levels below 100 ng/mL. About one-fourth of the patients had high levels, between 300 and 900 ng/mL; of this group 80% (12 of 15) improved (Biederman et al. 1989b).

Untoward effects were usually mild and were more frequent in subjects receiving DMI than in the placebo group ($P < .05$); overall, there was no discernible relationship between serum level and untoward effects. Symptoms included dry mouth (32%), decreased appetite (29%), headache (29%), abdominal discomfort (26%), tiredness (25%), dizziness (23%), and insomnia (23%). Although no subjects developed any clinically apparent cardiovascular signs or symptoms, cardiovascular and ECG untoward effects, such as increased diastolic blood pressure, tachycardia, and conduction abnormalities, were statistically more frequent in subjects receiving

DMI. There was a suggestion that ECG changes occurred more frequently at higher serum DMI levels. Although side effects were rated as mild, the authors noted that in 71% of patients (22 of 31) receiving DMI and 52% of patients (16 of 31) receiving placebo, untoward effects prevented the medication from being raised to the target dose of 5 mg/kg/day (Biederman et al. 1989b). Of special interest is the fact that in contrast to reports of rapid improvement of subjects with ADD in response to IMI, subjects in this study required 3 to 4 weeks to show significant clinical improvement with DMI as compared to placebo (Biederman et al. 1989b).

Biederman et al. (1989b) suggested that a steady-state serum DMI level between 100 ng/mL and a maximum of 300 ng/mL is probably efficacious and safe for most children and adolescents but that some patients will require daily doses > 3.5 mg/kg/day to reach these serum levels. They estimated that optimal doses range between 2.5 and 5 mg/kg/day. The authors (Biederman et al. 1989b) recommended the following parameters as being more clinically relevant in the titration of DMI than accepting an arbitrary maximum limit in dose (e.g., 5 mg/kg):

1. The DMI serum level should be kept under 300 ng/mL.
2. The PR interval on the ECG should be < 200 msec.
3. The QRS interval on the ECG should be < 120 msec.

Desipramine shows some promise as an alternative medication for children and adolescents diagnosed with ADHD who have unsatisfactory responses to stimulant medication. Gualtieri et al. (1991) reported that DMI improved long-term memory performance, analogous to that reported with stimulants, when used in treating children diagnosed with ADHD. Its use requires strict clinical monitoring, including ECG and serum levels, because of its pharmacokinetics and cardiotoxicity.

Coadministration of Desipramine Hydrochloride and Methylphenidate in the Treatment of Attention-deficit/Hyperactivity Disorder with Symptoms of Major Depressive Disorder or Comorbid MDD. Rapport et al. (1993) studied the separate and combined effects of methylphenidate and DMI on cognitive functions in 16 hospitalized children (aged 7 years, 9 months to 12 years, 10 months) diagnosed with ADHD and MDD, ADHD with symptoms of MDD, or MDD with symptoms of ADHD. Following a 2-week baseline period, subjects received placebo, DMI, three dose levels of methylphenidate (10, 15, and 20 mg), and combined methylphenidate and DMI at each of the methylphenidate levels. Desipramine was begun at 50 mg/day and increased by 25 mg every 2 days, unless untoward effects prevented the increase, until plasma levels between 125 and 225 mg/mL were reached, because earlier studies had suggested this to be the range of maximum therapeutic efficacy in prepubertal children. Methylphenidate alone improved vigilance, both drugs had positive effects on short-term memory and visual problem solving, and the combination of both drugs affected learning of higher-order relationships. The effects of these drug conditions on mood and behavior were not reported.

In a separate report concerning the same subjects, Pataki et al. (1993) detailed the untoward effects of methylphenidate and DMI alone and in combination in a subset of 13 patients. The mean final dose of DMI during combined administration with methylphenidate was 148 mg/day (range, 75 to 300 mg/day) or 4.4 mg/kg/day (range, 2.5 to 6.6 mg/kg/day). The mean plasma DMI level during combined administration with methylphenidate was 170 ng/mL (range, < 50 to 228 ng/mL for the 11 subjects for whom it was available). As methylphenidate is reported to inhibit hepatic enzymes that metabolize tricyclics, DMI plasma levels alone and when coadministered with methylphenidate were compared. The mean final plasma level of DMI when administered alone was 159 ng/mL, compared to a level of 170 ng/mL when administered in combination with methylphenidate, and the difference in plasma levels was not significant. On individual bases, however, the most extreme variations were found in a subject who received 75 mg of DMI daily (2.9 mg/kg/day) in combination with methylphenidate and had a plasma level of 158 ng/mL and another subject who received 300 mg of DMI daily (6.6 mg/kg/day) that resulted in a plasma level of 146 ng/day.

Untoward effects were more frequent in the combined DMI and methylphenidate treatment than in any of the other conditions: nausea (17% vs. 8% in the 40 mg/day methylphenidate group), dry mouth (42% vs. 8% in the 40 mg/day methylphenidate and the DMI alone groups), and tremor (8% vs. none in any other group). The combination of DMI and methylphenidate resulted in an increase in ventricular heart rate that was significantly greater than that in the other conditions; however, this increase was not in a range that would place the children at clinical risk according to the pediatric cardiologist. Three children had sinus tachycardia on ECG: all three occurred during the combined drug treatment but were not thought to be of clinical significance by the pediatric cardiologist.

The authors concluded that, clinically, the untoward effects of combined DMI and methylphenidate treatment were not significantly greater than those for DMI alone; untoward effects were similar to those during administration of DMI alone, and there was no evidence that the addition of methylphenidate increased DMI levels significantly (Pataki et al. 1993). This study was conducted on a very small number of patients, and much larger samples are needed before definitive conclusions may be reached.

Desipramine Hydrochloride in Comorbid Attention-deficit/Hyperactivity Disorder and Chronic Motor Tic Disorder or Tourette's Syndrome. Although stimulants are the treatment of choice in ADHD, they may exacerbate tics or precipitate them *de novo.* Hence problems arise when children have preexisting tic disorders, or when they develop tics while being treated with stimulants. Indeed, some authorities recommend not giving stimulants to children with a family history of tics or Tourette's disorder.

Riddle et al. (1988) noted that Tourette's disorder and ADHD coexist in approximately 50% of children who are referred for evaluation of Tourette's disorder and that between 20% and 50% of such patients develop worsening of their tics if treated with stimulants. The authors treated 7 children with DMI, aged 7 to 11 years, all of whom had diagnoses of ADHD and various tic disorders (one with Tourette's disorder, three with chronic multiple tics, and two with family histories of Tourette's disorder, four of whom had developed chronic tic symptoms when previously treated with methylphenidate). Five of the children had an additional diagnosis of oppositional disorder. Desipramine was begun at 25 mg daily and increased by 25 mg every 2 to 3 days to a maximum of 100 mg, or a lower level when clinical improvement was satisfactory or untoward effects prevented further increase. Four children improved "remarkably," and one child "moderately" when rated on the Clinical Global Impressions-Improvement Scale CGI-I Scale. Two children were considered nonresponders. Six children showed no change in the status or severity of their tics. One child's intermittent eyeblinking became persistent after 3 weeks of DMI; this had also occurred in this patient during a previous trial of methylphenidate (Riddle et al. 1988).

In a retrospective study of 33 children and adolescents (age range, 5 to 17 years; mean, 12.0 ± 0.6 years) diagnosed with chronic motor tic disorder or Tourette's syndrome, 30 of whom had comorbid ADHD, Spencer et al. (1993a) reported that 27 (82%) of the 33 had significant improvement ($P = .0001$) in their movement disorders and 24 (80%) of the 30 with ADHD had significant improvements ($P = .0001$) in their ADHD symptoms when treated with DMI. The average dose of DMI was 127 ± 9.8 mg/day or 3.5 ± 0.3 mg/kg/day. Mean serum DMI level was 132 ± 16 ng/mg for the 22 patients for whom such values had been determined. Untoward effects, rash (one) and abdominal pain (one), caused two patients to withdraw prematurely from the study, precluding their inclusion in the analysis of data. The study was discontinued in four patients because of untoward effects: nausea and vomiting (one), irritability and agitation (two), and worsening of a tic (one). Eight subjects (24%) had asymptomatic cardiac abnormalities including new onset of incomplete right bundle branch block (four), junctional rhythms (two), benign ectopic atrial contractions on Holter monitor (one), and an increase in the QTc interval (one).

It is unclear why none of the subjects in the study of Riddle et al. (1988) had improvement in their tic disorders, whereas subjects in the 1993 study of Spencer et al. showed very significant improvement. Although further experience is necessary to establish that DMI is both safe and efficacious in treating children and adolescents with coexisting ADHD and tic disorder, it appears to be a potentially useful alternative treatment for children whose ADHD is of sufficient severity to necessitate pharmacological intervention and for those diagnosed with ADHD who develop tics after the initiation of stimulant therapy.

Clomipramine Hydrochloride (Anafranil)

Clomipramine is an antiobsessional drug that belongs to the class of tricyclic antidepressants. Clomipramine itself has potent inhibitory effects on the neuronal reuptake of serotonin as compared with neuronal reuptake of norepinephrine; however, its primary metabolite, desmethylclomipramine, effectively inhibits norepinephrine uptake.

Flament et al. (1987) studied the actions of clomipramine on peripheral measures of serotonergic and noradrenergic function in children and adolescents diagnosed with obsessive-compulsive disorder. They compared 29 such children and adolescents (mean age, 13.9 ± 2.5 years; range, 8 to 18 years) with controls and found that a high pretreatment level of platelet serotonin was a strong predictor of a favorable clinical response and that clomipramine treatment produced a very marked decrease in platelet serotonin concentration in all patients ($P < .0001$). Clomipramine treatment also produced a trend toward reduction in platelet monoamine oxidase (MAO) activity ($P = .11$) and increased peripheral noradrenergic function. The plasma level of norepinephrine in standing subjects increased significantly ($P < .008$). These data suggest that clomipramine's inhibition of serotonin uptake may be essential to its antiobsessional effect (Flament et al. 1987).

Pharmacokinetics of Clomipramine Hydrochloride

Clomipramine has a long half-life. The mean half-life of a single 150-mg dose is 32 hours, and the mean half-life of its major metabolite, desmethylclomipramine, is 69 hours. Steady-state serum levels usually occur within 1 to 2 weeks at a given daily dosage. Children and adolescents < 15 years of age had significantly lower plasma concentrations for a given dose compared to adults (package insert). Dugas et al. (1980) reported that peak plasma clomipramine levels were achieved 3 to 4 hours after ingestion in the three children they studied and reported an apparent plasma terminal half-life of 11.9 to 17.3 hours. The bioavailability of clomipramine is not significantly affected by ingestion with food, and administering it during initial titration in divided doses with meals helps to reduce gastrointestinal side effects. Clomipramine is metabolized largely into its major bioactive metabolite, desmethylclomipramine; both compounds are ultimately metabolized into their glucuronide conjugates by the liver. The metabolites are excreted through the bile duct and the kidneys.

Contraindications for the Administration of Clomipramine Hydrochloride

Known hypersensitivity to clomipramine hydrochloride is a contraindication.

Untoward Effects of Clomipramine Hydrochloride

The most significant risk of clomipramine appears to be the development of seizures. Risk for seizures is cumulative and, for doses up to 300 mg/day, increased from 0.64% at 90 days to 1.45% at 1 year. Other untoward effects that occur in children and adolescents include somnolence, tremor, dizziness, headache, sleep disorders, increased sweating, dry mouth, gastrointestinal effects (constipation and dyspepsia), anorexia, fatigue, cardiovascular effects (postural hypotension, palpitations, tachycardia, and syncope), abnormalities of vision, urinary retention, dysmenorrhea in females, and ejaculation failure in males (package insert). Because of reports of blood dyscrasias, a complete blood cell count should be determined in patients who develop fever and sore throat during the course of treatment.

Dugas et al. (1980) reported in their study of 8 children and 28 adolescents who were administered clomipramine for enuresis or depressive symptomatology that the incidence of untoward effects was clearly related to the clomipramine plasma concentration. Untoward effects occurred in about 15% to 20% of patients with plasma clomipramine levels below 60 ng/mL and were present in more than 90% of cases with serum levels above 90 ng/mL. Hypotension occurred only in cases with serum levels above 80 ng/mL. No discernible relationship was found between untoward effects and plasma levels of desmethylclomipramine.

Indications for Clomipramine Hydrochloride in Child and Adolescent Psychiatry

Note: Review the Black Box Warning at the beginning of the chapter or in the package insert before prescribing.

Clomipramine has been approved by the FDA for the treatment of obsessions and compulsions in patients at least 10 years of age who have been diagnosed with obsessive-compulsive disorder.

Clomipramine Dosage Schedule for Children and Adolescents

- Children ≤ 9 years of age: Not recommended.

(continued)

Indications for Clomipramine Hydrochloride in Child and Adolescent Psychiatry *(Continued)*

- Children and adolescents 10 to 17 years of age: Initial dose of 25 mg/day, titrated upward to a daily maximum of 100 mg or 3 mg/kg/day, whichever is less, over the first 2 weeks. Subsequently, dosage may be increased gradually to a maximum of 200 mg/day or 3 mg/kg/day, whichever is less. After the optimal dose has been determined, clomipramine may be given in a single bedtime dose to minimize daytime sedation.
- Adolescents at least 18 years of age and adults: As above, but the maximum dose can be increased to 250 mg/day.

Clomipramine Withdrawal Syndrome

Abrupt withdrawal of clomipramine may result in withdrawal symptoms similar to those that occur when the tricyclics used in treating depression are suddenly discontinued. Symptoms may include dizziness, nausea, vomiting, headache, malaise, sleep disturbances, hyperthermia, irritability, and worsening of psychiatric status. Hence a gradual tapering of the dose over a period of 10 days to 2 weeks is recommended.

Clomipramine Hydrochloride Dose Forms Available

- Capsules: 25 mg, 50 mg, and 75 mg

Reports of Interest

Clomipramine Hydrochloride in the Treatment of Obsessive-Compulsive Disorder in Children and Adolescents. There are few published studies on the use of clomipramine in children and adolescents diagnosed with obsessive-compulsive disorder. Those of Flament et al. (1985, 1987) and of Leonard et al. (1989) include some children below the age of 10 years and are summarized below.

Clomipramine was found to be significantly superior to placebo in a placebo-controlled, double-blind, crossover study of 19 subjects whose ages ranged from 10 to 18 years (mean, 14.5 ± 2.3 years) who were diagnosed with severe primary obsessive-compulsive disorder (Flament et al. 1985). The dose range was 100 to 200 mg/day (mean, 141 ± 30 mg/day). The experimental data suggested that clomipramine has a direct antiobsessional action that is independent of any antidepressant effect. In fact, 10 of the subjects had been previously treated with other tricyclics without significant benefit. Flament et al. (1987) increased the number of their subjects to 29 (mean age, 13.9 ± 2.5 years; range, 8 to 18 years) and reported the continued efficacy of clomipramine; the mean daily dose of clomipramine was 134 ± 33 mg/day.

Leonard et al. (1989) compared the efficacy of clomipramine and DMI in the treatment of severe primary obsessive-compulsive disorder in 49 child and adolescent subjects (31 males and 18 females) (mean age, 13.86 ± 2.87 years; range, 7 to 19 years) in a 10-week crossover-design study. Administration of clomipramine was begun at 25 mg/day for children weighing 25 kg or less and at 50 mg/day for subjects weighing more than 25 kg. Dosage was increased weekly by an amount equal to each subject's initial dose. Maximum dosage did not exceed 250 mg/day or 5 mg/kg/day. The mean dose of clomipramine at week 5 was

150 ± 53 mg/day, with a range of 50 to 250 mg/day. Clomipramine was markedly superior to desipramine DMI in decreasing obsessive-compulsive symptoms on several rating scales. In addition, 64% of patients who improved significantly when initially on clomipramine experienced relapse following the crossover to DMI; this was a relapse rate similar to that for placebo in the preceding Flament (1985) study. The most common side effects reported were dry mouth, tremor, tiredness, dizziness, difficulty sleeping, sweating, constipation, poor appetite, and weakness.

Leonard et al. (1991) reported that, of the 48 children completing the preceding 1989 study, 28 (58%) were still receiving maintenance clomipramine 4 to 32 months later. Twenty-six of these patients agreed to participate in an 8-month double-blind study in which DMI was substituted for clomipramine. At the time of entry to the protocol, subjects' daily doses of clomipramine ranged from 50 to 250 mg (mean dose, 134.7 ± 58.2 mg/day or 2.4 ± 0.6 mg/kg/day). Subjects continued to receive clomipramine at their maintenance level for 3 months, at which time DMI was substituted for clomipramine for the next 2 months. For the final 3-month period, all subjects received clomipramine. Twenty subjects completed the study. Eight of nine patients (89%) randomly assigned to DMI relapsed during the 2-month period, whereas only 2 (18%) of 11 patients remaining on clomipramine relapsed. The authors noted that the eight patients who relapsed on DMI experienced symptom improvement to previous levels within 1 month after clomipramine was reinstituted. This is clinically important because it suggests that a significant percentage of children and adolescents need long-term drug treatment to prevent recurrence of obsessive-compulsive symptoms; however, if relapse occurs when an attempt to discontinue clomipramine is made, comparable clinical control can usually be regained upon reinstating clomipramine.

DeVeaugh-Geiss et al. (1992) reported a multicenter trial in which 60 children and adolescents, aged 10 to 17 years, diagnosed with obsessive-compulsive disorder were administered clomipramine in a 10-week, double-blind, fully randomized, parallel-groups, placebo-controlled study. Thirty-one patients were assigned to the clomipramine group and 29 to the placebo group; except for an excess of males in the clomipramine group, they were comparable. Placebo was administered to all patients under single-blind conditions for the first 2 weeks. During the active drug stage, the initial daily dose was 25 mg of active drug or placebo; over the next 2 weeks, this dose was titrated to either 75 mg or 100 mg daily based on weight. Subsequent increases to a maximum of 3 mg/kg/day or 200 mg were permitted at the discretion of the investigator. Twenty-seven subjects in each group completed the study. Untoward effects were typical of the tricyclic antidepressants. The patients receiving clomipramine improved significantly compared with those in the placebo group. On the Yale–Brown Obsessive-Compulsive Scale (Y-BOCS) the clomipramine group had a mean reduction in score of 37% and the placebo group a reduction of 8% ($P < .05$), and on the National Institute of Mental Health (NIMH) Global Scale the groups had reductions of 34% and 6%, respectively ($P < .05$).

Evidence suggests that clomipramine is effective for children and adolescents with severe obsessive-compulsive disorder, however, the FDA has not approved for advertising it as effective and safe in treating children < 10 years of age.

Clomipramine Hydrochloride in the Treatment of Attention-deficit/Hyperactivity Disorder. Garfinkel et al. (1983) compared the clinical efficacy of methylphenidate, DMI, and clomipramine in a double-blind, placebo-controlled, crossover study of 12 males (mean age, 7.3 years; range, 5.9 to 11.6 years) diagnosed with attention deficit disorder who required day hospital or inpatient treatment for severe impulsiveness, attention deficit, and aggression. The mean dose of clomipramine was 85 mg/day and did not exceed 100 mg or 3.5 mg/kg/day for any subject. Methylphenidate was significantly better than the other three conditions in improving overall classroom functioning as rated on the Conners Scale by teachers ($P < .005$) and program child care workers ($P < .001$). Clomipramine, however, was significantly better than DMI in reducing scores reflecting aggressivity, impulsivity, and depressive/affective symptoms. Based on these data, clomipramine would merit further study in treating children and adolescents with ADHD who do not respond satisfactorily to stimulant medication.

Clomipramine Hydrochloride in the Treatment of Autistic Disorder. Gordon et al. (1993) conducted a double-blind comparison of clomipramine, DMI, and placebo in 30 subjects (20 males and 10 females; age range, 6 to 23 years; mean, 10.4 ± 4.11 years) diagnosed with autistic disorder to assess the efficacy of clomipramine in treating obsessive-compulsive and stereotyped motor behaviors. During the initial 2-week, single-blind, placebo washout period, two patients were dropped, one because of positive response and the other because of a refusal to take pills. Fourteen subjects were randomly assigned to a 10-week, double-blind, crossover comparison of clomipramine and placebo, and the other 14 subjects were randomly assigned to a similar comparison of clomipramine and DMI. Two patients were dropped from each group—a 23-year-old man on placebo because of violent outbursts, a 7-year-old girl on clomipramine secondary to a grand mal seizure, and two others for extraneous reasons. The 12 patients in the clomipramine/placebo comparison group showed significantly reduced autistic behaviors ($P = .0001$), anger/uncooperativeness ($P = .0001$), hyperactivity ($P = .001$), but not speech deviance ($P = .27$) in week-5 ratings on the 14-item Autism Relevant Subscale of the Children's Psychiatric Rating Scale (CPRS) while receiving clomipramine. These subjects also had a significant improvement in obsessive-compulsive symptoms ($P = .001$) and overall improvement on the Efficacy Index of the Clinical Global Impressions Scale (CGIS) ($P = .0001$) during the period on the active drug. The 12 patients in the clomipramine/DMI comparison group improved significantly more during the period on clomipramine than during the period on DMI on week-5 ratings on the Autism Relevant Subscale of the CPRS ($P = .0003$) and anger/uncooperativeness ($P = .008$). The two drugs were not significantly different on the hyperactivity factor, but both were better than placebo; and clomipramine showed a trend toward improvement on the speech factor compared to DMI ($P = .08$). Obsessive-compulsive symptoms improved significantly more with clomipramine ($P = .001$), and clomipramine was superior to DMI on the Efficacy Index of the CGIS ($P = .005$). The authors noted that self-injurious behaviors (SIB) such as hitting, kicking, biting, and pinching, which were present in four patients who had not responded to intensive behavioral and drug interventions in two cases, improved significantly in all four subjects when they were receiving clomipramine. Untoward effects of clomipramine were usually minor, and they were not significantly different from placebo or DMI. However, dosage of clomipramine was reduced in one patient because of prolongation of QTc interval to 450 msec and in another because of severe tachycardia (Gordon et al. 1993).

Five patients who continued to be maintained on clomipramine underwent a double-blind placebo substitution for 8 weeks between months 5 and 12 of maintenance therapy. Four (80%) of the five worsened during the period on placebo but regained former clinical improvement when clomipramine was reinstated (Gordon et al. 1993).

Clomipramine Hydrochloride in the Treatment of Enuresis. Dugas et al. (1980) administered clomipramine to 10 enuretic children. A therapeutic effect was observed at plasma clomipramine concentrations of 20 to 60 ng/mL, whereas lower and higher levels were associated with lack of therapeutic efficacy or untoward effects. In a later report, the sample was increased to 31 enuretic children (Morselli et al. 1983). Of the 21 who had good therapeutic outcomes, 16 (76%) had plasma steady-state clomipramine concentrations > 15 ng/mL, whereas only 3 of the 10 nonresponders had such high plasma levels. The plasma level differences between the responders and the nonresponders were significant ($P < .05$).

Clomipramine Hydrochloride in the Treatment of Depressive Symptoms. Dugas et al. (1980) treated one boy, 8.5 years old, and 25 adolescents, 13 to 19 years old, who had significant depressive symptomatology with clomipramine. Clomipramine doses ranged from 0.24 to 2.93 mg/kg/day. Sixteen patients received other psychoactive medication simultaneously. Twelve of the 26 patients responded positively. Final diagnoses of these patients were school phobia (3), anorexia nervosa (6), manic-depressive psychosis (1), depression (5), and depressive reactions in behavior disorders or borderline personalities (11). Two patients had no therapeutic response, 1 had a minimal response, 11 had moderate improvement, 3 had "good" results, and 9 had excellent results. The patients diagnosed with anorexia responded least favorably; only two had a good response, whereas four of the five diagnosed with depression had excellent responses. Similar plasma levels of clomipramine were present in both responders and nonresponders; however, nonresponders had proportionally higher levels of desmethylclomipramine.

Clomipramine Hydrochloride in the Treatment of School Phobia (Separation Anxiety). Berney et al. (1981) treated 52 children diagnosed with school refusal, which consisted of a neurotic disorder with a marked reluctance to attend school for at least 4 weeks' duration and was frequently associated with depressive features. The study was double-blind and placebo controlled and lasted for 12 weeks. Forty-six patients, aged 9 to 14 years, completed the study; 19 were on placebo and 27 were on clomipramine. The total daily dosage of clomipramine was titrated slowly to 40 mg/day for 9- and 10-year-olds; 50 mg/day for 11- and 12-year-olds; and 75 mg/day for 13- and 14-year-olds. There was no evidence that clomipramine was superior to placebo in reducing separation anxiety and neurotic behavior or being specific for depression. The authors, however, noted that they used proportionally lower doses of clomipramine than the doses used in studies reporting its efficacy in treating school phobia/separation anxiety.

SELECTIVE SEROTONIN REUPTAKE INHIBITORS (SSRIs)

The selective serotonin reuptake inhibitors (SSRIs) approved by the FDA for the treatment of depression only in adults are sertraline hydrochloride (Zoloft), paroxetine hydrochloride (Paxil), citalopram hydrobromide (Celexa) and escitalopram oxalate (Lexapro). Fluoxetine hydrochloride (Prozac) is approved for treating depression in individuals 8 years of age or older. The FDA has approved for treating obsessive-compulsive disorder (OCD) the following SSRIs: sertraline for individuals 6 years of age or older, fluoxetine for individuals 7 years of age or older, fluvoxamine maleate (Luvox) for individuals 8 years of age or older and paroxetine only for adults. Fluoxetine, paroxetine, and sertraline are approved for treating panic disorder only in adults. Paroxetine and sertraline are approved for treating social anxiety disorder and posttraumatic stress disorder in adults. Fluoxetine is approved for treating bulimina nervosa disorder only in adults. Fluoxetine and sertraline are approved to treat premenstrual dysphoric disorder only in adults. Finally escitalopram and paroxetine are approved to treat generalized anxiety disorder only in adults. Table 7.3 summarizes the FDA-approved uses of these SSRIs.

With the exception of escitalopram, which is the S-enantiomer of racemic citalopram, these SSRIs are chemically unrelated to each other or to tricyclic or tetracyclic antidepressants, or to other antidepressants currently used in clinical practice (PDR, 2006). As the term SSRI suggests, at therapeutic levels, these drugs act primarily to inhibit serotonin reuptake; they also have relatively little effect on catecholaminergic (norepinephrine) reuptake mechanisms. At least five types and several subtypes of serotonin receptors with both distinct and overlapping functions have been identified in the central nervous system (Sussman, 1994a). These SSRIs have differing specificities in the serotonin receptors whose reuptake they inhibit, which explains their efficacy in treating disorders other than depression and the fact that they have somewhat different untoward effects. SSRI antidepressants also do not have clinically significant direct effects on the adrenergic, muscarinic, or histaminergic systems, resulting in fewer and less severe untoward effects than the tricyclic antidepressants. The most common untoward effects of the SSRIs parallel the symptoms caused by the administration of exogenous serotonin and include headache, nausea, vomiting, diarrhea, nervousness, sleep disturbance, and sexual dysfunction (Sussman, 1994a).

SSRI induced sexual dysfunction is of particular concern in adolescents. Sharko (2004) reviewed the literature and reported a paucity of reported cases of sexual dysfunction—only 1 male of 1,346 pediatric subjects in 31 clinical studies of SSRIs reported such an adverse event (AE), erectile dysfunction. During 11 years, only eight subjects, all male were reported to MedWatch for sexual dysfunction secondary to treatment with an SSRI: four reported loss of orgasm, three reported loss in interest, and one reported loss of physical arousal. Scharko noted that in adults on adequate doses of SSRIs, sexual dysfunction has been reported by 30% to 40% of patients and that this was probably a low estimate because of the difficulties many adults have in discussing sexual matters. He further speculated that the surprisingly low incidence reported was because it was even more difficult for adolescents to talk to their doctors/psychiatrists but also noted that only 3 of 15 controlled clinical trials cited used ratings to assess AEs (two studies used the Systematic Assessment for Treatment Emergent Events and one study the Side Effects Form for Children and Adolescents) and that neither measure asks directly about sexual dysfunction and relies on self-report. In adults treated with SSRIs, it is known that relying on spontaneous self-report greatly underestimates the actual frequency of SSRI-related sexual dysfunction (Sharko, 2004). It is likely that clinicians and researchers fail to adequately address this area and do not directly ask adolescents about sex and sexual functioning as a part of their medication management. Doing this is likely to be the best way to assess sexual dysfunction of our adolescent patients (Sharko, 2004) and neglecting to do so is a disservice to them and may also increase rates of noncompliance with treatment.

A discontinuation syndrome has been identified for the selective serotonin reuptake inhibitors (SSRIs). Rosenbaum et al. (1998) reviewed the literature

TABLE 7.3 ● Summary of Selective Serotonin Reuptake Inhibitor Indications by Age for FDA-approved Advertising

SSRI	Major Depressive Disorder	Obsessive-Compulsive Disorder	Panic Disorder	Social Anxiety Disorder	Posttraumatic Stress Disorder	Bulimia Nervosa	Premenstrual Dysphoric Disorder	Generalized Anxiety Disorder
Citalopram	≥ 18 y							
Escitalopram	≥ 18 y							≥ 18 y
Fluoxetine	≥ 8 y	≥ 7 y	≥ 18 y			≥ 18 y	≥ 18 y	
Fluvoxamine		≥ 8 y						
Paroxetine	≥ 18 y	≥ 18 y	≥ 18 y	≥ 18 y	≥ 18 y			≥ 18 y
Sertraline	≥ 18 y	≥ 6 y	≥ 18 y	≥ 18 y	≥ 18 y			

on discontinuation-emergent symptoms in adults taking SSRIs and noted that dizziness, headache, nausea, vomiting, diarrhea, movement disorders, insomnia, irritability, visual disturbances, lethargy, anorexia, tremor, electric shock sensations, and lowered mood have all been reported following SSRI discontinuation. Rosenbaum et al. conducted a 4-week, prospective double-blind, placebo-substitution, discontinuation study of 242 adults receiving long-term maintenance (duration 4 to 24 months) with SSRIs for remitted depression (81 subjects on fluoxetine, 79 subjects of sertraline, and 82 subjects on paroxetine). Effects of the abrupt withdrawal of medication were evaluated by baseline ratings on the Symptom Questionnaire (SQ), the Discontinuation-Emergent Signs and Symptoms (DESS) Checklist, and two depression rating scales, the Hamilton Depression Rating Scale and the Montgomery-Asberg Depression Rating Scale. Medication was abruptly interrupted for 5 to 8 days; 83% were randomly assigned to receive placebo and 17% to continue on their medication. Following this phase, all subjects on placebo resumed their usual maintenance dose of the SSRI they were previously taking. Two hundred twenty (91%) of the subjects completed the entire protocol. Following medication withdrawal during placebo, scores both on the DESS and the SQ increased significantly for patients who had been on sertraline or paroxetine ($P < .001$ for both) but not for patients who were receiving fluoxetine ($P = .578$). The authors noted the following spontaneously reported discontinuation-emergent effects in $> 10\%$ of patients: fluoxetine, headache (16%); sertraline, dizziness (18%), headache (18%), nervousness (18%), and nausea (11%); and paroxetine, dizziness (29%), nausea (29%), insomnia (19%), headache (17%), abnormal dreams (16%), nervousness (16%), asthenia (11%), and diarrhea (11%). There were many more discontinuation-emergent symptoms reported on the DESS under inquiry than reported spontaneously; fluoxetine-treated patients reported significantly fewer such symptoms than sertraline-treated patients ($P = .001$) or paroxetine-treated patients ($P < .001$). Reported symptoms (ranked from most to least frequent) that occurred in at least 10% of the 185 subjects who underwent withdrawal from medication in decreasing frequency were the following: worsened mood, irritability, agitation, dizziness, confusion, headache, nervousness, crying, fatigue, emotional lability, trouble sleeping, dreaming, anger, nausea, amnesia, sweating, depersonalization, muscle aches, unsteady gait, panic, sore eyes, diarrhea, shaking, muscle tension, and chills. Overall, a SSRI discontinuation syndrome occurred in 14% of patients withdrawn from fluoxetine, 60% of patients withdrawn from sertraline, and 66% of patients withdrawn from paroxetine. There appeared to be a relationship between a longer half-life and the development of fewer discontinuation-emergent symptoms (e.g., patients abruptly discontinued from fluoxetine developed fewer clinically significant such effects than patients withdrawn from sertraline or paroxetine). In addition, patients treated with either sertraline or paroxetine were rated as having a significant increase in depressive symptoms during the withdrawal period on placebo ($P < .001$). Subjects who were taking fluoxetine did not experience this reemergence of depressive symptoms. Following restabilization on medication, there were no significant rating scale differences among the three drugs (Rosenbaum et al. 1998).

SSRIs are of great interest to child and adolescent psychiatrists for several reasons:

1. Only one double-blind, placebo-controlled study conducted with prepubertal children and no such studies with adolescents have shown tricyclic

antidepressants to be superior to placebo in treating MDD. In that study (Preskorn et al. 1987), however, subjects receiving IMI had their dose of IMI adjusted by laboratory personnel to achieve plasma levels within the therapeutic range.

2. There have been several reports of sudden death in at least eight children and adolescents being treated with tricyclics, leading to particular concern about their cardiotoxicity in younger patients. SSRIs have a significantly safer untoward-effect profile, including decreased lethality in overdose.

3. Although significant, the untoward effects of SSRIs are more tolerable than those of tricyclic and MAOI antidepressants.

4. SSRIs may be administered once daily.

5. SSRIs appear to have potential in treating a spectrum of childhood psychiatric disorders in addition to depression, including obsessive-compulsive disorder with and without comorbid Tourette's disorder, ADHD, anxiety disorders, elective mutism, and eating disorders.

Fluoxetine was the first SSRI to be approved by the FDA and there are more published reports of its use in children and adolescents than for the SSRIs that were introduced later. As additional clinical experience with the SSRIs in this age group has continued to accumulate, the SSRIs have displaced the tricyclic antidepressants as the agents of choice in treating children and adolescents diagnosed with depression, OCD and other disorders where TCAs were used.

Fluoxetine Hydrochloride (Prozac, Sarafem)

Fluoxetine is a selective serotonin reuptake inhibitor (SSRI) that is chemically unrelated to any current antidepressant. Fluoxetine's antidepressant effect is thought to be related to its specific and selective inhibition of serotonin reuptake by central nervous system neurons. This action appears to take place at the serotonin reuptake pump, not at a neurotransmitter receptor site, and fluoxetine appears to have no significant pharmacological effect on norepinephrine or dopamine uptake (Bergstrom et al. 1988).

Fluoxetine binds to muscarinic, histaminergic, and alpha-1 adrenergic receptors significantly less than tricyclic antidepressants, which may account for the relative lack of anticholinergic, sedative, and cardiovascular effects of fluoxetine compared to tricyclic antidepressants.

Several studies, including some that were placebo controlled, have found fluoxetine's therapeutic efficacy to be comparable to that of the tricyclics (IMI, amitriptyline, and doxepine) in treating adults with MDD (for reviews see Benfield et al. 1986; Lader, 1988).

Pharmacokinetics of Fluoxetine Hydrochloride

Peak plasma levels of fluoxetine at usual clinical doses occur after 6 to 8 hours. Food does not significantly affect the bioavailability of fluoxetine; hence it may be administered with or without food. Fluoxetine is metabolized by the P450 2D6 system in the liver; active and inactive metabolites are excreted by the kidneys. About 95% of fluoxetine is bound to plasma proteins. The elimination half-life after chronic administration is 4 to 6 days for fluoxetine and 4 to 16 days for norfluoxetine, its active metabolite. It may take up to 4 to 5 weeks for steady-state plasma levels to be achieved, but once obtained they remain steady.

Sallee et al. (2000) reported the death of a 9-year-old male attributed to genetic polymorphism of the CYP2D6 gene, revealed upon genetic testing of autopsy material, which resulted in impaired metabolism of fluoxetine. The case was complicated with multiple psychiatric diagnoses treated with polypharmacy, including high doses of fluoxetine,methylphenidate, and clonidine.

Contraindications for the Administration of Fluoxetine Hydrochloride

Known hypersensitivity to the drug is a contraindication.

Fluoxetine should not be administered to any patient who has received a MAOI within the preceding 2 weeks. Because of the long half-lives of fluoxetine and its metabolites, a MAOI should not be administered sooner than 5 weeks (35 days) after discontinuing fluoxetine. The manufacturer notes that it may be advisable to wait even longer before giving a MAOI if fluoxetine has been prescribed chronically or at high doses (PDR, 2000).

The drug should be administered with caution if impaired liver function is present; if prescribed, a lower dose or a decrease frequency of administration should be used.

Fluoxetine is secreted in breast milk; nursing is not recommended while taking fluoxetine.

Interactions of Fluoxetine Hydrochloride with Other Drugs

The use of fluoxetine with other psychoactive drugs has not been systematically studied. However, because it is metabolized by the P450 2D6 enzyme system, the potential exists for interactions with other drugs metabolized by this system, including tricyclic antidepressants and other SSRIs.

When used with tricyclic antidepressants, their plasma levels may be significantly increased.

Agitation, restlessness, and gastrointestinal symptoms have occurred when used concurrently with tryptophan.

Diazepam clearance was significantly prolonged in some patients who were administered both drugs.

Elevated plasma levels and toxicity have occurred in some patients receiving carbamazepine or phenytoin when fluoxetine was added to their drug regimes.

Untoward Effects of Fluoxetine Hydrochloride

Wernicke (1985) and Cooper (1988) have reviewed the safety and untoward effects of fluoxetine. The most frequent troublesome untoward effects are nausea, weight loss, anxiety, nervousness, insomnia, and excessive sweating. They are reported more frequently, and anticholinergic effects and sedation less frequently, compared to the tricyclic antidepressants.

Many of the untoward effects may be described as behavioral activation. Riddle et al. (1990/1991) reported the behavioral side effects of fluoxetine in 24 children and adolescents of various diagnoses (age range, 8 to 16 years). Mean dose was 25.8 ± 9.0 mg/day for the 12 subjects (including the ADHD children) who developed fluoxetine-induced behavioral side effects, such as restlessness, hyperactivity, insomnia, an internal feeling of excitation, subtle impulsive behavioral changes, and suicidal ideation (Riddle et al. 1990/1991; King et al. 1991). Bangs et al. (1994) documented significant memory impairment in a 14-year-old who was receiving 20 mg/day of fluoxetine for treatment of MDD. Hypomania, mania, and transient psychosis have also been reported to occur in children and adolescents treated with fluoxetine (Hersh et al. 1991; Jafri, 1991; Jerome, 1991; Boulos et al. 1992; Rosenberg et al. 1992; and Venkataraman et al. 1992).

Simeon et al. (1990) reported that those subjects receiving fluoxetine who were depressed experienced a small but significant weight loss compared to subjects receiving placebo. As many teenagers, especially females, refuse to take tricyclic antidepressants because of frequently associated weight gain, this could be a clinically advantageous characteristic of fluoxetine for some patients.

Indications for Fluoxetine Hydrochloride in Child and Adolescent Psychiatry

Note: Review the Black Box Warning at the beginning of the chapter or in the package insert before prescribing.

Fluoxetine is approved for use in children at least 8 years of age, adolescents, and adults for the treatment of major depressive disorder; children at least 7 years of age, adolescents, and adults for the treatment of obsessive-compulsive disorder; and older adolescents and adults for treatment of bulimia nervosa, panic disorder, social anxiety disorder, and premenstrual dysphoric disorder (PMDD). Food does not seem to affect significantly the bioavailability of fluoxetine. It is recommended that once 20 mg/day is exceeded, particularly at higher doses, the medication be taken in divided portions twice daily, in the morning and at noon.

Fluoxetine Dosage Schedule

● Children and adolescents ≤ 17 years: Fluoxetine has been approved for the treatment of major depressive disorder in children aged 8 years and older and for the treatment of obsessive-compulsive disorder in children age 7 years and older. The safety and efficacy of fluoxetine in younger children with these disorders has not been established. At the present time, the safety and efficacy of fluoxetine for children and younger adolescents diagnosed with other disorders remains to be elucidated. However, studies including patients in this age range are appearing in the literature with increasing frequency. Riddle et al. (1992) noted that 20 mg/day may be too high a dose for some children and suggested that an initial dose of 10 mg/day of fluoxetine is the most common starting dose given to children by most clinicians. Boulos et al. (1992) found that an initial dose of 20 mg of fluoxetine too often causes unacceptable untoward effects and suggested beginning with 5 to 10 mg daily the first week; they noted that some of the subjects (ranging from 16 to 24 years of age) experienced good antidepressant response on doses as low as 5 to 10 mg daily. Gammon and Brown (1993) reported the optimal dose of fluoxetine to be between 2.5 and 7.5 mg/day in 22% (7 of 32) of their subjects who were receiving a combination of methylphenidate and fluoxetine.

Treatment of depression:

● Children < 8 years: Not approved.
● Children and adolescents ≥ 8 years through 17 years: An initial morning dose of 10 to 20 mg/day is recommended. Because of higher plasma levels in lower weight children both the starting and target doses should be 10 mg daily. If there is no improvement after several weeks, increasing the dose to 20 mg daily may be considered. Older and heavier children may initially be prescribed 20 mg daily;

(continued)

Indications for Fluoxetine Hydrochloride in Child and Adolescent Psychiatry *(Continued)*

there is evidence that this may frequently be the optimal dose (Altamura et al. 1988). The full antidepressant action may take 4 weeks or longer to develop.

● Adolescents ≥ 18 years and adults: An initial morning dose of 20 mg is recommended and this is usually the optimal dose. A dose increase may be considered after several weeks if there is inadequate clinical improvement. Such doses may be administered once or twice daily and should not exceed a maximum of 80 mg/day.

Treatment of Obsessive-Compulsive Disorder:

● Children < 7 years: Not approved.
● Children and adolescents ≥ 7 years through 17 years: In lower weight children, an initial morning dose of 10 mg/day is recommended; An increase to 20 mg may be considered after several weeks if there is inadequate clinical improvement. A dose range of 20 to 30 mg is recommended. In heavier children and adolescents, an initial dose of 10 mg is also recommended with an increase to 20 mg daily after 2 weeks. Further dose increases may be considered, if there is inadequate clinical improvement after several more weeks. A dose range of 20 to 60 mg/day is recommended.
● Adolescents ≥ 18 years and adults: An initial morning dose of 20 mg is recommended. Full therapeutic effect may take 5 weeks or longer to develop. A dose increase may be considered after several weeks if there is inadequate clinical improvement. A dose range of 20 to 60 mg/day is recommended; the maximum dose should not exceed 80 mg/day. Full therapeutic effect in the treatment of OCD may take 5 weeks or longer to develop. If adequate clinical response does not occur after several weeks, the dosage may be increased gradually to a maximum of 80 mg/day.

Treatment of Bulimia Nervosa:

● Children and adolescents ≤ 17 years: Not approved. At the present time, the safety and efficacy of fluoxetine for children and younger adolescents remains to be elucidated.
● Adolescents ≥ 18 years and adults:
● In clinical studies of fluoxetine in fixed doses of 20 or 60 mg/day versus placebo in subjects diagnosed with bulimia nervosa, only the 60-mg dose was significantly better than placebo; hence the recommended target dose is 60 mg/day administered in the morning. It is frequently helpful to begin at a lower dose and to reach the target dose by increments of dose over a period of several days.

Treatment of Panic Disorder:

● Children and adolescents ≤ 17 years old: Not recommended.
● Adolescents ≥ 18 years and adults: An initial dose of 10 mg/day with an increase to 20 mg/day after 1 week is recommended. Further increase in dose may be considered, if no significant clinical improvement has occurred after several weeks. Doses over 60 mg/day have not been systematically evaluated.

Treatment of Premenstrual Dysphoric Disorder:

The recommended daily dose is 20 mg.

(continued)

Indications for Fluoxetine Hydrochloride in Child and Adolescent Psychiatry *(Continued)*

Fluoxetine Hydrochloride Dose Forms Available

Eli Lilly who manufactures all four forms of the medications states that they are bioequivalent.
- Tablets: 10 mg (scored); Sarafem is available in 10 and 20 mg tablets.
- Pulvules: 10 mg, 20 mg, and 40 mg
- Weekly capsules (Prozac weekly capsules): 90 mg
- Liquid: 20 mg/5 mL

Reports of Interest

Fluoxetine in the Treatment of Child and Adolescent Major Depressive Disorder. Joshi et al. (1989) reported on their treatment with fluoxetine of 14 patients (eight males, six females) ranging in age from 9 to 15 years (average age, 11.25 years) who were diagnosed with major depression by DSM-III-R (APA, 1987) criteria and who had not responded adequately to tricyclic antidepressants, had serious untoward effects from tricyclics, or could not be treated with tricyclics for medical reasons. Ten (71.4%) of the subjects responded favorably within 6 weeks to fluoxetine 20 mg administered in the morning. Side effects were limited to transient nausea and hyperactivity in one patient each and did not require discontinuation of the drug.

Simeon et al. (1990) reported a 7-week, double-blind, placebo-controlled fluoxetine treatment study of 40 adolescents (22 females and 18 males), aged 13 to 18 years (mean age, 16 years), who met DSM-III criteria for major depression unipolar type and had baseline Hamilton Depression Scores (Ham-D) of at least 20. In addition, the Ham-D scores of all subjects improved < 20% during a preceding 1-week, single-blind placebo treatment protocol. Fluoxetine was begun at 20 mg/day, increased to 40 mg/day after 4 to 7 days, and increased to 60 mg/day during the second week. Further dosage changes were individually titrated.

At baseline, no significant differences were found between the groups. Thirty subjects completed the study divided equally between medication and control groups. About two-thirds of patients in each group showed moderate to marked clinical global improvement with significant improvement by week 3. With the exception of disturbances of sleep, all symptoms showed slightly greater improvement in subjects treated with fluoxetine than in those receiving placebo, but differences were not significant. Patients taking fluoxetine, however, experienced a small but significantly greater weight loss than those receiving placebo. Untoward effects were usually mild and transient, and none necessitated discontinuation of medication. Those most frequently reported were headache, vomiting, insomnia, and tremor. There were no significant differences in the effects of fluoxetine and placebo on heart rate or blood pressure.

Thirty-two patients were successfully followed up 8 to 46 months later (mean, 24 months) at ages 15 to 22 years (mean, 18 years). No significant differences were found between the fluoxetine and placebo groups, or between responders and nonresponders to the initial clinical trial. Both groups showed further overall improvement; however, psychosocial functioning was still poor in more than one-third of the patients, and 50% of the patients' parents felt their children still required professional help. The authors noted that 10 patients were still depressed and 7 of them were still in treatment. About half of the patients who did not respond to placebo or fluoxetine during the initial 8 weeks of treatment were thought to constitute a very-high-risk group and remained very disturbed at follow-up (Simeon et al. 1990).

Boulos et al. (1992) treated, with fluoxetine, 15 adolescents and young adults diagnosed with MDD who had responded unsatisfactorily to prior treatment with antidepressants, usually including tricyclics, for a minimum of 2 months at doses associated with clinical efficacy. Seven subjects were 18 years old or younger. Eleven patients completed at least 6 weeks of treatment. Of these, 64% showed at least a 50% improvement on the Hamilton Depression Rating Scale, and 73% achieved scores of "much" or "very much improved" on the Clinical Global Impressions Scale. Optimal doses ranged from 5 to 40 mg daily, and several patients received other medications concurrently. Untoward effects included headache, vomiting and other gastrointestinal complaints, insomnia, tremor, sweating, dry mouth, and hair loss.

Jain et al. (1992) conducted a retrospective chart review of 31 hospitalized subjects (age range, 9 to 18 years old) whose primary diagnosis was MDD ($N = 27$) or bipolar disorder ($N = 4$) and who were treated with fluoxetine. Twelve children were also diagnosed with a disruptive behavior disorder. The initial dose of fluoxetine was 20 mg/day. Nineteen patients (61%) continued at this dose for the duration of the hospitalization. The other subjects received maximum doses of 40 mg/day (eight patients, 26%), 60 mg/day (three patients, 10%), and 80 mg/day (one patient, 3%); no increased benefit was noted in patients receiving doses of more than 40 mg/day. After a mean treatment duration of 35 days, 74% of patients had improved ratings on the Clinical Global Impressions Scale; 54% were rated "much" or "very much" improved. The most common untoward effects included hypomanic symptoms (e.g., pervasive silliness, increased energy and activity, racing thoughts, insomnia, and socially intrusive or obnoxious behavior) (23%), irritability (19%), insomnia (13%), and gastrointestinal complaints (13%). All four bipolar patients developed hypomanic symptoms. Fluoxetine was discontinued in 8 (26%) of the patients, primarily because of increased irritability and hypomanic symptoms.

Emslie et al. (1997) reported an 8-week, double-blind, randomized (stratified for age, $\leq$ 12 years or $\geq$ 13 years, and sex), placebo-controlled study of 96 children and adolescents (52 males, 44 females; mean age, 12.35; range, 7 to 17 years), diagnosed by DSM-III-R (APA, 1987) criteria with nonpsychotic MDD. Following a 3-week evaluation period and a 1-week, single-blind, placebo run-in during which responders were dropped, the 96 remaining subjects were randomized to 8 weeks of treatment with placebo or fluoxetine; there were 48 in each group (24 subjects aged 12 years or younger and 24 subjects aged 13 years or older in each group). Overall effectiveness was rated on the Clinical Global Impressions-Improvement Subscale (CGI-I) and the Children's Depression Rating Scale-Revised (CDRS-R). In addition, the Brief Psychiatric Rating Scale-Children (BPRS-C) and the Children's Global Assessment Scale (CGAS) were used. Subjects were given 20 mg of fluoxetine or placebo daily for the entire 8 weeks unless they were dropped from the protocol because of failure to improve or untoward effects. Fourteen patients (29%) on fluoxetine discontinued the protocol, seven for lack of efficacy, four for untoward effects (three developed manic symptoms and one developed a severe rash), and three for protocol violation. Twenty-two patients

(46%) on placebo dropped out, 19 for lack of efficacy, one for an untoward effect, and two for protocol violations. Fluoxetine was statistically better than placebo on the CGI-I; using the intent-to-treat (ITT) sample, 27 (56%) of the fluoxetine group versus 16 (33%) of the placebo group were rated much or very much improved ($P = .02$). Using a last-observation-carried-forward (LOCF) analysis for all 96 subjects, there was a significant drug by time interaction in favor of fluoxetine ($P = .01$); there was no significant drug by age or sex interaction, meaning that males and females in both age groups responded equally well. After week 5, the mean CDRS-R score for the fluoxetine group became significantly lower than that for the placebo group ($P = .03$). Comparing initial and exit outcome LOCF scores on the CDRS-R for both groups, fluoxetine (initial score, 58.5 ± 10.5; exit score, 38.4 ± 14.8) was significantly better than placebo (initial score, 57.6 ± 10.4; exit score, 47.1 ± 17.0; $P = .002$). Subjects initially had relatively severe and chronic symptoms of depression and, despite their overall improvement, after 8 weeks, only 15 (31%) of the fluoxetine group and 11 (23%) of the placebo group had CDRS-R scores < 28, consistent with relatively complete remission of depressive symptoms. Scores on the BPRS-C and the CGAS improved for both groups and were not significantly different. The authors concluded that fluoxetine was significantly better than placebo in acute-phase treatment of children and adolescents diagnosed with severe, persistent MDD and encouraged further studies.

The Treatment for Adolescents with Depression Study (TADS) Team (2004) conducted a randomized controlled trial in 439 patients at 13 sites (age 12 to 17 years, mean age 14.6 years; 45.6% males and 73.8% white, 12.5% black, and 8.9% Hispanic) with a primary diagnosis of major depressive disorder by DSM-IV criteria (APA, 1994), which compared the efficacy of fluoxetine (10 to 40 mg/day) versus cognitive-behavior therapy (CBT) versus fluoxetine (10 to 40 mg/day) plus CBT versus placebo (equivalent to 10 to 40 mg/day) over a 12-week period. Medication in the fluoxetine and placebo group was administered in a double-blind fashion; fluoxetine was administered openly in the fluoxetine plus CBT group as CBT was administered unblindly.

The 439 subjects of the study were those remaining from an initial 2804 screened by telephone after inclusion and exclusion criteria were satisfied and those not interested in participation or withdrawing consent were eliminated. Major outcome measures were the Children's Depression Rating Scale-Revised (CDRS-R) and the Clinical Global Impressions-Improvement (CGI-I) Score. The Reynolds Adolescent Depression Scale total score and the Suicidal Ideation Questionnaire—Junior High School Version (SIQ-Jr) total score were used as secondary outcome measures. CBT was comprised of a possible 15 skills-orientated 50 to 60 minute sessions based on the premise that depression is "caused by or maintained by depressive thought patterns and a lack of active, positively reinforced behavioral patterns." The mean number of sessions completed was 11 in both groups with CBT. The mean fluoxetine dose in the fluoxetine only group was 28.4 ± 8.6 mg/day and in the fluoxetine plus CBT group was 33.3 ± 10.8 mg/day; the mean placebo dose was 34.1 ± 9.5 mg/day.

Based on the improvement on the CDRS-R, combined treatment with fluoxetine and CTB was superior ($P = 001$) to treatment with placebo, but treatment with fluoxetine alone ($P = .10$) and CBT alone ($P = .40$) were not. Fluoxetine with CBT was superior to fluoxetine alone ($P = .02$) and to CBT alone ($P = .001$). Fluoxetine alone was also superior to placebo ($P = .01$).

On the CGI-I Scale, rates of positive response (a rating of 1 [very much improved] or 2 [much improved]) were fluoxetine plus CBT, 71% (95% CI 62% to 80%); fluoxetine only, 60.6% (95% CI 51% to 70%); CBT only, 43.2% (95% CI 34% to 52%); and placebo 34.8% (95% CI 26% to 44%).

After patients at high-risk for suicide were eliminated from the study because of exclusion criteria, 29% of the subjects had scores of > 31, a level of suicidal thinking that requires prompt clinical attention on the SIQ-Jr at baseline; this decreased to 10.3% at 12 weeks and there was clinically significant improvement in suicidal thinking in all 4 groups. During the 12-week trial, 24 (5.5%) of the patients reported a suicide-related adverse event (worsening suicidal ideation or a suicide attempt) and 7 (1.6%) of patients attempted suicide but none was successful. Improvement in suicidality was greatest for the fluoxetine plus CBT group and least for the fluoxetine only group. The authors concluded that fluoxetine is effective in the treatment of MDD and that the addition of CBT increases both clinical improvement and protection from suicidality (TADS, 2004).

Fluoxetine in the Treatment of Children and Adolescents with Obsessive-Compulsive Disorder or Obsessive-Compulsive Disorder and Tourette's Disorder. In an open clinical study, Riddle et al. (1990) treated, with fluoxetine, 10 children (5 males, 5 females) ranging in age from 8 to 15 years (average age, 12.2 years) diagnosed with obsessive-compulsive disorder only or with both obsessive-compulsive disorder and Tourette's disorder. Dosage ranged from 10 to 40 mg/day, with 80% of the patients receiving 20 mg/day; duration of treatment ranged from 4 to 20 weeks. Four of the patients with Tourette's disorder received concomitantly additional medication for treatment of their tics. Fifty percent were considered responders to fluoxetine and were rated much improved; response rates were similar in patients with obsessive-compulsive disorder only and in those with both diagnoses. The most common untoward effect was behavioral agitation/activation, characterized by increased motor activity and pressured speech. It occurred in 40% of the patients and usually started within the first few days; symptoms were most severe during the first 2 to 3 weeks but remained until medication was discontinued. No significant changes in blood pressure, pulse, weight, laboratory tests, or ECG were observed (Riddle et al. 1990/1991).

Riddle et al. (1992) reported a randomized, 20-week, double-blind, placebo-controlled, fixed-dose study with crossover after 8 weeks of fluoxetine in treating 14 subjects (6 males and 8 females; age range, 8.6 to 15.6 years; mean, 11.8 ± 2.3 years) diagnosed with obsessive-compulsive disorder by DSM-III-R criteria. Subjects received 20 mg of fluoxetine or placebo. For various reasons, 13 subjects completed the first 4 weeks, 11 subjects completed the first 8 weeks, and only 6 subjects satisfactorily completed the entire 20 weeks. A comparison of between-group differences at 8 weeks was made for 13 subjects; this number of subjects was made possible by carrying the 4-week data forward to 8 weeks for the 2 subjects who dropped out during that time. The seven subjects receiving fluoxetine showed significant decreases on the Children's Yale–Brown Obsessive-Compulsive Scale (CY-BOCS) total score (mean decrease, 44%; $P = .003$), obsessions score (mean decrease, 54%; $P = .009$), and compulsions score (mean decrease, 33%; $P = .005$), and on the Clinical Global Impressions for Obsessive-Compulsive Disorder (CGI-OCD) (mean decrease, 33%, $P = .0004$). The six subjects on placebo also showed reductions in their obsessive-compulsive symptomatology on the CY-BOCS of 27% and on the CGI-OCD of 12%, but these reductions were not significant. When the two groups were compared, the improvement of subjects on fluoxetine was significantly greater than that of those on placebo on the CGI-OCD ($P = .01$) but not on the CY-BOCS ($P = .17$). The most frequently reported untoward effects were insomnia, fatigue, motoric activation, and nausea. Preexisting chronic motor tics worsened in two subjects; however, fluoxetine was continued and the tics subsided to negligible levels over the subsequent 2 years. A subject with comorbid diagnoses of MDD, separation anxiety, and oppositional disorder developed suicidal ideation, which resolved after fluoxetine was discontinued. The authors noted that 20 mg/day may be too high a dose for some children and that an initial dose of 10 mg/day of fluoxetine was the most common starting dose given to children by most child and adolescent psychiatrists.

Of the six subjects initially on fluoxetine who crossed over to placebo at 8 weeks, three dropped out at week 12 because of worsening of symptoms, with a mean increase of 53% ±37% in CY-BOCS scores. A fourth subject was worse at week 20 on the CY-BOCS, and the remaining two showed improvement (decrease) in their CY-BOCS scores. Although three of the four subjects who crossed over from placebo to fluoxetine had shown substantial reductions in their CY-BOCS scores during the placebo period, there was further reduction in these scores at 20 weeks. Overall, these results complement findings in adults and suggest that fluoxetine is both safe and effective in treating children and adolescents with obsessive-compulsive disorder for 20 weeks (Riddle et al. 1992).

Fluoxetine in the Treatment of Children and Adolescents with Anxiety Disorders. Birmaher et al. (1994) treated with fluoxetine 21 patients (age range, 11 to 17 years; mean, 14 years) diagnosed with overanxious disorder (OAD) only ($N = 6$); OAD, Social Phobia (SP), and separation anxiety disorder (SAD) ($N = 5$); or OAD and SP or SAD ($N = 10$), who had not responded to prior psychopharmacotherapy or psychotherapy. Subjects with a prior history of OCD, panic disorder, or current MDD were excluded. The mean fluoxetine dose after an average of 10 months (range, 1 to 31 months) on fluoxetine was 25.7 mg/day; the following distribution of doses was reported: 10 mg/day (1); 20 mg/day (15); 30 mg/day (1); 40 mg/day (2); and 60 mg/day (2).

Twenty subjects (95%) showed some improvement in anxiety, with 17 (81%) rated as moderately to markedly improved on the severity and improvement subscales of the Clinical Global Impressions Scale (CGIS) ($P = .0001$). It is important to note that in most cases improvement did not begin until 6 to 8 weeks after initiation of fluoxetine. Although no subject fulfilled diagnostic criteria for MDD or dysthymia, 10 patients did have depressive symptoms. These symptoms also improved significantly ($P = .0001$); analysis suggested that the improvements in depressive symptoms and anxiety were independent. Only a few untoward effects, which were usually mild and transient, were reported: mild headache (one), nausea (three), insomnia (one), and stomachache (one). No significant changes in pulse, blood pressure, or ECG were found, and no subject experienced agitation, manic, or hypomanic symptoms, or suicidal ideation. These data suggest that fluoxetine may be a useful treatment for children and adolescents with anxiety disorders (Birmaher et al. 1994).

Fairbanks et al. (1997) treated with fluoxetine monotherapy on an open-label basis, 16 outpatients (8 males, 8 females; mean age, 13.0 ± 2.9 years; age range, 9 to 17 years) diagnosed by DSM-III-R (APA, 1987) criteria with mixed anxiety disorders and who were unresponsive to psychotherapy. Eleven subjects (69%) had a mean of 2.5 ± 1.5 coexisting anxiety disorders, including separation anxiety disorder ($N = 11$), social phobia ($N = 10$), generalized anxiety disorder (GAD)

($N = 7$), specific phobia ($N = 6$), and panic disorder ($N = 5$). Efficacy was assessed by ratings on the Children's Global Assessment Scale, the modified Liebowitz Social Anxiety Scale, the modified social behavior scale, the Clinical Global Impressions Scale (CGIS), and a side effects checklist. Fluoxetine was initiated at a dose of 5 mg/day and subsequently increased weekly by 5 or 10 mg/day for 6 to 9 weeks until clinical improvement occurred or to a maximum of 40 mg for subjects < 12 years of age or 80 mg/day for subjects ≥ 12 years of age.

The mean fluoxetine dose for all subjects was 35.0 ± 17.1 mg/day or 0.71 ± 0.28 mg/kg/day. The mean mg/kg/day dose was almost identical for subjects of all ages; subjects < 12 years had lower optimal doses because they weighed less. Subjects with only one anxiety disorder responded to lower doses than subjects with two or more anxiety disorders. The CGIS ratings showed significant improvement in the severity of anxiety in ratings by psychiatrists, mothers, and subjects. Mean duration of time on medication until a rating of "improved," "much improved," or "completely recovered" on the CGIS was 5 weeks, with a range of 1 to 9 weeks. According to diagnoses, improvements on the CGIS were as follows: separation anxiety ($N = 10$): six much improved, four improved; social phobia ($N = 10$): one much improved, seven improved; generalized anxiety disorder ($N = 6$): one much improved, four improved; panic disorder with or without agoraphobia ($N = 5$): one much improved, three improved. Fluoxetine did not appear to aggravate the anxiety of any of the patients. The authors state that their outcome assessments found that separation anxiety disorder, social phobia, specific phobia, and panic disorder all responded favorably to fluoxetine but that generalized anxiety disorder did not. The most common untoward effects were drowsiness, difficulty falling asleep or staying asleep, decreased appetite, nausea, abdominal pain, and a state of being easily excited or keyed up. None of the subjects was reported to have disinhibition, akathisia, suicidal or violent reactions, or hypomania. The authors concluded that fluoxetine is potentially effective in the short-term treatment of anxiety disorders (excluding generalized anxiety disorder) in children and adolescents who do not have comorbid MDD, obsessive-compulsive disorder, substance abuse, or medical complications and that further studies are needed.

Birmaher et al. (2003) conducted a 12-week, randomized, placebo-controlled, double-blind study to assess the efficacy and tolerability of fluoxetine in the outpatient treatment of 74 children and adolescents (age range 7 to 17 years; mean age 11.8 ± 2.8 years; 34 (45.9%) males and 40 (54.1%) females) diagnosed by DSM-IV (APA, 1994) criteria with Generalized Anxiety Disorder (GAD), Social Phobia (SP) and/or Separation Anxiety Disorder (SAD); most subjects were diagnosed with more than one anxiety disorder and 24 (32%) were also diagnosed with other nonanxiety psychiatric disorders. Fluoxetine was initiated at a dose of 10 mg/day for the first week and, if tolerated, was increased to 20 mg/day for the remaining 11 weeks of the study. No other psychiatric medications were permitted for the duration of the study.

At the end of the study, on the Clinical Global Impressions-Improvement (CGI-I) Scale, using an intent-to-treat (ITT) analysis for all subjects, 61% (22/36) of subjects taking fluoxetine and 35% (13/37) of subjects taking placebo had scores of 1 "very marked improvement" or 2, "marked improvement" ($P = .03$) although the analysis for completers was even more positive for the fluoxetine group: 75% for fluoxetine versus 38.7% for the placebo group ($P = .005$). The authors noted that compared to SP subjects on placebo ($N = 19$) the subgroup with a diagnosis of SP on fluoxetine ($N = 21$) had significantly better outcomes on the CGI-I (12% vs.

76%, $P = .001$). Regarding adverse events AEs during the first 2 weeks, subjects on fluoxetine had significantly more AEs than those on placebo for abdominal pain and nausea, 46% versus 22%, $P = .04$; drowsiness and headaches 44% versus 14%, $P = .004$. For the entire duration of the study only abdominal pain and nausea were significantly more frequent in the fluoxetine group: 44% versus 22%, $P = .04$. The authors also noted that during the study 11 patients (7 on fluoxetine and 4 on placebo p = NS) experienced 20 incidents of excitement, giddiness or disinhibition and 5 of these, all receiving fluoxetine were dropped from the study as a result. Subjects were more severely ill at intake (scores of > 30) on the Screen for Child Anxiety Related Emotional Disorders, Child (SCARED-C) and those with positive family histories for anxiety had a poorer clinical response to fluoxetine than subjects without such histories. The authors concluded that fluoxetine is clinically effective and safe for the acute treatment of anxiety in this age group. They suggested that an increase in dose is indicated for patients with no or only partial clinical response after 4 to 6 weeks of treatment. In addition, they noted that mild to moderate agitation/disinhibition may be successfully treated by lowering the dose of fluoxetine in many cases (Birmaher et al. 2003).

In a 1-year follow-up of the 74 subjects in Birmaher et al.'s (2003) 12-week acute, controlled study of fluoxetine, an open-label, l-year extension was conducted (Clark et al. 2005). Fifty-six completed the 1-year follow up; of these 4 were not included in the analysis as they received other medications as well. Of the 52 analysed completers, 42 were assigned to fluoxetine (of this group, 22 had been on fluoxetine during the acute 12-week trial and 20 had been on placebo) and 10 received no medication (of these 4 had been on fluoxetine during the 12-week acute study and 6 had been on placebo). Those subjects on fluoxetine were rated as significantly more improved than those on no medication on the SCARED-parent report ($P =< .01$), the SCARED-C ($P < .05$); the Pediatric Anxiety Rating Scale-Parent Report (PARS-P), and the PARS-rater report (PARS-R) ($P = .05$). The PARS-child report (PARS-C) was not significantly different between the fluoxetine and the placebo groups. The group showing the greatest improvement in CGI-S was the group that was on placebo during the 12-week acute trial and on fluoxetine during the 1 year open-label extension period. The results suggest that fluoxetine continues to be of benefit for the treatment of anxiety in this group of subjects for up to 15 months (Clark et al. 2005).

Fluoxetine in the Treatment of Children and Adolescents with Attention-deficit/Hyperactivity Disorder. Barrickman et al. (1991) reported on 19 children and adolescents (age range, 7 to 15 years) diagnosed with ADHD who were treated for 6 weeks in an open study with fluoxetine hydrochloride. Fourteen subjects had comorbid diagnoses of either conduct disorder ($N = 6$) or oppositional defiant disorder ($N = 8$). Most subjects had prior psychopharmacologic treatment that was unsatisfactory or had untoward effects on stimulants (e.g., tics) or antidepressants (e.g., sedation). Initial daily dose was 20 mg in the morning; subsequent doses were individually adjusted. Average daily dose was 27 mg (0.6 mg/kg) (range, 20 to 60 mg). Nine subjects took 20 mg/day, eight took 40 mg/day, and two took 60 mg/day. Most subjects improved within 1 week after a therapeutic dose was reached. Ratings were made on a large number of standardized instruments. Eleven subjects (58%) were rated moderately improved or very much improved after 6 weeks; eight had minimal improvement. Side effects were minimal and all remitted spontaneously or with dose reduction except mild sedation in one case. In particular, there were no reports of loss of appetite or significant changes in weight.

Only one subject experienced nervousness, and none had insomnia or developed suicidal ideation.

All three children diagnosed with ADHD showed worsening of ADHD symptoms on fluoxetine in the Riddle et al. (1990/1991) study of behavioral side effects of fluoxetine discussed earlier.

Gammon and Brown (1993) reported the use of fluoxetine augmentation of methylphenidate in an 8-week open trial with 32 patients (9 to 17 years old) who were diagnosed with ADHD and one or more comorbid disorders—that is, dysthymia (78%), oppositional defiant disorder (59%), MDD (18%), anxiety disorders (18%), and conduct disorder (13%)—and who had inadequate therapeutic responses to methylphenidate alone. Addition of fluoxetine was begun with an initial dose of 2.5 or 5.0 mg/day for subjects < 12 years of age and 12 years of age or older, respectively. Dose was titrated upward every 3 to 4 days in increments equal to the initial dose, to a maximum of 20 mg/day. Optimal daily dose of fluoxetine at 8 weeks ranged from 2.5 to 20 mg. The majority of subjects (19, or 59%) required 20 mg/day; 6 subjects (18%) received 10 to 15 mg/day; 4 subjects (12.5%) received 5 to 7.5 mg/day; and 3 subjects (9%) had optimal fluoxetine doses of 2.5 mg/day. No significant or lasting untoward effects were reported.

After 8 weeks of combined drug treatment, all 32 subjects showed statistically significant improvements on assessments rating attention, behavior, and affect. These improvements were also rated clinically significant in 94% (30) of the subjects. Scores on the Children's Global Assessment Scale dramatically improved ($P < .0001$). Mean scores on the Children's Depression Inventory declined from 22, which is in the clinical range for depressive symptoms, to 8, which is below that range ($P < .0001$). On the Conners' Parents Rating Scale, group means improved on all six scales; on five scales improvement was significant ($P < .001$ to $P < .0001$). There was also a marked jump in student grade point average within one marking period. Parents reported substantial improvement in hyperactivity, impulsivity, anxiety, conduct, and learning problems. Augmentation with fluoxetine also produced significant further improvement in sustaining attention and concentration, and helped to alleviate symptoms of anxiety, depression, irritability, and oppositionalism that had not responded adequately to methylphenidate alone. More seriously affected children showed the most significant improvements (Gammon and Brown, 1993).

Fluoxetine in the Treatment of Children Diagnosed with Selective (Elective) Mutism. Black and Uhde (1994) treated 15 subjects (age range of 6 to 11 years) who were diagnosed with elective mutism with fluoxetine in a double-blind, 12-week study. During a single-blind, 2-week placebo period preceding the study, a sixteenth subject who responded to placebo was dropped. Three boys and three girls (mean age, of 9.1 ± 2.3 years) were randomly assigned to fluoxetine. Three boys and six girls (mean age, of 8.1 ± 1.6 years) were assigned to placebo. Fluoxetine was given at a dose of 0.2 mg/kg/day for the first week, increased to 0.4 mg/kg for the second week, and further increased to 0.6 mg/kg for the final 10 weeks of the study. The mean maximum dose of fluoxetine was 0.60 to 0.62 mg/kg/day or 21.4 mg/day (range, 12 to 27 mg/day). The fluoxetine group improved more than the placebo group on 28 or 29 rating scales, but most of the differences were not significant. Both groups showed significant improvement from baseline over time in elective mutism, anxiety, and social anxiety as rated by parents, teachers, and clinicians. The fluoxetine group improved significantly more than the placebo group on parents', but not on teachers' or clinicians', ratings of mutism and clinical global improvement. This was consistent with earlier findings that children with elective mutism show improvements in the home setting before school and clinic settings. The authors noted that, although statistically significant, the improvements were modest and that the subjects continued to show serious impairments in their functioning. Untoward effects were minimal (Black and Uhde, 1994).

Dummit et al. (1996) reported a 9-week, open-label study of fluoxetine in the treatment of 21 children (five males, 16 females; mean age, 8.2 ± 2.6 years; range, 5 to 14 years) who met DSM-IV (APA, 1994) criteria for selective mutism and comorbid avoidant disorder or social phobia. Efficacy was assessed by ratings of the Children's Global Assessment Scale (CGAS) and the Lebowitz Social Anxiety Scale (LSAS). Subjects rated themselves on the social behavior scale, and parents rated their children on the same scale. Initially, fluoxetine was begun at a dose of 1.25 mg/day and gradually increased. As the authors found that none of the first 10 subjects improved on < 20 mg/day and there were no problematic untoward effects at that dose, for subsequent subjects the initial dose was increased to 5 mg/day for the first week, 10 mg/day for the second week, and 20 mg/day for the third week. It was permissible to increase the dose to 40 mg/day for the sixth week and to 60 mg/day at the eighth week if clinically indicated. The mean optimal daily dose of fluoxetine was 28.1 mg/day or 1.1 mg/kg/day, and the dose ranged from 20 to 60 mg/day, with 15 subjects receiving 20 mg/day, 4 receiving 40 mg/day, and 2 requiring 60 mg/day. Overall scores on all indicators indicated significant improvement on all rating scales ($P < .001$ for clinicians' and subjects' self-ratings and $P < .005$ for parental ratings). After 9 weeks, 16 of 21 (76%) subjects were rated improved by their psychiatrist. Treatment outcome was inversely related to age, with 14 of 15 children < 10 years improving to a clinically meaningful degree and only 2 of the 6 children ≥ 10 years old doing so. Four children developed excitement and behavioral disinhibition, which resulted in three of them discontinuing the medication and dose reduction in the fourth child. Most untoward effects were transient and none was reported during the final week of treatment. The authors recommended a relatively low initial dose of 5 to 10 mg/day because of the possibility of behavioral activation and also noted that complete remission of the elective mutism often required more than 9 weeks of treatment, even in the marked treatment responders.

Sertraline Hydrochloride (Zoloft)

Sertraline hydrochloride is a selective serotonin reuptake inhibitor (SSRI) that is chemically unrelated to other antidepressants currently in use. Its antidepressant effect is presumed to be related to its inhibition of neuronal serotonin uptake. Sertraline has also been approved for the treatment of obsessive-compulsive disorder in patients 6 years of age and older, and for the treatment of panic disorder, social anxiety disorder and posttraumatic stress disorder in adults. It has only very weak effects on norepinephrine and dopamine reuptake. *In vitro*, sertraline has no significant affinity for alpha-1, alpha-2, or beta adrenergic, cholinergic, gamma aminobutyric acid (GABA), dopaminergic, histaminergic, $5HT_{1A}$, $5HT_{1B}$, or $5HT_2$ serotonergic, or benzodiazepine receptors. Chronic administration of sertraline is thought to down-regulate norepinephrine receptors.

Pharmacokinetics of Sertraline Hydrochloride

Peak plasma levels of sertraline hydrochloride are reached between 4.5 and 8.4 hours after ingestion. Food increases the availability of sertraline slightly and peak blood levels are higher and are reached more quickly. Dosage, however, does not require adjusting and sertraline may be taken with or without food. During the first pass, sertraline undergoes extensive N-demethylation in the liver to form N-desmethylsertraline, which has a half-life of 62 to 104 hours but is significantly less pharmacologically active than sertraline. Both drug and metabolite subsequently undergo oxidative deamination followed by reduction, hydroxylation, and glucuronide conjugation. The average termination half-life of plasma sertraline is about 26 hours. Steady-state plasma levels at a given dose occur within about 7 days. Drug and metabolites are excreted in about equal amounts in the feces and urine, although all unmetabolized sertraline (about 13%) is found in the urine.

Data provided by the manufacturer suggest that patients in the pediatric age range, 6 through 17 years old, metabolize sertraline with slightly greater efficacy than adults. Nevertheless, because of their lower body weights, lower doses than that prescribed for adults may be advisable (PRD, 2000).

Alderman et al. (1998) explored single 50-mg-dose and steady-state (200 mg/day) pharmacokinetics of sertraline in 61 patients (age range, 6 to 17 years of age). The authors found that all pharmacokinetic parameters for serum sertraline and desmethylsertraline levels were similar for their patients and those reported for adults when corrected for weight. They conclude that the titration regime recommended for adults was suitable and safe.

In their study of 92 children and adolescents prescribed sertraline for the treatment of obsessive-compulsive disorder, March et al. (1998) reported that trough plasma levels of sertraline and its active metabolite desmethylsertraline, normalized for body weight, did not correlate significantly with age, sex, or clinical response.

Axelson et al. (2002) reported that the pharmacokinetics of sertraline varied significantly in adolescents (mean age 15.1; range 13.1 to 17.9 years) according to dose. The mean steady-state half-life at 50 mg/day was 15.3 ± 3.5 hours compared to 20.4 ± 3.4 hours at a dose of 100–150 mg/day. Because of this, they recommended that sertraline should be administered twice daily if adolescents were receiving < 200 mg daily. The authors also measured platelet serotonin reuptake inhibition. They found that after 2 weeks' treatment with 50 mg/day of sertraline, platelet serotonin uptake was less that 70% in 6 of 9 subjects and concluded that most adolescents need sertraline doses higher than 50 mg daily to achieve an adequate therapeutic response.

Contraindications for the Administration of Sertraline Hydrochloride

Known hypersensitivity to sertraline hydrochloride is a contraindication.

Because of a possibility for serious, life-threatening reactions when administered simultaneously with a MAOI, the use of sertraline in combination with a MAOI is contraindicated. At least 14 days should elapse after stopping a MAOI before administering sertraline. Based on the half-life of sertraline, at least 14 days should elapse following its discontinuation before administering a MAOI.

Untoward Effects of Sertraline Hydrochloride

The most common side effects of sertraline in premarketing controlled studies included nausea, insomnia, diarrhea, ejaculatory delay, and somnolence. March et al. (1998) reported in a multicenter, 12-week, placebo-controlled trial of 187 children and adolescents (age range, 6 to 17 years) that 4 untoward effects occurred significantly more frequently in the subjects receiving sertraline: insomnia

(37% vs. 13%; $P = <.001$); nausea (17% vs. 7%, $P = .05$); agitation (13% vs. 2%, $P = .005$); and tremor (7% vs. 0, $P = .01$) Additional untoward effects that occurred in at least 2% of the patients of the March et al. study and at least at twice the rate reported in patients on placebo were hyperkinesia, twitching, fever, malaise, purpura, weight loss, impaired concentration, manic reaction, emotional lability, abnormal thinking, and epistaxis (PDR, 2000).

Effects of Sertraline Upon the Heart

Wilens et al. (1999) prospectively assessed cardiovascular functions (vital signs and ECG parameters) of the 187 children and adolescents diagnosed with obsessive-compulsive disorder and treated with sertraline ($N = 92$) or placebo ($N = 95$) as discussed later in the report by March et al. (1998). Baseline data were contrasted with data from weeks 1, 4, and 12 of the study. There were no clinically significant differences in supine or standing heart rates or systolic or diastolic blood pressures between the two groups. There were no significant differences in PR, QRS, or QTc, and no significant new developments of sinus arrhythmias, nodal abnormalities, or intraventricular conduction abnormalities with the exception of two subjects on sertraline who developed a QTc interval of > 440 msec ($P = .05$); no subject developed a QTc interval of > 460 msec. The authors concluded that monotherapy with sertraline in doses of up to 200 mg/day in healthy children and adolescents was not associated with any symptomatic or asymptomatic clinically significant cardiovascular untoward effects but cautioned that the sample size precluded conclusions regarding small differences or rare events.

Indications for Sertraline Hydrochloride in Child and Adolescent Psychiatry

Note: Review the Black Box Warning at the beginning of the chapter or in the package insert before prescribing.

Sertraline has been approved for the treatment of depression, obsessive-compulsive disorder, panic disorder, posttraumatic stress disorder, premenstrual dysphoric disorder and social anxiety disorder in adults. It has been approved for the treatment of obsessive-compulsive disorder in children 6 years of age and older, but its safety and efficacy for treating the other adult indications in the pediatric age group have not been established or approved by the FDA.

Sertraline Dosage Schedule

- Children < 6 years of age: Not recommended.
- Children ≥ 6 and adolescents through 17 years of age:

  Treatment of obsessive-compulsive disorder: In children 6 to 12 years of age, a single initial daily dose of 25 mg either in the morning or in the evening is recommended. Although the manufacturer recommends a single initial daily dose of 50 mg for adolescents aged 13 to 17 years, it is often prudent to begin with 25 mg daily, particularly in younger, less heavy adolescents, to avoid possible activation. Effective doses in clinical trials of patients 6 to 17 years of age ranged from 25 to 200 mg daily. Because of sertraline's relatively long

(continued)

Indications for Sertraline Hydrochloride in Child and Adolescent Psychiatry *(Continued)*

(24-hour) elimination half-life, titration based on clinical response is recommended at intervals of at least 7 days to permit adequate assessment of clinical response at a given dosage. (See also recommendations of March et al. 1998, in the following text.)

Treatment of major depressive disorder, panic disorder, posttraumatic stress disorder, social anxiety disorder, and premenstrual dysphoric disorder: not recommended. The safety and efficacy of sertraline have not been established for the pediatric age group.

● Adolescents at least 18 years of age and adults:

Treatment of MDD and obsessive-compulsive disorder: An initial daily dose of 50 mg given either in the morning or at night is recommended. Full antidepressant response may be delayed for up to several weeks in some patients. Some patients may benefit from increases to a maximum of 200 mg/day. Because of sertraline's 24-hour elimination half-life, increments should be made at least 7 days apart to permit adequate assessment of clinical response at a given dosage.

Treatment of panic disorder, posttraumatic stress disorder, and social anxiety disorder: An initial daily dose of 25 mg is recommended with an increase to 50 mg daily after 7 days. Dose may be gradually increased in patients who do not have an adequate response. Effective dose range is usually between 50 mg and 200 mg daily. Because of sertraline's 24-hour elimination half-life, increments should be made at least 7 days apart to permit adequate assessment of clinical response to a given dosage.

Treatment of premenstrual dysphoric disorder: An initial dose of 50 mg/day is recommended to be given either throughout the menstrual cycle or during the luteal phase depending on the physician's assessment and judgment. Patients with inadequate clinical response may benefit from a 50-mg dose increase at the onset of each menstrual cycle to a maximum of 150 mg/day throughout the menstrual cycle or up to 100 mg/day if administered only during the luteal phase. If 100 mg/day is given during the luteal phase, it should be initiated with 50 mg/day and increased to 100 mg/day after 3 days of each luteal phase. Sertraline should be administered in a single morning or evening dose.

Sertraline Hydrochloride Dose Forms Available

● Tablets (scored): 25 mg, 50 mg, and 100 mg
● Oral concentrate: 20 mg/mL

Reports of Interest

Sertraline in the Treatment of Children and Adolescents with Obsessive-Compulsive Disorder. March et al. (1998) reported a multicenter randomized double-blind, placebo-controlled 12-week, parallel-group trial of sertraline versus placebo in 187 patients diagnosed with obsessive-compulsive disorder (OCD) by DSM-III-R criteria. There were 107 children aged 6 to 12 years, of whom 53 received active drug and 54 were given placebo, and 80 adolescents aged 13 to 17 years, of whom 39 received active drug and 41 were given placebo. The four main dependent-outcome measures for efficacy were the Children's

Yale-Brown Obsessive Compulsive Scale (CY-BOCS), the National Institute of Mental Health Global Obsessive-compulsive Scale (NIMH GOCS), and the NIMH Clinical Global Impressions-Severity of Illness (CGI-S) and Improvement (CGI-I) rating scales. Subjects were required to have a baseline score of at least seven on the NIMH GOCS indicative of at least moderate impairment and absence of significant depression. In addition, none of the subjects responded to a week-long, single-blind placebo lead-in that was to eliminate placebo responders. Sertraline was initiated at 25 mg/day for children and 50 mg/day for adolescents and titrated upward by 50 mg weekly for 4 weeks, until a maximum of 200 mg/day or the maximum tolerated dose was achieved. Patients then continued to receive this dosage for weeks 5 through 12 of the study. Mean dose of sertraline at end point was 167 mg/day for the 92 subjects on sertraline. The number of adolescents tolerating 200 mg/day was greater than that tolerated by children: 39 (82%) versus 30 (57%).

Patients receiving sertraline improved significantly more than patients on placebo on the CY-BOCS ($P = .005$), the NIMH GOCS ($P = .02$), and the CGI-I Scale ($P = .002$), but only a trend was seen on the CGI-S Scale. Of the subjects receiving sertraline, 49/92 (53%) showed at least a 25% decrease in their CY-BOCS scores at end point versus baseline and 39/92 (42%) were rated as very much or much improved on the CGI-I rating at end point. These results were significantly better than that of the subjects receiving placebo, of whom 35/95 (37%) ($P = .03$) showed at least a 25% decrease of the CY-BOCS and 25/95 (26%) ($P = .02$) were rated as very much or much improved on the CGI-I rating at end point. Despite the significant clinical improvement, the average subject in the sertraline group was rated in the mildly ill range on the CY-BOCS at the end of the 12-week study. Untoward effects reported are described earlier; the authors note they may have increased because the protocol required the dose to be titrated upward so rapidly. There was no evidence that sertraline caused clinically significant changes in vital signs, laboratory values, or electrocardiogram.

March et al. (1998) concluded that sertraline appears to be a safe and effective short-term treatment for OCD in this age group. There was no significant difference in the untoward effects of sertraline in children compared to adolescents. The authors recommended an initial sertraline dose of 50 mg/day, titrated over a period of 6 to 8 weeks to reach maximum doses in partial or nonresponders. For an adequate clinical trial, sertraline should be taken for at least 10 to 12 weeks.

Sertraline in the Treatment of Children and Adolescents with Obsessive-Compulsive Disorder or Depression. Alderman et al. (1998) treated 29 children (mean age, 10.4 ± 1.7 years; age range, 6 to 12 years) and 32 adolescents (mean age, 14.9 ± 1.4 years; age range, 13 to 17 years) who were diagnosed by DSM-III-R (APA, 1987) criteria with obsessive-compulsive disorder ($N = 16$), MDD ($N = 44$), or both ($N = 1$) for 5 weeks with sertraline. All 61 subjects received an initial morning 50-mg dose of sertraline to determine single-dose pharmacokinetic parameters, followed by a 7-day washout. Following this (on day 8), subjects received either 25 mg/day of sertraline, which was force-titrated in 25-mg increments every 3 to 4 days to reach 200 mg/day on day 32, or 50 mg/day of sertraline, which was force-titrated in 50-mg increments every 7 days to reach 200 mg/day on day 29. After the titration period, both groups received 200 mg/day through day 42. Efficacy was assessed by ratings of the Children's Yale-Brown Obsessive-Compulsive Scale (CY-BOCS), the National Institute of Mental Health-Global Obsessive Compulsive Scale (NIMH GOCS), and the Clinical Global Impressions-Severity of Illness (CGI-S) and Improvement (CGI-I) scales.

At the end of the 5 weeks on sertraline, scores on the CY-BOCS for the 17 patients diagnosed with OCD decreased significantly from baseline (24.9 vs. 12.9; $P < .001$), scores on the NIMH GOCS declined significantly from baseline (10.2 vs. 6.7; $P < .001$), and scores on the CGI-S declined from 4.8 to 2.8 ($P < .001$). Ratings on the CGI-S for the 41 depressed patients who completed the 5-week period on sertraline declined significantly from 4.8 to 2.8 ($P < .001$). Changes in the children's and adolescents' groups were similar. The mean CGI-S for all subjects improved by 2.26, a rating signifying "much improved." Overall, 51 subjects reported at least one untoward effect but most were mild or moderate. The most commonly reported were headache (21%), nausea (21%), insomnia (21%), somnolence (15%), dyspepsia (12%), and anorexia (12%). There was no significant difference in incidence of untoward effects between children and adolescents except for dyspepsia, which was more frequent in children. Medication was discontinued in three of the depressed children because of the development of moderate hyperactivity in one, nervousness attributed to family stress in another, and severe self-mutilation in the third. The development of untoward effects did not correlate with any pharmacokinetic parameter or dose titration schedule. The authors concluded that their results suggest that sertraline, administered as recommended for adults, is safe and effective in the treatment of subjects 6 to 17 years of age diagnosed with obsessive-compulsive disorder or MDD.

Sertraline in the Treatment of Children and Adolescents with Major Depression. Tierney et al. (1995) reported a retroactive chart study of 33 inpatients and outpatients (14 males, 19 females; mean age, 13.25; range, 8.1 to 18.1 years) who were diagnosed with MDD by DSM-III-R (APA, 1987) criteria and treated with sertraline monotherapy on an open basis. Efficacy was determined by chart review ratings on the Clinical Global Impressions-Severity of Illness Scale (CGI-S) and the CGI-Improvement Scale (CGI-I). Data were analyzed only for patients who completed 2 to 10 weeks of treatment in an attempt to eliminate those who had positive responses to hospitalization or spontaneous improvement. Twelve patients (including 10 inpatients) were treated for < 2 weeks. The 21 patients included in the data analysis of efficacy were 9 males (mean age, 13.2; age range, 12.0 to 15.3 years) and 12 females (mean age, 14.3; age range, 9.5 to 18.1 years). Several had comorbid diagnoses but none had a history of mania or hypomania at the time of treatment. Untoward effects were tabulated for all 33 subjects. The usual initial dose of sertraline was 25 mg, with an increase to 50 mg/day within 1 week and subsequently titrated individually based on clinical response. At the end of 10 weeks, the optimal dose for one subject was 25 mg/day, with the other 20 patients ranging from 50 to 200 mg/day. The mean daily dose of sertraline at the end of treatment was 100 ± 53 mg or 1.6 ± 0.7 mg/kg.

The overall ratings on the CGI-S decreased significantly, from 5.83 ± 0.69 at baseline to 3.44 ± 0.17 at endpoint ($P < .01$). On the CGI-I Scale, 11 of 17 patients treated with sertraline for 2 to 10 weeks had ratings of "very much improved" or "much improved" over baseline; no subject's depression worsened. Older patients showed significantly greater improvement in depressive severity than younger patients ($P < .01$). Untoward effects were reported by 16 (48%) of the initial 33 patients. Four of the 12 who dropped out during the first 2 weeks did so because of untoward effects; three had behavioral activation (one with intent to self-injure, one with mood lability, and one with symptoms [mania] consonant with bipolar I disorder) and one had nausea. Of the 33 subjects, 5 (15%) reported gastrointestinal symptoms (nausea, stomachache, vomiting, decreased appetite); 5 (15%), fatigue and sedation; 3 (33%), headaches; 7 (21%), behavioral activation, including 2 who developed mania (one at 3 days and one after 94 days). The authors concluded that their data suggested that sertraline was clinically beneficial in some children and adolescents but noted that the potential for inducing behavioral activation and mania was of concern (Tierney et al. 1995).

McConville et al. (1996) treated with open-label sertraline 13 inpatients (three males, 10 females; mean age, 15.1 years; range, 12 to 18 years) who were diagnosed with MDD by DSM-III-R criteria. No patient had received a psychotropic medication for at least 5 months before beginning sertraline at a mean of 6.75 days after admission. The hospitalizations of patients averaged a mean of 19 days (range, 9 to 38 days); patients were followed-up after discharge and evaluated after a total of 12 weeks on medication. Of the 20 subjects who were there at the beginning of the study, 6 were dropped because of poor compliance with outpatient follow-up and 1 was dropped because he developed a manic episode after 8 days of sertraline. Efficacy was assessed by ratings on the Hamilton Rating Scale for Depression (Ham-D), the Montgomery-Asberg Depression Scale (M-ADS), the Clinical Global Impressions Scale Adapted for Depression (CGI-D), the Children's Global Assessment Scale (CGAS), and the Family Global Assessment Scale (FGAS).

Sertraline was initiated at 50 mg/day and titrated weekly in increments of 50 mg based on clinical response. Two patients developed untoward effects on the initial dose and required a reduction in dosage. Mean sertraline dose at time of discharge from the hospital was 77 ± 26 mg/day or 1.5 ± 0.45 mg/kg/day. At the 12-week outpatient follow-up the mean dose was 110 ± 50 mg/day or 2.0 ± 0.85 mg/kg/day; final optimal dose range was 25 to 200 mg/day.

Mean ratings on the three scales (Ham-D, M-ADS, and CGI-D) measuring depressive symptoms decreased significantly from premedication baseline to 12 weeks ($P < .001$ in all cases), with 11 of the 13 patients experiencing a decrease of more than 50% in their Ham-D scores. The authors noted a sharp drop in depressive symptoms during the first week on the drug, which they attributed to placebo or nondrug effects (e.g., hospitalization), so they also analyzed changes from the end of treatment week 1 to the end of treatment week 12. All were still significant (Ham-D, $P = .027$; M-ADS, $P = .022$; and CGI-D, $P = .029$). The CGAS showed a significant improvement from baseline to 12 weeks ($P = .011$) but not from week 1 to week 12, and the FGAS ratings did not improve significantly for either time interval. The most frequent untoward effects at 12 weeks were insomnia (69%), drowsiness (61%), weight change (46%), nightmares (39%), loss of appetite (31%), and headache (31%). The authors concluded that sertraline was a promising drug for the treatment of adolescent MDD (McConville et al. 1996).

Ambrosini et al. (1999) reported the combined data of six university-affiliated outpatient clinics that treated 53 adolescents (26 males and 27 females; mean age, 16 ± 2 years; range, 12.2 to 19.8 years), diagnosed with MDD with sertraline in a 10-week, open-label, acute-phase study. Thirty-seven subjects (70%) had a single episode and 16 (30%) had recurrent MDD; the mean duration of the index depressive episode was 78 ± 79 weeks, and most subjects had moderate ($N = 29$ [55%]) or severe ($N = 22$ [42%]) symptoms by DSM-III-R criteria (APA, 1987). Sixty-eight subjects participated in a 2-week, single-blind placebo washout period before beginning the protocol. Fifteen were eliminated from the study during this period, usually because they had improved clinically and no longer met study criteria for severity. Forty-one subjects completed at least 6 weeks of the study and 34 completed the initial 10 weeks. The 26 "responders," defined as much or very much improved on the CGI-I, were eligible to continue receiving sertraline for an additional 12 weeks.

Severity of illness and efficacy were rated on the Schedule for Affective Disorders and Schizophrenia (SADS), Hamilton Depression Rating Scale (HDRS), the Children's Global Assessment Scale (CGAS), Beck Depression Inventory (BDI), and the Clinical Global Impressions-Severity (CGI-S) and CGI-Improvement (CGI-I) Scales. The initial dose of sertraline was 50 mg/day. Subjects were seen for evaluation of efficacy, untoward effects, and titration of medication at weeks 2, 3, 4, 6, 8, 10, and for responders, at weeks 14, 16, 18, 20, and 22. Dose could be decreased at any time for untoward effects and, beginning with week 3, could be increased by 50 mg each visit to a maximum of 200 mg. The mean sertraline dose at week 6 was 93.3 ± 20 mg/day and at week 10 was 127.2 ± 45 mg/day.

By week 2 there was significant improvement over baseline ($P = .0001$) in scores on the HDRS, the 17-item depression rating scale (part of the Mini-SADS), the BDI, and the CGI-S. Response rates improved with time throughout the study. The response rate on the 17-item scale, the most sensitive indicator of depressive symptoms, increased from 55% of subjects at 6 weeks to 76% by 10 weeks. On the HDRS, 26 (55.3%) subjects had a reduction in their scores by at least 50% by week 10. Response did not correlate with the age of the subject or baseline severity of depressive symptoms. Twenty-two of the 26 responders completed the additional 12-week period on sertraline, during which they maintained their improvement or improved further. Maximum clinician ratings of improvement occurred after the initial 10-week period. There were no clinically significant changes in vital signs, CBC, laboratory values, or ECGs. Untoward effects occurred in about 10% of the patients and were usually mild to moderate in severity. The most common were headache (36%), insomnia (26%), nausea (17%), dizziness (15%), flu-like symptoms (13%), diarrhea (13%), fatigue (11%), agitation (11%), and somnolence (11%). No patient developed manic symptoms. The only patient to discontinue sertraline did so because of akathisia.

The authors concluded that their data suggested that sertraline in doses of up to 200 mg/day was efficacious and safe in treating chronically depressed adolescent outpatients with moderate to severe MDD. They emphasized that, in the acute phase of treatment, it is important to administer sertraline for at least 10 weeks and that improvement can continue even after 10 weeks (Ambrosini et al. 1999).

Sertraline Hydrochloride in the Treatment of Children Diagnosed with Selective Mutism. Carlson et al. (1999) treated five outpatients (1 male, 4 females; age range, 5 to 11 years) diagnosed with selective mutism by DSM-IV (APA, 1994) criteria in a 16-week, double-blind, placebo-controlled trial of sertraline within a replicated multiple-baseline/across-participants research design. There were 4 randomly ordered treatment phases: no drug for 2 weeks, placebo for 2 to 6 weeks, 50 mg/day of sertraline for 2 weeks, and 100 mg/day of sertraline for 6 to 10 weeks (subjects who were assigned to longer placebo periods had a respectively shorter time on 100 mg/day of sertraline). Selective mutism had been present from 2 to 7 years in the subjects. Subjects had no comorbid psychiatric conditions, no prior drug treatment of their selective mutism, or ongoing psychotherapy, although all five had previously had behavioral therapy and three had had individual psychotherapy. Efficacy was determined by ratings on goal attainment scaling to quantify the progress toward a target behavior, for example, speaking; both parents and teachers rated children on this scale. Clinical Global

Impressions Severity of Illness (CGI-S) ratings adapted for mutism, anxiety, and shyness were completed by parent, teacher, and psychiatrist. Improvement in speaking occurred within a few days of beginning sertraline in four of the five subjects as rated by parents. Two of the five subjects were speaking in school and no longer met criteria for selective mutism after < 10 weeks of receiving sertraline. Parents of a third subject taking 50 mg/day of sertraline reported that their daughter was speaking in school and in other settings at follow-up 20 weeks after the study. Untoward effects were minimal and did not require dose reduction. The results suggest that sertraline may be useful in treating selective mutism in this age group.

Paroxetine Hydrochloride (Paxil); Paroxetine Mesylate (Pexeva)

Paroxetine hydrochloride, a selective serotonin reuptake inhibitor (SSRI), is the hydrochloride salt of a phenylpiperazine compound. Its chemical structure is unrelated to other SSRIs and antidepressants currently in use. Studies suggest that its antidepressant action and clinical efficacy in obsessive-compulsive, panic, and social anxiety disorders are related to its being a highly potent selective inhibitor of neuronal serotonin reuptake. In addition, paroxetine has only a very weak effect on the neuronal reuptake of norepinephrine and dopamine. Paroxetine has little affinity for muscarinic alpha-1-, alpha-2-, beta-adrenergic; dopamine (D_2); $5HT_1$, $5HT_2$; and histamine (H_1) receptors.

Pharmacokinetics of Paroxetine Hydrochloride

Food slightly increases bioavailability of paroxetine; it increases maximum plasma levels and decreases the time to reach peak plasma concentration from about 6.5 hours to about 5 hours. Paroxetine may be administered with or without food without dosage adjustment. Paroxetine is extensively metabolized in the liver; in part by the P450 2D6 enzyme system; its principal metabolites have only one-fiftieth the potency of the parent compound in inhibiting serotonin reuptake. About two-thirds of the drug is excreted in the urine and one-third in the feces. Serum half-life ($T_{1/2}$) is approximately 21 hours. Steady-state plasma levels usually occur within 10 days.

Findling et al. (1999) studied paroxetine pharmacokinetics in 30 children and adolescents (age range, 6 to 17 years; mean age, 11.2 ± 2.9 years), 15 of each sex, who were being treated for a diagnosis of MDD. The mean half-life of paroxetine in this age group was 11.1 ± 5.2 hours, considerably shorter than that in adults; however, steady-state plasma levels were still achieved with once-daily dosing.

Contraindications for the Administration of Paroxetine Hydrochloride

Known hypersensitivity to paroxetine hydrochloride is a contraindication.

Because of a possibility of serious, life-threatening reactions when administered simultaneously with a MAOI, the use of paroxetine in combination with a MAOI is contraindicated. At least 14 days should elapse after stopping a MAOI before administering paroxetine. Based on the half-life of paroxetine, at least 14 days should elapse following its discontinuation before administering a MAOI.

Paroxetine hydrochloride is secreted in breast milk; nursing is not recommended while taking paroxetine.

Untoward Effects of Paroxetine Hydrochloride

In clinical trials, between 16% and 20% of patients discontinued taking paroxetine for the following reasons: asthenia, sweating, nausea, decreased appetite, somnolence, dry mouth, dizziness, insomnia, tremor, nervousness, ejaculatory and other male sexual disturbances, and female sexual disorders.

Findling et al. (1999) reported that two (6.7%) of their 30 subjects (mean age, 11.2 ± 2.9 years) diagnosed with MDD and treated with paroxetine developed hypomania requiring discontinuation of the medication. In both cases, the hypomanic symptoms remitted without complications following discontinuation.

Indications for Paroxetine Hydrochloride or Paroxetine Mesylate in Child and Adolescent Psychiatry

Note: Review the Black Box Warning at the beginning of the chapter or in the package insert before prescribing.

Paroxetine hydrochloride has been approved for the treatment of major depressive disorder, obsessive-compulsive disorder, panic disorder, social anxiety disorder, generalized anxiety disorder, and posttraumatic stress disorder in adults. Its safety and efficacy for use in the pediatric age group have not been established. One manufacturer notes that three placebo-controlled studies of paroxetine in the treatment of major depressive disorder in pediatric patients did not adequately support its use in this age group (PDR, 2006).

Paroxetine Dosage Schedule

Paroxetine may be administered with or without food. It is recommended that it be given in a single daily dose, usually in the morning.

- Children and adolescents ≤ 17 years of age: Not recommended. Safety and efficacy have not been established in this age group.
- Adolescents at least 18 years of age and adults:

    Treatment of major depressive disorder: An initial single dose of 20 mg, usually administered in the morning, is recommended. Full antidepressant response may be delayed for up to several weeks. Although 20 mg/day is adequate for many patients, others may benefit from higher doses. Based on clinical response, weekly increments of 10 mg/day may be made at intervals of at least 1 week to a maximum daily dose of 50 mg.

    Treatment of obsessive-compulsive disorder: The usual target dose for the treatment of OCD is 40 mg daily. The recommended initial daily dose is 20 mg, usually administered in the morning. Increments of 10 mg/day are suggested at weekly intervals to reach the recommended dose of 40 mg/day. Some patients may benefit from higher doses and further increments at least 1 week apart, may be made to a maximum of 60 mg/day.

    Treatment of panic disorder: The usual target dose for the treatment of panic disorder is 40 mg daily. The recommended initial daily dose is 10 mg, usually administered in the morning. Increments of 10 mg/day are suggested at weekly intervals to reach the recommended dose of 40 mg/day. Some patients may benefit from higher doses, and further increments at least 1 week apart may be made to a maximum of 60 mg/day.

(continued)

Indications for Paroxetine Hydrochloride or Paroxetine Mesylate in Child and Adolescent Psychiatry (Continued)

Treatment of social anxiety disorder: An initial single dose of 20 mg, usually administered in the morning, is recommended. Available information shows no additional benefit to patients treated with higher doses (up to 60 mg/day) for this disorder.

Treatment of generalized anxiety disorder: An initial single dose of 20 mg, usually administered in the morning, is recommended. Available information shows no additional benefit to patients treated with higher doses (up to 50 mg/day) for this disorder.

Treatment of posttraumatic stress disorder: An initial dose of 20 mg is recommended, which is the established effective dose. In there is an inadequate clinical response, weekly increases in increments of 10 mg, to a maximum of 50 mg, may be considered.

Paroxetine Hydrochloride Dose Forms Available

- Tablets: 10 mg (scored), 20 mg (scored), 30 mg, and 40 mg
- Oral suspension: 10 mg/5 mL
- Controlled release tablets (Paxil CR): 12.5 mg, 25 mg, and 37.5 mg

Paroxetine Mesylate Dose Forms Available

- Tablets: 10 mg and 20 mg

Reports of Interest

Paroxetine in the Treatment of Children and Adolescents with Major Depressive Disorder. In an open-label study, Rey-Sanchez and Gutierrez-Casares (1997) treated 45 outpatients (23 males and 22 females) < 14 years of age (mean age, 10.7 ± 2.0 years) who were diagnosed with MDD, with paroxetine. Ratings on the Clinical Global Impressions-Severity (CGI-S) Scale were used to assess efficacy. Paroxetine was initiated at a dose of 10 mg/day and individually titrated. The optimal mean dose was 16.22 mg/day. At baseline, the mean CGI-S was 3.02 ± 0.78 (profound [CGI-S = 4] in 14 subjects, severe [CGI-S = 3] in 18 subjects, and moderate [CGI-S = 2] in 13 subjects). After 1 month, the mean CGI-S was 2.2 ± 0.87, and after 3 months the mean CGI-S score had improved to 1.22 ± 0.71. All subjects were treated until the depressive symptoms had resolved, that is, for a minimum of 6 months and a mean time of 8.4 ± 1.38 months. The authors noted that the females improved significantly more slowly than the males. Sixteen of the subjects were treated simultaneously with benzodiazepine for insomnia or acute anxiety that appears to have existed before treatment with paroxetine and was not considered an untoward effect. Four subjects (8.9%) were reported to have mild to moderate untoward effects, including vomiting, anxiety and nervousness, abdominal pains, cramps, and nausea that remitted following dose adjustments. No patient developed decreased appetite or excited, disinhibited, or hypomanic behavior. The 12 patients who had ECGs showed no significant changes.

Berard et al. (2006) conducted a 12-week, prospective, international (10 different countries), multicenter (33 centers), randomized, double-blind, placebo-controlled, flexible-dose, parallel-group study of the safety and efficacy of paroxetine in the treatment of outpatient adolescents, age range 12 to 19 years, diagnosed with unipolar major depression by DSM-IV criteria and confirmed by the Kiddie-Schedule for Affective Disorders and Schizophrenia for School-age Children-Life-time (K-SADS-L), a score of > 16 on the Montgomery-Åsberg Depression Rating Scale (MADRS) at screening and baseline (average score at baseline was 25.9), and a rating of < 69 on the Children's Global Assessment Score (C-GAS). At baseline 33.7% of the paroxetine group and 39.3% of the placebo group were rated as markedly or severely ill. Of the 324 subjects who were screened, 286 met study criteria and were randomly assigned at a 2:1 ratio to paroxetine ($N = 187$) or to placebo ($N = 99$). This was the first major depressive episode for approximately 83% of the subjects. Analyses, based on intention-to-treat (ITT), comprised 275 subjects (age range 12–19 years; 92 males, 183 females) with at least 1 dose of study medication, and one postbaseline safety or efficacy assessment included 182 subjects in the paroxetine group and 93 in the placebo group.

All subjects received single-blind placebo for a 2-week run-in period before the 12-week study. Following this, subjects in the paroxetine group were initially prescribed 20 mg daily in the morning with food. Dosage was flexible and could be increased or decreased at a maximum of 10 mg/week but had to remain between 20 and 40 mg/day. The mean maximum paroxetine dose at the end of the 12-week study was 25.8 mg/day; 59% of subjects received 20 mg/day, the lowest permitted dose. During the study, 55 (30.2%) of the paroxetine group (including 11.8% because of Adverse Events (AEs) and 4.9% for lack of efficacy) and 24 (25.8%) of the placebo group (including 7.1% because of AEs and 6.5% for lack of efficacy withdrew from the study.

The primary outcome measures necessary for a positive response were at least a 50% decrease from baseline in both the Montgomery-Åsberg Depression Rating Scale (MADRS) score and the Kiddie-Schedule for Affective Disorder and Schizophrenia for School-age Children-Life-time(K-SADS-L) depression subscale. Subjects meeting "responder" criteria on the MADRS included 60.5% of the paroxetine group and 58.2% of the placebo group, which did not differ significantly ($P = .70$) or clinically. On the K-SADS-L, the paroxetine group had a decrease of 9.3 points and the placebo group of 8.9 points, which did not differ significantly ($P = .62$) or clinically. Regarding secondary measures of efficacy, the two groups did not differ significantly on the Clinical Global Impressions-Severity (CGI-S), the Mood and Feelings Questionnaires (MFQs), or the Beck Depression Inventory (BDI); however, the Clinical Global Impressions-Improvement (CGI-I) Scale showed a significant difference between the groups. A rating of 1 (very much improved) or 2 (much improved) was present at endpoint for 69.2% of the paroxetine group versus 57.3% of the placebo group ($P = .045$).

Berard et al. (2006) noted that older adolescents treated with paroxetine had a greater response than younger adolescents so treated. This was indicated by the fact that although the CGI-I responder rate was significant for the entire group, when it was analysed by age subgroups, it was significant only in the older (> 16 years old) adolescent group ($P = .040$).

Adverse events (AEs) were not statistically different between the paroxetine and placebo groups, being reported in 69% of the paroxetine group and 59.1% of the placebo group. The most frequent AEs reported in the paroxetine group were nausea (24.2%), headache (18.7%), dizziness (10.4%), somnolence (9.3%) decreased appetite (7.7%), infection (7.7%) and asthenia (6.6%); however, only decreased appetite was statistically more frequent compared to the placebo group (7.7% vs. 3.2%). AEs related to suicidality occurred in 4.4% of the paroxetine group (4 in adolescents ≤ 16 years and 4 in adolescents > 16 years) and 2.1% of the placebo group (2 adolescents ≤ 16 years), which was not statistically different (P = .502). Suicidal attempts were reported in 3 (1.7%) of the paroxetine group (1 adolescent < 16 years and 2 adolescents > 16 years) and 2 (2.1%) of the placebo group with no statistical difference between the groups (P = 1.000).

The authors concluded that there were no significant statistical or clinical differences between paroxetine and placebo in treating this group of adolescents diagnosed with major depressive disorder on the primary outcome variables; however, the CGI-I rate was significantly greater for the paroxetine group. They also suggested that adolescents > 16 years may respond more favorably to paroxetine than younger adolescents. The authors thought that paroxetine in the doses used (20 to 40 mg/day) was generally well tolerated in this age group (Berard et al. 2006).

Paroxetine in the Treatment of Children and Adolescents Diagnosed with Dysthymia. Nobile et al. (2000) treated 7 subjects (5 males, 2 females; mean age, 14.4 ± 2.6 years; age range, 11 to 18 years) diagnosed by DSM-III-R (APA, 1987) criteria with dysthymia, primary type, without comorbidity for MDD, for 3 months in an open-label study. Efficacy was assessed by ratings on the Hamilton Depression Rating Scale (Ham-D), the Clinical Global Impressions-Severity of Illness Scale (CGI-S), and the CGI Improvement Scale (CGI-I). The initial dose of paroxetine was 10 mg daily. Dosage was titrated based on clinical response. A 10-mg increment was permissible after 1 week, with possible further increases to a daily maximum of 40 mg. Dose reduction was possible at any time. Clinical improvement of responders was noted within the first month of treatment and the improvement continued over the course of treatment. The mean dose of paroxetine after 3 months was 20.12 mg/day. Responders were *a priori* decided to have > 50% improvement on the Ham-D and/or a CGI-I score of 1 ("very much improved") or 2 ("much improved"). Five (71%) of the seven completers (two subjects withdrew during the first month, one female was noncompliant and another female stopped because of nausea and stomach pains) were "responders." The 5 responders were maintained on medication and reassessed 6 months after beginning paroxetine; all 5 showed further improvement on the Ham-D (mean 6-month score was 1.2 ± 2.17) and all 5 were rated with "no disease" on the CGI-S and "very much improved" on the CGI-I. The most common untoward effects were nausea and stomachache (28.6%). Sedation, insomnia, behavioral activation, and inappropriate behavior were reported by one patient each. The authors noted that their data suggest that paroxetine is effective in the treatment of dysthymia in this age group and merits further study.

Paroxetine in the Treatment of Children and Adolescents Diagnosed with Obsessive-Compulsive Disorder. Rosenberg et al. (1999) conducted a 12-week, open-label trial of paroxetine in treating 20 outpatients (9 males, 11 females; ages 8 to 17 years) diagnosed with obsessive-compulsive disorder by DSM-IV criteria (APA, 1994) and having a Children's Yale-Brown Obsessive-Compulsive Scale (CY-BOCS) rating of > 16. Twelve subjects had comorbid diagnoses but only two were given additional medication (lorazepam for anxiety) during the study. Ratings on the Hamilton Anxiety Scale (Ham-A), the Yale Global Tic Severity Scale (YGTSS), the Children's Global Assessment Scale (CGAS), and the Clinical Global Impressions Scale (CGI) were also used to assess efficacy. The criterion for a positive response was a reduction of OCD symptom severity by $> 30\%$ on the CY-BOCS.

The initial dose of paroxetine was 10 mg/day and could be titrated upward by a maximum increase of 10 mg every 2 weeks to a daily maximum of 60 mg or until good clinical response or until untoward effects prevented further increase. At the end of the study, subjects showed significant $(P = .001)$ improvement on the CY-BOCS, the CGAS, and the CGI. Patients also showed a significant decrease in anxiety $(P = .008)$. Of clinical interest, one of the two subjects with tic-related OCD failed to improve and the other, diagnosed with Tourette's disorder, had a worsening of OCD symptoms and a doubling of tic severity consonant with the earlier studies suggesting that tic-related OCD may be less responsive to specific serotonin reuptake inhibitors. Serious untoward effects occurred in two subjects (suicidal ideation in one and increased tics in one). Mild untoward effects included hyperactivity/behavioral inhibition that required dosage reduction in some cases (30%), headache (25%), insomnia (15%), gastrointestinal distress (15%), increased anxiety (10%), drowsiness (5%), and dry mouth (5%). There were no manic-like untoward effects or allergic reactions. Overall paroxetine was considered safe and effective in treating these particular subjects.

Gilbert et al. (2000) used volumetric magnetic resonance imaging (MRI) to measure and compare thalamic volumes in 21 psychotropic drug-naive subjects (7 males, 14 females; mean age, 12.35 ± 2.93 years; range, 8.08 to 17.33 years) diagnosed by DSM-IV (APA, 1994) criteria with obsessive-compulsive disorder whom they were treating with paroxetine with 21 matched healthy controls. After baseline assessment, including MRI, 13 of the 21 subjects were treated with paroxetine 10 mg/day that was titrated to a maximum of 60 mg/day based on clinical response; mean dose of paroxetine after 12 weeks was 51.00 ± 8.76 mg/day (range, 40 to 60 mg/day). Subjects did not receive cognitive behavior therapy or psychotherapy other than supportive or family therapy. The other eight subjects elected not to participate in the protocol. Ten of the 13 subjects had a second MRI at time 12 weeks. (Two of the others refused a second MRI and the MRI of the third subject could not be used because of excess motion artifact.)

Based on CY-BOCS ratings, 7 of the 10 subjects were considered responders, having a 30% or greater improvement in their scores. At baseline, thalamic volumes of treatment-naive patients with OCD were significantly greater than those of controls $(P = .01)$. Thalamic volume in the 10 patients with OCD decreased significantly (19% mean reduction in volume) after 12 weeks' treatment with paroxetine $(P = .01)$ and was no longer significantly different from that of the controls $(P = .76)$. Reduction in thalamic volume correlated with significantly lower scores on the CY-BOCS, but the dose of paroxetine did not correlate with final thalamic volume. Repeat MRIs were also obtained in 8 medication-free controls about 12 weeks after baseline; they showed less variation (a mean of $\pm 5.6\%$ of baseline) in volume, suggesting that the greater change in the paroxetine group was a real phenomenon. The authors' preliminary findings suggest that treatment-naive children diagnosed with OCD have serotonergic abnormalities that result in increased thalamic volumes. During the 12-week period of treatment with paroxetine, significant reduction in thalamic volume and clinical improvement in OCD symptomatology occurred.

Geller et al. (2004) conducted a prospective, multicenter, 10-week, randomized, double-blind, placebo-controlled, flexible-dose, parallel-group trial to evaluate the efficacy and safety of paroxetine hydrochloride in treating 203 children and adolescents who were diagnosed with obsessive-compulsive disorder (OCD) by DSM-IV criteria. Comorbid psychiatric diagnoses were made in 35.5% (72) of the patients; the most common were attention-deficit/hyperactivity disorder (9.4%), generalized anxiety disorder (6.9%), and enuresis (6.9%). Of the 203 patients, 56.7% (115) were children aged 7–11 years and 43.3% (88) were adolescents aged 12 to 17 years; 57.6% (117) were male and 42.4% (86) were female; 88.2% were white.

The primary measure of efficacy was the change from baseline to the week 10 last observation carried forward (LOCF) end point in total score on the Children's Yale-Brown Obsessive-Compulsive Scale (CY-BOCS). Six secondary measures of efficacy were used: (i) Reduction > 25% on the CY-BOCS; (ii) a score of 1 (very much improved) or 2 (much improved) on the Clinical Global Impressions-Improvement (CGI-I) score (iii and iv) changes from baseline to endpoint scores on the Compulsions Subtest and the Obsessions Subtest of the CY-BOCS; (v) the CGI-Severity (CGI-S) score and (vi) Global Assessment of Functioning (GAF) rating. Safety was assessed by monitoring adverse effects and vital signs at each visit, laboratory tests, physical examinations and ECGs at baseline and endpoint.

The intention-to-treat (ITT) population, consisting of the randomized patients who had at least one dose of study medication and one postbaseline assessment ($N = 203$) were assigned to paroxetine ($N = 98$) or placebo ($N = 105$). During week 1, patients received paroxetine 10 mg daily or placebo. Dose was then titrated in 10-mg increments based on the clinical response with a weekly maximum permitted increase of 10 mg/day. The maximum total dose permitted was 50 mg/day. The mean baseline CY-BOCS total score was 24.8 (moderate to severe OCD symptomatology); baseline CGI-S ratings were 52% moderately ill, 34% markedly ill and 11.8% severely or among the most extremely ill.

About one-third (33.7%) of the paroxetine group and 23.8% of the placebo group did not complete the study. Adverse effects (10.2%; $N = 10$) were the most common reason for this in the paroxetine group and lack of efficacy (13.3%; $N = 14$) the most common reason in the placebo group. The average length of treatment for the paroxetine group was 60 days and for the placebo group 64 days. The final (week 10 LOCF end point) mean dose of paroxetine for children was 25.4 mg/day and for adolescents was 36.5 mg/day.

The paroxetine group improved significantly more than the placebo group on the CY-BOCS total score (-8.75 points vs. -5.34 points, $P = .002$). Patients with higher initial CY-BOCS scores had greater changes from baseline than patients with lower initial scores ($P = .002$) and children had greater changes from baseline than adolescents ($P < .001$). In addition, the three secondary measures utilizing the CY-BOCS for paroxetine were all statistically superior to those for placebo and the other three were numerically but not significantly superior.

The most frequently reported adverse effects in the paroxetine group were headache (24.5%), abdominal pain (17.3%), nausea (16.3%), upper respiratory infection (12.2%), somnolence (12.2%), motor hyperactivity (12.2%), and trauma (physical and accidental injuries) (10.2%); of these, only hyperactivity and trauma occurred at least twice as frequently as in the placebo group. Overall, 10.2% (8 children and 2 adolescents) of the paroxetine group and 2.9% of the placebo group discontinued treatment because of an adverse effect. Serious adverse effects (SAEs) were reported in three children in the paroxetine group; two exhibited aggressive behavior and one was hospitalized for suicidal thoughts, which were closely related in timing to the patient's being forced out of his home by his guardian and his being sent to a youth shelter, and not related to the medication. One patient in the placebo group exhibited aggressive behavior.

During treatment discontinuation, that is the period of drug taper or follow-up during the first 2 weeks off the drug, patients who were taking paroxetine experienced nausea (2.5%) and vomiting (3.8%) compared to 1.1% and 0%, respectively, of patients who were on placebo.

The authors concluded that paroxetine had a modest overall effect in reducing symptoms on the CY-BOCS and was significantly more efficacious that placebo. Its tolerability and safety profile were similar to those observed with other SSRIs in children and adolescents being treated for OCD.

Paroxetine in the Treatment of Children and Adolescents Diagnosed with Social Anxiety Disorder. Wagner et al. (2004) conducted a 38-center, randomized, double-blind, placebo-controlled 16-week study of paroxetine in a total of 322 children (age 8 to 11) and adolescents (age 12 to 17) who met DSM-IV (1994) criteria for social anxiety disorder. The exclusion criteria for subjects included having a clinically prominent Axis I diagnosis other than social anxiety disorder, or a history of a psychotic disorder. The ITT population for statistical analysis consisted of the 319 subjects who had had at least one dose of study medication and one postbaseline follow-up assessment; of these 28.5% (91) were children and 71.5% (228) were adolescents. The paroxetine group ($N = 163$) was 43.6% male and the placebo group ($N = 156$) was 57.1% male.

Paroxetine was begun at a dose of 10 mg and could be increased at weekly intervals to a maximum of 50 mg/day; after week 2, dose could be reduced to the prior dose in the event of an adverse effect (AE). At the end of the study, subjects whose daily dose was 20 mg or more were tapered off by reducing the dose by 10 mg weekly. The primary outcome measure (efficacy end point) was a rating of 1 "very much improved" or 2 "much improved" on the Clinical Global Impressions-Improvement (CGI-I) Scale.

At week 16, the mean dose of paroxetine for all subjects was 32.6 mg/day; for children it was 26.5 mg/day and for adolescents it was 35.0 mg/day. Of the subjects in the paroxetine group, 77.6% (125/161) met criteria for responders versus 38.3% (59/154) of subjects in the placebo group ($P < .001$). The benefit of paroxetine was apparent within 4 weeks. Paroxetine also showed statistically more clinical benefit than placebo ($P < .001$) on all five secondary outcome measures: The Clinical Global Impression-Severity Scale; the Global Assessment of Functioning; the Liebowitz Social Anxiety Scale for Children and Adolescents (LSAS-CA); the Kutcher Generalized Social Anxiety Disorder Scale for Adolescents; and the Social Phobia and Anxiety Inventory (SPAI) or the SPAI for Children (SPAI-C). Remission was defined as either a > 70% reduction on the LSAS-CA or a rating of "1" very much improved on the GCI-I; 34.6% of the paroxetine group met both criteria, whereas only 8% of the placebo group did so.

Most adverse events were of mild to moderate intensity. AEs that possibly occurred as a result of treatment in > 5% of subjects on paroxetine and at a rate at least twice that of placebo were: insomnia, 14.1% versus 5.8% ($P = .02$); decreased appetite, 8.0% versus 3.2% ($P = .11$); and vomiting 6.7% versus 1.9% ($P = .07$). Rates of nervousness, hyperkinesia, asthenia, and hostility also met the preceding criteria in children but not in adolescents; rates of somnolence and insomnia met these criteria in adolescents but not in children (P values were not given.) The authors concluded that paroxetine was effective in treating children and adolescents diagnosed with social anxiety disorder (Wagner et al. 2004)

Fluvoxamine Maleate (Luvox)

Fluvoxamine maleate is an SSRI that belongs to a new chemical series, the 2-aminoethyloxime ethers of aralkylketones. It is chemically unrelated to other SSRIs and clomipramine. In *in vitro* studies, the drug exhibited no significant affinity for histaminergic, alpha- or beta-adrenergic, muscarinic, or dopamine receptors.

Fluvoxamine has been approved for the treatment of obsessive-compulsive disorder in patients at least 8 years of age.

Pharmacokinetics of Fluvoxamine Maleate

Food does not significantly affect the bioavailability of fluvoxamine. In volunteers, peak plasma concentrations at steady state occurred between 3 and 8 hours after ingestion of the drug and revealed nonlinear pharmacokinetics for single doses of 100, 200, and 300 mg, with higher doses resulting in disproportionately higher plasma levels (e.g., plasma levels of 88, 283, and 546 ng/mL, respectively). The mean plasma half-life at steady state for young adults taking 100 mg/day was 15.6 hours.

Labellarte et al. (2004) reported on the multiple-dose pharmacokinetics of fluvoxamine maleate in 16 children (9 males, 7 females) and 18 adolescents (9 males, 9 females) being treated for obsessive-compulsive disorder. They measured serum levels > 12 hours after 12 or more consecutive doses of 25, 50, 100 and 150 mg of fluvoxamine. Maximum daily dose was 200 mg/day for children and 300 mg/day for adolescents, given in 2 doses 12 hours apart. Compared to adolescents, children had higher mean peak plasma concentrations, higher mean area under the plasma concentration-time curve, and lower apparent oral clearance; at a dose of 50 mg twice daily adjusted mean serum level for children was 182.45 versus 67.50 ng/mL for adolescents ($P = <.05$). Compared to male children, female children had higher mean peak plasma concentration, higher mean area under the plasma concentration-time curve and reported more adverse effects. Adolescents had similar pharmacokinetics to those reported for adults on 150 mg, twice daily doses. These data suggest that children, especially female children, have a higher exposure to fluvoxamine at a given dose than adolescents and adults.

Smokers metabolize fluvoxamine maleate about 25% faster than nonsmokers.

Contraindications for Fluvoxamine Maleate Administration

Known hypersensitivity to fluvoxamine maleate is a contraindication.

Coadministration of terfenadine, astemizole, or cisapride with fluvoxamine maleate is contraindicated. This is because fluvoxamine maleate is likely to be a potent inhibitor of P450 3A4 isoenzyme, which would cause increased levels of the previously mentioned drugs and result in the lengthening of the QT interval, which has been associated with torsade de pointes–type ventricular tachycardia and fatalities.

Because of a possibility for serious, life-threatening reactions when administered simultaneously with a MAOI, the use of fluvoxamine maleate in combination with a MAOI is contraindicated. At least 14 days should elapse after stopping a MAOI before administering fluvoxamine maleate. Based on the half-life of fluvoxamine maleate, at least 14 days should elapse following its discontinuation before administering a MAOI.

Interactions of Fluvoxamine Maleate with Other Drugs

Benzodiazepines should be coadministered with great caution. Plasma levels and half-life of alprazolam were approximately doubled when it was given together with fluvoxamine, resulting in decreased psychomotor performance and memory; if coadministered, the dose of alprazolam should be reduced by at least 50% and gradually titrated to the lowest effective dose. Coadministration of diazepam is not recommended, as fluvoxamine maleate reduces its clearance and that of its major metabolite N-desmethyldiazepam and clinically significant increases would be expected.

Many other potential interactions, particularly with drugs that inhibit or are metabolized by cytochrome P450 isoenzymes, have been reported (package insert).

Untoward Effects of Fluvoxamine Maleate

The most frequently reported untoward effects were somnolence, insomnia, dry mouth, nervousness, tremor, nausea, dyspepsia, anorexia, vomiting, abnormal ejaculation, asthenia, and sweating. As decreased appetite and weight loss can occur with fluvoxamine, these parameters should be monitored.

Indications for Fluvoxamine Maleate in Child and Adolescent Psychiatry

Note: Review the Black Box Warning at the beginning of the chapter or in the package insert before prescribing.

Fluvoxamine is approved only for the treatment of obsessions and compulsions in children 8 years of age and older, adolescents, and adults diagnosed with obsessive-compulsive disorder. Its safety and efficacy have not been established in children < 8 years.

Fluvoxamine Dosage Schedule

Treatment of Obsessive-Compulsive Disorder:

- Children < 8 years of age: Not recommended. Safety and efficacy have not been established for this age range.
- Children at least 8 and adolescents up to 17 years of age: An initial bedtime dose of 25 mg is recommended. The dose may be titrated upward every 4 to 7 days as clinically indicated in 25-mg increments to a maximum of 200 mg to achieve maximal therapeutic response. Daily doses totaling more than 50 mg should be given in two doses; if the two doses are unequal, the larger dose should be taken at bedtime.
- Adolescents at least 18 years of age and adults: An initial bedtime dose of 50 mg is recommended. The dose may be titrated upward every 4 to 7 days as clinically indicated in 50-mg increments to a maximum of 300 mg to achieve maximal therapeutic response. Daily doses totaling more than 100 mg should be given in two doses; if the two doses are unequal, the larger dose should be taken at bedtime. Usual optimal doses range from 100 to 300 mg.

Fluvoxamine Maleate Dose Forms Available

- Tablets: 25 mg, 50 mg (scored), and 100 mg (scored).

Reports of Interest

Fluvoxamine Maleate in the Treatment of Adolescents Diagnosed with Major Depressive Disorder or Obsessive-Compulsive Disorder. Apter et al. (1994) reported treating 20 adolescent inpatients 13 to 18 years of age who were diagnosed with MDD ($N = 6$) or obsessive-compulsive disorder (OCD) ($N = 14$) with fluvoxamine in an 8-week, open-label protocol. Inclusion criteria for the six depressed patients included lack of response to a tricyclic antidepressant, additional symptoms of suicidality, impulsivity or affective instability, or a comorbid major psychiatric diagnosis. Four had comorbid diagnoses of both borderline personality and conduct disorders, one had comorbid bulimia, and the sixth was diagnosed with MDD only. Eleven of the 14 patients with OCD also had comorbid diagnoses: Tourette's syndrome (TS) (four), schizophrenia (four), and anorexia nervosa (three). All eight subjects diagnosed with comorbid TS or schizophrenia also received haloperidol; in addition, three of them received benzhexol, an anticholinergic drug. Fluvoxamine was increased by 50 mg weekly until either a therapeutic result was obtained or untoward effects prevented further increase. Doses ranged from 100 to 300 mg/day (mean, 200 mg/day). Sixteen patients completed the study, and four dropped out because of untoward effects; for the latter four patients, the last ratings while on medication were used in analyzing the data.

All six patients with MDD improved significantly on the Beck Depression Inventory ($P < .0002$), but only two of the four patients with comorbid MDD and borderline personality disorder showed clinically significant decreases in impulsivity and suicidality.

As a group, the 14 patients with OCD improved significantly on the Yale-Brown Obsessive Compulsive Scale (Y-BOCS) ($P < .0001$). However, one of the three patients with comorbid anorexia nervosa developed confusion and delirium and another developed hallucinations; both were dropped from the study at week 6. Of note, statistically significant improvement over baseline ratings on the Y-BOCS did not occur until week 6, and there was further improvement at week 8.

All subjects developed at least some mild untoward effects compared with baseline ratings on the Dosage Record Treatment Emergent Symptom Scale (DOTES). Fluvoxamine initially caused some activating untoward effects, such as insomnia, hyperactivity, agitation, excitement, anxiety, and hypomania. These were mild and transient in most cases; however, one patient with a family history of bipolar disorder who developed hypomania was dropped during the fifth week. Nausea, tremor, and dermatitis occurred in about 75% of subjects; in one case the drug had to be discontinued because of itchy maculopapular dermatitis. No changes in heart rate, blood pressure, ECG, or routine laboratory tests were reported. No patient showed a significant increase in ratings on the Suicide Potential or Overt Aggression Scales (Apter et al. 1994).

Fluvoxamine Maleate in the Treatment of Children and Adolescents Diagnosed with Anxiety Disorders. Vitiello (2000) reported preliminary findings of a multisite, double-blind, placebo-controlled trial of fluvoxamine in the treatment of 128 subjects (age range, 6 to 17 years) who were diagnosed with social phobia, separation anxiety disorder, or generalized anxiety disorder and treated for 8 weeks with fluvoxamine or placebo. Fluvoxamine was titrated on an individual basis to a maximum of 300 mg/day. Efficacy was determined by ratings on the Pediatric Anxiety Rating Scale (PARS) and the Clinical Global Impressions-Improvement (CGI-I) Scale. Fluvoxamine-treated subjects had significantly improved ratings on the PARS compared with subjects on placebo ($P < .001$); on the CGI-I, 76% of subjects on fluvoxamine were rated as responders versus only 29% on placebo ($P < .001$). These initial data suggest that fluvoxamine may be an effective treatment for children and adolescents diagnosed with these three anxiety disorders.

Citalopram Hydrobromide (Celexa)

The SSRI citalopram hydrobromide is a racemic bicyclic phthalane derivative that is chemically unrelated to other SSRIs or to tricyclic, tetracyclic, and other antidepressants.

Citalopram has minimal effects on the neuronal reuptake of norepinephrine and dopamine. It has no or very low affinity for $5HT_{1A}$, $5HT_{2A}$, dopamine D_1, and D_2, alpha-1, alpha-2, or beta adrenergic, histamine H_1, gamma aminobutyric acid (GABA), muscarinic, cholinergic, and benzodiazepine receptors.

Pharmacokinetics of Citalopram Hydrobromide

Food does not affect the bioavailability of citalopram hydrobromide. Peak serum levels occur about 4 hours after ingestion. With once-daily dosing, steady-state plasma levels occur in approximately 1 week and are about 2.5 times the concentration observed after a single dose.

Metabolism occurs primarily by N-demethylation in the liver, with CYP3A4 and CYP2C19 being the primary enzymes involved. The parent compound is at least eight times more active than its metabolites, suggesting that they do not play a significant role clinically. Mean terminal half-life is about 35 hours.

Contraindications for Administration of Citalopram Hydrobromide

Known hypersensitivity to citalopram hydrobromide is a contraindication.

Because of a possibility of serious, life-threatening reactions when administered simultaneously with a MAOI, it is recommended that the drug is not used in combination with a MAOI. At least 2 weeks should elapse after stopping citalopram before administering a MAOI and conversely, after stopping a MAOI before administering citalopram.

Untoward Effects of Citalopram Hydrobromide

Dry mouth, increased sweating, nausea, diarrhea, somnolence or insomnia, ejaculatory disturbance (in 6%, usually ejaculatory delay) have been reported in individuals taking citalopram.

Advantages of Citalopram Hydrobromide

There was no clinically significant difference between placebo and citalopram on cardiac parameters, including electroconductivity from baseline ECG. The only significant difference was a mean decrease in cardiac rate of 1.7 beats/minute.

Indications for Citalopram Hydrobromide in Child and Adolescent Psychiatry

Note: Review the Black Box Warning at the beginning of the chapter or in the package insert before prescribing.

(continued)

Indications for Citalopram Hydrobromide in Child and Adolescent Psychiatry (Continued)

Citalopram is approved for the treatment of depression. The safety and efficacy for use in children and adolescents has not been determined. One manufacturer notes that the data from 2 placebo-controlled studies in which a total of 407 subjects in the pediatric age group who were diagnosed with major depressive disorder were not adequate to report a claim for citalopram's use in this age group. Citalopram is usually administered once daily, in the morning or evening, and may be taken with or without food.

Citalopram Dosage Schedule

Treatment of Major Depressive Disorder:

- Children and adolescents ≤ 17 years of age: Not recommended. Safety and efficacy have not been established for this age group.
- Adolescents at least 18 years of age and adults: An initial morning or evening dose of 20 mg is recommended. An increase to 40 mg daily is usual after 1 week. Doses of more than 40 mg daily are not usually recommended as increased efficacy with higher doses has not been demonstrated. A maximum dose of 60 mg/day.

Citalopram Hydrobromide Dose Forms Available

- Tablets: 10 mg, 20 mg (scored), and 40 mg (scored)
- Oral solution: 10 mg/5 mL (10 mg/tsp)

Report of Interest

Citalopram Hydrobromide in the Treatment of Children and Adolescents Diagnosed with Obsessive-Compulsive Disorder

Thomsen (1997) treated 23 subjects (11 males, 12 females; mean age, 13.1 ± 2.5 years; age range, 9 to 18 years) diagnosed with obsessive-compulsive disorder (OCD) by DSM-III-R (APA, 1987) criteria with citalopram in a 10-week, open-label study. Fifteen had comorbid diagnoses, including four with MDD. Nine subjects were inpatients, two of whom were followed-up after discharge, and 14 were outpatients. An initial dose of 10 mg of citalopram was given approximately 2 weeks after referral and gradually titrated to a target dose of 40 mg/day for 20 subjects. Because of untoward effects, the final dose for two subjects was 20 mg/day and for one subject was 10 mg/day. The mean dose of citalopram at the end of the 10 weeks was 37.0 ± 0.8 mg/day; dose range, 10 to 40 mg/day. Efficacy was assessed by ratings on the Yale-Brown Obsessive-Compulsive Scale (Y-BOCS) or its version for children (CY-BOCS) < 15 years old, the Children's Assessment Schedule (CAS) and the Children's Global Assessment Scale (CGAS). Posttreatment (10-week) ratings on the Y-BOCS or CY-BOCS improved significantly over baseline (mean scores declined from 30.1 to 20.9; $P = .001$). Four subjects (17%) were rated as markedly improved with a > 50% decrease in the rating, 14 patients (61%) were rated as moderately improved (a 20% to 43% reduction in scores), four patients (17%) were slightly improved (5% to 20% reduction in scores), and one patient showed no change. Improvement in social functioning was reflected by scores on the CGAS, which improved significantly from baseline to posttreatment ratings (mean scores increased from 59.1 to 71.0; $P = .001$). Overall, however, only six patients improved sufficiently so as to no longer meet the diagnostic criteria for OCD, and they continued to have symptoms of subclinical OCD. Mild untoward effects were reported by 13 subjects. Most, including all cases of dry mouth, headache, and tremor, were transient, resolving within a few weeks. Restlessness occurred in four patients, increased anxiety in two patients, and erectile dysfunction in one patient. In no case did untoward effects necessitate discontinuation of citalopram. The findings suggested that citalopram may be effective and well tolerated in children and adolescents diagnosed with OCD at doses of up to 40 mg/day.

Escitalopram Oxalate (Lexapro)

Escitalopram oxalate is the pure S-enantiomer, the active isomer, of racemic citalopram, a selective serotonin reuptake inhibitor (SSRI).

Pharmacokinetics of Escitalopram Oxalate

Escitalopram oxalate may be taken with or without food. Maximum plasma levels occur about 5 hours after ingestion of the drug. Escitalopram oxalate has a half-life of about 27 to 32 hours. Steady-state plasma levels occur in approximately one week at a given dose. Escitalopram oxalate is metabolized primarily through demethylation by the hepatic enzymes CYP3A4 and CYP2C19. About 18% is excreted in the urine.

Contraindications for the Administration of Escitalopram Oxalate

Hypersensitivity to escitalopram oxalate, any of its inactive ingredients, or citalopram is a contraindication to its administration. As escitalopram is the active isomer of racemic citalopram, the two drugs should not be administered together.

Escitalopram oxalate should not be coadministered with a monoamine oxidase inhibitor (MAOI) or within 14 days of treatment with a MAOI being discontinued. At least 14 days should elapse after stopping escitalopram oxalate therapy before administering a MAOI.

Untoward Effects of Escitalopram Oxalate

Untoward effects included gastrointestinal disorders, especially nausea (15%), insomnia (9%), somnolence (6%), increased sweating (5%), fatigue (5%), and decreased appetite (3%). Sexual untoward effects in males: ejaculation disorder (12%, most of which was accounted for by delayed ejaculation), decreased libido (6%) and impotence (3%); and in females: decreased libido (3%), anorgasmia (3%). Of note, untoward effects were approximately twice as frequent in patients treated with 20 mg of escitalopram daily compared to patients treated with 10 mg daily.

No significant ECG changes were reported.

Indications for Escitalopram Oxalate in Child and Adolescent Psychiatry

Note: Review the Black Box Warning at the beginning of the chapter or in the package insert before prescribing.

(continued)

Indications for Escitalopram Oxalate in Child and Adolescent Psychiatry (Continued)

Escitalopram oxalate is indicated for the treatment of major depressive disorder and generalized anxiety disorder in adults. Safety and efficacy have not been established for pediatric patients.

Escitalopram Oxalate Dosage Schedule

Children and Adolescents: Not recommended. Safety and efficacy has not been established for this age group.

Adults: The recommended dose is 10 mg, once daily. An increase to 20 mg daily can be considered after a minimum of 1 week; however, a fixed-dose trial showed no increased benefit for 20 mg compared to 10 mg.

Escitalopram Oxalate Dose Forms Available

● Coated tablets (scored): 10 mg and 20 mg

Oral solution (peppermint flavored): 5 mg/5 mL

Report of Interest

Escitalopram Oxalate in the Treatment of Children and Adolescents Diagnosed with Pervasive Developmental Disorders

Owley et al. (2005) assessed the effectiveness of escitalopram in the treatment of 28 subjects (25 [89%] males, 3 [11%] females; age range 6 to 17 years; mean age 125.1 ± 33.5 months) who were diagnosed with pervasive developmental disorders [PDDs]; autistic disorder 20 [71%], Asperger's disorder 5 [18%], and pervasive developmental disorder not otherwise specified [PDDNOS] 3 [11%]) in a 10-week, open-label forced titration study. Inclusion criteria included a score of > 12 on the Irritability Subscale of the Aberrant Behavior Checklist-Community Version (ABC-CV). The Primary outcome measures were the Clinical Global Impressions-Severity (CGI-S) Scale and the ABC-CV. A subject with a reduction of > 50% on the ABC-CV irritability subscale was defined as a "responder."

Escitalopram was initiated at a dose of 2.5 mg daily with forced weekly increases to 5, 10, 15 and 20 mg as of the fifth week. If predetermined problems with sleep or significant increases in irritability or hyperactivity on the subscales of the ABC-CV occurred, the dose was reduced to that of the preceding week and maintained there for the duration of the study. Twenty-three of the subjects completed the study. Of the five withdrawals, two were for continued significant hyperactivity, one for obsessions/compulsions that required additional medications, and two subjects secondary to their developing disinhibition and aggression. At endpoint, the mean daily dose of escitalopram was 11.1 ± 6.5 mg with a range of 0 mg/day (a subject who developed disinhibition and aggression on the lowest permitted dose of 2.5 mg was dropped from the study) to 20 mg/day. Subjects' endpoint doses were unrelated to weight and corresponded only weakly to age. Five subjects had no adverse effects and tolerated the 20 mg/day dose. The authors noted that some patients might be able to tolerate only doses as low as 1 mg/day without developing adverse effects. Of the 18 subjects for whom adverse effects were reported who required reduction in dose to that of the preceding week, irritability was primarily responsible in 7, hyperactivity in 6, and both irritability and hyperactivity in 5. No subjects reported suicidal ideation and there was no evidence of increased self-injurious behavior or sleep difficulties.

The responder rate was 17/28 (61%); 7 had an optimal response at < 10 mg/day and 10 had optimal responses at doses of ≥ 10 mg/day. On the ABC-CV Rating Scale, scores at week 10 were significantly improved on the Irritability, Lethargy, Stereotypy, Hyperactivity subscales at $P < .001$ and on the Inappropriate Speech subscale at $P = .035$; the ABC-CV total score was also significant at $P < .001$. CGI-S mean score at baseline was 5.2 ± 1.0 and at endpoint was 4.6 ± 1.2 ($P < .001$). The authors concluded that escitalopram was useful in treating some common symptoms present in PDD and that controlled studies should be undertaken for such subjects.

OTHER ANTIDEPRESSANTS

Trazodone Hydrochloride (Desyrel)

Trazodone hydrochloride is chemically unrelated to tricyclic, tetracyclic, and other currently approved antidepressant agents. Although it is a serotonin reuptake inhibitor, it is unlike the SSRIs in that its metabolites have significant effects on other neurotransmitter systems and their receptors (Cioli et al. 1984). It is approved for the treatment of patients diagnosed with major depressive episode, both with and without prominent symptoms of anxiety. Although trazodone's antidepressant activity is not fully understood, it inhibits serotonin reuptake in the brain in animals and potentiates behavioral changes induced by 5-hydroxytryptophan.

Pharmacokinetics of Trazodone Hydrochloride

It is recommended that trazodone be ingested soon after eating. When taken in this manner, up to 20% more of the drug may be absorbed than when taken on an empty stomach, and maximum serum concentration is achieved more slowly (in about 2 hours rather than 1 hour) and with a lesser peak. This appears to diminish the likelihood of developing dizziness and/or lightheadedness.

Trazodone is eliminated through the liver (about 20% biliary) and the kidneys (about 75%). Elimination is biphasic: the initial half-life is between 3 and 6 hours, which is followed by a second phase with a half-life of between 5 and 9 hours.

Contraindications for Trazodone Hydrochloride Administration

Known hypersensitivity to the drug is a contraindication.

Interactions of Trazodone Hydrochloride with Other Drugs

Increased phenytoin levels have been reported when administered concomitantly with trazodone.

Trazodone should not be administered with MAOIs because the effects of their interaction are unknown.

Untoward Effects of Trazodone Hydrochloride

The most common side effects include drowsiness, dizziness or lightheadedness, dry mouth, and nausea or vomiting.

Priapism, which has necessitated surgical intervention and resulted in some cases of permanent impairment of sexual functioning, has been reported (incidence, about

1:15,000). Male patients with a prolonged or inappropriate erection should be told to discontinue trazodone immediately and contact their physician or, if it persists, to go to an emergency room.

Indications for Trazodone Hydrochloride in Child and Adolescent Psychiatry

Note: Review the Black Box Warning at the beginning of the chapter or in the package insert before prescribing.

Trazodone is approved only for the treatment of major depressive disorder in individuals at least 18 years old.

The drug is not recommended for use in the pediatric age group because its safety and effectiveness have not been established for this age range.

Trazodone Dosage Schedule

USPDI (2005) reports the following pediatric dosage guidelines when trazodone is used as an antidepressant:
- Children < 6 years: Not determined.
- Children 6 to 18 years of age: Begin with 1.5 to 2 mg/kg/day in divided doses. Titrate dosage gradually at 3- to 4-day intervals to a maximum of 6 mg/kg/day.

Trazodone Hydrochloride Dose Forms Available

- Tablets: 50 mg (scored), 100 mg (scored), 150 mg (quadrisected), and 300 mg (scored to divide into three equal parts or two equal parts)

Reports of Interest

Trazodone in the Treatment of Children and Adolescents with Significant Aggressivity

Fras (1987) reported successfully treating a 15-year-old male hospitalized for recurrent violence with a daily dose of 200 mg of trazodone. Because of a misunderstanding, following discharge the dose was significantly decreased and at times omitted altogether. Repeated angry outbursts and threats of violence developed within 1 week and the patient became morose. Upon resumption of a daily dose of 200 mg, the patient returned to the previous stability and cooperativeness, and remained so for 8 months of follow-up.

Zubieta and Alessi (1992) reported an open study of 22 inpatients (18 males and 4 females; age range, 5 to 12 years; mean age, 9 ± 2 years) with severe, treatment-refractory, behavioral disturbances. They were diagnosed with disruptive behavioral and mood disorders often with comorbidity. Six of the children continued to receive neuroleptic drugs for psychotic symptoms during the trial of trazodone. An initial dose of 50 mg of trazodone at bedtime was begun on an average of 23 ± 20 days after admission. It was titrated over a period of about 1 week to the maximum dose tolerated and given three times daily. The

13 children designated as responders received a mean dose of 185 ± 117 mg/day (4.8 ± 1.7 mg/kg/day) of trazodone for a mean of 27 ± 13 days. The 7 nonresponders received a mean dose of 158 ± 70 mg/day (4.7 ± 2.0 mg/kg/day) for a mean of 24 ± 11 days. One patient was dropped from the study for severe orthostatic hypotension and a second for reported painful erections (not priapism). The other children tolerated any untoward effects that occurred. The most frequent was orthostatic hypotension (50%), but this effect diminished over a few days and did not require clinical intervention; 27% of children reported drowsiness; 9%, nervousness; and 9%, anger. Dizziness, increased fatigue, and nocturnal enuresis each occurred in one child (4.5%).

Target symptoms that improved most frequently were impulsivity, hyperactivity, "involvement in dangerous activities," cruelty to people, frequency of physical fights, arguing with adults, and losing one's temper. Improvement of symptoms usually occurred within a few days of the initial administration of trazodone, as contrasted with the several weeks of continuous administration typically required for its antidepressant effects to occur. In a telephone follow-up 3 to 14 months later (mean, 8.8 ± 4.2 months), nine of the 13 responders were successfully contacted. Eight of the children continued to receive a mean trazodone dose of 241 ± 128 mg/day (range, 100 to 800 mg/day). Trazodone was the only medication being taken at follow-up, the neuroleptics that three children were taking at discharge having been withdrawn within 2 months after discharge. The ninth child had an unsatisfactory response and his medication was changed to a combination of carbamazepine and pemoline. Overall, parents rated their children's improvement at 70 ± 20 (range, 50 to 90) on a subjective overall rating of efficacy scale ranging from 0 to 100 (Zubieta and Alessi, 1992). Trazodone appears to be a potentially useful drug in treating acute and chronic behavioral disorders that have not responded to other treatments and merits further investigation.

Ghaziuddin and Alessi (1992) noted the relationship of the expression of aggression and decreased levels of serotonin in the central nervous system and the successful use of trazodone to control aggressive behavior in adults with organic mental disorders. They administered trazodone to 3 boys who were 7, 8, and 9 years old with primary diagnoses of severe disruptive behavioral disorders; 2 of the boys were hospitalized. Trazodone was initiated at doses of 25 mg once or twice daily and increased gradually. Improvement of symptoms was noted within 7 to 10 days at a mean dose of 3.5 mg/kg/day of trazodone (about 75 mg/day). In all three cases, marked deterioration of behavior occurred upon discontinuing the medication and aggressiveness decreased to former treatment levels once medication was resumed. One boy had no reported untoward effects; one experienced mild sedation during the first week, but this remitted with no change in dosage. The third experienced spontaneous erections on 100 mg/day; because of concerns about reported priapism, dosage was reduced to 75 mg daily and behavioral control deteriorated. When 1,000 mg daily of L-tryptophan (which has been subsequently withdrawn from the commercial market) was added, behavior markedly improved again. No ECG changes were noted in any of the boys. The authors note that further studies will be needed to determine the efficacy and safety of trazodone in treating aggressive children.

Bupropion Hydrochloride (Wellbutrin, Zyban)

Bupropion hydrochloride is an antidepressant of the aminoketone class. It is not related chemically to the tricyclics, tetracyclics, or other known antidepressants.

Pharmacokinetics of Bupropion Hydrochloride

Peak plasma concentrations are usually reached in about 2 hours. The metabolism of bupropion is extensive and complex. Following peak serum levels there is a biphasic decline; average half-life of the second (postdistributional) phase is 14 hours (range, 8 to 24 hours). Several metabolites are pharmacologically active and have long half-lives. Six hours after a single dose, plasma bupropion levels are about 30% of peak concentration.

Based on a study of 19 subjects (11 males, 8 females; age range 11 to 17, mean age 15.2 ± 1.8 years) who were treated with bupropion SR for diagnoses of ADHD ($N = 16$) and depressive disorders ($N = 16$) which were comorbid in 13 subjects, Daviss et al. (2005) reported that youths metabolize bupropion SR to active metabolites faster than adults and that bupropion SR should be given to subjects in this age group in divided doses.

Contraindications for Bupropion Hydrochloride Administration

Known hypersensitivity to bupropion hydrochloride and seizure disorders are contraindications.

A current or prior diagnosis of bulimia or anorexia nervosa is also a contraindication because a higher incidence of seizures is reported when bupropion is administered to such patients.

Bupropion should not be administered concurrently with a MAOI. At least a 14-day period off MAOIs should precede initiation of treatment with bupropion hydrochloride.

Concurrent administration with any drug that reduces the seizure threshold is a relative contraindication.

Interactions of Bupropion Hydrochloride with Other Drugs

Relatively few data are available on interactions of bupropion hydrochloride with other drugs. Increased adverse experiences were reported when the drug was administered concomitantly with L-dopa. MAOIs may increase the acute toxicity of bupropion.

Although bupropion is not metabolized by the CYP2D6 enzyme, the drug and its metabolite, morpholinol, inhibit this enzyme *in vitro*. Therefore extreme caution should be exercised when coadministering any drug metabolized by that enzyme, and initial dosage of the drug should be as low as possible.

Untoward Effects of Bupropion Hydrochloride

Of particular clinical concern is the finding that seizures have been associated with about 4 (0.4%) per 1,000 patients treated with bupropion at doses of 450 mg/day or less. This is about four times the incidence of seizures reported with other approved antidepressants, and the incidence of seizures increases with higher daily doses. Conversely, Clay et al. (1988) note that the positive effects of bupropion on memory performance may be unique among antidepressants and that other antidepressants either have no effect or a negative effect on memory performance.

During the first few days of treatment, agitation, motor restlessness, and insomnia frequently occur; starting at a lower dose and making increments gradually helps to minimize these effects.

The most common untoward effects were reported to be agitation, dry mouth, insomnia, headache, nausea, vomiting, constipation, and tremor.

Ferguson and Simeon (1984) reported no adverse (or positive) effects on cognition on a cognitive battery in 17 children with attention deficit disorder or conduct disorders who were treated in an open trial with bupropion.

Indications for Bupropion Hydrochloride in Child and Adolescent Psychiatry

Note: Review the Black Box Warning at the beginning of the chapter or in the package insert before prescribing.

Bupropion hydrochloride is indicated for the treatment of major depressive disorder. Bupropion hydrochloride SR (sustained release, Zyban) is indicated as an aid to smoking cessation treatment.

Bupropion Dosage Schedule

- Children and adolescents ≤ 17 years of age: Not recommended. Safety and efficacy have not been established for this age group.
- Adolescents at least 18 years of age and adults:

Standard-release tablets: An initial dosage of 100 mg twice daily is suggested. Based on clinical response, this may be increased to 100 mg three times daily but not before day 4 of treatment. During the first few days of treatment, agitation, motor restlessness, and insomnia frequently occur; starting at a lower dose and making increments slowly helps to minimize these effects. When insomnia is problematic, administer divided doses earlier in the day and not at bedtime. If no or insufficient clinical improvement occurs within 4 weeks, dosage may gradually be increased. Because of increased risk of seizure, a dose of 150 mg should not be exceeded within a 4-hour time period. The maximum daily dosage should not exceed 450 mg.

Sustained-release tablets: Sustained S-release tablets should be swallowed whole and there should be at least an 8-hour interval between successive doses. See preceding text regarding pharmacodynamics of bupropion SR in older children and adolescents.

Sustained-release tablets (in treating major depressive disorder): an initial morning dose of 150 mg is recommended. If tolerated, an additional 150 mg may be added after four or more days to reach the target dose of 300 mg. Sustained-release tablets should be administered at least 8 hours apart. If no or insufficient clinical improvement occurs within 4 weeks, dosage may be increased to a maximum daily dose of 400 mg (administered as 200 mg bid).

Sustained-release tablets (Zyban, as a smoking cessation aid): an initial daily dose of 150 mg is recommended for the initial 3 days, followed by an increase to the target and maximum recommended daily dose of 150 mg twice daily.

Extended-release tablets (in treating major depressive disorder): an initial morning dose of 150 mg is recommended. If tolerated, an increase to a single,

(continued)

Indications for Bupropion Hydrochloride in Child and Adolescent Psychiatry (Continued)

morning target dose of 300 mg/day may be made at day 4. There should be an interval of at least 24 hours between doses (PDR, 2006).

Bupropion Hydrochloride Dose Forms Available

- Tablets: 75 mg and 100 mg
- Sustained-release tablets (Wellbutrin SR): 100 mg, 150 mg, and 200 mg; (Zyban) 150 mg
- Extended-release tablets (Wellbutrin XR): 150 mg and 300 mg

Reports of Interest

Bupropion Hydrochloride in the Treatment of Children Diagnosed with ADHD. Simeon et al. (1986) treated 17 male subjects (age range, 7 to 13.4 years; mean, 10.4 years) with bupropion in a 14-week, single-blind, uncontrolled study. Fourteen subjects were diagnosed with attention-deficit disorder with hyperactivity (ADDH); of these, eight were also diagnosed with conduct disorder, undersocialized aggressive type, and two with overanxious disorder. Eleven of the subjects had prior drug treatment; of these, eight had shown no improvement. Four weeks of placebo were followed by 8 weeks of bupropion and then by 2 weeks of placebo. The initial dose of bupropion was 50 mg/day; this was increased to 50 mg twice daily during the second week and to a maximum of 50 mg three times daily during the third week. None of the subjects responded to the baseline placebo. Of the subjects who were on the drug, five patients showed marked improvement, seven moderate improvement, and two mild improvement on the Clinical Global Impressions-Improvement (CGI-I) ratings. Significant improvements also occurred on the Children's Psychiatric Rating Scale (CPRS), Conners' Parents and Teachers Scales, and self-ratings. Although not significant, group means for all nine cognitive test variables showed improvement. Optimal dose was 150 mg/day in 15 cases and 100 mg/day and 50 mg/day in the other two subjects. Untoward effects were reported to be infrequent, mild, and transient.

Clay et al. (1988) reported that bupropion hydrochloride was safe and efficacious in treating prepubertal children diagnosed with ADHD. The authors' clinical impression was that children with additional prominent symptoms of conduct disorder responded particularly well to bupropion.

Thirty prepubertal children diagnosed with ADHD were enrolled in a double-blind, placebo-controlled study and individually titrated to optimal doses of bupropion (Clay et al. 1988). Optimal doses ranged from 100 to 250 mg/day (3.1 to 7.1 mg/kg/day; mean, 5.3 ± 1 mg/kg/day). Subjects receiving bupropion showed statistically significant improvement on the Clinical Global Impressions-Improvement and Severity Rating Scales, on the Self-Rating Scale, and on digit symbol and delayed recall on the Selective Reminding Test. No significant improvement was reported was also reported on the Conners Parent Questionnaire and the Conners Teacher Questionnaire. The only serious side effect noted was an allergic rash in two children.

Clay et al. (1988) also noted that some children who had previously not responded satisfactorily to stimulants had a good response to bupropion. On the other hand, some subjects who had never received stimulants and who did not respond well to bupropion responded well when methylphenidate was openly prescribed at a later time.

Casat et al. (1989) administered bupropion to 20 children and placebo to 10 children in a parallel-groups design, double-blind comparison study. All subjects were diagnosed with attention deficit disorder with hyperactivity. Decreases in symptom severity and overall clinical improvement were noted in physician ratings, and there was a significant decrease in hyperactivity in the classroom settings on the Conners Teacher Questionnaire.

Barrickman et al. (1995) conducted a 16-week, double-blind crossover-design study comparing bupropion with methylphenidate (MPH) in the treatment of 15 outpatients (12 males, 3 females; mean age, 11.8 ± 3.3 years; range, 7 to 16 years) who were diagnosed with ADHD by DSM-III-R (APA, 1987) criteria. Following an initial 2-week washout period, subjects were randomly assigned to bupropion or MPH for a 6-week treatment period. This was followed by another 2-week washout; subjects then received the alternative medication for the next 6 weeks. Efficacy was determined by ratings on the Iowa-Conners Abbreviated Parent and Teacher Questionnaires (ICQ-P and ICQ-T), the Clinical Global Impressions (CGI) Improvement Scale (CGI-I), the CGI-Severity Scale (CGI-S), and side effects scale. Bupropion was administered at a dose of 1.5 mg/kg/day for the first week, increased to 2.0 mg/kg/day for the second week, and individually titrated clinically during the third week to achieve an optimal dose, which was then held constant for the final 3 weeks. Active doses of bupropion were usually given twice daily in the morning and at 4:00 PM. The final mean dose of bupropion was 140 ± 146 mg/day (range, 50 to 200 mg/day) or 3.3 ± 1.2 mg/kg/day (range, 1.4 to 5.7 mg/kg/day). Methylphenidate was given at a dose of 0.4 mg/kg/day for the first week and individually titrated to the optimal dose over the next 2 weeks; this dose was then maintained for the final 3-week period on the drug. The final mean dose of MPH was 31 ± 11 mg/day (range, 20 to 60 mg/day) or 0.7 ± 0.2 mg/kg/day (range, 0.4 to 1.3 mg/kg/day).

Treatment with both bupropion and MPH resulted in significantly lower scores on the ICQ-Parent ratings and the ICQ-Teacher ratings when compared with baseline ($P < .001$). There was no significant difference between the two drugs, and the order in which they were given was not significant. Ratings on some of the individual factors on the ICQ improved significantly more on methylphenidate (e.g., attention on the ICQ-parent), and all the rating scales except the R-CMAS, which had nonsignificant trends, suggesting that MPH was slightly more effective than bupropion. Untoward effects were minimal, were usually transient, and occurred primarily during the first 2 weeks of treatment. While on bupropion, nine (60%) subjects reported nine untoward effects: drowsiness (four), fatigue (three), nausea (three), anorexia (two), dizziness (two), "spaciness" (two), anxiety (one), headache (one), and tremor (one). Only five (33%) reported nine untoward effects during the period they were on MPH: anxiety (one), anger/crying (one), drowsiness (one), headache (one), insomnia (one), irritability (one), low mood (one), nausea (one), and stomachache (one). Bupropion appears to be a useful treatment option for treating ADHD but may be slightly less effective than MPH overall and have somewhat more, although usually mild, untoward effects.

Conners et al. (1996) conducted a multisite, 6-week, parallel-group random-ized, double-blind comparison of bupropion hydrochloride ($N = 72$) and placebo

($N = 37$) in 109 children diagnosed with attention deficit disorder with hyperactivity (ADDH) by DSM-III criteria (APA, 1980); none of the subjects had comorbid MDD. Subjects were 90% male and 75% were white; their average age was about 8.5 years (range, 6 to 12 years); two-thirds were in the third grade or below.

Following an initial 1-week single-blind placebo phase, bupropion or placebo was administered at 7:00 AM and 7:00 PM daily over the 4-week flexible-dose treatment phase. Dose was initiated at 3 mg/kg/day and titrated to reach 6 mg/kg/day during days 15 to 28. Daily maximum doses of 150, 200, and 250 mg were permitted for subjects weighing 20 to 30 kg, 31 to 40 kg, and > 40 kg, respectively. The sixth week was again a 1-week placebo washout for all subjects. Efficacy was assessed on several scales, including the Conners Parent and Teacher Questionnaires, the Abbreviated Parent and Teacher Questionnaire (Conners 10-item "Hyperactivity Index"), Clinical Global Impressions-Severity (CGI-S) and CGI-Improvement Scales, a short-term memory test and a continuous performance test.

Teachers noted significant improvement in hyperactivity and conduct problems after the third day on medication. Parents rated restless-impulsive behavior and conduct problems as significantly improved only at the end of the 4-week treatment period. GCI ratings by clinicians at the four settings were not significant when their data was pooled. At the end of the study, when all subjects had completed a week on placebo, teachers' ratings showed no difference between the placebo and medication groups. The authors also reported modest improvement in cognitive functions of attention and memory retrieval. Although the bupropion group improved below the subject selection cutoff of 15 points on the hyperactivity index, the degree of improvement was less than that typically found with the treatment of the standard stimulants.

Overall untoward effects were infrequent. There were no clinically important differences in vital signs, ECG, or laboratory values between the two groups. EEGs at day 28 compared with baseline found that six patients on bupropion developed abnormal EEGs, including three who developed spike-and-wave discharges. No patient had evidence of clinical seizure activity during treatment. Four (6%) patients receiving bupropion developed apparent allergic skin rashes with urticaria and were dropped from the study. Bupropion hydrochloride appears to be a possible second-line treatment for children diagnosed with ADHD, although the magnitude of clinical improvement appears to be less than what is typical for standard stimulants, and there is some concern about adverse effects on the EEG and increased seizure potential (Conners et al. 1996).

Although confirmation of these findings is needed, bupropion may be an alternative treatment for ADHD that does not respond to standard therapies.

Bupropion Treatment of Adolescents Diagnosed with ADHD and Comorbid Substance Abuse and Conduct Disorder. Riggs et al. (1998) treated in a 5-week, open-label study using bupropion, 13 nondepressed adolescent males (mean age, 15.5 years; range, 14 to 17 years) diagnosed with ADHD by DSM-IV (APA, 1994) criteria, who were residing in a long-term, unlocked facility for treatment of their comorbid substance abuse and conduct disorders. Efficacy was determined by ratings on the Conners' Teacher Rating Scale-39 (CTRS-39), the Clinical Global Impressions-Severity of Illness (CGI-S) and the CGI-Improvements (CGI-I) Scales. Bupropion was started at a dose of 100 mg twice daily and increased to 100 mg given three times daily after 7 days for the final 4 weeks of the study. Final dose of all subjects was 300 mg/day (dose range, 3.9 to 5.6 mg/kg/day). Subject mean score on the CTRS-39 declined significantly by 13% ($P = <.01$); the mean CGI-S score improved by 39% ($P < .002$); and the mean CGI-I score was rated "much" or "very much improved" for seven subjects and "minimally improved" for the remaining six. Untoward effects were reported by seven (54%) of the adolescents; most were mild and transient. One subject, however, developed hypomanic symptoms during the fifth week of the study. The symptoms resolved within 1 week after discontinuing bupropion. These initial data suggest that bupropion may be a useful treatment for such adolescents.

Bupropion in the Treatment of Comorbid ADHD and Chronic Motor Tic Disorder or Tourette's Syndrome. Spencer et al. (1993b) reported that bupropion exacerbated tics in four children with ADHD and comorbid Tourette's syndrome (TS). All four patients had been initially treated with stimulants, when two patients with preexisting symptoms of ADHD and TS experienced worsening of their tics and the other two developed tics and TS. Bupropion was subsequently prescribed as a possibly effective alternative treatment for children diagnosed with ADHD who did not respond satisfactorily to stimulants or could not tolerate their untoward effects. All four children experienced an exacerbation of tics over a period ranging from almost immediately to 2 months. The tics rapidly improved to pretreatment levels when bupropion was discontinued. The authors suggest that bupropion may not be a useful alternative to stimulants in treating patients with comorbid ADHD and TS.

Bupropion in the Treatment of Adolescents with Comorbid ADHD and Nicotine Dependency. In an open-label study, Upadhyaya et al. (2004) administered bupropion SR to 16 adolescents (10 males, 6 females, age range, 12 to19 years), with nicotine dependency, 11 of whom had comorbid ADHD. Over the first week, subjects weighing 90 or more pounds were titrated to 150 mg bupropion SR b.i.d.; this dose was maintained for the next 6 weeks. Subjects weighing less than 90 pounds remained on a total daily dose of 150 mg of bupropion SR for the entire 7-week period. All subjects also received two 30-minute individual sessions on smoking cessation. Nine subjects completed at least 4 weeks on medication. Three subjects withdrew because of untoward effects; 2 withdrew because of pregnancy and one subject took an overdose of study medication. Five subjects (31.25%) had stopped smoking within 4 weeks of taking bupropion Sr. Some subjects did not stop smoking but did reduce the number of cigarettes smoked, suggesting that bupropion SR might have a harm reduction effect. The weights of the subjects did not change significantly; the authors noted the potential importance of this as the possibility of gaining weight was a frequent concern, especially among girls, before entering the study. Finally, ADHD symptoms did not change significantly; this is relevant as bupropion has been shown to be effective in the treatment of ADHD and there is also some evidence that nicotine may improve ADHD symptoms in adults—both smokers and nonsmokers.

SELECTIVE SEROTONIN AND NOREPINEPHRINE REUPTAKE INHIBITORS (SSNRIs)
Venlafaxine Hydrochloride (Effexor)

Venlafaxine hydrochloride is chemically unrelated to other available antidepressants. Its antidepressant effects are thought to be due to its potent inhibition of the reuptake of neuronal serotonin and norepinephrine and weak inhibition of dopamine uptake (a serotonergic noradrenergic reuptake inhibitor [SNRI]). Venlafaxine does not have significant affinity for muscarinic, histaminergic, or alpha-1 adrenergic receptors.

Pharmacokinetics of Venlafaxine Hydrochloride

Food has no significant effect on the bioavailability of venlafaxine. The drug is extensively metabolized by the liver to O-desmethylvenlafaxine (ODV), the major metabolite, which is clinically active. Mean terminal elimination half-life is approximately 11 hours. Steady-state serum concentrations are achieved within approximately 3 days of multidose administration. The primary route of excretion of venlafaxine and its metabolites is through the kidneys.

Contraindications for Venlafaxine Hydrochloride Administration

Known hypersensitivity to the drug is a contraindication.

Because of a possibility of serious, life-threatening reactions when administered simultaneously with a MAOI, it is recommended that the drug not be used in combination with a MAOI. At least 2 weeks should elapse after stopping a MAOI before administering venlafaxine. Based on the half-life of venlafaxine, at least 7 days should elapse following its discontinuation before administering a MAOI.

Significant hepatic or renal disease may markedly decrease elimination of the drug and increase serum levels. If the clinician elects to use venlafaxine, adjustment of dosage may be necessary.

Use with caution in depressed patients with a history of hypomania or mania, as activation of either could occur.

Untoward Effects of Venlafaxine Hydrochloride

Among the most commonly reported untoward effects are anxiety, nervousness, somnolence or insomnia, nausea, anorexia, initial dose-dependent weight loss, constipation, increased sweating, dry mouth, dizziness, abnormal ejaculation/orgasm, and impotence. A sustained increase in supine diastolic blood pressure, which appeared to be dose related has been reported in some patients treated with venlafaxine. Many other untoward effects have been reported.

ECG Changes

Administration of regular venlafaxine resulted in no treatment emergent conduction abnormalities compared with placebo, but the mean heart rate was increased by 4 beats/minute compared with baseline. On Effexor XL (brand name extended-release preparation), however, the QTc interval increased by 4.7 msec over baseline, compared to a decrease of 1.9 msec for placebo. Heart rate increased by 4 beats/minute over baseline on Effexor XL compared to an increase of 1 beat/minute over baseline for placebo.

Indications for Venlafaxine Hydrochloride in Child and Adolescent Psychiatry

Note: Review the Black Box Warning at the beginning of the chapter or in the package insert before prescribing.

(continued)

Indications for Venlafaxine Hydrochloride in Child and Adolescent Psychiatry (Continued)

Venlafaxine hydrochloride in its immediate release form is indicated for the treatment of major depressive disorder only. Venlafaxine hydrochloride in its extended-release capsule form (Effexor XR) has been approved for the treatment of major depressive disorder, generalized anxiety disorder, and social anxiety disorder. Venlafaxine's efficacy and safety in patients < 18 years of age have not been established. One manufacturer notes that data from two placebo-controlled trials with extended-release venlafaxine (Effexor XR) in a total of 766 pediatric patients (ages 6 to 17 years) diagnosed with major depressive disorder and from two placebo-controlled studies in a total of 793 pediatric patients diagnosed with general anxiety disorder were not sufficient to support a claim for use in this age group (PDR, 2006). Data from these studies suggest that venlafaxine may adversely effect weight and height, which should be monitored if used in children. It was also noted that elevations in blood pressure and in serum cholesterol that were considered clinically relevant occurred in these subjects and that they were similar to those reported in adult patients (PDR, 2006).

Venlafaxine Dosage Schedule

- Children and adolescents ≤ 17 years of age: Not recommended. Safety and efficacy have not been established in this age group.
- Adolescents at least 18 years of age and adults:

Treatment of major depressive disorder with immediate release tablets: The initial recommended starting dose is 75 mg divided into two or three doses and taken with food. If clinically indicated, the dose may be titrated up to 225 mg/day for moderately depressed patients and up to a maximum of 375 mg/day in severely depressed patients. Increments of up to 75 mg may be made at intervals of at least 4 days.

Treatment of major depressive disorder, generalized anxiety disorder and social anxiety disorder with extended-release capsules: Should be swallowed whole and taken with food in a single morning or evening dose at about the same time each day. Initial recommended daily dose is 75 mg, but 37.5 mg/day initially is an option. Steady-state serum levels usually occur by the fourth day. If adequate clinical response does not occur, dose may be raised by 75 mg increments at intervals of 4 days or more to a maximum of 225 mg/day.

Venlafaxine Hydrochloride Dose Forms Available

- Tablets: 25 mg, 37.5 mg, 50 mg, 75 mg, and 100 mg
- Extended-release capsules: 37.5 mg, 75 mg, and 150 mg

Report of Interest

Venlafaxine Hydrochloride in the Treatment of Attention-deficit/Hyperactivity Disorder in Children and Adolescents

Olvera et al. (1996) conducted a 5-week, open-label trial of venlafaxine in the treatment of 16 subjects (15 males, 1 female; mean age, 11.6 ± 2.3 years; age range, 8 to 16 years) diagnosed with ADHD without comorbid depression by DSM-IV (APA, 1994) criteria to assess efficacy, dose range, and untoward effects. Efficacy was determined by ratings on the Conners' Parent Rating Scale (CPRS) and the Conners Continuous Performance Test (CPT). Venlafaxine was given at a daily dose of 12.5 mg for the first week. Dose was subsequently increased by 25 mg/week to reach a target dose of 75 mg/day unless prevented by untoward effects; subjects weighing < 40 kg had weekly increases of 12.5 mg to a maximum of 50 mg/day. Ten subjects completed the 5-week study. Of the six noncompleters, three had behavioral activation (increased hyperactivity), one had severe nausea, and two were lost to follow-up. The mean dose of venlafaxine for the 10 completers was 60 mg/day or 1.4 mg/kg/day given in two or three divided doses.

Overall, seven (44%) of the 16 subjects improved on the CPRS. At the end of 5 weeks, mean ratings on the CPRS impulsivity factor improved significantly ($P = .008$), and mean ratings on the CPRS hyperactivity index improved significantly ($P = .003$); there were no significant changes in mean ratings on the CPRS conduct factor. Cognitive symptoms of ADHD as reflected in omission or commission errors or reaction time on the CPT showed no significant improvement. The most common untoward effects were drowsiness (8/16, 50%), nausea (6/16, 37.5%), irritability (5/15, 33%), and behavioral activation (worsening of hyperactivity in 5/15, 33%). The authors concluded that low doses of venlafaxine appeared to be effective in reducing behavioral but not cognitive symptoms of ADHD but that behavioral activation may be of concern (Olvera et al. 1996).

Mirtazapine (Remeron)

Mirtazapine is a selective serotonin and norepinephrine reuptake inhibitor (SSNRI) belonging to the piperazine/azepine group. It has a tetracyclic chemical structure unrelated to other antidepressants in use. Preclinical studies showed that it acts as an antagonist at central presynaptic alpha-2-adrenergic inhibitory autoreceptors and heteroreceptors, resulting in an increase in central noradrenergic and serotonergic activity. Mirtazapine is a potent antagonist of $5HT_2$ and $5HT_3$ receptors but has no significant affinity for $5HT_{1A}$ and $5HT_{1B}$ receptors. It also is a potent antagonist of histamine (H_1) receptors, which may cause its prominent sedative effects. Mirtazapine is a moderate peripheral alpha-1-adrenergic antagonist, which may cause the orthostatic hypotension that sometimes occurs. The drug also has moderate antagonistic properties at muscarinic receptors, which may explain the relatively low incidence of anticholinergic effects associated with its use.

Pharmacokinetics of Mirtazapine

Food has a clinically insignificant effect on the rate and bioavailability of mirtazapine. It is rapidly absorbed, with peak plasma concentrations occurring about 2 hours after ingestion. It is extensively metabolized in the liver by demethylation and hydroxylation followed by glucuronide conjugation. Serum half-life ranges between 20 and 40 hours and is significantly longer in females (mean, 37 hours) than in males (mean, 26 hours). Steady-state plasma levels occur within 5 days at a given dose. Elimination is about 75% via urine, with most of the remainder being excreted in the feces.

Contraindications for the Administration of Mirtazapine

Known hypersensitivity to the drug is a contraindication.

Because mirtazapine was associated with the development of severe neutropenia in about 0.1% of patients in premarketing clinical trials, whenever a patient develops sore throat, fever, stomatitis, or other signs of infection and has a low white blood cell count, mirtazapine should be discontinued and the patient closely monitored.

Because of a possibility of serious, life-threatening reactions when administered simultaneously with a MAOI, it is recommended that the drug not be used in combination with a MAOI. At least 2 weeks should elapse after stopping a MAOI before administering mirtazapine. Likewise, based on the half-life of mirtazapine, at least 2 weeks should elapse following its discontinuation before administering a MAOI.

Untoward Effects of Mirtazapine

Somnolence occurred in more than one-half of patients administered mirtazapine and resulted in discontinuation of treatment in 10.4% of 453 subjects in a controlled 6-week trial (package insert). Other untoward effects included increased appetite, weight gain, dizziness, dry mouth, and constipation. Many other untoward effects have been reported.

Indications for Mirtazapine in Child and Adolescent Psychiatry

Note: Review the Black Box Warning at the beginning of the chapter or in the package insert before prescribing.

Mirtazapine is approved for the treatment of depression in adults. Its safety and efficacy in pediatric patients have not been established.

Mirtazapine Dosage Schedule

- Children and adolescents ≤ 17 years of age: Not established.
- Adolescents at least 18 years of age and adults: An initial daily dose of 15 mg at bedtime is recommended. Effective daily doses usually range between 15 and 45 mg. Dose should be titrated upward based on clinical response but, because of the relatively long serum half-life of mirtazapine (20 to 40 hours), increments should not be made at intervals of < 1 to 2 weeks in order to permit adequate assessment of therapeutic response at each dose.

Mirtazapine Dose Forms Available

- Tablets: 15 mg (scored), 30 mg (scored), and 45 mg

Duloxetine Hydrochloride (Cymbalta)

Duloxetine hydrochloride is a selective serotonin and norepinephrine reuptake inhibitor (SSNRI).

Pharmacokinetics of Duloxetine Hydrochloride

Duloxetine may be taken with or without food which does not affect the maximum plasma concentration but delays it and decreases the amount absorbed by about 10%. Because the capsules contain enteric-coated pellets that prevent the drug from degrading in the stomach, there is a median delay of about 2 hours until absorption begins. Evening doses are absorbed up to 3 hours more slowly and cleared up to 33% more rapidly than morning doses. Maximum plasma levels occur about 6 hours after ingestion of the drug.

Duloxetine hydrochloride has a half-life of about 12 hours (range 8 to 17 hours). Steady-state plasma levels occur after about 3 days at a given dose. Duloxetine is extensively metabolised primarily by the hepatic P450 enzymes CYP2D6 and CYP1A2. About 70% is eliminated in the urine and 20% through the feces.

Contraindications for the Administration of Duloxetine Hydrochloride

Hypersensitivity to duloxetine hydrochloride or its components is a contraindication to its administration. Concomitant use with monoamine oxidase inhibitors is contraindicated. It should not be prescribed to patients with uncontrolled narrow-angle glaucoma. Duloxetine should not be coadministered with thioridazine.

Duloxetine should not be coadministered with a monoamine oxidase inhibitor (MAOI) or within 14 days after treatment with an MAOI has been discontinued. At least 5 days should elapse after stopping duloxetine therapy before administering a MAOI.

Interactions of Duloxetine Hydrochloride with Other Drugs

CYP1A2 inhibitors are expected to increase duloxetine plasma levels; for example, fluvoxamine increases maximum plasma levels by $2\frac{1}{2}$ times and the serum concentration by up to 6 times. Quinolone antibiotics should also be avoided for the same reason.

Potent CYP2D6 inhibitors also are expected to increase duloxetine plasma levels, for example, 20 mg of paroxetine daily reportedly increased plasma levels caused by 40 mg daily of duloxetine by 60%; fluoxetine and quinidine would also be expected to increase plasma levels of duloxetine.

Duloxetine, itself, is a moderate inhibitor of CYP2D6. Coadministration of duloxetine with other drugs that are extensively metabolized by CYP2D6, which have a narrow therapeutic index such as the tricyclic antidepressants (TCAs) nortriptyline, amitriptyline, imipramine, and desipramine; phenothiazines, and type 1C antiarrhythmics should be avoided if possible because of potentially dangerous increases in their serum levels. If coadministered, TCA serum levels should be monitored closely. Coadministration with thoridizine is contraindicated because of the risk of ventricular arrhythmias and sudden death that has been associated with elevated thioridazine levels.

Untoward Effects of Duloxetine Hydrochloride

The most common untoward effects reported in adult placebo-controlled clinical trails were nausea (20% vs. 7%), dry mouth (15% vs. 6%), constipation (11% vs. 4%), fatigue (8% vs. 4%), decreased appetite (8% vs. 2%), somnolence (7% vs. 3%) and increased sweating (6% vs. 2%). Duloxetine was associated with a mean blood pressure increase of 2 mm Hg systolic and 0.5 mm Hg diastolic compared to levels with placebo.

Indications for Duloxetine Hydrochloride in Child and Adolescent Psychiatry

Note: Review the Black Box Warning at the beginning of the chapter or in the package insert before prescribing.

(continued)

Indications for Duloxetine Hydrochloride in Child and Adolescent Psychiatry *(Continued)*

Duloxetine is indicated for the treatment of major depressive disorder in adults. Safety and efficacy have not been established for pediatric patients.

Duloxetine Hydrochloride Dosage Schedule

- Children and adolescents < 18 years of age: Not recommended.
- Adolescents ≥ 18 years of age and adults: The recommended target dose is 60 mg, given in a single daily dose. Administration may be begun at 20 mg, twice daily and titrated upwards. If discontinuing duloxetine, a gradual tapering down of dose is recommended to avoid possible serious untoward effects that may occur with abrupt cessation.

Duloxetine Hydrochloride Dose Forms Available

- Delayed-release capsules 20 mg, 30 mg, and 60 mg

SELECTIVE NOREPINEPHRINE REUPTAKE INHIBITORS (SNRIs)

Atomoxetine Hydrochloride (Strattera)

Atomoxetine hydrochloride is a selective norepinephrine reuptake inhibitor (SNRI); it inhibits the presynaptic norepinephrine transporter. Its receptor occupancy profile shows minimal affinity for cholinergic, histaminic, serotonergic, or alpha-adrenergic receptors (Spencer et al. 1998).

Pharmacokinetics of Atomoxetine Hydrochloride

Taken orally, atomoxetine hydrochloride is rapidly absorbed; absorption is minimally affected by food but taking it with meals does result in an average 9% lower maximum plasma concentration in children and adolescents. Peak plasma concentrations occur within 1 to 2 hours. Mean elimination half-life is about 5.2 hours. Atomoxetine is metabolized primarily through the CYP2D6 enzymatic pathway. The major metabolite is 4-hydroxyatomoxetine, which is equipotent to atomoxetine but circulates at a much lower plasma concentration. Atomoxetine is excreted primarily as 4-hydroxyatomoxetine-O-glucuronide about 80% of which is excreted in urine and 17% in feces. Less than 3% of atomoxetine is excreted unchanged.

About 7% of Caucasians and 2% of Afro–Americans are poor metabolizers of atomoxetine because they have reduced ability to metabolize CYP2D6 substrates. Such individuals have a net increase of about five times (500%) in maximum plasma concentration of atomoxetine, compared to extensive (normal) metabolizers of the drug. The elimination half-life of atomoxetine for poor metabolizers is about 21.6 hours, about four times that of extensive metabolizers.

Interactions of Atomoxetine with Other Drugs

Drugs such as quinine, which inhibit CYP2D6 can result in significant increases in plasma levels and require downward adjustment of the dose of atomoxetine. Fluoxetine and paroxetine, both potential CYP2D6 inhibitors, may increase the maximum plasma concentration of atomoxetine by up to three or four times in extensive metabolizers.

Contraindications for Atomoxetine Administration

Atomoxetine is contraindicated in patients with known hypersensitivity to the drug. It should not be taken concomitantly with a MAOI, within 2 weeks of discontinuing a MAOI, and a MAOI should not be administered within the 2-week period after discontinuing atomoxetine.

Untoward Effects of Atomoxetine

In clinical trials, the most common untoward effects of atomoxetine with an incidence of 5% or more and occurring at least twice as frequently as in patients treated with placebo were dyspepsia, nausea, vomiting, fatigue, decreased appetite, dizziness, and mood swings.

Indications for Atomoxetine in Child and Adolescent Psychiatry

Note: Review the Black Box Warning at the beginning of the chapter or in the package insert before prescribing.

Atomoxetine is indicated for the treatment of attention-deficit/hyperactivity disorder in individuals at least 6 years of age.

Atomoxetine Hydrochloride Dosage Schedule

- Children < 6 years of age: Not recommended. The safety and efficacy of atomoxetine have not been established for this age group.
- Children and adolescents 6 years of age and over and weighing 70 pounds or less: Atomoxetine should be administered as a single morning dose or in two divided doses, in the morning and late afternoon/early evening. The initial total daily dose should be approximately 0.5 mg/kg. After a minimum of three days, the dose should be increased to reach a total target daily dose of 1.2 mg/kg. No additional benefit has been demonstrated for doses over 1.2 mg/kg/day and the maximum recommended total daily dose should not exceed 1.4 mg/kg or 100 mg, whichever is less.
- Children and adolescents weighing over 70 pounds and adults: Atomoxetine should be administered as a single morning dose or in two divided doses, in the morning and late afternoon/early evening. The initial total daily dose should be 40 mg. After a minimum of 3 days, the dose should be increased to reach a total target daily dose of approximately 80 mg/kg. After 2 to 4 additional weeks, the dose may be increased to a recommended maximum of 100 mg.

Atomoxetine Hydrochloride Dose Forms Available

- Capsules: 10, 18, 25, 40, and 60 mg.

Reports of Interest

Atomoxetine versus Stimulants in the Treatment of Attention-deficit Hyperactivity Disorder in Children and Adolescents. In head-to-head studies comparing stimulant drugs with atomoxetine, stimulants have been more efficacious than atomoxetine in treating subjects with ADHD. In a multicenter, randomized, double-blind, forced-dose-escalation laboratory school study, Wigal et al. (2005) compared mixed amphetamine salts extended release (MAS XR; Adderall XR) to atomoxetine in 203 children aged 6 to 12 years who were diagnosed with attention-deficit disorder, combined or hyperactive/impulsive type by DSM-IV criteria. The MAS XR group ($N = 102$) demonstrated significantly greater improvement from baseline on the Swanson, Kotkin, Agler, M-Flynn and Pelham (SKAMP) Rating Scale than did the atomoxetine group ($N = 102$), $-.056$ versus -0.13, $P < .0001$. The authors noted that adverse events were similar in both groups and that their data suggested that with its extended duration of action and greater therapeutic efficacy, MAS XR was more effective that atomoxetine in children diagnosed with ADHD.

The Formal Observation of Concerta versus Strattera (FOCUS) study (funded by the maker of OROS methylphenidate) was presented at the 102nd Annual Convention and Scientific Assembly of the National Medical Association (NMA, San Diego CA, August 3, 2004). In a multicenter, community based, 3-week, open label, parallel-design, 1323 subjects, age range 6 to 12 years and diagnosed with ADHD by DSM-IV criteria, were randomly assigned to receive OROS methylphenidate (Concerta) ($N = 850$) or atomoxetine (Strattera) ($N = 473$). Subjects were either newly diagnosed with ADHD or had an unsatisfactory response to prior treatment with medication. OROS methylphenidate was begun at a once-daily dose of 18 mg and atomoxetine at a dose of 0.5 mg/kg/day. Titration based on clinical response was permitted over the study. Outcome measures were the Attention-deficit/Hyperactivity Disorder Rating Scale (ADHD-RS) and the physician rated, Clinical Global Impressions-Improvement (CGI-I) Scale made at baseline and weekly throughout the study. OROS methylphenidate: weekly ADHD-RS scores for the OROS methylphenidate group showed a significantly greater rate of improvement in inattentive and hyperactive behavior ($P < .001$) than the atomoxetine group. Improvement in CGI-I scores for the OROS methylphenidate group was also significantly greater compared to the atomoxetine group. This study was later published as Kemner et al. 2005.

Starr and Kemner (2005) reported on the treatment outcomes for the African–American children who participated in the FOCUS study summarized above; this subgroup comprised 183 (13.8%) subjects of whom 125 were assigned to OROS methylphenidate and 58 to atomoxetine. At 3 weeks, the mean daily dose of OROS methylphenidate was 32.8 ± 10.9 mg and the mean dose of atomoxetine was 1.1 ± 0.4 mg/kg. The authors noted that both drugs were associated with significant improvement in ADHD symptoms from baseline but that the group receiving OROS methylphenidate demonstrated significantly greater improvement in total ADHD symptoms, inattentiveness and Clinical Global Impressions-Improvement ratings than the atomoxetine group.

Atomoxetine in the Treatment of Attention-deficit/Hyperactivity Disorder in Children and Adolescents. Michelson et al. (2001) showed in a randomized, placebo-controlled dose-response study, that atomoxetine was effective and safe in treating ADHD in children and adolescents when administered twice daily. In 2002, Michelson et al. conducted a study showing that for most subjects atomoxetine could also be administered once daily with good clinical results (Michelson et al. 2002). They reported a 6-week, double-blind, placebo-controlled study of once-daily treatment with atomoxetine in 171 children and adolescents (age range 6 to 16 years, mean age 10.3 years) who were diagnosed with ADHD by DSM-IV criteria and who had a symptom severity score of at least 1.5

SDs above age and sex norms on the Attention-deficit/Hyperactivity Disorder Rating Scale-IV-Parent Version:Investigator administered and scored (ADHDRS-IV-Parent:Inv). The most common comorbid diagnosis was oppositional defiant disorder (34, 20%).

Following a minimum of 5 medication-free days, subjects in the atomoxetine group received a single morning dose of 0.5 mg/kg/day, which was increased to 0.75 mg/kg/day on day 4, and 1.0 mg/kg/day on day 8. At time 4-weeks, subjects who had a CGI-S score of > 2 (more than minimum symptoms) had their doses of atomoxetine increased to 1.5 mg/kg/day.

Ratings on the ADHDRS-IV-Parent:Inv were significantly better for subjects on atomoxetine beginning at week-1 and remained so throughout the study. Positive clinical response, defined as > 25% reduction from baseline to endpoint, was significantly better in the atomoxetine group (59.5%) than in the placebo group (31.3%)(P < .001). The atomoxetine group also showed significantly greater improvement that the placebo group on the ADHD Index scores of the Conners' Parent Rating Scale (P < .001), the Conners' Teacher Rating Scale (P < .001) and the CGI-S score (P < .001). The authors noted that this study suggested that once-daily dosing with atomoxetine is an effective treatment for ADHD and despite the fact that its half-life is only about 4 hours, beneficial effects of one morning dose lasted into the evening for many subjects.

Weiss et al. (2005) conducted a multicenter, randomized, placebo-controlled 7-week study of the efficacy of once-daily atomoxetine in the school setting in treating 153 subjects (123 [80.4%] male, 30 [19.6%] female; age range 8 to 12 years, mean age 9.9 ± 1.3 years) diagnosed with Attention-deficit/hyperactivity disorder by DSM-IV criteria. One hundred and one (101) subjects were assigned to the atomoxetine group and 52 to the placebo group. Subjects in the atomoxetine group were initially prescribed a morning dose of 0.8 mg/kg of atomoxetine. On day 4, the dose was increased to 1.2 mg/kg/day. An increase to 1.8 mg/kg/day was permitted for subjects with inadequate symptom control after 3 weeks on atomoxetine. At endpoint (time 7-weeks), the mean once-daily dose of atomoxetine was 1.33 ± 0.30 mg/kg.

The primary measure of clinical improvement was the 18-item Attention-deficit/Hyperactivity Disorder Rating Scale-IV-Teacher Version:Investigator administered and scored (ADHDRS-IV-Teacher:Inv). A baseline score on at least 1.0 SD above age and sex norms was required for admission to the study. Enrolled subjects were also required to have a Conners' Parents Rating Scale-Revised: Short Form (CPRS-R:S) ADHD index score of at least 1.5 SDs above age and sex norms. A positive response was defined as a 20% or greater reduction in the ADHDRS-IV-Teacher:Inv score; 69 (69%) of the atomoxetine group versus 22 (43%) of the placebo group were rated as responders (P = .003). The atomoxetine group also had significantly greater improvement in the ADHD Index of the parent-rated CPRS-R:S (P < .001) and as rated by clinicians on the Clinical Global Impressions-Improvement (CGI-I) Scale. The atomoxetine group also showed significantly more improvement than the placebo group on several secondary measures of response.

Regarding Adverse Events (AEs), decreased appetite (24.0% vs. 3.8%; P = .001) and somnolence (17.0% vs. 3.8%, P = .020) were significantly more frequent in the atomoxetine group. Six subjects in the atomoxetine group discontinued the drug because of AEs: abdominal pain (two), emotional disturbance (one), feeling abnormal (one), irritability (one), and vomiting (one); no subjects in the placebo group discontinued because of AEs. As a group, subjects in the atomoxetine group lost a mean of 0.67 ± 1.21 kg compared with a mean gain of 1.21 ± 1.38 kg in the placebo group ($P < .001$) over the 7-week study. The subjects in the atomoxetine group experienced an increase in heart rate of 3.3 ± 11.33 beats per minute but this was not significantly different from the mean decrease of 0.1 beat per minute in the placebo group ($P = .067$) (Weiss et al. 2005).

Atomoxetine in the Treatment of ADHD or Comorbid Attention-deficit/ Hyperactivity Disorder and Oppositional Defiant Disorder in Children and Adolescents. Newcorn et al. (2005) reported the treatment of 293 subjects (age range 8 to 18 years; mean age 11.15 years) diagnosed with ADHD only ($N = 178$, 61%) or ADHD comorbid with oppositional defiant disorder (ODD) ($N = 115$, 39%) with atomoxetine in a 13-outpatient-site, approximately 8-week, randomized, double-blind, placebo-controlled study. Those who enrolled were required to have a symptom severity score of > 1.5 SDs above age and gender norms on the Attention-deficit/Hyperactivity Disorder Rating Scale-IV-Parent version, investigator administered and scored (ADHDRS-IV-Parent:Inv) for the total score or on the Inattentive or Hyperactive/Impulsive subscale and to have an IQ > 80. Medication was randomly assigned at doses of 0.5, 1.2, and 1.8 mg/kg/day, or placebo and was administered in divided doses given in the morning and late afternoon. All subjects receiving atomoxetine were begun at a dose of 0.25 mg/kg twice daily; subjects assigned to higher doses were titrated upward at weekly intervals, the first increase being to 0.8 mg/kg/day and the second increase to 1.2 mg/kg/day at week 3. The subjects assigned to 1.8 mg/kg/day were increased to that dosage at the beginning of week 4. The primary outcome measure was the ADHDRS-IV-Parent:Inv. Other outcome measures were the Connors' Parent Rating Scale-Revised Short Form (CPRS-R:S), the Clinical Global Impressions-Severity Scale Keyed to ADHD Severity (CGI-ADHD-S) and the Child Health Questionnaire (CHQ) in which parents rate their child's physical and psychosocial well-being.

The authors noted that high comorbidity of ADHD and ODD is a consistent finding in published studies. The severity of ADHD and symptoms was greater in the comorbid group ($P < .001$); depressive symptoms were also greater in the comorbid group but were not severe enough to warrant a diagnosis of any depressive disorder. In the ADHD/ODD group, atomoxetine was superior to placebo in reducing ADHD symptoms as rated on the ADHDRS-IV-Parent:Inv total score ($P = .030$) and the Inattentive subscale ($P = .020$) for the 1.8 mg/kg/day dose but not for either of the lower doses; no atomoxetine dose was rated significantly better than placebo on the Hyperactive/impulsive subscale. Subjects with ADHD only showed significantly more improvement on atomoxetine than the placebo group in the reduction of ADHD symptoms at both the 1.2 and 1.8 mg/kg/day doses, whereas patients with ADHD/ODD showed a greater response at 1.8 mg/kg/day. On the CPRS-R:S ADHD Index, all doses of atomoxetine compared to placebo resulted in significant reduction of ADHD symptoms for subjects with or without comorbid ODD except for the 0.5 mg/kg/day dose, which was not significant in patients in the ADHD only group. Quality of life scores as measured by the CHQ also showed significant improvement with atomoxetine treatment. The authors concluded that atomoxetine resulted in statistically and clinically significant improvement in subjects in this age group diagnosed with ADHD or ADHD/ODD and that their results suggested that higher doses are required when ODD is comorbid with ADHD.

Atomoxetine in the Treatment of Children and Adolescents Diagnosed with Pervasive Developmental Disorders. Jou et al. (2005) assessed the effectiveness and tolerability of treatment with atomoxetine in a retrospective chart review of all 20 outpatients (mean age 11.5 ± 3.5 years, age range 6 to 19 years; 16 males, 4 females) diagnosed with autistic disorder ($N = 16$), Asperger's disorder ($N = 2$) or pervasive developmental disorder not otherwise specified (PDDNOS; $N = 2$) and other comorbid disorders, including 10 with varying degrees of mental retardation, who had been prescribed atomoxetine to treat ADHD-like symptoms over a 1-year period during which the doses of any other medications they were taking were unchanged.

An initial 18 mg daily dose of atomoxetine was prescribed; after 1 week, atomoxetine was titrated upward on a weekly basis to a target dose of 1.2 mg/kg/day. If this did not result in satisfactory clinical response, the dose could be further titrated up to a maximum of 1.4 mg/kg/day. Duration of treatment with atomoxetine averaged 19.5 ± 10.5 weeks; range 1 to 36 weeks. Subjects were rated on the Conners' Parent Rating Scale (CPRS) and the Global Improvement item of the Clinical Global Impressions Scale (CGI-GI).

The mean atomoxetine dose was 43.3 ± 18.1 mg/day; there was no significant difference in the mean daily dose of the 12 responders, 47.5 ± 18.5 mg; range 25 to 80 mg and that of the 8 nonresponders, 37.0 ± 16.7 mg. On the CPRS, there were significant improvements on subscales for conduct ($P = .01$); hyperactivity ($P = .001$); inattention ($P = .01$); learning ($P = .01$); but not for psychosomatic or anxiety. The authors noted, however, that the existing symptoms of anxiety that were present (10 subjects had codiagnoses of anxiety disorder NOS) were not aggravated by atomoxetine and that there was a nonsignificant decrease on the anxiety scale, which appears to be a major advantage over stimulant medications. Adverse events were generally of mild to moderate intensity and included constipation, decreased appetite, ear ringing, mood swings, and sedation. Effect on weight varied; the overall mean weight change was $0.36 + 2.41$ kg (range -3.18 to 9.09 kg; 5 subjects lost weight, 8 had no weight change, and 7 gained weight.) The one patient who terminated treatment secondary to an adverse event probably related to atomoxetine experienced mood swings. The authors noted that their study suggested that atomoxetine was potentially useful in addressing secondary symptoms of PDD including inattention and hyperactivity and that further more rigorous studies are needed (Jou et al. 2005).

MONOAMINE OXIDASE INHIBITORS (MAOIs)

There are two forms of monoamine oxidase (MAO), which are distinguished by their substrate specificity. Type A MAO deaminates or deactivates norepinephrine, serotonin, and normetanephrine, and type B MAO deaminates dopamine and phenylethylamine (Zametkin and Rapoport, 1987).

MAOIs are primarily used in treating adults with depressive disorders that are unresponsive to antidepressant drugs of other classes. MAOIs presently FDA approved and marketed in the United States include phenelzine sulfate (Nardil), which has been approved for use only in individuals at least 16 years of age, and tranylcypromine sulfate (Parnate), which has been approved only for adults.

MAOIs that have been used in children and adolescents include clorgyline (a selective MAO-A inhibitor), tranylcypromine sulfate and phenelzine sulfate (mixed MAO-A and MAO-B inhibitors), and L-deprenyl or selegiline hydrochloride (Eldepryl) (a selective central MAO-B inhibitor). Because of the potentially very serious drug interactions and untoward effects of MAOIs, their use in children and adolescents is not usually recommended, and only a few reports in this age group are reviewed.

Special Considerations in Using MAOI

It is critical to have a minimum of a 2-week washout period after stopping a MAOI and beginning a tricyclic or when changing from one MAOI to another MAOI. It is also contraindicated to add a tricyclic antidepressant when a MAOI is already being used, although the reverse has been done; that is, a MAOI can be added to an ongoing treatment regimen to augment a tricyclic that has been only partially effective (Ryan et al. 1988b). If patients are on MAOIs and are in areas that are not rapidly accessible to medical treatment, they may be given several 25-mg chlor-promazine tablets to be taken should they accidentally ingest tyramine and become symptomatic (Ryan et al. 1988b). Pare et al. (1982) suggested that a combination of tricyclics and MAOIs might provide relative protection against tyramine-induced hypertension, or "cheese effect," which may occur with dietary indiscretions while taking MAOIs; however, this is not common practice at the present time.

Contraindications for Monoamine Oxidase Inhibitor Administration

Note: Review the Black Box Warning at the beginning of the chapter or in the package insert before prescribing.

Known hypersensitivity to a MAOI, pheochromocytoma, congestive heart fail-ure, liver disease, or abnormal liver function are contraindications.

MAOIs must not be prescribed if a tricyclic antidepressant (however, see Ryan et al. 1988b, for a different opinion), another MAOI, or buspirone hydrochloride has been taken within the preceding 2 weeks.

Other contraindications usually found more frequently in older patients also exist. In addition, the patient must not be unreliable or be unable to keep to a strict diet (i.e., avoiding foods with high tyramine or dopamine concentrations).

Interactions of MAOIs with Other Drugs

Ingestion of tyramine can cause a hypertensive crisis. Hence foods rich in tyramine, such as cheese, wine, beer, yeast derivatives, some beans, and others, must be avoided.

Concomitant use with tricyclic antidepressants should be avoided because hypertensive crises or severe seizures have been reported with such combinations (see Ryan et al. 1988b, for a different opinion).

Use with sympathomimetic drugs such as amphetamines, methylphenidate, cocaine, dopamine, caffeine, epinephrine, norepinephrine, and related compounds may cause a hypertensive crisis.

Other drug interactions occur as well.

Untoward Effects of MAOIs

MAOIs may cause significant orthostatic hypotension, dizziness, headache, sleep disturbances, sedation, fatigue, weakness, hyperreflexia, dry mouth, and gastroin-testinal disturbances; other untoward effects occur as well.

Reports of Interest

MAOIs in the Treatment of Adolescent Depression. Ryan et al. (1988b) reported an open clinical trial of tranylcypromine sulfate and phenelzine sulfate, both alone and in combination with a tricyclic antidepressant, in which 23 adolescents diagnosed with MDD who had responded inadequately to tricyclic antidepressants were treated with these MAOIs. Seventy-four percent (17) had a fair to good antidepressant response; however, because of dietary noncompliance the MAOI was discontinued in four subjects and only 57% (13) of the subjects continued on the medication. The authors concluded that MAOIs appeared to be useful in treating some adolescents with major depression who had not responded satisfactorily to tricyclic antidepressants. During the study, a total of seven (30%) had purposeful or accidental dietary noncompliance, and the authors emphasized that only very reliable adolescents are suitable for treatment with MAOIs (Ryan et al. 1988b).

MAOIs in the Treatment of Attention-deficit/Hyperactivity Disorder. Zametkin et al. (1985) conducted a double-blind crossover study of 14 boys (mean age, 9.2 ± 1.5 years) who were diagnosed with attention deficit disorder with hyperactivity. The authors compared dextroamphetamine to either clorgyline, a selective MAO-A inhibitor (six subjects), or tranylcypromine sulfate, a mixed MAO-A and MAO-B inhibitor (eight subjects). Both MAOIs had immediate, clinically significant effects (in contrast to delayed effects when used as an antidepressant), which were clinically indistinguishable from those of dextroamphetamine.

Zametkin and Rapoport (1987) reported that M. Donnelly had administered 15 mg/day of L-deprenyl, a selective MAO-B inhibitor, to 14 hyperactive children with relatively little therapeutic effect. The authors suggested that the fact that a type A MAOI and a mixed MAOI showed therapeutic efficacy in children with ADHD, whereas a type B MAOI did not support the hypothesis that dysregulation of the noradrenergic system is important in the etiology of ADHD (Zametkin and Rapoport, 1987).

At the present time, the use of MAOIs in the treatment of ADHD is not recommended because of necessary dietary constraints.

CHAPTER 8

Mood Stabilizers: Lithium Carbonate and Antiepileptics

LITHIUM CARBONATE (Lithotabs, Eskalith, Lithane, Lithobid) and LITHIUM CITRATE (Cibalith-S)

Currently, lithium carbonate is approved by the FDA only for the treatment of manic episodes of bipolar disorders and for maintenance therapy of bipolar patients with a history of mania; the drug is approved only for persons 12 years of age and older. Over the past three decades, however, lithium carbonate has been investigated in the treatment of many child and adolescent disorders, but especially in the treatment of children with severe aggression directed toward self or others, children with bipolar or similar disorders, and behaviorally disturbed children whose parents are known lithium responders. One major impetus for this research was that standard antipsychotic agents, which were frequently used to control severe behavioral disorders and sometimes mania, not only could cause cognitive dulling when used in sufficient dosage to control symptoms, but also carried significant risk of causing tardive dyskinesia when used on a long-term basis (Platt et al. 1984).

Pharmacokinetics of Lithium Carbonate

The lithium ion is readily absorbed from the gastrointestinal tract and is most commonly administered in the form of lithium carbonate (Li_2CO_3), a highly soluble salt. Peak plasma concentrations occur within 2 to 4 hours, and complete absorption takes place within approximately 8 hours (Baldessarini, 1990). Approximately 95% of a single dose of lithium is excreted by the kidneys, with up to two-thirds of an acute dose being excreted within 6 to 12 hours. The serum half-life is approximately 20 to 24 hours. Depletion of the sodium ion causes a clinically significant degree of lithium retention by the kidneys. Steady-state serum lithium levels typically occur within 5 to 8 days of repeated identical daily doses of lithium carbonate. Although lithium pharmacokinetics differ considerably among individuals, they are fairly stable over time for a given person (Baldessarini and Stephens, 1970).

Vitiello et al. (1988) studied the pharmacokinetics of lithium carbonate in nine children aged 9 to 12 years. The children had a trend toward a shorter elimination half-life of lithium and a significantly higher total renal clearance of lithium. The clinical significance of this rate is that a steady state of lithium serum levels is reached more rapidly in children than in adults, and therapeutic levels can be achieved more quickly.

Contraindications for Lithium Carbonate Administration

Administration of lithium carbonate is relatively contraindicated in individuals with significant renal or cardiovascular disease, severe debilitation, severe dehydration, or sodium depletion, because these conditions are associated with a very high risk of lithium toxicity. Patients with such disorders should be thoroughly assessed, usually in consultation with the person providing medical care, before beginning lithium therapy.

Except under urgent circumstances, adolescents who are likely to become pregnant should not be administered lithium; this is particularly true of those in early pregnancy. Lithium carbonate is associated with a significant increase in cardiac teratogenicity, especially with Ebstein's anomaly. A significantly increased incidence of other cardiac anomalies has also been reported. Kallen and Tandberg (1983) reported that 7% of the infants of women who used lithium in early pregnancy had serious heart defects other than Ebstein's anomaly.

Significant thyroid disease is a relative contraindication to lithium carbonate therapy; however, with careful monitoring of thyroid function and the use of supplemental thyroid preparations when necessary, it may be used when other drugs are not effective and the potential benefits outweigh the risks.

Interactions of Lithium Carbonate with Other Drugs

There are several reports that increased neuroleptic toxicity with an encephalopathic syndrome or neuroleptic malignant syndrome may occur when lithium and neuroleptics are used concomitantly, but this has usually been seen with high doses. The simultaneous use of lithium and neuroleptic agents, however, may be indicated in some cases of mania or schizoaffective psychoses, and many patients have received both a neuroleptic and lithium with no untoward effects.

Elevations in lithium serum concentration and increased risk of neurotoxic lithium effects may occur when carbamazepine and lithium are used simultaneously, because carbamazepine decreases lithium renal clearance.

Many other drugs may increase or decrease serum lithium levels by influencing its absorption or excretion by the kidneys; for example, tetracyclines increase lithium levels.

Lithium Toxicity

One major difficulty associated with the administration of lithium carbonate is its low therapeutic index; lithium toxicity is closely related to serum lithium levels and may occur at doses of lithium carbonate close to those necessary to achieve therapeutic serum lithium levels. Adverse or side effects are those unwanted symptoms that occur at therapeutic serum lithium levels, whereas toxic effects occur when serum lithium levels exceed therapeutic levels. However, this is not an absolute, as patients who are unusually sensitive to lithium may develop toxic signs at serum levels below 1.0 mEq/L (PDR, 2000).

Lithium toxicity may be heralded by diarrhea, vomiting, mild ataxia, coarse tremor, muscular weakness and fasciculations (twitches), drowsiness, sedation, slurred speech, and impaired coordination. Patients and/or their caretakers must be made familiar with the symptoms of early lithium toxicity and instructed to discontinue lithium immediately and contact their physician if such signs occur. Increasingly severe and life-threatening toxic effects, including cardiac arrhythmias and severe central nervous system difficulties such as impaired consciousness, confusion, stupor, seizures, coma, and death, may occur with further elevations in serum lithium levels.

No specific treatment for lithium toxicity is available. If signs of early lithium toxicity appear, the drug should be withheld, lithium levels determined, and the medication resumed at a lower dosage only after 24 to 48 hours. Severe lithium toxicity is life-threatening and requires hospital admission, treatments to reduce the concentration of the lithium ion, and supportive measures.

Lithium's low therapeutic index and its pharmacokinetics make it necessary to administer lithium carbonate tablets or immediate-release capsules in divided doses, usually three or four times daily, to maintain therapeutic serum levels without toxicity. Even controlled-release tablets must be administered every 12 hours. It is essential that a laboratory capable of determining serum lithium levels rapidly and accurately be readily available to the clinician. For accuracy and serial comparisons, determinations of serum lithium levels should be made when lithium concentrations are relatively stable, and at the same time each day. Typically, blood is drawn 12 hours after the last dose of lithium and immediately before the morning dose (trough level).

Saliva lithium levels have also been used to monitor lithium levels in children, which avoids the necessity of repeated venipunctures, an upsetting experience for some children and adolescents. Perry et al. (1984) reported that saliva lithium levels in 15 children diagnosed with undersocialized aggressive conduct disorder averaged approximately 2.5 times higher than serum lithium levels, with saliva/serum ratios for individual children ranging from 1.56 to 3.99. Weller et al. (1987) found that saliva lithium levels were approximately 1.82 times those of serum levels in 14 prepubertal children receiving lithium for treatment of bipolar disorder. Saliva/serum lithium ratios in these children ranged from 1.50 to 2.32. Vitiello et al. (1988) reported saliva lithium levels to be 2.84 times those of serum lithium levels in nine children, six of whom were diagnosed with conduct disorder and three of whom were diagnosed with adjustment disorders. Saliva/serum lithium ratios in these children ranged from 2.08 to 3.88. Bernstein (1988) found that in adults the ratio of saliva lithium levels to serum lithium levels varied from 1:1 to as high as 3:1. Despite the rather marked interindividual variability in the saliva/serum ratio, it appears to be relatively constant for a given individual. Therefore, to be clinically useful, a stable saliva/serum lithium level ratio must be calculated for each patient.

Although some patients who are unusually sensitive to lithium may exhibit toxic effects at serum levels below 1 mEq/L, for most patients mild-to-moderate toxic effects occur at serum levels between 1.5 and 2 mEq/L, and moderate-to-severe reactions occur at levels of 2 mEq/L and above. Younger subjects may be at greater risk than adults for developing adverse effects at lower serum lithium levels. Many adverse effects have been reported to occur in children at serum levels well below 1 mEq/L (Campbell et al. 1984a). The most common adverse effects of lithium carbonate in 36 children, aged 3 to 13 years and diagnosed with conduct disorder ($N = 24$), infantile autism ($N = 8$), or other ($N = 4$) were weight gain in 44.4%, excessive sedation in 27.8%, decreased motor activity in 25%, and stomachache, vomiting, tremor, and/or irritability in 19.4% of patients (Campbell et al. 1984a).

Lithium decreases sodium reuptake by the renal tubules; hence adequate sodium intake must be maintained. This is especially important if there is significant sodium loss during illness (e.g., sweating, vomiting, or diarrhea) or because of changes in diet or elimination of electrolytes. The importance of adequate ingestion of ordinary table salt and fluids should be emphasized. Caution during hot weather or vigorous exertion has been advised, because additional salt loss and concomitant dehydration secondary to pronounced diaphoresis may cause the serum lithium levels of patients on maintenance lithium to increase and move into the toxic range. This may also be true of sweating caused by elevated body temperature secondary to infection or heat without exercise (e.g., sauna), but some evidence suggests that heavy sweating caused by exercise may result in lowered rather than elevated serum lithium levels. Jefferson et al. (1982) studied four healthy athletes who were stabilized on lithium for 1 week before running a 20-km race. At the end of the race, the subjects were dehydrated but their serum lithium levels had decreased by 20%. The authors found that the sweat-to-serum ratio for the lithium ion was approximately four times greater than that for the sodium ion. These authors concluded that strenuous exercise with extensive perspiration was more likely to decrease rather than increase serum lithium levels, and patients were more likely to require either no change or an increase, rather than a decrease, in dosage of lithium to maintain therapeutic levels. The authors do caution, however, that any conditions that significantly alter fluid and electrolyte balance, including strenuous exercise with heavy sweating, should be carefully monitored with serum lithium levels.

Untoward Effects of Lithium Carbonate

Lithium carbonate is frequently reported to have adverse effects early in the course of treatment. Most of these diminish or disappear during the first weeks of treatment.

These early adverse effects include fine tremor (unresponsive to antiparkinsonism drugs), polydipsia, and polyuria that may occur during initial treatment and persist or be variably present throughout treatment. Nausea and malaise or general discomfort may initially occur but usually subside with ongoing treatment. Weight gain, headache, and other gastrointestinal complaints such as diarrhea may also occur. Taking lithium with meals or after meals or increasing the dosage more gradually may be helpful in controlling gastrointestinal symptoms.

Later adverse effects are often related to serum level, including levels in the therapeutic range; these include continued hand tremor that may worsen, polydipsia, polyuria, weight gain and edema, thyroid and renal abnormalities, dermatologic abnormalities (including acne), fatigue, leukocytosis, and other symptoms. As serum levels increase, toxicity increases and other, more severe untoward effects, discussed earlier under toxicity, appear.

Abnormalities in renal functioning (diminution of renal concentrating ability) and morphologic structure (glomerular and interstitial fibrosis and nephron atrophy) have been reported in adults on long-term lithium maintenance. Occasional proteinuria was reported in a 14-year-old girl (Lena et al. 1978). Vetro et al. (1985) reported that after 1 year of lithium treatment, one child developed polyuria with daytime enuresis and impaired renal concentration. Other parameters of renal function did not change, and polyuria ceased within a few days of lithium's being discontinued. Five other children on long-term lithium therapy showed transient albuminuria that remitted spontaneously, and discontinuation of treatment was not necessary (Vetro et al. 1985).

Lithium may also interfere with thyroid function, with decreased circulating thyroid hormones and increased thyroid-stimulating hormone (TSH). Vetro et al. (1985) reported that two children developed goiter with normal function after 1.5 to 2 years of lithium therapy.

Neuroleptic malignant syndrome has been reported in a few patients who were administered neuroleptic drugs and lithium simultaneously.

Dostal (1972) reported specific adverse effects of lithium in 14 retarded adolescent males, that interfered with patient management despite significant therapeutic gains. Polydipsia, polyuria, and nocturnal enuresis were so severe as to alienate staff who cared for the youngsters. These symptoms remitted within 2 weeks of discontinuing lithium (Dostal, 1972).

Premedication Workup and Periodic Monitoring for Lithium Treatment

Routine Laboratory Tests

Complete Blood Cell Count with Differential. Lithium frequently causes a clinically insignificant and reversible elevation of white blood cells, with counts commonly between 10,000 and 15,000 cells/mm^3. The lithium-induced leukocytosis characteristically shows neutrophilia (increased polymorphonuclear leukocytes) and lymphocytopenia (Reisberg and Gershon, 1979). Thus leukocytosis can usually be differentiated from one caused by infection, because the increase in neutrophils is in more mature forms, whereas in infection younger forms predominate. Lithium may also increase platelet counts.

Serum Electrolytes. Serum electrolyte levels should be determined in particular to verify that sodium ion levels are normal, because hyponatremia decreases lithium excretion by the renal tubules.

Pregnancy Test. Lithium crosses the placenta, and data from birth registries suggest teratogenicity with increased abnormalities, including cardiac malformations, especially Ebstein's anomaly. Lithium is relatively contraindicated during pregnancy but especially during the first trimester. Infants born to mothers taking lithium appear to be at increased risk for hypotonia, lethargy, cyanosis, and ECG changes (USPDI, 1990). All females who could be pregnant should be tested before initiation of lithium therapy and warned that, because of lithium's teratogenic potential for the fetus, they should take care not to become pregnant while taking the medication.

Renal Function Tests. Baseline assessment of renal functioning is essential, because the kidney is the primary route of elimination of lithium. For healthy children and adolescents, a baseline serum creatinine, blood urea nitrogen (BUN) level, and urinalysis are usually adequate (Jefferson et al. 1987). If kidney disease is suspected or abnormalities are found, a more thorough evaluation, including tests such as urinalysis (including specific gravity), 24-hour urine volume, and 24-hour urine for creatinine clearance and protein, should be performed and the patient referred to a renal consultant if necessary.

Thyroid Function Tests. Lithium causes thyroid abnormalities primarily by decreasing the release of thyroid hormones. This causes such findings as euthyroid goiter; hypothyroidism; decreased triiodothyronine (T_3), thyroxine (T_4), and protein-bound iodine (PBI) levels; and elevated ^{131}I and thyroid-stimulating hormone (TSH) levels between 5% and 15% of patients receiving long-term lithium therapy (Jefferson et al. 1987). Hypothyroidism resulting from lithium treatment is thought to be related to preexisting Hashimoto's thyroiditis, suggesting that determining antithyroid antibodies as part of the workup may be useful (Rosse et al. 1989). Recommended baseline studies include thyroxine (T_4), triiodothyronine resin uptake (T_3RU), and TSH levels.

Cardiovascular Function Tests. Various cardiac conduction and repolarization abnormalities (e.g., bradycardia) and reversible ECG abnormalities have been reported in a large percentage of adults receiving lithium. ECG changes commonly include benign, reversible T-wave changes (flattening, isoelectricity, and inversion of T waves), which are dose-dependent, and an increase in the PQ interval (Jefferson et al. 1987). It has been hypothesized that lithium's cardiotoxic effects result from its displacing and substituting for intracellular potassium. A baseline ECG should be obtained routinely in patients > 40 years of age or those who have any history or clinical suggestions of cardiovascular disease. Although not considered mandatory in young, healthy patients, a baseline ECG is justifiable and useful to have for comparison, should cardiovascular abnormalities develop at some later time. If patients have or develop cardiac abnormalities, frequent ECG monitoring should be done and the advice of a cardiac consultant sought. In other patients it is prudent to repeat the ECG at the time of scheduled routine physical examinations.

Calcium Metabolism Tests. Lithium may increase renal calcium reabsorption, resulting in hypocalcuria (Jefferson et al. 1987). Lithium may also cause hyperparathyroidism with hypercalcemia and hypophosphatemia, with resulting decreased bone formation or density in children. If abnormal results occur, parathyroid hormone (parathormone) levels may be determined. Lithium may also replace calcium in bone formation, especially in immature bones (USPDI, 1990). A baseline calcium level should be determined in children and adolescents, but a baseline parathormone level is not usually recommended.

Electroencephalogram. Bennett et al. (1983) reported that optimal doses of lithium caused worsening of conduct-disordered children's EEGs in statistically significant numbers. Paroxysmal and focal EEG abnormalities, in particular, were increased over pretreatment EEGs. EEG worsening, however, did not correlate with clinical symptoms of toxicity, and children receiving lithium showed significantly more behavioral improvement than those receiving placebo.

Although an EEG is not required as a baseline workup for normal healthy youngsters, if EEG abnormalities or a seizure disorder is known to exist, a baseline EEG should be obtained and the EEG periodically monitored. Lithium levels should be determined the morning that the EEG is performed, to facilitate correlation of EEG changes and serum lithium levels.

Periodic Monitoring

Because there is little information on the long-term effects of lithium on the development and maturation of children and adolescents, periodic monitoring of thyroid, kidney, and cardiac functioning is particularly important. It is recommended that

TSH, BUN, and serum creatinine levels be determined at approximately 6-month intervals. When there is a concern about renal function, 24-hour urine volume, creatinine clearance, and protein excretion should also be determined. If a suggestion of thyroid abnormality arises, T_3 and T_4 levels should also be determined (Rosse et al. 1989).

Lithium Carbonate (Lithotabs; Eskalith, Lithane, Lithobid); Lithium Citrate Syrup (Cibalith-S)

Indications for Lithium Carbonate in Child and Adolescent Psychiatry. The following boxed warning appears in the package insert.

Note: Warning: Lithium toxicity is closely related to serum lithium levels, and can occur at doses close to therapeutic levels. Facilities for prompt and accurate serum lithium determinations should be available before initiating therapy.

Lithium carbonate is FDA approved for the treatment of manic episodes of manic-depressive illness and maintenance therapy of manic-depressive patients, with a history of mania, who are at least 12 years of age. Significant normalization of manic symptomatology may require up to 3 weeks of lithium carbonate therapy; hence concomitant use of antipsychotic medication may be initially required for more rapid control of manic symptoms. See subsequent text regarding titration of dose and recommended serum lithium levels.

Lithium Dosage Schedule

- Children up to 11 years of age: Not recommended (see later under section "Reports of Interest").
- Adolescents at least 12 years of age and adults: Dosage must be individually regulated according to clinical response and serum lithium levels. As noted earlier, the pharmacokinetics of lithium carbonate makes it necessary to administer the total daily dose in smaller doses administered three or four times daily if immediate-release tablets or syrup is used, or twice daily if controlled-release capsules are used, to minimize risk of reaching toxic serum levels of lithium. (More detailed information on administering, titrating, and monitoring lithium in children and adolescents is found in subsequent text.)

Lithium Carbonate Dose Forms Available

- Tablets (Lithotabs): 300 mg
- Capsules: (Eskalith) 150 mg, 300 mg, 600 mg
- Controlled-release tablets (Eskalith CR): 450 mg (scored)
- Slow-release tablets (Lithobid) 300 mg
- Syrup (lithium citrate): 8 mEq/5 mL (equivalent to one 300 mg tablet)

Titration of Lithium Dosage

Schou (1969) noted that early untoward effects, such as nausea, diarrhea, muscle weakness, thirst, urinary frequency, hand tremor, and a dazed feeling, may be caused by a too rapid rise in serum lithium levels. Lithium is also a gastric irritant. A low initial dose of lithium taken after meals, which slows absorption, and gradual increases in dose will often avert the development of these symptoms. When they develop, they usually subside spontaneously within a few days.

Serum lithium levels should be monitored twice weekly during the acute manic phase and until both serum level and clinical condition have stabilized. In the maintenance phase of therapy during remission, serum lithium levels and thyroid, kidney, and cardiac functions should be periodically monitored. The National Institute of Mental Health/National Institutes of Health (NIMH/NIH) Consensus Development Panel (1985) recommends that serum lithium levels be determined at intervals of 1 to 3 months and that TSH and serum creatinine values be determined every 6 to 12 months. Because there is less experience in long-term administration of lithium carbonate to children and adolescents than that to adults, the author recommends monitoring at the shorter recommended intervals; that is, determining the lithium level at least bimonthly and TSH and serum creatinine levels every 6 months.

Typically, doses of approximately 1,800 mg/day will achieve the serum lithium levels between 1 and 1.5 mEq/L necessary to control symptoms during acute mania. During long-term maintenance, serum lithium levels usually range between 0.6 and 1.2 mEq/L; this usually requires a divided daily dose between 900 mg and 1,200 mg (PDR, 2000). Berg et al. (1974), however, reported that a 14-year-old girl and her father, who were both diagnosed with bipolar manic-depressive disorder, required daily doses of lithium as high as 2,400 mg to achieve therapeutic levels.

Kutcher et al. (1990) reported differences in lithium responsiveness in adolescents with bipolar disorder only and with comorbid personality disorder. When assessed during a period of relative euthymia following discharge from an inpatient unit, 35% ($N = 7$) of 20 adolescents (mean age, 17.5 years) diagnosed with bipolar disorder and having had at least one manic and one depressive episode were diagnosed with at least one comorbid personality disorder. None of the subjects diagnosed with comorbid personality disorder improved on lithium, whereas 6 of the 13 subjects with bipolar disorder only improved on lithium ($P = .05$).

The NIMH/NIH Consensus Development Panel (1985) notes that criteria for prophylactic use of lithium in children and adolescents do not yet exist, and thus the preventive use of lithium must be based on clinical judgment. The risks versus the benefits for this age range are not yet firmly established, although available data suggest that the potential problems are similar to those encountered in adults (NIMH/NIH, 1985).

Use of Lithium Carbonate in Children Under 12 Years of Age

The therapeutic dosages of lithium carbonate used in treating children over 5 years of age with various disorders do not differ significantly from those used in treating older adolescents and adults, and the principles of administration are essentially the same (Campbell et al. 1984a). This higher dose per body weight ratio may reflect the fact that higher renal lithium clearance may occur in children and adolescents than in adults.

Weller et al. (1986) published a guide for determining the initial total daily lithium dose for prepubertal children 6 to 12 years of age. The guide and summary of how it is used are presented in Table 8.1. Lower initial doses should be used for children diagnosed with mental retardation or organicity (central nervous system damage) (E.B. Weller, personal communication, 1990).

The purpose of this guide is to reach therapeutic serum lithium levels (0.6 to 1.2 mEq/L) as rapidly as possible using currently available tablet strengths without

TABLE 8.1 ● **Lithium Carbonate Dosage Guide for Prepubertal School-Aged Children[a,b]**

Weight	8 AM Dose	12 Noon Dose	6 PM Dose	Total Daily Dose
< 25 kg	150 mg	150 mg	300 mg	600 mg
25–40 kg	300 mg	300 mg	300 mg	900 mg
40–50 kg	300 mg	300 mg	600 mg	1,200 mg
50–60 kg	600 mg	300 mg	600 mg	1,500 mg

[a]Dose specified in schedule should be maintained at least 5 days with serum lithium levels drawn every other day 12 hours after ingestion of the last lithium dose until two consecutive levels appear in the therapeutic range (0.6–1.2 mEq/L). Dose may then be adjusted based on serum level, side effects, or clinical response. Do not exceed 1.4 mEq/L serum level.
[b]Lower initial dose should be used for children diagnosed with mental retardation or organicity.
From Weller EB, Weller RA, Fristed MA. Lithium dosage guide for prepubertal children: A Preliminary report. *J Am Acad Child Psychiatry* 1986:25;92–95.

undue risk of reaching toxic serum levels. The authors administered lithium to ten subjects diagnosed with manic-depressive illness and five subjects diagnosed with conduct disorder, following these guidelines. Thirteen of the 15 subjects had serum lithium levels in the therapeutic range after only 5 days of treatment. Side effects were reported to be minimal, primarily mild nausea, abdominal pain, polydipsia and polyuria, and increase in preexisting enuresis. Most were transient and none required discontinuation of lithium. As discussed earlier, some adverse effects of lithium appear to be related to excessively rapid increases in serum lithium level. It remains to be determined whether the use of the proposed lithium dosage guide will cause significantly more adverse effects or will increase their severity more than would a more gradual titration of lithium. In cases where very rapid control of symptoms is critical, however, it may be prove to be especially useful.

Reports of Interest

Lithium Carbonate in the Treatment of Mood Disorders (Mania, Bipolar Disorder), Behavioral Disorders with Mood Swings, and/or Patients Whose Parent(s) are Lithium Responders. DeLong and Aldershof (1987) reported successful treatment with lithium carbonate in 66% of 59 children diagnosed with bipolar affective disorder; 82% of 11 children with emotionally unstable character disorder; and 71% of seven offspring of a lithium-responsive parent.

Varanka et al. (1988) treated ten prepubertal children (nine males, one female; mean age, 9 years, 6 months ± 2 years; range, 6 years, 9 months to 12 years, 7 months) with lithium carbonate. All ten children were diagnosed with manic episode with psychotic features. Doses ranged from 1,150 to 1,800 mg/day (32 to 63 mg/kg/day). Therapeutic lithium levels of 0.6 to 1.4 mEq/L were reached in all cases within 3 to 5 days. Substantial improvement was observed in all the children within an average of 11 days (range, 3 to 24 days) after therapy was begun.

All psychotic symptoms remitted, and mood normalized. The children became less irritable and destructive; their thought processes, motor activity, and attention spans improved remarkably. Untoward effects, such as fatigue, diminished appetite, abdominal discomfort, nausea, urinary frequency, and tremor, were infrequent and so mild that they did not necessitate discontinuation of lithium.

Carlson et al. (1992) reported data on 11 hospitalized children (age range, 5 years, 11 months to 12 years) whom the authors thought were likely to be lithium responders. Diagnoses and symptomatology varied but included bipolar disorder (two), manic episode (three), bipolar not otherwise specified (four); disruptive behavior disorders (nine), exhibited psychotic symptoms (seven), and multiple placements in the seclusion room for explosive behaviors (six). Four subjects had first-degree relatives with histories of bipolar illness. Seven of the subjects participated in a double-blind, placebo-controlled protocol, whereas the other four received lithium on an open basis. Lithium dosage ranged from 600 to 1,500 mg/day, resulting in serum lithium levels that ranged between 0.7 and 1.1 mEq/L. In general, positive clinical responses increased with time, and improvements in self-control, aggression, and anxiety/agitation were greater at 8 weeks than at 4 weeks in all the subjects. These improvements, however, could not be distinguished from the effects of a longer time in the hospital, because the seven children in the double-blind crossover study maintained their gains on placebo. Only three subjects improved sufficiently on lithium to be discharged on that drug. Three patients diagnosed with bipolar disorder or bipolar disorder not otherwise specified (NOS) and one diagnosed with major depressive disorder did not have adequate therapeutic responses to lithium; however, they improved and were discharged when given an open trial of desipramine. There was no evidence that lithium caused worsening or improvement in attention, cognitive functioning, or learning performance on several rating scales (Carlson et al. 1992).

Lithium Carbonate in the Treatment of Acute Mania in Adolescents. Kafantaris et al. (2003) conducted a 4-week, open trial of lithium carbonate in treating acute mania in 100 adolescents (mean age 15.23 years, age range, 12 to 18 years; 50 males, 50 females) who had been diagnosed with bipolar I disorder and met DSM-IV criteria for a current manic or mixed episode and had a score of ≥ 16 on the Young Mania Rating Scale (YMRS). ADHD was a codiagnosis in 31% of patients. Immediate-release lithium was rapidly titrated to therapeutic serum levels between 0.6 and 1.2 mEq/L using Cooper's technique (Cooper et al. 1973). Subjects with severe aggression and/or psychosis were treated concomitantly with antipsychotics. Mean lithium serum level at the end of week 1 was 0.90 ± 0.25 mEq/L; at endpoint (week 4), the mean serum level was 0.93 ± 0.21 mEq/L and the mean dose was $1,355 \pm 389$ mg/day.

Subjects were rated weekly on the YMRS, Hamilton Depression Rating Scale (HDRS, 17 item), Brief PsychiatricRating Scale (BPRS), Clinical Global Impressions-Improvement (CGI-I) Scale, and the Children's Global Assessment Scale (CGAS). Responders were defined as having both a decrease of > 33% from baseline YMRS score and a ≤ 2 rating (much or very much improved) on the CGI-I. At the end of week 4, all the ratings showed significant improvement ($P < .001$). Sixty-three patients met responder criteria by the end of week 2. Remission of manic symptoms (YMRS score < 6) occurred in 26 patients by week 4 and only 4 of the 23 patients with suicidal ideation at baseline had such symptoms by week 4. The authors reported that the presence of baseline psychotic features (with antipsychotic treatment), prominent depressive symptoms, comorbid diagnoses including ADHD, early onset of mood disorders, severity of mania at initial presentation and hospitalization did not impact significantly on response to lithium at week 4.

Adverse events present at week 4 ratings in > 10% of patients included weight gain (1 to 12 pounds), 55.3%; polydipsia, 33.3%; polyuria 25.5%; headache 23.5%; tremor 19.6%; gastrointestinal pain, 17.6%; nausea, 15.7%; vomiting 13.7%; anorexia 13.7%; and diarrhea 13.7%.

This study suggests that lithium is an effective treatment for moderate-to-severe acute mania in adolescents (Kafantaris et al. 2003).

Lithium Carbonate versus Valproic Acid in the Maintenance Treatment of Children and Adolescents Diagnosed with Bipolar Disorder. The paper by Findling et al. (2005), which found no clinically significant differences between the two drugs for this indication is summarized in the section on valproic acid.

Lithium Carbonate in the Treatment of Adolescents Diagnosed with Bipolar Disorder and Substance Dependency. Geller et al. (1998) conducted a 6-week, double-blind, placebo-controlled, parallel-groups study comparing lithium and placebo in the treatment of 25 outpatients (16 males, 9 females; mean age, 16.3 ± 1.2 years) diagnosed by DSM-III-R (APA, 1987) criteria with a bipolar disorder or major depressive disorder with one or more predictors of future bipolar disorder and substance dependency disorder. The mean age of onset of substance abuse disorders was approximately 6 years after the mean age of onset of subjects' mood disorders. Subjects did not have to agree to stop their substance abuse to participate in the study. Thirteen subjects were assigned to the lithium group; of these, ten completed the study. Twelve were assigned to the placebo group and 11 completed the study.

Efficacy was determined by ratings on the Children's Global Assessment Scale (CGAS) and random weekly urine drug assays. "Responders" were required to have a score of ≥ 65. Lithium was initiated with a 600-mg dose; serum lithium levels were determined 24 hours later, and an initial target dose was calculated for each subject using a nomogram to yield a serum lithium level between 0.9 and 1.3 mEq/L. The dose was further individually adjusted as necessary; total dose was divided and given at 7:00 AM and 7:00 PM daily. The subjects on lithium improved significantly more than those on placebo. Six (60%) of the 10 completers on lithium were "responders," compared with 1 (9.1%) of the 11 completers on placebo ($P = .024$). The mean daily lithium dose for the ten completers was $1,733 \pm 428$ mg; the responders' daily dose was significantly higher ($1,975 \pm 240$ mg) than that of the nonresponders ($1,368 \pm 399$ mg; $P = .02$), but there was no significant difference in their serum lithium levels (responders, 0.88 ± 0.27 mEq/L vs. nonresponders, 0.85 ± 0.3 mEq/L). After 3 weeks, the percentage of the weekly random urine tests that was positive for drug assays was significantly lower in the lithium group than that in the placebo group ($P = .042$) for the 21 completers. The ratings of untoward effects on the acute lithium side effects scale showed that lithium was well tolerated. Only polyuria and polydipsia occurred significantly more frequently in the lithium group than in the placebo group. The authors concluded that the results after 6 weeks in their sample were encouraging but further research for these chronic disorders was needed with larger samples and long-term maintenance on the lithium.

Lithium Carbonate in the Treatment of Disorders with Severe Aggression, Especially When Accompanied by Explosive Affect, Including Self-Injurious Behavior. In a double-blind, placebo-controlled study of 61 treatment-resistant hospitalized children (age range, 5.2 to 12.9 years) diagnosed with undersocialized aggressive conduct disorder, both haloperidol and lithium were found to be superior to placebo in ameliorating behavioral symptoms (Campbell et al. 1984b). Optimal doses of lithium carbonate ranged from 500 to 2,000 mg/day (mean, 1,166 mg/day); corresponding serum levels ranged from 0.32 to 1.51 mEq/L (mean, 0.99 mEq/L), and saliva levels ranged from 0.81 to 5.05 mEq/L (mean, 2.52 mEq/L). The authors noted that lithium caused fewer and milder untoward effects than did haloperidol and that these effects did not appear to interfere significantly with the children's daily routines. There was also a suggestion that lithium was particularly effective in diminishing the explosive affect and that other improvements followed (Campbell et al. 1984b).

In 1995, Campbell et al. (1995) reported a double-blind, placebo-controlled study that was designed to replicate their 1984 study. Fifty treatment-resistant inpatients (46 males, 4 females; mean age, 9.4 ± 1.8 years; age range, 5.1 to 12.0 years) diagnosed with conduct disorder, undersocialized aggressive type by DSM-III (APA, 1980a) criteria and having chronic severe explosive aggressiveness were treated with lithium carbonate only or placebo. Following a 2-week, placebo baseline period during which baseline assessments were conducted and placebo responders were eliminated, the 50 remaining subjects were randomly assigned to placebo ($N = 25$) or lithium ($N = 25$) for a 6-week period; this was followed by 2 weeks of posttreatment placebo. Efficacy was assessed by ratings on the Global Clinical Judgments (Consensus) Scale, Children's Psychiatric Rating Scale (CPRS), Clinical Global Impressions (CGI), Clinical Global Impressions-Severity (CGI-S), and Improvement (CGI-I) Scales, Conners Teacher Questionnaire (CTQ), and the Parent-Teacher Questionnaire (PTQ). Lithium carbonate was begun at 600 mg/day and titrated individually over a 2-week period with a maximum permitted dose of 2,100 mg/day or serum lithium of 1.8 mEq/L or equivalent saliva lithium level. The mean optimal dose of lithium was 1,248 mg/day (range, 600 to 1,800 mg/day); the mean serum lithium level was 1.12 mEq/L (range, 0.53 to 1.79 mEq/L; and the mean saliva lithium level was 2.5 mEq/L (range, 1.45 to 4.44 mEq/L).

On the Global Clinical Judgments (consensus) Scale, 68% (17/25) of subjects on lithium were rated as moderately or markedly improved while only 40% (10/25) of subjects on placebo were so rated ($P = .003$). Further refining this measure, 40% (10/25) of the subjects of lithium were "markedly" improved versus only 4% (1/25) of the subjects on placebo. The CGI-I scores after 6 weeks were also significantly better for the lithium group ($P = .044$); although it was not significant whether the lithium group improved more on the CGI-S. The authors concluded that these data supported the conclusions of their earlier study and that lithium carbonate can be efficacious in treating children with conduct disorder and explosive aggressiveness who have not responded to psychosocial treatments or medication with methylphenidate or standard neuroleptics.

Vetro et al. (1985) treated 17 children, aged 3 years to 12 years, with lithium, who were hospitalized for hyperaggressivity, active destruction of property, severely disturbed social adjustment, and unresponsiveness to discipline. Ten of the children had not responded to prior pharmacotherapy, including haloperidol and concomitant individual and family therapy. Lithium carbonate was titrated slowly over 2 to 3 weeks to achieve serum levels in the therapeutic range (0.6 to 1.2 mEq/L). Mean serum lithium level was 0.68 mEq/L ± 0.30 mEq/L. The authors reported that 13 of the children improved enough that their abilities to adapt to their environment could be described as good, and their aggressivity had been reduced to tolerable levels. Three of the four cases that did not improve had poor compliance in taking the medication at home. The authors also noted that these children usually required continuous treatment with lithium for longer than 6 months.

DeLong and Aldershof (1987) reported that rage, aggressive outbursts, and, interestingly, encopresis responded favorably to lithium pharmacotherapy in children with behavioral disorders associated with a variety of neurologic and medical diseases, including mental retardation.

Lithium Carbonate in the Treatment of Children and Adolescents Diagnosed with Conduct Disorder. Malone et al. (2000) conducted a 6-week, double-blind, placebo-controlled, parallel-groups study comparing lithium carbonate and placebo in the treatment of 40 inpatients (33 males, seven females; mean age, 12.5 years; age range, 9.5 to 17.1 years) who were diagnosed with conduct disorder by DSM-III-R (APA, 1987) criteria and hospitalized for chronic, severe aggressive behavior. Eighty-six inpatients entered the study, however, 46 were eliminated during the initial 2-week single-blind placebo baseline; 40 of this group did not meet the protocol's aggression criteria. All 40 remaining subjects entered the 4-week treatment phase and completed the protocol; 20 subjects were assigned randomly to each group.

Efficacy was determined by ratings on the Global Clinical Judgments (Consensus) Scale (GCJCS), the Clinical Global Impressions (CGI), and the Overt Aggression Scale (OAS). Lithium was initiated with a 600-mg dose; serum lithium levels were determined 24 hours later and an initial target dose was calculated for each subject using a nomogram. Subsequent lithium doses were increased by 300 mg daily and given in three equal doses to reach the target dose. At the end of the study, optimal mean lithium dose was $1,425 \pm 321$ mg/day (range, 900 to 2,100 mg/day) with a mean steady-state therapeutic lithium level of 1.07 ± 0.19 mmol/L (range, 0.78 to 1.55 mmol/L).

On the GCJCS, 16 (80%) of the lithium group versus six (30%) of the placebo group were rated as "marked" or "moderately" improved on the criterion for responders ($P = .004$). Significantly more of the lithium group were also rated as responders on the CGI (17 [30%] vs. four [20%] of the placebo group; $P = .004$). On the OAS, the lithium group continued to show improvement over the 4-week period, whereas the placebo group showed an initial decline at week 1 but then remained rather stable. The lithium group's mean decrease from baseline was significantly greater than that of the placebo group, with a significant interaction between treatment group and time ($P = .04$). Although untoward effects were frequent, they were usually mild and similar for both placebo and lithium groups. Only three adverse effects occurred significantly more on lithium: nausea in 12 of 20, vomiting in 11 of 20, and urinary frequency 11 of 20 ($P \leq .05$ in all cases). The authors noted that the aggressive behavior of 40 (47.1%) of their initial 85 subjects improved significantly during the first 2 weeks secondary to hospitalization and treatment with placebo alone. For the 40 subjects who remained aggressive and entered the medication phase of the protocol, lithium was a safe and effective treatment. The authors noted that determining the long-term efficacy and safety of lithium in such subjects will require further research.

Lithium Carbonate in the Treatment of ADHD. Greenhill et al. (1973) and DeLong and Aldershof (1987) reported that lithium was not effective or worsened symptoms in the treatment of children with earlier equivalent diagnoses of ADHD.

ANTIEPILEPTICS/MOOD STABILIZERS

The use of antiepileptic drugs for the treatment of psychiatric disorders in children and adolescents was reviewed by Stores, 1978. He concluded that "while some of the antiepileptic drugs show possibilities as psychotropic agents, their use in children with nonepileptic conditions such as behavior or learning disorders of childhood cannot be justified except as a carefully controlled research exercise" (p. 314).

Currently, most clinical interest in the off-label use of antiepileptic drugs to treat psychiatric disorders in children and adolescents is focused on valproic acid (valproate) and carbamazepine; their safety and efficacy in treating these disorders remains to be elucidated. Carbamazepine and valproic acid are being used with increasing frequency to treat many psychiatric and neuropsychiatric disorders that have failed to respond satisfactorily to more standard therapies. Both drugs have been used independently and as adjunctive agents to treat adults and children with bipolar disorder and mania as mood stabilizers and to treat patients with aggressiveness directed either toward self or others, and behavioral dyscontrol. Some mentally retarded persons with concomitant affective symptomatology and disordered behavior have also shown significant clinical benefit from these drugs, allowing decrease or cessation of antipsychotic drugs. Further research is necessary to determine which specific disorders, symptoms, and patients or subgroups of patients are most likely to respond well (e.g., patients with various abnormal EEG findings and patients who are mentally retarded or have other evidence of abnormal central nervous system functioning compared with affectually or behaviorally disordered patients without signs of central nervous system dysfunction). It will also be important to ascertain further the adverse effects in children and adolescents when these drugs are used for off-label indications rather than to treat seizure disorders. Both have rare but potentially fatal adverse effects and must be used cautiously and monitored carefully.

Valproic Acid (Depakene); Divalproex Sodium (Valproic Acid and Valproate Sodium [Depakote; Depacon])

Note: The FDA has directed the manufacturers of Valproic Acid and its derivatives [e.g., Divalproex sodium and Valproate sodium] to label their products with the following Black Box Warning. HEPATOTOXICITY: Hepatic failure resulting in fatalities has occurred in patients receiving valproic acid. Experience has indicated that children under the age of 2 year are at a considerable increased risk of developing fatal hepatotoxicity, especially those with congenital metabolic disorders, those with severe seizure disorders accompanied by mental retardation and those with organic brain disease. When valproic acid products are used in these patient groups, they should be used with extreme caution and as a sole agent. The benefits of therapy should be weighed against the risks. Above this age-group, experience in epilepsy has indicated that the incidence of fatal hepatotoxicity decreases

considerably in progressively older patient groups. These incidents usually have occurred during the first six months of treatment. Serious or fatal hepatotoxicity may be preceded by nonspecific symptoms such as malaise, weakness, lethargy, facial edema, anorexia, and vomiting. In patients with epilepsy, a loss of seizure control may also occur. Patients should be monitored closely for appearance of these symptoms. Liver function tests should be performed prior to therapy and at frequent intervals thereafter, especially during the first six months. TERATOGENICITY: Valproate can produce teratogenic effects such as neural tube defects (e.g., spina bifida). Accordingly, the use of valproate products in women of childbearing potential requires that the benefits of its use be weighed against the risk of injury to the fetus. PANCREATITIS: Cases of life-threatening pancreatitis have been reported in both children and adults receiving valproate. Some of the cases have been described as hemorrhagic with a rapid progression from initial symptoms to death. Cases have been reported shortly after initial use as well as after several years of use. Patients and guardians should be warned that abdominal pain, nausea, vomiting, and/or anorexia can be symptoms of pancreatitis that require prompt medical evaluation. If pancreatitis is diagnosed valproate should ordinarily be discontinued. Alternative treatment for the underlying medical condition should be initiated as clinically indicated.

Valproic acid and divalproex sodium (a stable coordination compound of valproic acid and valproate sodium) both dissociate to the valproate ion in the gastrointestinal tract and have antiepileptic properties. These drugs are indicated for the treatment of simple and complex absence seizures and adjunctively in patients with multiple seizure types, which include absence seizures. Divalproex sodium has also been approved by the FDA for advertising as safe and effective in the treatment of manic episodes associated with bipolar disorder for up to 3 weeks and the prophylaxis of migraine headaches in adults (PDR, 2006).

Pharmacokinetics of Valproic Acid

Following oral administration, valproic acid and divalproex sodium dissociate to the valproate ion, which is the active agent, in the gastrointestinal tract. Administration of valproic acid with food may slow the absorption rate but does not interfere with clinical efficacy. Food does not significantly affect the total amount of valproate absorbed and may be helpful in reducing gastrointestinal irritation in some patients.

Peak plasma concentration after a single dose usually occurs between 1 and 4 hours after ingestion of valproic acid, 4 hours after ingestion of sodium valproate tablets, and 3.3 hours after taking sodium valproate "sprinkles." Valproic acid is metabolized almost entirely by the liver; the metabolites are excreted primarily in the urine. Plasma valproate half-life is between 6 and 16 hours; the more rapid metabolism rates occur most frequently in patients receiving valproic acid and other antiepileptics that induce enzymes that increase the metabolism rate of valproate.

In a retroactive chart review of 16 males (age range, 5 to 14 years; mean age, 9.3 years) hospitalized for mood stabilization, Good et al. (2001) found that a relatively conservative total loading dose of 15 mg/kg/day of divalproex sodium given in two equal doses resulted in therapeutic trough plasma valproate levels on day 5 of therapy in 13 (81.3%) cases. The initial dose was calculated for one subgroup using actual weight and for a second subgroup using adjusted ideal body weight (IBW). For the latter group, Adjusted IBW = IBW + 40% (Current Weight–IBW). All subjects were also taking atypical antipsychotics, and some were taking stimulants as well during this period. The authors noted several findings of clinical interest: of the eight patients experiencing untoward effects (mostly sedation and nausea), six (75%) had valproate plasma levels of > 90 µg/mL. Patients who were ≥ 15%

over IBW and who were dosed according to actual body weight were significantly more likely to have supratherapeutic (> 120 µg/mL) valproate plasma levels than normal-weight subjects or overweight subjects whose doses were determined by adjusted IBW. Based on this study, it would seem prudent to calculate and use adjusted IBW for significantly overweight children and adolescents if it is decided to administer a loading dose of valproate to rapidly achieve therapeutic plasma levels.

Contraindications for Valproic Acid Administration

Valproic acid can cause severe hepatotoxicity, including fatal hepatic failure. Children under 2 years of age are at increased risk. It should not be administered to anyone with hepatic disease, significant liver dysfunction, or known hypersensitivity to the drug.

Because valproic acid has been reported to cause teratogenic effects in the fetus, it should be administered with caution to women who are likely to become pregnant, and they should be warned to notify their physician immediately if they become pregnant.

Interactions with Other Drugs

Valproate may potentiate the action of central nervous system depressants such as alcohol and benzodiazepines.

Coadministration with clonazepam may induce absence seizures in patients with a history of absence-type seizures.

Coadministration with risperidone (4 mg/day) did not affect the predose or average plasma concentrations and exposure area under the curve (AUC) of valproate (a total of 1,000 mg administered in three divided doses) but there was a 20% increase in valproate peak plasma concentration after concomitant administration of risperidone.

Ambrosini and Sheikh (1998) have reported two cases in which coadministration of valproic acid and guanfacine resulted in significantly increased levels of valproic acid. It was suggested that this was secondary to drug-drug competition at the level of hepatic glucuronidation.

Other drug interactions have been reported.

Untoward Effects of Valproic Acid

The most serious side effect of valproic acid is hepatic failure, which can be fatal; it occurs most frequently within the first 6 months of treatment. Children under 2 years of age are at increased risk. The risk of hepatotoxicity decreases considerably as patients become progressively older. Hence liver function must be monitored carefully and frequently, especially during the first 6 months of treatment.

Nausea, vomiting, and indigestion may occur early in treatment with valproic acid and usually are transient. Sedation may occur, and untoward psychiatric effects such as emotional upset, depression, psychosis, aggression, hyperactivity, and behavioral deterioration have been reported. Thrombocytopenia, other hematologic abnormalities, and many other untoward effects have been reported.

Valproate and Polycystic Ovaries

Isojarvi et al. (1993) published an article noting that there was an association between valproate use in treating epileptic women and polycystic ovaries and hyperandrogenism (elevated serum testosterone concentrations). The finding was more pronounced in women who had begun treatment with valproate before 20 years of age than in women who began valproate treatment at 20 years of age or older. Sussman and Ginsberg (1998) published a critical review of valproate and polycystic ovary syndrome (PCOS), concluding that the available evidence suggests that early and long-term treatment with valproic acid is a causal or precipitating factor in the development of polycystic ovary syndrome in epileptic women, particularly if they are overweight; relative risk factors for nonepileptic adolescents are at present unknown. Johnston (1999) basically concurs. Piontek and Wisner (2000) have suggested clinical guidelines for the appropriate clinical management of women with reproductive capacity who are treated with valproate. Although risk of PCOS does not preclude the use of valproic acid/divalproex sodium in adolescent females, risks and benefits must be discussed, informed consent obtained, and careful monitoring maintained. Further research is urgently needed to clarify this issue.

Indications for Valproic Acid/Divalproex Sodium in Child and Adolescent Psychiatry. *Prior to prescribing review the Boxed Warning at the beginning of this Chapter*

Valproic acid, valproate sodium, and divalproex sodium are approved for use alone or in combination (see exception to this in patients less than two years of age in boxed warning at beginning of chapter) with other drugs in treating patients with simple and complex absence seizures or as an adjunctive agent in patients with multiple-type seizures, which include absence seizures.

Divalproex sodium is additionally approved for the treatment of acute mania in bipolar disorder and the prophylaxis of migraine headache in patients at least 16 years of age. Of note, there is no evidence that it is useful in the acute treatment on migraine headaches. (Valproic acid has not been evaluated for safety and efficacy in treating mania or in the prophylactic treatment of migraine headache and is not approved by the FDA for such advertizing.)

Dosage Schedule

- Children < 2 years of age: Contraindicated for any indication.

Treatment of Epilepsy:

- Children ≥ 2 years of age, adolescents and adults:
  An initial daily dose of 15 mg/kg is recommended. Weekly increases of 5 to 10 mg/kg/day until seizures are controlled or untoward effects prevent further increases are recommended. The maximum recommended daily dose is 60 mg/kg. Amounts > 250 mg/day should be administered in divided doses.

Treatment of Acute Mania (Divalproex Sodium Only)

- Children and Adolescents < 18 years of age: Not recommended.
- Adolescents at least 18 years of age and adults:

  An initial divided daily dose of 750 mg is recommended, followed by rapid titration to achieve satisfactory clinical response or reach total (trough) plasma

(continued)

Indications for Valproic Acid/Divalproex Sodium in Child and Adolescent Psychiatry. *Prior to prescribing review the Boxed Warning at the beginning of this Chapter* (Continued)

valproate levels of 50 to 125 µg/mL, which are usually associated with clinical efficacy. The maximum recommended dosage is 60 mg/kg/day. Titration can usually be completed within 14 days.

Plasma levels of total valproate between 50 and 100 µg/mL are usually considered to be the therapeutic range for epilepsy (and for off-label psychiatric uses); however, in the treatment of acute mania, levels up to 125 µg/mL are recommended.

Prophylactic Treatment of Migraine Headache (Divalproex Sodium Only):

Children and Adolescent < 16 years old: Not recommended.

Adolescents at least 16 years of age and adults: An initial 250-mg dose of divalproex sodium administered twice daily is recommended. Some patients have benefitted from doses as high as 1,000 mg/day, however, higher doses showed no evidence of increased benefit in clinical trials.

Dosage Forms Available (Valproic Acid, Depakene)

- Capsules: 250 mg
- Syrup: 250 mg/5 mL dispensed in 16 ounce bottles

Dosage Forms Available (Divalproex Sodium, Depakote)

- Sprinkle capsules: 125 mg
- Delayed-release tablets (Depakote): 125 mg, 250 mg, 500 mg

Extended-release tablets (Depakote-ER): 250 mg, 500 mg. This formulation permits once-a-day dosing.

Dosage Forms Available (Valproate Sodium)

Injectable (Depacon): 100 mg/mL dispensed in 5 mL single dose vials

Reports of Interest

Valproic Acid in the Treatment of Adolescents Diagnosed with Mania. West et al. (1994) treated 11 adolescents (nine males and two females; age range, 12 to 17 years; mean, 14.5 years) with valproate, on an open basis, who were diagnosed with bipolar disorder (five were manic type and six were mixed type) and hospitalized for acute mania. Seven patients had comorbid diagnoses of ADHD. All the patients had unsatisfactory responses to antipsychotic drugs alone ($N = 5$) or in combination with lithium ($N = 6$). Valproate was added to the medications already being prescribed and was begun at a dose of 250 mg twice daily and titrated upward based on clinical response and adverse effects. Optimal doses ranged from 500 to 2,000 mg/day (mean, 1,068 mg/day), and serum levels ranged from 38 to 94 µg/mL (mean, 74 µg/mL). The length of inpatient valproate administration ranged from 6 to 26 days, with a mean of 17 days. Three patients showed marked improvement, with virtual or complete remission of manic symptoms; six patients improved moderately, with significant reduction of symptoms; and two showed only slight improvement. The only adverse effects reported were sedation in two patients.

Papatheodorou et al. (1995) reported an open-label, 7-week study in which the efficacy and safety of divalproex sodium was assessed in the treatment of 15 subjects (two males, 13 females; mean age, 17.3 years, with 10 subjects being 15 to 18 years old and 5 being 19 or 20 years old) who were diagnosed by DSM-III-R (APA, 1987) criteria with bipolar disorder, in an acute manic phase. Efficacy was evaluated using ratings on the Modified Mania Rating Scale (MMRS), the Brief Psychiatric Rating Scale (BPRS), the Global Assessment Scale (GAS), the Clinical Global Impressions Scale (CGI), and the Valproic Acid Side Effects Scale (VA-SES). Following a 2-day entry phase during which baseline evaluations were performed, subjects began 7 weeks of treatment with divalproex sodium. Medication was administered in three divided doses and individually titrated. Thirteen patients completed the 7-week study; one patient was discontinued for lack of clinical response and one patient withdrew because of "subjectively intolerable sedation and dizziness." All 13 completers required some additional medication for symptom control (e.g., agitation) during the study. Mean dose at the end of 7 weeks was 1,423.08 mg/day (range, 750 to 2,000 mg/day) and the mean serum valproic acid level (12 to 14 hours after the evening dose and before the morning dose) was 642.85 ± 183.08 μmol/L (range, 360 to 923 μmol/L).

The 13 completers' ratings on the MMRS, BPRS, GAS, and CGI were all very significantly lower ($P < .0001$ for all four scales) than at baseline. An analysis of variance (ANOVA) found a significant reduction in the MMRS within 1 week on valproex ($P < .016$), which continued to increase throughout the treatment period. Overall untoward effects were benign and their frequency was reported to decrease over the duration of the study, with a very low number being reported at the end of the study. The most significant adverse effect was the development of hypocortisolemia and hypothyroidism in one patient. Liver function tests remained normal except for one patient with transiently elevated enzyme levels that reverted to normal without change in dosage. The data suggest that divalproex sodium is safe and efficacious in the acute (short-term) treatment of mania in adolescents; further research is indicated.

Valproic Acid versus Lithium in the Maintenance Treatment of Children and Adolescents Diagnosed with Bipolar Disorder. Findling et al. (2005) conducted a double-blind study to determine whether Divalproex sodium (DVPX) or lithium was superior as the only drug in maintenance treatment of 139 subjects (age range 5 to 17 years; mean age 10.8 ± 3.5 years, 93 (66.9%) males 46 (33.1%) females) who were diagnosed with Bipolar I (131, 94.2%) or Bipolar II (8, 5.8%) disorder and stabilized on a combination of lithium carbonate and valproex sodium during acute treatment. Sixty subjects who met remission criteria (Children's Depression Rating Scale score < 40, Young Mania Rating Scale score < 12.5 and a Children's Global Assessment Scale score > 51) for a minimum of 4 weeks were than randomized to monotherapy with either lithium ($N = 30$) or divalproex ($N = 30$) for up to 76 weeks; subjects were dropped from the study if they violated protocol or required additional clinical intervention. Subjects were tapered off the nonmaintenance/discontinued drug over a period of 8 weeks to minimize discontinuation rebound relapse. Subjects maintained on lithium were maintained at lithium serum concentrations between 0.6 and 1.2 mmol/L and those on valproex were maintained with valproate plasma concentrations between 50 and 100 μg/mL. Primary measures of effectiveness were time to premature discontinuation because of emerging mood symptoms of relapse and premature discontinuation for any reason.

Median survival time to mood relapse for subjects on lithium was 114 ± 57.4 days for lithium and 112 ± 56 days for subjects on valproex and was not statistically different ($P = .55$); overall, 38 (63.3%) subjects relapsed. There was also no significant difference between the lithium and valproex groups in the 12 (20%) who dropped out for any reason ($P = .72$). At the study's conclusion, the mean lithium serum level was 0.84 ± 0.3 mmol/L and the mean valproate plasma level was 75.3 ± 29.4 µg/mL (Findling et al. 2005). Only six subjects (10%), three in each treatment group completed the 76-week protocol, a vivid indication of the chronic and debilitating course of pediatric bipolar disorder.

Regarding adverse events, comparing lithium to valproex, emesis (30% vs. 3%), enuresis (30% vs. 6.7%), and increased thirst (16.5% vs. 0%) were significantly more frequent in the lithium group; other frequent adverse events, which were not significantly different between lithium and valproex were headache (13.3% vs. 23.3%), tremor (20.0% vs. 16.7%), stomach pain (10.0% vs. 23.3%), nausea (16.7% vs. 6.7%), diarrhea (13.3% vs. 6.7%) and decreased appetite (10% vs. 10%).

The authors concluded that there was no clinically significant difference between lithium and valproex monotherapy in maintaining the youth who were stabilized on combination lithium/valproex therapy for bipolar disorder (Findling et al. 2005).

Valproic Acid in the Treatment of Children and Adolescents Diagnosed with Mental Retardation and Mood Disorders. Kastner et al. (1990) reported treating three patients with valproic acid, a 16-year-old moderately retarded male and 13- and 8-year-old profoundly retarded girls, all of whom also had symptoms of mood disorder. These symptoms included self-injurious behaviors such as face gouging and head banging, irritability, aggressiveness, hyperactivity, sleep disturbance, and paroxysms of crying. All had unsatisfactory responses to several trials of other medications. All three patients showed excellent response to valproic acid and at follow-up had maintained their gains for 7 to 10 months. Maintenance doses were 2,700 mg/day (plasma level, 109 µg/mL) for the 16-year-old, 3,000 mg/day (plasma level, 75 µg/mL) for the 13-year-old, and 1,500 mg/day (plasma level, 111 µg/mL) for the 8-year-old. The authors noted that the plasma levels were high or just above the typical therapeutic upper range and that no hepatic abnormalities developed in their patients.

In a 2-year prospective study, Kastner et al. (1993) administered valproic acid to 21 patients diagnosed with mental retardation who also had behavioral symptoms of irritability, sleep disturbance, aggressive or self-injurious behavior, and behavioral cycling that were interpreted as symptomatic of an affective disorder. Eighteen patients completed the study. (Two could not be followed up and one developed acute hyperammonemia and was dropped from the study.) Twelve of the patients completing the study were 18 years old or younger; the degree of their retardation ranged from moderate to profound. Valproic acid was titrated upward until symptoms remitted or untoward effects prevented further increase to plasma levels between 50 and 125 µg/mL. Patients' ratings on the Clinical Global Impressions of Severity (CGI-S) Scale after 2 years on medication were significantly improved ($P < .001$) from ratings at baseline. Patients with a diagnosis of epilepsy or a suspicion of seizures correlated with a positive response ($P < .005$). Of note, nine of the ten patients who were receiving neuroleptic drugs at the beginning of the study were no longer being prescribed these drugs at the study's completion.

Divalproex Sodium in the Treatment of Adolescents with Explosive Mood Disorder. In an open-label, 5-week study, Donovan et al. (1997) treated with divalproex sodium ten outpatient adolescents (eight males, two females; age range, 15 to 17 years) who were diagnosed by DSM-III-R (APA, 1987) criteria with disruptive behavioral disorders (seven, conduct disorder; two, oppositional defiant disorder; and one, ADHD). Most had comorbid drug abuse or dependency (five, marijuana abuse; three, marijuana dependency; and one, alcohol abuse). All ten subjects had severe unpredictable mood swings and a low threshold/high amplitude for dyscontrol once irritable with frequent and severe temper tantrums ("explosive mood disorder"), which preceded drug abuse by at least 1 year. Efficacy was determined based on multiple informants' (subjects, parents, and teachers) reports of temper outbursts and mood lability and the Global Assessment of Functioning (GAF; Axis V of the DSM-III-R diagnoses) Scale.

Divalproex sodium was initiated at a dose of 250 mg/day and titrated to 1,000 mg/day over a period of 2 to 4 weeks. The mean plasma valproate level after receiving 1,000 mg/day of divalproex for 1 week was 75 µg/mL, range 45 to 113 µg/mL. At the end of the fifth week, all ten subjects showed very significant improvement on all three measures; nine subjects had no temper outbursts during the fifth week and six subjects had no significant mood lability. Their mean number of temper outbursts decreased from 6.5 ± 4.5 at baseline to 0.1 ± 0.3 after 5 weeks ($P < .001$). The mean mood lability score (0 = least to 4 = greater frequency, duration, and autonomy of mood swings) decreased from 3.8 ± 0.4 at baseline to 0.5 ± 0.7 after 5 weeks ($P < .000$). The mean GAF score improved from 37.8 ± 7.0 at baseline to 65.7 ± 10.2 after 5 weeks ($P < .000$). Divalproex was well tolerated with only two patients reporting mild sedation and transient nausea. There were no serious untoward effects, and liver function tests showed no significant changes. Improvements were maintained while on medication during follow-up; however, five subjects independently discontinued medication for at least 5 days and rapidly relapsed; improvement recurred within a few days of resuming medication. A sixth patient took medication sporadically during follow-up and maintained gains for approximately 6 weeks, when partial relapse occurred. The data suggest that divalproex sodium may be safe and efficacious in such adolescents; further studies should be undertaken (Donovan et al. 1997).

Donovan et al. (2000) conducted a 12-week, randomly assigned, double-blind, placebo-controlled, crossover study of divalproex sodium in the treatment of 20 outpatients (16 males, 4 females; mean age, 13.8 ± 2.4 years; age range, 10 to 18 years), all of whom were diagnosed with conduct disorder or oppositional defiant disorder by DSM-IV (APA, 1994) criteria and chronic explosive temper (more than four episodes monthly of rage, property destruction, or fighting with minimal provocation) and mood lability (multiple daily unpredictable shifts in mood from normal to irritable and withdrawn to boisterous behavior). Four subjects were diagnosed with comorbid ADHD and six with marijuana abuse. Efficacy was assessed by ratings on the Modified Overt Aggression Scale and on six items from the anger-hostility subscale of the Symptom Checklist-90 (SCL-90); it was decided *a priori* that "responders" had to have a $\geq 70\%$ reduction from baseline scores on both rating scales. The first 6 weeks of the study consisted of a parallel-groups design, with ten subjects randomly assigned to valproate or placebo. Divalproex was gradually titrated to 10 mg/lb/day over the first 2 weeks; if the plasma level of valproate was < 90 µg/mL at that time, a single increase of 250 mg/day was added. (To preserve the blind, a similar number of increases were made in the placebo group.) Doses ranged from 750 to 1,500 mg/day, and the mean plasma valproate level was 82.2 ± 19.1 µg/mL. At the end of this 6-week phase, eight (80%) of the ten patients receiving divalproex were rated as responders versus no responders in the ten subjects on placebo ($P < .001$). Seventeen subjects completed phase I (during the first 2 weeks, one subject on divalproex dropped out as he was incarcerated for parole violation and two subjects on placebo dropped out for lack of clinical improvement). Fifteen subjects (eight responders to divalproex and seven nonresponders to placebo) entered the crossover phase of the study (weeks 7 to 12) and all completed it. Six (86%) of the seven placebo nonresponders during phase I responded to divalproex during phase II. Six of the eight responders to divalproex during phase I began relapsing between 1 and 2 weeks into phase II, and at the end of week 12, their average Modified Overt Aggression Scale score had worsened to only 33% over baseline and their average anger-hostility scores on the subscale of the SCL-90 declined to 27% over baseline. Of the 15 subjects completing the entire study, 12 met "responder" criteria only during the medication phase, indicating that divalproex is significantly better than placebo ($P = .003$) in this population.

Divalproex Sodium in the Treatment of Aggression in Children and Adolescents Diagnosed with Pervasive Developmental Disorders. Hellings et al. (2005) conducted a double-blind, placebo-controlled study to evaluate the efficacy of valproate (VPA) in treating aggressive symptoms in 30 subjects (20 male and 10 female; age range 6 to 20 years) who were diagnosed with a pervasive developmental disorder (PDD) by DSM-IV criteria (27 were diagnosed with autistic disorder, 1 with PDDNOS and 2 with Asperger's disorder). Comorbid diagnoses, with the exception of Tourette's disorder were permitted. No other psychotropic medications or antiseizure medications were permitted. Subjects exhibited significant aggression toward themselves or others, or to property, a minimum of three times weekly. Twenty-six subjects had IQs in the mentally retarded range. Subjects were randomly assigned to liquid placebo ($N = 14$) or liquid VPA ($N = 16$) for a period of 8 weeks, following a 1-week lead-in on placebo. In the VPA group, the liquid placebo was gradually replaced by liquid VPA beginning with a 250 mg/5 mL dose. VPA liquid (250 mg/5 mL) was added every 3 days to reach a target dose of 20 mg/kg/day. A psychiatrist not involved in ratings, adjusted the VPA to achieve trough plasma levels of 70 to 100 µg/mL after measurement at the end of 2 and 4 weeks. Mean VPA trough plasma levels were 75.5 µg/mL at week 4 and 77.8 µ/mL at week 8.

There were no statistically significant differences between the two groups on the primary outcome measure, the Aberrant Behavior Checklist—Community Scale (ABC-C; $P = .65$), or the secondary outcome measures, the Clinical Global Impressions-Improvement Subscale (CGI-I; $P = .16$) and the Overt Aggression Scale (OAS; $P = .96$). The CGI-Severity Subscale (CGI-S) also showed no statistical difference between the groups ($P = .96$).

Adverse effects were usually mild. One subject on VPA developed a rash and dropped out of the study. Increased appetite was the only adverse effect that was significantly greater in the VPA group ($P = .03$). Gastrointestinal complaints, sedation, headache, chills, and fever did not differ. Two subjects on VPA had elevations of ammonia above the normal range of 21 to 50 µmol/L and the parent of one of these subjects reported cognitive slowing and slurred speech at times (ammonia was 98 μmol/L at the end of the study).

The authors noted that there was high intrasubject variability with large differences in the frequency and severity of aggression in different weeks, and high intersubject variability with large standard deviations for each of the outcome measures, which weakened study power. Following completion of the study, ten subjects on VPA elected to continue on the drug and six on placebo elected to an open trial of VPA. Ten of these 16 subjects continued to demonstrate a positive and sustained response. The authors concluded that although this study did not demonstrate efficacy of VPA, there might be a subgroup of aggressive children and adolescents with PDD who respond favorably to VPA and that a larger, multisite study is indicated.

Carbamazepine (Tegretol; Carbatrol, Equetro)

Note: The FDA has directed that a Black Box Warning be added to the labeling of carbamazepine products indicating that the risk of developing aplastic anemia and agranulocytosis is 5 to 8 times greater than in the general population, although the incidence is very low. Most cases of leukopenia do not progress to the more serious aplastic anemia or agranulocytosis. However, complete pretreatment hematologic testing should be obtained as a baseline. If low or decreased white blood cell or platelet count occurs during treatment, close monitoring should be implemented and discontinuing carbamazepine should be seriously considered if there is any evidence of bone marrow depression.

Carbamazepine is an anticonvulsant indicated for the treatment of psychomotor and grand mal seizures. It is also a specific analgesic for trigeminal neuralgia.

Pharmacokinetics of Carbamazepine

Peak serum levels occur 4 to 5 hours after ingestion of standard carbamazepine tablets. Initial serum half-life values range from 25 to 65 hours; however, carbamazepine is an autoinducer of its own metabolism. Autoinduction stabilizes over 3 to 5 weeks at a fixed dose, with half-life decreasing to 12 to 17 hours. In children there is a poor correlation between dose and serum level of carbamazepine.

Contraindications for Carbamazepine Administration

Known hypersensitivity to carbamazepine or tricyclic antidepressants, a history of previous bone marrow depression, and the ingestion of an MAOI within the previous 14 days are contraindications.

Interactions of Carbamazepine with Other Drugs

Carbamazepine has been reported to decrease the serum half-lives of haloperidol, phenytoin, theophylline, and other drugs.

When coadministered with risperidone (6 mg/day) over a 3-week period, plasma concentrations of risperidone and 9-hydroxyrisperidone were decreased by approximately 50%. Plasma levels of carbamazepine did not appear to be effected.

When coadministered with olanzepine, carbamazepine in doses of 200 mg twice daily caused approximately 50% increase in the clearance of olanzapine. This was thought to be secondary to carbamazepine's being a potent inducer of CYP1A2 activity. Higher daily doses of carbamazepine may cause an even greater increase in olanzapine clearance.

Carbamazepine serum levels are markedly reduced by the simultaneous use of phenobarbital, phenytoin, or primidone.

Increased lithium serum concentrations and increased risk of neurotoxic lithium effects may occur when carbamazepine and lithium are used simultaneously, because carbamazepine decreases lithium renal clearance.

The FDA has advised that carbamazepine may lose up to one-third of its potency if stored under humid conditions such as in a bathroom. Supplies should be kept tightly closed and in a dry location.

Untoward Effects of Carbamazepine

Evans et al. (1987) attributed the increased interest in the use of carbamazepine in child and adolescent psychiatry in part to both the increased awareness of the serious untoward long-term complications of standard neuroleptic drugs and the finding that the untoward effects of carbamazepine are less formidable than initially thought. In particular, the serious blood dyscrasias, agranulocytosis, and aplastic anemia are very rare. The risk of developing these disorders when treated with carbamazepine is five to eight times that of the general population. Agranulocytosis occurs in approximately six per million and aplastic anemia in approximately two per million of the untreated general population (PDR, 2000).

The most frequently reported untoward effects are dizziness, drowsiness, unsteadiness, nausea, and vomiting. These are more likely to occur if treatment is not begun with the low doses recommended. As noted earlier, aplastic anemia and agranulocytosis, although rare, have been reported. Hence a complete baseline hematologic evaluation must be done and complete blood cell count with differential and platelets must be repeated and monitored closely throughout the treatment.

Pleak et al. (1988) reported that adverse behavioral and neurologic reactions developed in 6 of their 20 male subjects, aged 10 to 16, who were diagnosed with various disorders, but primarily with ADHD and conduct disorder, and who were participating in an ongoing protocol evaluating the efficacy of carbamazepine in treating severe aggressive outbursts in child and adolescent inpatients. The untoward effects included a severe manic episode in a 16-year-old, hypomania in a 10-year-old, and increased irritability, impulsivity, and aggressiveness and/or worsening of behavior in two subjects aged 14 and 15. Two 11-year-old boys developed EEG abnormalities, with sharp waves and spikes. One of these boys improved behaviorally but had his first two absence seizures in several years. The authors caution that patients must be monitored carefully for the development of adverse neuropsychiatric effects.

Carbamazepine and the Induction of Mania

Three additional cases of carbamazepine-induced mania have been reported in children (Reiss and O'Donnell, 1984; Myers and Carrera, 1989). Myers and Carrera speculated that when adverse behavioral effects such as irritability, insomnia, agitation, talkativeness, and prepubescent hypersexuality occur with carbamazepine administration, they may be symptoms of an unrecognized hypomania or mania.

Indications for Carbamazepine in Child and Adolescent Psychiatry

Carbamazepine is approved for use in patients at least 6 years of age for the treatment of various seizure types. Patients diagnosed with partial seizures with complex symptomatology (psychomotor or temporal lobe) tend to benefit the most from carbamazepine, but patients with generalized tonic-clonic (grand mal) seizures or a mixed seizure pattern may also improve. Absence (petit mal) seizures are not controlled by carbamazepine. Patients with trigeminal and glossopharyngeal neuralgias have shown reduction in pain when treated with carbamazepine. There are no FDA-approved psychiatric indications for carbamazepine.

Carbamazepine Dosage Schedule

The following are doses recommended for treatment of epilepsy. It is recommended that carbamazepine be taken with meals.

- Children under 6 years of age: Not recommended.
- Children 6 through 12 years of age: Begin with a dose of 100 mg twice daily (or 50 mg four times daily if suspension is used). The dose may be increased weekly by increments of 100 mg as clinically indicated to obtain optimal response. Daily doses of 300 mg or more should be administered in three or four doses. The daily dose should not usually exceed 1,000 mg. Usual maintenance daily dose is 400 to 800 mg.
- Patients > 12 years old: Begin with a dose of 200 mg twice daily (or 100 mg four times daily if suspension is used). The dose may be increased weekly by increments of 200 mg as clinically indicated to obtain optimal response. Daily doses of 400 mg or more should be administered in three or four doses. The daily dose should not usually exceed 1,200 mg. Usual maintenance daily dose is 800 to 1,200 mg. Usual therapeutic carbamazepine plasma levels are 4 µg/mL to 12 µg/mL.

Carbamazepine Dose Forms Available

- Tablets: 200 mg
- Chewable tablets: 100 mg
- Suspension: 100 mg/5 mL
- Extended-release tablets (Tegretol-XR): 100 mg, 200 mg, 400 mg
- Extended-release capsules (Carbatrol; Equetro): 100 mg, 200 mg, 300 mg

Reports of Interest

Evans et al. (1987) reviewed the use of carbamazepine in treating children and adolescents with psychiatric disorders, including hyperkinesis, aggression, impulsivity, and emotional lability. They noted the lack of systematic, well-controlled studies. These authors also addressed the important issue of the behavioral toxicity of carbamazepine and noted that, in their clinical experience in treating hyperactive and conduct-disordered children with carbamazepine, untoward effects on mood and behavior such as irritability, aggressiveness, increased hyperactivity, emotional lability, angry outbursts, and insomnia commonly occurred and sometimes resembled the target symptoms for which the drug was being prescribed. Although a few studies have appeared since then, many of their concerns remain valid today.

Carbamazepine in the Treatment of Children and Adolescents with Various Diagnoses. Although approved only for treating certain kinds of seizure disorders and neuralgias, carbamazepine has been used to treat many psychiatric disorders. In adults, perhaps the best known of these is the treatment of lithium-resistant bipolar disorder. There is evidence that carbamazepine has acute antimanic and antidepressive effects as well as longer-term prophylactic action in treating bipolar disorder (Post, 1987). Post notes that more severe and dysphoric mania and a rapidly cycling course, variables associated with a poor response to lithium, appear to correspond to better responses to carbamazepine. It has been suggested that the efficacy of carbamazepine in psychiatric disorders may be secondary to its hypothesized ability to inhibit limbic system kindling. Kessler et al. (1989) reported that three psychotic adults improved markedly when carbamazepine was substituted for their neuroleptic medication and suggested criteria to identify effectively ill patients who may have a primary or superimposed organic mood disorder and who might benefit from carbamazepine.

There are many reports, particularly in the European literature, of the use of carbamazepine on an open basis to treat children and adolescents with psychiatric disorders; however, few placebo-controlled studies have been published. In 1988, Pleak et al. noted that carbamazepine was so frequently chosen to treat aggressive children and adolescents who did not respond satisfactorily to standard treatments that it had become "somewhat of a 'vogue' medication" (p. 502).

Remschmidt (1976) reviewed data from 28 clinical trials (seven double-blind and 21 open studies) with a total of > 800 nonepileptic child and adolescent subjects who were treated with carbamazepine. Positive clinical results were found for target symptoms of hyperactivity or hypoactivity, impaired concentration, aggressive behavioral disturbances, and dysphoric mood disorders. In addition to these behavioral effects, Remschmidt suggested that these patients experienced positive mood changes, increased initiative, and decreased anxiety.

Groh (1976) reported on 62 nonepileptic children treated with carbamazepine for various abnormal behavioral patterns. Of the 27 who showed improvement, most had a "dysphoric or dysthymic syndrome," the most important features of which were emotional lability and moodiness, which were thought to cause most of the other behavioral abnormalities.

Kuhn-Gebhart (1976) reported symptom improvement in a large number of nonepileptic children who were treated with carbamazepine for a wide variety of behavioral disorders. The author reported that 30 of the last 50 patients treated showed good or very good responses, 10 had discernible improvement, 9 had no change in behavior, and 1 deteriorated. The author noted that the more abnormal the EEGs of these nonepileptic patients are in general, the better the response; that many of the good responders came from stable homes; and that poorer results were more frequent in subjects from unfavorable homes.

Puente (1976) reported an open study in which carbamazepine was administered to 72 children with various behavioral disorders who did not have evidence of neurologic disease. Fifty-six children completed the study. The usual optimal dose was 300 mg/day (range, 100 to 600 mg/day). Carbamazepine was given for an average of 12 weeks (range, 9 to 23 weeks). Twenty symptoms were rated on a severity scale at the beginning and end of the treatment. Individual symptoms were present in as many as 55 and in as few as 2 of the 56 children. Over the course of treatment, a decrease in symptom expression of 70% or more occurred in 17 of 20 symptoms in at least 60% of the subjects. Interestingly, all 6 children (100%) with night terrors responded positively, as did 16 (94%) of the 17 children with other sleep disturbances. Anxiety, present in 47 children, improved in 34 (72%). Enuresis improved in 8 of 9 children (89%), and aggressiveness, present in 46 children, improved in 32 (70%). The most frequent untoward effects were transient drowsiness (20%), nausea and vomiting (4%), and urticaria (4%).

Carbamazepine in the Treatment of Juvenile-Onset Bipolar I Disorder. Woolston (1999) reported three cases diagnosed with bipolar I disorder whom he treated successfully with carbamazepine. One case, a 16-year-old female, had experienced several cycles of mania followed by depression that had been managed with various neuroleptics and lithium for approximately 4 years. The patient was noncompliant with lithium at least three times, resulting in manic episodes within a month that were followed by severe depression. Following the last of these episodes, she was begun on carbamazepine, 150 mg/day, which was increased to 300 mg/day 3 weeks later and continued at that dosage. Her serum carbamazepine level was 7 μg/mL. The patient became euthymic within 3 weeks and remained so on 300 mg/day of carbamazepine over the next 4 years, with the exception of three brief hypomanic episodes that responded to the addition of a short course of haloperidol 1 mg/day. No untoward effects were reported and blood counts and liver function remained within normal limits.

A 14-year-old male who had been treated for his mania with lithium for approximately 2 years was seen after he discontinued his lithium because it made him tired and dysphoric and he subsequently developed another manic episode. Carbamazepine was begun at a dose of 100 mg/day and increased to 200 mg/day, 5 days later. His mania improved significantly within 15 days and he did not experience the unpleasant symptoms he associated with lithium. His carbamazepine serum level was 8 μg/mL. He remained euthymic on carbamazepine 200 mg/day for the next 3 years with serum levels ranging from 6 μg/mL to 9 μg/mL. No untoward effects were reported and blood counts and liver chemistries remained normal throughout his treatment.

The third case was a 12.5-year-old girl also diagnosed with spastic cerebral palsy and mild mental retardation. She was treated briefly with risperidone for persistent euphoric mood, decreased need for sleep, and intermittent hallucinations. After 3 weeks, she had increased manic symptoms with flight of ideas, pressured speech, motor restlessness, and nearly continuous visual hallucinations with poor reality testing. Risperidone was discontinued and carbamazepine 100 mg/day was begun. After 1 week she showed improvement in sleep and reality testing and no untoward effects. Carbamazepine was then increased to 200 mg/day. Six days later, hallucinations had totally remitted, she was euthymic, had no evidence of a thought disorder, and had her normal sleep pattern. Her serum carbamazepine level was 8 μg/mL. The patient was continued on maintenance carbamazepine, 200 mg/day. Over the next 2 years she developed two brief periods of hypomania, both of which responded rapidly to an additional 50 mg of carbamazepine. She remained euthymic on her final maintenance daily dose of 300 mg of carbamazepine.

Carbamazepine in the Treatment of Children Diagnosed with Conduct Disorder. Kafantaris et al. (1992) reported an open pilot study in which ten children (nine male, one female; age range, 5.25 to 10.92 years; mean, 8.27 years) diagnosed with conduct disorder and hospitalized for symptoms of explosive aggressiveness were treated with carbamazepine. Five of the subjects had previously failed to respond to a trial of lithium. After a 1-week baseline period, carbamazepine was administered in three divided doses, beginning at a total of 200 mg/day and titrated to a maximum of 800 mg/day, or a serum level of 12 μg/mL over a period of 3 to 5 weeks. Optimal dose range was 600 to 800 mg/day (mean, 630 mg/day) with serum levels from 4.8 to 10.4 μg/mL (mean, 6.2 μg/mL). Target symptoms of aggressiveness and explosiveness declined significantly on all measures compared with baseline ratings. On the Global Clinical Consensus Ratings, four subjects were rated as markedly improved, four as moderately improved, one as slightly improved, and one as not improved. Three of the lithium nonresponders showed marked improvement, and one showed moderate improvement; the fifth did not respond to either drug. Untoward effects during regulation and at optimal dose included fatigue (2 of 10 cases), blurred vision (2 of 10), and dizziness (1 of 10). Untoward effects above optimal dose included diplopia (2 of 10), mild ataxia (2 of 10), mild dysarthria (1 of 10), headache (2 of 10), and lethargy (1 of 10). One child experienced worsening of preexisting behavioral symptoms and loosening of associations, which were thought to be manifestations of behavioral toxicity. Overall, the untoward effects were transient and were decreased to tolerable levels or eliminated by reduction in dose. White blood cell counts remained within normal limits, although four children had reductions from baseline determinations.

Cueva et al. (1996) reported a 9-week, double-blind, placebo-controlled study comparing carbamazepine and placebo in 22 children (20 males, 2 females; mean age, 8.97 years; age range, 5.33 to 11.7 years) who were diagnosed with conduct disorder, solitary aggressive type, by DSM-III-R (APA, 1987) criteria and hospitalized for treatment-resistant aggressiveness and explosiveness. Thirty-eight children who met protocol criteria entered the initial 2-week placebo washout period. At the end of this period, 14 were eliminated because they no longer met study or aggression criteria. Of the 24 subjects who entered the treatment phase of the study, 13 were assigned to carbamazepine and 11 to placebo; 22 subjects completed the study. Efficacy was measured using the Children's Psychiatric Rating Scale (CPRS), the NIMH Clinical Global Impressions-Severity (CGI-S) and, CGI-Improvement (CGI-I) scales, the Overt Aggression Scale (OAS), and the Global Clinical Judgments (Consensus) Scale, with a blind rating by all clinical staff occurring just before the code is broken. Medication was dispensed in two capsules given three times daily throughout the study. Carbamazepine was initiated at a dose of 200 mg/day and increased over a 2-week period in predetermined steps of 200 mg/dose to a maximum of 1,000 mg/day or until therapeutic effects were observed or untoward effects prevented further increase. Mean optimal dose of carbamazepine was 683 mg/day (range, 400 to 800 mg/day), with a mean serum carbamazepine level of 6.81 μg/mL (range, 4.98 to 9.1 μg/mL), for the 11 subjects for whom values were available.

The results showed no significant differences in the clinical improvement of aggression between carbamazepine and placebo on any of the rating scales. Both groups improved on the aggression factor of the CPRS over time and both improved similarly on the Global Clinical Judgments (Consensus) Scale as rated by clinical staff. Carbamazepine treatment resulted in significantly more untoward effects than placebo. Twelve of the 13 subjects on carbamazepine reported a total of 57 untoward effects, whereas only 6 of 11 subjects on placebo reported six untoward effects. Two subjects on carbamazepine developed marked leukopenia with between 2,000 and 3,000 WBC/mm^3, and four developed moderate leukopenia with between 3,000 and 3,500 WBC/mm^3; one subject on placebo also developed moderate leukopenia. The leukopenia was transient in all seven cases. Other untoward effects experienced by subjects on carbamazepine included dizziness ($N = 7$, 54%), rash ($N = 6$, 46%), headache (46%), diplopia ($N = 5$, 38%), drowsiness ($N = 4$, 31%), nausea (31%), ataxia ($N = 3$, 23%), and vomiting (23%) (Cueva et al. 1996).

Carbamazepine in the Treatment of Children and Adolescents with Symptoms of ADHD. Silva et al. (1996) searched the world literature for reports in which carbamazepine was used to treat children and adolescents with behavioral problems and hyperactivity. Twenty-nine such reports were located; ten of them provided information suitable for a meta-analysis. Seven studies, with a total of 189 patients, were open; 70% of subjects experienced at least a marked improvement in target symptoms (significance ranged from $P < .001$ to $P = .05$). There was a significant correlation between longer treatment and positive outcome. In the three double-blind studies, 53 subjects were assigned to carbamazepine and 52 to placebo. Thirty-eight (72%) subjects on carbamazepine and 14 (27%) subjects on placebo were rated as moderately to markedly improved. Meta-analysis of these three studies found carbamazepine significantly ($P = .018$) more efficacious than placebo in diminishing target symptoms. The most common untoward effects in the studies reviewed were sedation and rash. The authors concluded that carbamazepine merited further study as a possible second-line treatment for children and adolescents with ADHD that is not responsive to stimulant medication or when stimulant medication cannot be tolerated.

Phenytoin, Diphenylhydantoin (Dilantin)

Contraindications for Phenytoin Administration

Known hypersensitivity to the phenytoin or a related drug is a contraindication.

Interactions of Phenytoin with Other Drugs

Acute alcohol intake may increase serum phenytoin levels, whereas chronic alcohol use may decrease levels.

Tricyclic antidepressants may precipitate seizures in susceptible patients, necessitating increased phenytoin doses.

Specific drugs have been reported to increase, decrease, or either increase or decrease phenytoin levels. Obtaining serum phenytoin levels may help clarify the situation when necessary. Some drugs that increase phenytoin levels are alcohol (when acutely ingested), benzodiazepines, phenothiazines, salicylates, and methylphenidate. Some drugs that decrease phenytoin levels are carbamazepine, alcohol (with chronic abuse), and molindone.

Interactions of phenytoin and phenobarbital, valproic acid, and sodium valproate are unpredictable, and serum levels of the drugs involved may either increase or decrease.

Use of Phenytoin in Child and Adolescent Psychiatry

Reports of Interest. Three double-blind, placebo-controlled studies that treated children and adolescents with phenytoin (diphenylhydantoin) reported that it was not significantly better than placebo.

Lefkowitz (1969) reviewed some of the earlier literature in which phenytoin was administered, primarily on an open basis, to nonepileptic children with psychiatric disorders with discrepant results. Lefkowitz compared the efficacy of placebo and phenytoin in treating disruptive behavior in male juvenile delinquents (mean age, 14 years, 11 months; range, 13 years to 16 years, 3 months) in a residential treatment center. Each group contained 25 subjects. Phenytoin or placebo was administered in doses of 100 mg twice daily for 76 days. Both groups showed marked reductions in disruptive behavior. Phenytoin, however, was not significantly better than placebo on any of the 11 behavioral measures. In fact, placebo was significantly more efficacious than phenytoin in diminishing distress, unhappiness, negativism, and aggressiveness. The author suggested that mild toxic effects of phenytoin, such as insomnia, irritability, quarrelsomeness, ataxia, and gastric distress, may have accounted for the superiority of placebo.

Looker and Conners (1970) administered phenytoin to 17 children and adolescents (mean age, 9.1 years; range, 5.5 years to 14.5 years) who had severe temper tantrums and suspected minimal brain dysfunction. Eleven subjects had normal EEGs, three had mildly abnormal EEGs, and three had abnormal EEGs, but no subject had clinical seizures. Subjects were placed on a 9-week, double-blind, placebo-controlled, crossover protocol, and phenytoin was titrated to achieve blood levels of at least 10 µg/mL. Twelve of the 13 subjects who had final blood levels determined had adequate levels to suppress epileptic discharge. Scores on the Continuous Performance Test, the Porteus Maze Test, parent questionnaires for all subjects, and school questionnaires for 11 subjects showed no statistically significant differences between phenytoin and placebo. The authors noted, however, that some individual subjects appeared to respond positively and rather dramatically to phenytoin.

Conners et al. (1971) treated 43 particularly aggressive or disturbed delinquent males (mean age, 12 years; range, 9 to 14 years) living in a residential training school with phenytoin (200 mg/day), methylphenidate (20 mg/day), or placebo administered for 2 weeks in a double-blind protocol. Although the authors noted some limitations in their study, they found no significant difference between drugs and placebo on ratings by cottage parents, teachers, clinicians, and scores on the Rosenzweig Picture Frustration Test and Porteus Maze Test.

Overall, although there are individual patients without seizure disorder who appear to benefit from phenytoin, as yet there is no convincing evidence from double-blind placebo-controlled studies attesting to the effectiveness of phenytoin prescribed for psychiatric symptoms.

Gabapentin (Neurontin)

Gabapentin is an anticonvulsant whose mechanism of action is unknown. Gabapentin is indicated as adjunctive therapy in the treatment of partial seizures with and without secondary generalization in adults with epilepsy.

Pharmacokinetics of Gabapentin

Gabapentin is not significantly metabolized in humans. It is eliminated unchanged by renal secretion, which is directly proportional to creatinine clearance. Half-life is 5 to 7 hours, and food has no effect on its absorption or excretion. Bioavailability of gabapentin decreases with dose, with a greater percentage of lower doses being available; at doses of approximately 600 mg/day and higher, it stabilizes at approximately 60% of the dose being available.

Contraindications for the Administration of Gabapentin

Gabapentin is contraindicated for patients with known hypersensitivity to the drug.

Interactions of Gabapentin with Other Drugs

There are no significant interactions of gabapentin with other commonly used antiepileptic drugs.

Untoward Effects of Gabapentin

The most common untoward effects reported somnolence, dizziness, ataxia, fatigue, and nystagmus. Many other effects have been reported.

Indications for Gabapentin in Child and Adolescent Psychiatry

Gabapentin is approved only for the treatment of partial seizures and Postherpetic Neuralgia and it is not approved for any psychiatric indication at this time. The manufacturer notes that it is not necessary to monitor serum levels to optimize therapy (PDR, 2006).

- *Gabapentin Dosage Schedule*: Because of its short serum half-life, gabapentin should be given three times daily, with the time interval between any two doses no longer than 12 hours.
- *Children < 3 years of age*: Not recommended. Safety and efficacy have not been evaluated in this age-group.
- *Children 3 years through 12 years of age*: A starting dose of of 10 to 15 mg/kg/day in three divided doses is recommended. This should be titrated over approximately 3 days to a recommended effective dose of 40 mg/kg/day for 3- and 4-year-old patients and between 25 and 35 mg/kg/day for patients 5 years of age or older.
- *Adolescents > 12 years of age and adults*: An initial daily dose of 900 mg (300 mg t.i.d.) is recommended. The usual effective dose is between 900 and 1,800 mg/day. Based on clinical response the dose may be titrated upward to 2,400 mg/day. Higher doses have been tolerated by some patients with epilepsy.

Gabapentin Dose Forms Available

- Capsules: 100 mg, 300 mg, 400 mg
- Tablets (scored): 600 mg, 800 mg
- Oral Solution: 250 mg/5 mL dispensed in 470 mL bottles.

Lamotrigine (Lamictal)

Note: The FDA has directed that a Black Box Warning be added to the labeling of lamotrigine indicating that serious rashes requiring hospitalization and discontinuation of treatment have been reported in association with the use of lamotrigine. The incidence of these rashes which have included Stevens-Johnson Syndrome, is approximately 8/1,000 (0.8%) in patients less than 16 years old receiving lamotrigine as adjunctive therapy for epilepsy... because the rate of serious rash is greater in pediatric patients than in adults, it bears emphasis that lamictal is approved only for use in pediatric patients below the age of 16 years who have seizures associated with the Lennox-Gastaut syndrome or in patients with partial seizures. [This is a summary; see the package insert or current PDR for the complete warning.]

Lamotrigine is an antiepileptic drug of the phenyltriazine class and is chemically unrelated to antiepileptic drugs currently in use. Its mechanism of action is unknown. Lamotrigine is approved for use in the adjunctive treatment of partial seizures and in the adjunctive treatment of the generalized seizures of Lennox-Gastaut syndrome in patients ≥ 2 years old. Lamotrigine is also approved for use in adult patients diagnosed with partial seizures who are being treated with a single hepatic enzyme-inducing antiepileptic drug (EIAED; e.g., carbamazepine, phenytoin, phenobarbital, primidone, or valproate) to convert them to monotherapy with lamotrigine. Lamotrigine has also been approved for the maintenance treatment of bipolar I disorder to decrease the frequency of mood episodes (depression, amnia, hypomania, mixed episodes) in patients at least 18 years old who are being treated for acute mood episode with standard therapy. Lamotrigine has not been proved effective in treating acute mood episodes.

Safety and efficacy in patients under 16 years of age (except for Lennox-Gastaut syndrome) have not been established. A boxed warning notes that serious rashes, including Stevens-Johnson syndrome, requiring hospitalization and discontinuation of lamotrigine occur in approximately 8/1,000 (0.8%) of patients under 16 years of age. Because the rate of serious rash is greater in pediatric patients than in adults (approximately threefold greater), it bears emphasis that due to the preceding considerations, currently lamotrigine cannot be recommended for use in child and adolescent psychiatry, although its use as an adjunctive mood stabilizer is being explored.

Indications for Lamotrigine in Child and Adolescent Psychiatry:

Lamotrigine is approved for use in patients aged ≥ 2 years old who have seizures associated with the Lennox-Gastaut syndrome or as an adjunctive therapy for partial seizures

Lamotrigine Dosage Schedule:

Treatment of Lennox-Gastaut syndrome or as adjunctive therapy for partial seizures.

Children < 2 years old: Not recommended. See boxed warning!

Children ≥ 2 years old, adolescents and adults: The initial, titration, and target doses for lamotrigine vary considerably according to age and which other medications the patient is taking for treatment of the seizure disorder. The package insert or current PDR should be consulted for the appropriate medication protocol.

Maintenance Treatment of Bipolar Disorder

- *Children and adolescents < 16 years of age:* Not recommended. Safety and efficacy have not been evaluated in this age-group. [See boxed warning, in the preceding text]
- *Adolescents ≥ 16 years of age and adults:* The initial, titration, and target doses for lamotrigine vary considerably according to which other medications the patient is taking for treatment of the acute episode. The package insert or current PDR should be consulted for the appropriate medication protocol.

(continued)

Indications for Lamotrigine in Child and Adolescent Psychiatry: *(Continued)*

Lamotrigine Dose Forms Available

- Tablets (scored): 25 mg, 100 mg, 150 mg, 200 mg

    Chewable Dispersible Tablets: 2 mg, 5 mg, 25 mg

Oxcarbazepine (Trileptal)

Oxcarbazepine is an antiepileptic drug; pharmacologic activity is exerted primarily through its 10-monohydroxy metabolite (MHD). Its mechanism of action is unknown; however, *in vitro* studies have indicated that oxcarbazepine and MHD produce blockade of voltage-sensitive sodium channels resulting in stabilization of hyperexcited neural membranes.

Pharmacokinetics of Oxcarbazepine

Oxcarbazepine taken orally is completely absorbed and extensively metabolized to MHD. The half-life of oxcarbazepine is approximately 2 hours and the half-life of MHD is approximately 9 hours. Food does not appear to affect the bioavailability of either oxcarbazepine or MHD. The median peak plasma level is 4.5 hours (range, 3 to 13 hours) for film-coated tablets and 6 hours for the oral suspension preparation; both preparations have similar bioavailability. Steady-state plasma concentrations are achieved in 2 to 3 days when a given dose is administered twice daily. Clearance of oxcarbazepine and its metabolites is primarily (over 95%) through the kidneys. Clearance in children under 8 years of age is 30% to 40% greater than in older children and adults, and in a controlled clinical trial such patients had the highest maintenance doses.

Contraindications for the Administration of Oxcarbazepine

Hypersensitivitity to oxcarbazepine or its components is a contraindication to the administration of oxcarbazepine. Approximately 25% to 30% of patients who had hypersensitivity reactions to carbamazepine are likely to do so with oxcarbazepine, hence they should be asked about any such prior exposure.

Interactions of Oxcarbazepine with Other Drugs

Oxcarbazepine can inhibit CYP2C19 and induce CYP3A4 and CYP3A5, which can potentially significantly effect plasma concentrations of other drugs. Drugs that induce cytochrome P450, including some other antiepileptic drugs, can result in decreases in plasma levels of oxcarbazepine and MHD. Plasma levels of phenytoin increased by up to 40% when oxcarbazepine was give in doses > 1,200 mg/day, however, phenobarbital levels increased by only 15%. Carbamazepine, phenytoin, and phenobarbital, which are all strong inducers of cytochrome P450 enzymes decreased the plasma level of MHD by 29% to 40%.

Coadministration of oxcarbazepine with an oral hormonal contraceptive decreased plasma concentrations of ethinylestradiol and levonorgestrel, which may decrease the effectiveness of the contraceptive.

Untoward Effects of Oxcarbazepine

The most common untoward effects reported in pediatric patients being treated for a partial seizure disorder include: fatigue, vomiting, nausea, headache, somnolence, dizziness, ataxia, nystagmus, diplopia, vision abnormalities, and emotional liability. One manufacturer noted that approximately 9.2% (14) of 152 pediatric patients who were treated with oxcarbazepine but had not been treated previously with antiepileptic drugs discontinued the drug because of untoward effects. Although relatively infrequent as total untoward effects ($< 1\%$), "rash" was responsible for 5.3% (8) and "maculopapular rash" for 1.3% (2) of those discontinuing. In a second group of 456 pediatric patients who were being treated with oxcarbazepine as a monotherapy or adjunctive therapy and who had been previously treated with antiepileptic drugs, 11% (50) discontinued the drug because of untoward effects. Patients discontinued for the following reasons: somnolence 2.4% (11), vomiting 2.0% (9), ataxia 1.8% (8), diplopia 1.3% (6), dizziness 1.3% (6), fatigue 1.1% (5), and nystagmus 1.1% (5).

Oxcarbazepine has a reduced risk for leukopenia, rashes, drug interactions, and enzyme autoinduction compared with carbamazepine (see references sited by Teitelbaum, 2001).

Hyponatremia

Clinically significant hyponatremia (sodium < 125 mmol/L) may occur during treatment with oxcarbazepine. This usually occurs within 3 months of initiation of therapy but may also occur after over a year of treatment. In 14 studies with a total of 1,524 patients, 38 (2.5%) developed a sodium of < 125 mmol/L sometime during treatment compared with no patients on placebo or active control (other antiepileptic drugs). Symptoms that may reflect hyponatremia such as nausea, malaise, headache, lethargy, confusion, obtundation, or increase in seizure frequency or severity should be the cause for determining sodium plasma levels. Monitoring of sodium levels during treatment should be considered.

Indications for Oxcarbazepine in Child and Adolescent Psychiatry

Oxcarbazepine is indicated as monotherapy or adjunctive therapy in the treatment of partial seizures in children and adolescents 4 to 16 years old and adults.

Oxcarbazepine Dosage Schedule Initiation of Monotherapy

- Total daily dose should always be administered in two divided doses (b.i.d.) Children under 4 years of age: Not recommended. Safety and efficacy have not been evaluated in this age-group.
- Children 4 years of age through adolescents 16 years of age (not taking other antiepileptic drugs): An initial daily dose of 8 to 10 mg/kg given in two divided doses (b.i.d.) is recommended. The dose should be increased by 5 mg/kg every third day to reach the following target maintenance doses based on the patient's weight. 20 kg, 600 to 900 mg/day; 25 kg, 900 to 1,200 mg/day; 30 kg, 900 to 1,200 mg/day; 35 kg, 900 to 1,500 mg/day; 40 kg, 900 to 1,500 mg/day; 45 kg, 1,200 to 1,500 mg/day; 50 kg, 1,200 to 1,800 mg/day; 55 kg, 1,200 to 1,800 mg/day;

(continued)

Indications for Oxcarbazepine in Child and Adolescent Psychiatry (Continued)

60 kg, 1,200 to 2,100 mg/day; 65 kg, 1,200 to 2,100 mg/day and 70 kg, 1,500 to 2,100 mg/day.

Adolescents 17 years of age and above and adults (not taking other antiepileptic drugs): An initial dose of 300 mg twice daily (600 mg/day) is recommended. Dose may be increased by 300 mg/day every third day to a dose of 1,200 mg/day. Many patients are unable to tolerate doses of 2,400 mg/day.

For using oxcarbazepine as an adjunctive treatment for epilepsy or to convert patients being treated with other drugs to monotherapy with oxcarbazepine, see the package insert or the current PDR.

Oxcarbazepine Dose Forms Available

● Film-coated tablets: 150 mg, 300 mg, 600 mg

Oral suspension: 300 mg/5 mL (store in original container; shake well before using) The oral suspension preparation and film-coated tablets are interchangeable at equal doses.

Reports of Interest

Teitelbaum (2001) reported that a 6-year-old female diagnosed with bipolar I disorder who had been hospitalized four times in the preceding year for out-of-control behavior with extreme aggression toward others and destruction of property and who did not have an adequate clinical response to trials with lithium, lamotrigine (some benefit but discontinued because of rash), valproate, gabapentin, clonidine, guanfacine, risperidone, olanzepine, quetiapine, fluoxetine, and methylphenidate (worsened symptoms), improved significantly when oxcarbazepine was added to her medication regime of 3 months, which consisted of lithium carbonate 150 mg three times daily (0.7 mEq/L serum level) and guanfacine 0.5 mg three times daily. Oxcarbazepine was added to these medications at an initial dose at 150 mg twice daily with full mood stabilization after 6 weeks. Three months after the initiation of oxcarbazepine, the lithium dose was decreased to 150 mg twice daily; good control continued to be maintained for 7 months. The author noted that the girl experienced some transient mild exacerbation of symptoms during a school vacation and again during a viral illness, but was being maintained on lithium 150 mg twice daily; guanfacine 0.5 mg twice daily and oxcarbazepine 150 mg twice daily (Teitelbaum, 2001).

Staller et al. (2005) conducted a retrospective chart review of 14 outpatients (age range, 6 to 17 years; 6 males and 8 females) to whom oxcarbazepine was prescribed to address their moderate-to-severe problems with anger, irritability, and aggression but many subjects had additional symptoms including depression, mania, anxiety, disruptiveness, oppositionality, and psychosis. Subjects were rated as moderately ill (6), markedly ill (7); and severely ill (1) on the Clinical Global Impressions-Severity scale. Subjects' Axis I diagnoses, including multiple diagnoses in 11, included bipolar disorder (5); other mood disorders (3); ADHD (4); disruptive behavior disorder (3); and PDD spectrum disorders (2). Ten (71.4%) of the subjects had failed to respond adequately to prior drug trials. During treatment with oxcarbazepine, three subjects received oxcarbazepine only; three subjects were already receiving one additional medication; and seven subjects were receiving two additional medications and one subject was receiving three additional medications; the medications included atypical antipsychotics (7); SSRIs (4); stimulants (2), alpha agonists (2) antihistamines (2) beta blocker (1) and valproate (1). The average daily dose of oxcarbazepine was 878 mg with a range from 600 to 1,800 mg/day. Duration on oxcarbazepine averaged 9.8 months with a range of 0.5 to 30 months. Clinical improvement was rated on the CGI-I scale. The ratings were "much improved" in seven subjects; "minimally improved" in two and unchanged in five. AEs including dizziness, muscle aches, and tremors resulted in discontinuation in two (14%) of the subjects, but they were not considered to be serious AEs.

Topiramate (Topamax)

Topiramate, an antiepileptic drug, is a sulfamate-substituted monosacharide. The mechanisms responsible for its antiepileptic and migraine prophylaxis effects have not been elucidated; however, preclinicial studies suggest that at clinically effective concentrations, topiramate blocks voltage-dependent sodium channels, augments the activity of the neurotransmitter gamma-aminobutyrate at some subtypes of the GABA-A receptor, antagonizes the AMPA/kainate subtype of the glutamate receptor, and inhibits the carbonic anhydrase enzyme, particularly isoenzymes II and IV (package insert).

Pharmacokinetics of Topiramate

The bioavailability of topiramate is not affected by food. Peak plasma concentrations occur in approximately 2 hours. Mean plasma elimination half-life is 21 hours after single or multiple doses and steady state occurs in approximately 4 days at a given dose. Topiramate is not extensively metabolized and approximately 70% is eliminated unchanged through the kidneys. Pediatric patients, aged 4 to 17 years, have approximately a 50% higher clearance than adults. Consequently such patients have a shorter elimination half-life than adults and their plasma concentration of topiramate may be lower than that of adults receiving the same dose.

Contraindications for the Administration of Topiramate

Topiramate is contraindicated in patients with a history of sensitivity to topiramate or any of the components included in the pill. Clearance may be significantly reduced in patients with renal or hepatic impairment.

Interactions of Topiramate with Other Drugs

Hyperammonemia with or without encephalopathy has been associated with the combined use of topiramate and valproic acid in patients who have not developed these symptoms when treated with either drug alone. Patients who develop symptoms such as acute alterations in the level of consciousness or cognitive functioning in combination with lethargy or vomiting, which may be associated with hyperammonemic encephalopathy should have their serum ammonia levels determined.

Topiramate can decrease the AUC and maximum serum concentration of Lithium by up to 20%.

Many other drug interactions are possible; see package insert.

Untoward Effects of Topiramate

Topiramate is associated with metabolic acidosis, which if chronic and untreated may cause osteomalacia/rickets and may reduce growth rate and maximal stature in pediatric patients. Treatment-emergent adverse events in children in the age-group 10 through 16 years who were being treated with monotherapy (400 mg/day) for epilepsy that occurred with an incidence of at least 5% and which were more frequent than those at lower doses (50 mg/day) included: fever (9%), paresthesias (16%), diarrhea (11%), weight loss (21%), anorexia (14%), mood problems (11%), difficulty with concentration/attention (9%), and alopecia (5%).

Indications for Topiramate in Child and Adolescent Psychiatry:

Topiramate is approved for use as a monotherapy treatment in patients ≥ 10 years of age with partial onset or primary generalized tonic-clonic seizures; as an adjunctive therapy in patients ≥ 2 years of age with partial onset seizures, primary generalized tonic-clonic seizures, or seizures associated with Lennox-Gestaut syndrome; and for the prophylaxis of migraine headache in adults.

Topiramate Dosage Schedule for monotherapy:

Children < 10 years of age: Not recommended.

Children ≥ 10 years of age, adolescents, and adults: An initial dose of 25 mg, twice daily is recommended. Dose should be increased as tolerated by 50 mg weekly to reach a recommended target dose of 200 mg, twice daily (total dose, 400 mg/day).

Topiramate Dosage Schedule for prophylaxis of migraine headache:

Children and Adolescents < 18 years of age: Not recommended

Adolescents ≥ 18 years of age and adults: An initial evening dose of 25 mg is recommended. Dose should be increased as tolerated by 25 mg weekly (week 2, 25 mg b.i.d., week 3, 25 mg in the morning and 50 mg in the evening to a recommended target dose of 50 mg b.i.d. during week 4 (total dose, 100 mg/day).

For dosage schedule for use of topiramate as an adjunct in treating partial onset seizures, primary generalized tonic-clonic seizures or Lennox-Gastaut syndrome see package insert.

Topiramate Dose Forms Available

Tablets: 25 mg, 50 mg, 100 mg, 200 mg,

Sprinkle capsules: 15 mg, 25 mg sprinkle capsules may be swallowed whole or opened and put on a small amount of soft food, which should be swallowed without chewing immediately and not stored for future use.

Report of Interest

DelBello et al. (2005) reported a 4-week, multicenter, randomized, double-blind, placebo-controlled, parallel group trial of topiramate in treating mania in 56 children and adolescent means age 13.8 ± 2.56 years, age range 6 to 17 years, who were diagnosed with bipolar disorder type I; 33 subjects (58.9%) had codiagnoses of ADHD. The primary outcome measure of efficacy was the Young Mania Rating Scale (YMRS) scores at baseline and 4, 7, 14, 21, and 28 days of treatment. Secondary outcome measures included baseline and weekly scores on the Clinical

Global Impressions-Improvement Scale (CGI-I), the Brief Psychiatric Rating Scale for Children (BPRS-C), the Children's Global Assessment Scale (C-GAS) and the Childrens' Depression Rating Scale (CDRS).

Although the study was designed to enroll approximately 230 subjects, only 56 were enrolled; 29 subjects were assigned to topiramate and 27 to placebo. This was because a study of topiramate in adult subjects hospitalized with acute mania showed no benefit of topiramate over placebo and hence it was thought topiramate would be unlikely to benefit younger subjects and that it was not ethical to continue and the study was stopped at that time. Because of this, the study was inconclusive as it was not adequately powered to detect treatment differences. The baseline YMRS score for the topiramate group was 31.7 ± 5.53 and it was decreased by -9.7 ± 9.65 at endpoint. The baseline YMRS score for the placebo group was 29.9 ± 6.01 and it was decrease by -4.7 ± 9.79 at endpoint, less than one-half the improvement seen in the topiramate group. However, there was no significant group difference at any visit for the change in YMRS score, the total BPRS-C score, total CDRS score, or CGAS score.

Treatment-emergent adverse events occurring in > 10% of subjects and greater for topiramate than for placebo included decreased appetite (27.6% vs. 0%), nausea (24.1% vs. 0%), diarrhea (13.8% vs. 7.4%), paresthesia (13.8% vs. 3.7%), somnolence (13.8% vs. 3.7%), insomnia (10.3% vs. 3.7%) and rash (10.3% vs. 3.7%). Mean change in body weight from baseline to endpoint was significantly different, with the topiramate group losing a mean of -1.76 ± 2.03 kg and the placebo group gaining a mean of 0.95 ± 1.45 kg ($P < .001$). No subject experienced a serious adverse event. The authors noted that this study suggests that topiramate may be effective in treating bipolar disorder type I in children and adolescents, although it was not so in adults, and that adequately powered, controlled studies in this age-group are needed to determine whether this is the case.

CHAPTER 9

Antianxiety Drugs

BENZODIAZEPINES

Benzodiazepines, introduced into clinical practice in the early 1960s, were the most frequently prescribed drugs in the United States for the 12 years before 1980. In 1978 alone, 68 million prescriptions for benzodiazepines were written for approximately 10 million individuals; more than half of these were for diazepam (Ayd, 1980). Greenblatt et al. (1983) noted that by 1980 the trend toward the increasing use of benzodiazepines had reversed, perhaps subsequent to publicity about abuse of and addiction to the benzodiazepines. The abuse and addiction potential of the benzodiazepines continue to be of concern, and in 1989 New York State began requiring all prescriptions for benzodiazepines to be written on triplicate forms, as for other controlled drugs. It should be noted, however, that many experts think that compared with other drugs of abuse the dangers of benzodiazepines have been "greatly exaggerated" (Simeon and Ferguson, 1985). The American Psychiatric Association (APA) Task Force on Benzodiazepines in a summary statement noted that "overall, the APA Task Force found that benzodiazepines, when prescribed appropriately, are therapeutic drugs with relatively mild toxic profiles and low tendency for abuse" (Salzman, 1990, p. 62). Benzodiazepines are poor self-reinforcers of use and tend to be taken alone for pleasure rarely. An exception to this occurs among substance abusers. Benzodiazepine abuse is very frequent among alcoholics; cocaine, narcotic, and methadone abusers frequently abuse benzodiazepines as well. These groups use benzodiazepines to "augment the euphoria (narcotics and methadone users), to decrease anxiety and withdrawal symptoms (alcoholics), or to ease the 'crash' from cocaine-induced euphoria" (Salzman, 1990, p. 62).

Surprisingly little is known about the use of benzodiazepines in child and adolescent psychiatric disorders. In their important 1974 monograph, Greenblatt and Shader, after reviewing the use of benzodiazepines in children and adolescents, stated, "At present it is doubtful that the benzodiazepines have a role in the pharmacotherapy of psychoses or in the treatment of emotional disorders in children" (p. 88).

Werry concluded that if pharmacotherapy is necessary for certain childhood sleep disturbances, including insomnia, night waking, night terrors, and somnambulism, "probably" benzodiazepines are indicated and that they are "possibly" indicated for some kinds of anxiety (Rapoport et al. 1978b).

In 1983, Coffey et al. reported that benzodiazepines appeared to be prescribed to both older adolescents and adults for relief of anxiety and tension, muscle relaxation, sleep disorders, and seizures. In children, however, they were used primarily for treatment of sleep and seizure disorders and were used much less commonly for their anxiolytic and muscle-relaxant qualities.

The literature concerning their use in children has been reviewed by Campbell et al. (1985) and by Simeon and Ferguson (1985). Most published reports in the literature appeared in the 1960s and were open studies. Many of the studies comprised diagnostically heterogeneous subjects; results were discrepant. Diazepam and chlordiazepoxide were the drugs most frequently employed.

Currently, the psychiatric conditions occurring in childhood for which there is the most convincing rationale for the use of a benzodiazepine as the drug of choice are sleep terror disorder (pavor nocturnus) and sleepwalking disorder (somnambulism); however, these conditions are not usually treated with pharmacotherapy unless they are unusually frequent or severe. Both sleep terror disorder and sleepwalking disorder usually occur "during the first third of the major sleep period (the interval of nonrapid eye movement [NREM] sleep that typically contains EEG delta activity, sleep stages 3 and 4)" (APA, 1987, pp. 310–311). Because benzodiazepines decrease stage 4 sleep, they theoretically might be of therapeutic value in these conditions. Conversely, benzodiazepines are theoretically contraindicated in treating sleep disturbance in psychosocial dwarfism (psychosocially determined short stature) because they would further compromise nocturnal secretion of growth hormone, which occurs maximally during sleep stages 3 and 4, slow-wave sleep (Green, 1986). Reite et al. (1990) suggested that either 2 mg of diazepam or 0.125 mg of triazolam at bedtime may decrease the frequency of night terrors or somnambulism in children with severe cases.

Coffey et al. (1983) have emphasized that the infant has an immature liver and that the newborn's capacity for hydroxylation, demethylation, and especially glucuronide conjugation is limited until approximately 5 months of age, when the necessary liver enzymes reach and begin to exceed adult capacities. During childhood and until pubescence, enzyme activity levels may exceed those of adults, causing the rate of metabolism to exceed that in adults and necessitating more frequent administration of benzodiazepines than in adolescents and adults (Coffey et al. 1983).

If a benzodiazepine is used as a hypnotic, consideration of the serum half-life of the drug is important. For example, flurazepam (Dalmane), temazepam (Restoril), and triazolam (Halcion) are used for treating sleep disorders. Flurazepam is a long-acting benzodiazepine with a half-life (for it and its metabolites) of 47 to 100 hours. The manufacturer notes that this pharmacokinetic profile may explain the clinical observation that flurazepam is increasingly effective on the second or third night of use and, similarly, that after discontinuing the drug, both sleep latency and total wake time may still be decreased. Hence flurazepam appears to be most useful in persons with both significant daytime anxiety and insomnia. In contrast, temazepam and triazolam, also effective hypnotics, are short-acting benzodiazepines with a relatively rapid onset of action and half-lives of 9.5 to 12.4 hours (temazepam) and of 1.5 to 5.5 hours (triazolam). These data suggest that triazolam is the drug of choice for sleep-onset insomnia and is preferable in terms of reduced risk of any unwanted daytime sedation. The manufacturer of triazolam reports that all benzodiazepines used to induce sleep can cause an anterior-grade amnesia, in which the person may not recall events occurring for several hours after taking the drug. Triazolam is more likely than other benzodiazepines to cause such amnesia if a person is awakened before the drug has been metabolized sufficiently and/or excreted to eliminate the effect. Because many travelers, especially on long flights, may take medication to induce sleep and subsequently are awakened before the effects of the drug wear off, this phenomenon has commonly been called "traveler's amnesia." Triazolam should not be used in such situations. Also, because of triazolam's short half-life there can be a withdrawal effect, resulting in increased wakefulness during the last third of the night and subsequent increased daytime anxiety or nervousness.

Wysowski and Barash (1991) compared postmarketing adverse behavioral reactions of triazolam and temazepam reported through the FDA's spontaneous reporting system. Triazolam was associated with significantly more frequent reports of confusion than temazepam (133 vs. 2), of amnesia (109 vs. 3), of bizarre behavior (59 vs. 2), of agitation (58 vs. 4), and of hallucinations (40 vs. 1). Overall, the incidence was quite small because, during the period of comparison, 13.5 million prescriptions were written for triazolam and 19.1 million prescriptions were written for temazepam. The authors noted that adverse reactions to triazolam tended to occur at higher doses (0.25 mg and higher) and in the elderly.

Klein et al. (1980) suggested that a supplemental low dose of a benzodiazepine (e.g., diazepam 5 mg) might be useful in treating residual anticipatory anxiety in school-phobic youngsters whose separation anxiety had been alleviated by treatment with imipramine.

Simeon and Ferguson (1985) reported that some overly inhibited children may show lasting behavioral improvement following a brief (not exceeding 4 to 6 weeks) treatment with a benzodiazepine. They attributed the improvement to an interaction between disinhibition facilitated by the medication and social learning. Consistent with this finding, they noted that children and adolescents with impulsivity and aggression who were under significant environmental stress should not be treated with benzodiazepines because the disinhibition could result in the worsening of behavior (Simeon and Ferguson, 1985).

Most of the literature suggests that benzodiazepines usually worsen symptoms in psychotic children. In studies comparing dextroamphetamine, placebo, and chlordiazepoxide or diazepam in treating hyperactive children, chlordiazepoxide and diazepam were both less effective than dextroamphetamine, and placebo was rated better than diazepam (Zrull et al. 1963, 1964).

Contraindications for Benzodiazepine Administration

Known hypersensitivity to benzodiazepines and acute narrow-angle glaucoma are usually considered absolute contraindications.

Persons predisposed to substance abuse or alcoholism should be prescribed benzodiazepines with caution because they may cause physical and psychological dependence and interact additively with sedative or hypnotic drugs.

Adolescents who are likely to become pregnant or who are known to be pregnant should rarely, if ever, be prescribed benzodiazepines, because there are suggestions of increased risk for congenital malformations. Also, maternal abuse of benzodiazepines may cause a withdrawal syndrome in the newborn (Rall, 1990). Simeon and Ferguson (1985) concluded that benzodiazepines are relatively contraindicated in children and adolescents with significant impulsivity, aggressiveness, and environmental stress as negative disinhibiting drug effects may occur.

Interactions of Benzodiazepines with Other Drugs

The most clinically important drug interactions of the benzodiazepines are associated with additive effects when combined with other sedative or hypnotic drugs, including alcohol (ethanol). Phenothiazines, narcotics, barbiturates, monoamine oxidase inhibitors (MAOIs), tricyclic antidepressants, and cimetidine (Tagamet) have been reported to potentiate benzodiazepines. The rate of absorption of benzodiazepines and the resulting central nervous system depression are both increased by ethanol (Rall, 1990). Benzodiazepines are relatively safe drugs, and even large overdoses are infrequently fatal unless taken in combination with other drugs (Rall, 1990).

Flumazenil (Romazicon) is a benzodiazepine receptor antagonist that is specific for the reversal of the sedative effects of benzodiazepines; however, it does not reverse hypoventilation or respiratory suppression caused by benzodiazepines. The manufacturer does not recommend its use in children because no clinical studies have been done in this age group to determine risks, benefits, or dosage. In cases of overdose in adolescents and adults, flumazenil is administered intravenously in doses of 0.2 mg (2 mL) over a 30-second period. If the desired level of consciousness is not obtained, a second dose of 0.3 mg may be administered over 30 seconds, and additional doses of 0.5 mg over 30 seconds at 1-minute intervals to a maximum of 3 mg. Only rarely do patients benefit from higher doses. Resedation may occur because flumazenil has a relatively short half-life compared with many benzodiazepines; in such cases additional flumazenil may be administered. Risk of precipitating seizures is of particular concern in patients who have been administered benzodiazepines on a long-term basis or in patients who show evidence of concomitant tricyclic antidepressant overdose.

Untoward Effects of Benzodiazepines

The most common untoward effects of benzodiazepines are manifestations of their being central nervous system depressants: oversedation, fatigue, drowsiness, ataxia, and confusion progressing to coma may occur at high doses. When anxiety is the target symptom, benzodiazepines should be administered in divided doses to minimize sedation.

"Paradoxical reactions," episodes of marked dyscontrol and disinhibition, have been reported in children and adolescents. Symptoms have included acute excitation, increased anxiety, increased aggression and hostility, rage reactions, loss of all control and "going wild," hallucinations, insomnia, and nightmares.

Use of Benzodiazepines in Child and Adolescent Psychiatry

In general psychiatry, the benzodiazepines are indicated in the management of anxiety disorders or for the short-term relief of symptoms of anxiety and the short-term treatment of some sleep disorders. They are also used to treat acute symptoms of alcohol withdrawal. Several manufacturers note that they are not usually indicated for anxiety or tension associated with the everyday stresses of life. The effectiveness of benzodiazepines in treatment lasting > 4 months has not been assessed by systematic clinical studies.

TABLE 9.1 ● **Some Representative Benzodiazepines**

Benzodiazepine (Trade Name) (Estimated Serum Half-life)	Minimum Age Approved for Any Use	Usual Daily Dosage
Alprazolam (Xanax) (12–15 h)	18 y	See text
Chlordiazepoxide (Librium) (24–48 h)	6 y	5 mg 2–4 times/d, maximum 30 mg/d
Clonazepam (Klonopin) (18–50 h)	Not specified	See text
Clorazepate (Tranxene) (approximately 48 h)	9 y	For children 9–12 y old, maximum initial dose of 7.5 mg twice daily. Maximum weekly increase, 7.5 mg. Maximum total dose, 60 mg
Diazepam (Valium) (30–60 h)	6 mo	0.1–0.3 mg/kg/d for infants and young children. 1–2.5 mg 3–4 times/d for older children and adolescents; titrate as needed and tolerated
Estazolam (ProSom) (10–24 h)	18 y	1–2 mg at bedtime
Flurazepam (Dalmane) (47–100 h)	15 y	15–30 mg at bedtime
Lorazepam (Ativan) (12–18 h)	12 y	1–6 mg/d
Oxazepam (Serax) (5.7–10.9 h)	6 y	Not established for children 6–12 y old; adolescents usual dose is 10 mg 3 times daily to maximum of 30 mg 4 times daily
Quazepam (Doral) (73 h)	18 y	7.5–15 mg at bedtime
Temazepam (Restoril) (9.5–12.4 h)	18 y	15–30 mg at bedtime
Triazolam (Halcion) (1.5–5.5 h)	18 y	0.125–0.25 mg at bedtime. See text also

Currently, there are no specific clinical guidelines for treating any of the childhood psychiatric disorders with benzodiazepines. If used, manufacturers' clinical recommendations for children should not be exceeded. Table 9.1 gives usual daily dosages for some representative benzodiazepines, an estimate of the serum half-life of the parent compound and/or its significant active metabolites, the youngest age for which the FDA has approved their use for any purpose, and, when available, suggested dosages for their use in child and adolescent psychiatric disorders.

The need for benzodiazepines should be reassessed frequently, and they should be discontinued within a relatively short period, usually within a few weeks.

Because of the relative paucity of information available on the use of benzodiazepines in children and young adolescents, most of the available studies are reviewed in the following discussion, although many are older, uncontrolled studies or case reports.

Chlordiazepoxide (Librium)

Reports of Interest

Chlordiazepoxide in the Treatment of Behaviorally Disordered Children and Adolescents of Various Diagnoses

Krakowski (1963) treated 51 emotionally disturbed children and adolescents 4 to 16 years of age with chlordiazepoxide. Criteria for inclusion were the presence of anxiety (especially with coexisting hyperactivity), irritability, hostility, impulsivity, and insomnia. Nine children had concurrent individual therapy, and seven received other medications, mainly antiepileptics. Chlordiazepoxide was administered initially in divided doses totaling 15 mg, and individually titrated. Maintenance dosage for periods of up to 10 months ranged from 15 to 40 mg/day (mean, 26 mg/day). Twelve patients (23.5%) showed complete remission of psychiatric symptoms, and 22 (43.1%) improved moderately. Children with adjustment disorders were particularly likely to improve; specifically, 11 of 18 with conduct disorders, 2 of 3 with habit disturbances, and all 4 with neurotic traits showed marked or moderate remission of symptoms. Of 12 mentally deficient patients, 3 improved moderately and 3 improved markedly. Untoward effects were relatively infrequent and included drowsiness, fatigue, muscular weakness, ataxia, anxiety, and depression. These effects were alleviated to a satisfactory degree by dosage reduction in all but one case.

Kraft et al. (1965) prescribed chlordiazepoxide to 130 patients (99 males, 31 females) who ranged in age from 2 to 17 years (112 were between 7 and 14 years of age). The most common diagnoses were primary behavior disorder (50), school phobia (18), adjustment reaction of adolescence (17), and chronic brain damage (14). Most subjects had marked hyperactivity and neurotic traits. Dosage ranged from 20 to 130 mg/day and was administered in divided doses; 94 subjects (72%) received 40 mg or more daily. Moderate or marked improvement occurred in 53 subjects (40.8%). Forty subjects (30.8%) had either no or insignificant improvement, and 37 (28.5%) worsened. The diagnostic group showing the greatest improvement was school phobia (77%). Only 38% of the primary behavior disorder subjects and 41.2% of the adolescent adjustment disorder subjects improved to a moderate or marked degree. Of those with organic brain damage, 50% worsened, 28.6% showed minimal or no benefit, and none had an excellent response. Across diagnoses, symptoms of hyperactivity, fears, night terrors, enuresis, reading and speech problems, truancy, and disturbed or bizarre behavior were moderately or markedly improved in 40.8% of the 130 subjects. The authors concluded that chlordiazepoxide was effective in decreasing anxiety and "emotional overload" (Kraft et al. 1965). The authors also reported that 22 of the 130 had untoward effects of sufficient severity to interfere with treatment results and that 14 other subjects had milder untoward effects that were transient or responded to a lowering of the dose.

Breitner (1962) administered chlordiazepoxide, 20 to 50 mg/day, to more than 50 juvenile delinquents between 8.5 and 24 years of age. He reported that the drug produced cooperativeness, released tension, created a feeling of well-being, and made the subjects more accessible to psychotherapy.

D'Amato (1962) treated nine children 8 to 11 years of age, who were diagnosed with school phobia, with 10 to 30 mg/day of chlordiazepoxide for 5 to 30 days. The children were also seen in psychotherapy. Only one child did not attend school regularly after the second week of treatment. The author compared these nine children with 11 others, aged 5 years to 12 years, also diagnosed with school phobia, who were treated over the six preceding years with psychotherapy only. Only 2 of these 11 children returned to school within 2 weeks, and 9 remained out of school for 1 month or longer. The author thought that this strongly suggested that chlordiazepoxide was an effective adjunct to psychotherapy in mobilizing children with school phobia to return to school.

Petti et al. (1982) treated nine boys (7 to 11 years of age) with chlordiazepoxide who had failed to respond to 3 weeks of hospitalization and treatment with placebo. The subjects' diagnoses were conduct disorder (five, three of whom had borderline features), personality disorder (three, one of whom had borderline features), and schizophrenia (one). Verbal IQs on the Wechsler Intelligence Scale for Children (WISC) ranged from 71 to 110. Target symptoms were anxiety, depression, impulsivity, and explosiveness. The initial dose of chlordiazepoxide was 15 mg, administered in divided doses. The optimal dose was determined by individual titration and ranged from 15 to 120 mg/day (0.58 to 5.28 mg/kg/day). Children's ratings on optimal dose were compared with baseline ratings. Marked improvement was noted in two boys, improvement in four, and no change or worsening in three. The major improvements were increased verbal production, increased rapidity of thought associations, and a shift from blunted affect or depressed mood to a more animated appearance and feeling subjectively better. The authors noted that chlordiazepoxide had the most positive effect on children who were withdrawn, inhibited, anergic, depressed, or anxious. The child with schizophrenia had worsening of psychotic symptoms, and two children with severe impulsive aggressiveness had worsening of behavior; the authors suggest that chlordiazepoxide's use may be contraindicated in such children (Petti et al. 1982).

Diazepam (Valium)

Reports of Interest

Diazepam in the Treatment of Children and Adolescents with Various Psychiatric Diagnoses. Lucas and Pasley (1969), in one of the few double-blind, placebo-controlled studies of benzodiazepines in this age group, administered diazepam to 12 subjects, 7 to 17 years of age (mean, 12.3 years) who were diagnosed as psychoneurotic ($N = 10$) or with schizophrenia ($N = 2$). All subjects were inpatients or in a daycare program. Target symptoms included moderate to high anxiety levels, highly oppositional behavior, poor peer relationships, and aggression. The initial dose of diazepam was 2.5 mg twice daily. The drug was increased until a satisfactory therapeutic response or untoward effects occurred. The maximum dose achieved was 20 mg/day. The study lasted 16 weeks, during which subjects were assigned randomly to four different sequences of drug and placebo. Subjects were rated on 10 items: hyperactivity, anxiety and tension, oppositional behavior, aggressiveness, impulsivity, relationship to peers, relationship to adults, need for limit setting, response to limit setting, and participation in program. There was no significant difference between diazepam and placebo on any item for the nine patients who completed the study (the two patients with schizophrenia and one other patient dropped out). However, when scores on all 10 items were combined, diazepam scored significantly better than placebo ($P < .05$); although clinically the difference was not very apparent. Eleven of the 12 children participated in the study long enough to be rated on a global rating scale. Five subjects showed no change, two were somewhat more anxious, and four were definitely worse, with increased anxiety and deterioration in their behavior on diazepam compared with placebo. From this study and their clinical experience with diazepam, the authors concluded that diazepam was not clinically effective in reducing anxiety or acting-out behavior in children and young adolescents. Older adolescents appeared to react similar to adults, and diazepam was thought to be useful in treating their anxiety.

Diazepam in the Treatment of Enuresis. In a double-blind study, Kline (1968) administered diazepam or placebo to 50 children and adolescents (3 to 15 years of age) with nightly enuresis. Organic uropathy and mental retardation were exclusion criteria. Initially, 5 mg of diazepam was given in the morning and 10 mg at night. This was increased up to a total of 25 mg if no positive response occurred at a lower dosage. If the child had at most two wet nights weekly at time 4 weeks, he or she continued on the same condition for a total of 12 weeks, when the code was broken. If the subject had three or more wet nights nightly at time 4 weeks, diazepam was given on an open basis for weeks 5 through 12. After the code was broken, it was determined that at time 4 weeks the 28 children who were assigned to diazepam improved significantly more than those assigned to placebo ($P < .05$). Of the 28 children on the drug, 22 became dry, 2 were wet one or two nights per week, 3 continued to wet six or seven nights per week, and 1 worsened. Only 1 subject of the 22 on placebo became dry. The others were unchanged, except for one who worsened. Of 21 children on placebo at time 4 weeks who were doing poorly and were switched to known diazepam, 12 became dry (Kline, 1968).

Diazepam, with its relatively low toxicity, may be a useful alternative to tricyclic antidepressants in cases of enuresis in which pharmacologic intervention is clinically indicated.

Diazepam in the Treatment of Sleep Disorder. In an open study, three children with somnambulism and pavor nocturnus and four children with insomnia were treated with 2 to 5 mg of diazepam near bedtime; all seven responded favorably (Glick et al. 1971). However, no controlled study of benzodiazepines in these disorders has yet been published.

Alprazolam (Xanax)

Reports of Interest

Alprazolam in the Treatment of Pavor Nocturnus. Cameron and Thyer (1985) successfully treated a 10-year-old girl with severe nightly attacks of pavor nocturnus, with alprazolam. Initially, 0.5 mg of alprazolam was given at bedtime for 1 week; the dose was increased to 0.75 mg nightly for the next 4 weeks, and then the medication was tapered off. Attacks of night terrors ceased on the first night and had not recurred at follow-up 9 months later.

Alprazolam in the Treatment of Anxiety Disorders. Pfefferbaum et al. (1987) used alprazolam to treat anticipatory and acute situational anxiety and panic in 13 patients, aged 7 to 14 years, who were being treated for concomitant cancer. Treatment was initiated 3 days before and continued through the day of the stressful procedures. This study was conducted under an Investigational New Drug permit and the maximum dosage allowed was 0.02 mg/kg/dose or 0.06 mg/kg/day. The highest dosage reported was on a single child for whom the FDA granted permission to increase doses incrementally by 0.25 mg to a maximum of 0.05 mg/kg/dose or 0.15 mg/kg/day. Initial doses were 0.005 mg/kg or lower and were titrated upward based on efficacy while monitoring untoward effects. Total daily dose ranged from 0.375 to 3 mg (0.003 to 0.075 mg/kg/day). Subjects were rated on four scales measuring anxiety, distress, and panic. The subjects' improvement was statistically significant ($P < .05$) on three scales and reached borderline significance on the fourth scale. Untoward effects were minimal, mild drowsiness being the most frequently reported.

Simeon and Ferguson (1987) administered alprazolam openly to 12 children and adolescents (8.8 to 16.5 years of age; mean, 11.5 years) who were diagnosed with overanxious and/or avoidant disorder. After a 1-week placebo baseline period, to which none of the subjects responded, alprazolam was titrated individually over a 2-week period to maximum daily dosages ranging from 0.50 to 1.5 mg. The total period of active treatment with alprazolam was 4 weeks. Seven of the 12 showed at least moderate improvement on several rating scales; no child worsened. Ratings by clinicians showed significant improvement of anxiety, depression, and psychomotor excitation; parents reported significant improvement of anxiety and hyperactivity on questionnaires, and teachers reported significant improvement on an anxious–passive factor. Improvement in the subjects' sleep problems was frequently reported by parents. The few untoward effects were mild and transient. Ferguson and Simeon (1984) reported no adverse effects of alprazolam on cognition or learning at therapeutically effective doses.

Simeon and Ferguson (1987) also noted that the subjects who responded best to alprazolam and who continued on it improved after the drug was stopped had good premorbid personalities and prominent symptoms of inhibitions, shyness, and nervousness. Patients with poor premorbid personalities and poor family backgrounds tended to develop negative symptoms of disinhibition such as increased aggressiveness and impulsivity, especially at higher doses, and relapsed following drug withdrawal.

Simeon et al. (1992) reported a double-blind placebo-controlled study of alprazolam in 30 children and adolescents (23 males and 7 females; age range, 8.4 to 16.9 years; mean, 12.6 years) who had primary diagnoses of overanxious disorder ($N = 21$) or avoidant disorder ($N = 9$). Clinical impairment ranged from moderate to severe.

Placebo was administered for 1 week and was followed by random assignment to a 4-week period of either placebo or alprazolam. Medication was tapered with placebo substitution during the fifth week. During the sixth week all subjects received only placebo. Patients who weighed under 40 kg received an initial dose of 0.25 mg of alprazolam; heavier patients were given an initial dose of 0.5 mg of alprazolam. The maximum daily dosage permitted was 0.04 mg/kg. Medication was increased at 2-day intervals until optimal dose was achieved. At completion of the active drug phase, the average daily maximum dose was 1.57 mg (range, 0.5 to 3.5 mg). Untoward effects were few and minor (e.g., dry mouth and feeling tired), and at these doses did not appear to interfere with academic performance.

There was a strong treatment effect in both groups. At the time of completion of the double-blind period, alprazolam was superior to placebo based on clinical global ratings, but the differences were not significant. There were strong individual responders in both groups. After tapering off medication and the final week of placebo, there was a slight relapse with recurrence of original symptoms among the subjects on alprazolam, whereas subjects on placebo showed no further change, or continued to improve. The authors noted that doses employed were relatively low and were administered for only 4 weeks and suggested that higher doses and longer trials be investigated in the future. They also recommended that alprazolam be tapered more gradually over a period of several weeks.

Klein and Last (1989) reported Klein's unpublished data from a clinical trial of alprazolam in children and adolescents whose separation anxiety disorder did not respond to psychotherapy. Alprazolam was clinically effective when administered to 18 subjects, aged 6 to 17 years, for 6 weeks in daily doses of 0.5 to 6 mg/day (mean, 1.9 mg/day). Parents and the psychiatrist judged that > 80% of the subjects improved significantly, whereas 65% of the subjects rated themselves as improved.

Clonazepam (Klonopin)

Clonazepam is approved for use alone or as an adjunct in treating various seizure disorders.

Reports of Interest

Clonazepam in the Treatment of Panic Disorder. In an open clinical trial, Kutcher and MacKenzie (1988) treated four adolescents (three females and one male; average age, 17.2 years; range, 16 to 19 years) who were diagnosed with panic disorder by DSM-III criteria with a fixed dose of clonazepam (0.5 mg twice daily). Average ratings on the Hamilton Anxiety Rating Scale fell from 32 at baseline, to 7.5 at 1 week, and to 5.7 after 2 weeks. The number of panic attacks fell from an average of three per week to 0.5 per week after 1 week and to 0.25 per week after 2 weeks. One adolescent complained of initial drowsiness that resolved within 4 days; no other untoward effects were reported. At follow-up examinations 3 to 6 months later, all four patients continued to take clonazepam with improved functioning in school and interpersonal relations.

Clonazepam in the Treatment of Childhood Anxiety Disorders. Graae et al. (1994) treated 15 subjects (eight males, seven females; age range, 7 to 13 years; mean, 9.8 ± 2.1 years), who were diagnosed with various anxiety and comorbid disorders, with clonazepam in a double-blind, placebo-controlled, crossover study of 8 weeks' duration. Diagnoses included separation anxiety disorder $(N = 14)$, overanxious disorder $(N = 6)$, social phobia $(N = 5)$, oppositional disorder $(N = 3)$, avoidant disorder $(N = 2)$, conduct disorder $(N = 1)$, and attention-deficit/hyperactivity disorder $(N = 1)$. Clonazepam was initiated with a 0.25-mg dose at breakfast time and increased by 0.25 mg every third day to reach a dose of 1.0 mg/day. Subsequent increments of 0.25 mg were made every other day until a dose of 2 mg/day was reached unless untoward effects or compliance issues prevented it. After 4 days at a maximum of 2 mg/day, clonazepam was tapered to reach zero by the end of the 4-week period.

Three boys dropped out during the period on active medication, two because of serious disinhibition—including marked irritability, tantrums, aggressivity, and self-injurious behavior—and the other because of noncompliance. Nine children were rated as clinically improved (five had good/marked improvement and four had some/moderate improvement), and three children showed no improvement of symptoms of anxiety or overall functioning while on clonazepam. Although there was no statistically significant difference between periods on clonazepam and placebo for the 12 subjects, the authors thought that individual patients made significant clinical improvements while on clonazepam. The most common untoward effects of clonazepam were drowsiness, irritability or lability, and oppositional behavior. Overall, 10 (83%) children had untoward effects during the period on clonazepam compared with 7 (53%) while on placebo; the difference, however, was not statistically significant. Disinhibition occurred only while on clonazepam, and the two boys who dropped out because of this effect were not included in the data analysis. It was suggested that a slower dosage increase might reduce some untoward effects, including disinhibition (Graae et al. 1994).

Clonazepam in the Treatment of Obsessive-Compulsive Disorder. Ross and Piggot (1993) treated a 14-year-old male with clonazepam who had been hospitalized with severely disabling obsessive-compulsive disorder. The patient had not responded adequately to prior trials of clomipramine, thioridazine, alprazolam, fluoxetine, or diazepam, either alone or in various combinations. Clonazepam was administered at an initial dose of 0.5 mg twice daily and increased to 1.0 mg twice daily after 1 week. Behavior began to improve after 2 weeks, and he could be discharged on that dose after 11 weeks.

Leonard et al. (1994) reported the use of clonazepam as an augmenting agent in a 20-year-old who had severely disabling obsessive-compulsive disorder with onset at age 7. He was treatment-resistant to prior trials of clomipramine, desipramine, fluoxetine, fluvoxamine, and buspirone augmentation, either alone or in various combinations. He experienced marked clinical improvement with at least 75% reduction in symptom severity on a combination of 60 mg/day of fluoxetine and 4 mg/day of clonazepam, which had been maintained for approximately 1 year. The authors suggested that clonazepam might be an efficacious and safe augmentation agent to specific serotonin reuptake inhibitors in treating obsessive-compulsive disorder in children and adolescents.

AZASPIRODECANEDIONES
Buspirone Hydrochloride (Buspar)

Buspirone hydrochloride, a drug with anxiolytic properties, is not pharmacologically related to the benzodiazepines or barbiturates. Buspirone has a high affinity for $5\text{-}HT_{1A}$ serotonin receptors, which is associated with anticonflict activity in animals and predicts clinical anxiolytic activity (Sussman, 1994b). Buspirone has moderate affinity for brain D_2-dopamine receptors. It does not appear to have significant affinity for benzodiazepine receptors or to affect gamma-aminobutyric acid (GABA) binding (PDR, 2000). Buspirone does not have cross-tolerance with the benzodiazepines, does not suppress panic attacks, and lacks anticonvulsant activity (Sussman, 1994b); hence it does not block the withdrawal syndrome that may occur when benzodiazepines and other common sedative hypnotic drugs are abruptly discontinued. At therapeutic doses it is less sedating than the benzodiazepines. In addition, no evidence of physical or psychological dependence or a withdrawal syndrome has been reported, and it appears to have low abuse potential even by individuals at increased risk for drug dependency. It is not classified as a controlled (Schedule II) substance.

Buspirone has been approved by the FDA for advertising as clinically effective for the management of anxiety disorders or the short-term relief of the symptoms of anxiety. It has been reported that, unlike benzodiazepines which have an immediate anxiolytic effect, buspirone may take as long as 1 to 2 weeks for its antianxiety effect to develop fully (Sussman, 1994b). Symptom improvement may continue for at least 4 weeks with psychic symptoms of anxiety improving sooner than somatic symptoms of anxiety (Feighner and Cohen, 1989).

Pharmacokinetics of Buspirone Hydrochloride

Peak plasma levels occur between 40 and 90 minutes after an acute oral dose of buspirone. Average elimination half-life after single doses of 10 to 40 mg of buspirone is usually between 2 and 3 hours.

Contraindications for Buspirone Hydrochloride Administration

Known hypersensitivity to buspirone is a contraindication. It is not recommended to use buspirone concomitantly with MAOIs.

Interactions of Buspirone Hydrochloride with Other Drugs

The knowledge of the effects of concomitant administration of buspirone and other drugs is very limited; hence buspirone should be used cautiously with other drugs. There are reports that patients receiving MAOIs have developed elevated blood pressure when given buspirone.

Untoward Effects of Buspirone Hydrochloride

The untoward effects most frequently reported by adults taking buspirone include dizziness (12%), drowsiness (10%), nausea (8%), headache (6%), insomnia (3%), and lightheadedness (3%). Of note, however, drowsiness and insomnia were reported to occur with approximately equal frequency in subjects taking placebo; hence these effects may not have been related to buspirone per se (PDR, 2000).

Indications for Buspirone Hydrochloride in Child and Adolescent Psychiatry

Buspirone is approved only for treatment of anxiety disorders and the short-term relief of anxiety in individuals at least 18 years of age. Its safety and efficacy in children and adolescents remain to be determined.

Buspirone Dosage Schedule

- Children and adolescents up to 17 years of age: Not approved. Coffey (1990), however, has cautiously suggested the following doses if a clinician elects to use buspirone in this age group:

    Prepubescent children: An initial total daily dose of 2.5 to 5 mg with increases of 2.5 mg every 3 to 4 days to a maximum of 20 mg/day.

    Younger adolescents: An initial total daily dose of 5 to 10 mg with increases of 5 to 10 mg every 3 to 4 days to a maximum of 60 mg/day.

- Adolescents at least 18 years of age and adults: Initiate treatment with 5 mg three times daily. Titrate to optimal therapeutic response by increases of 5 mg every 2 to 3 days to a maximum daily dose of 60 mg. Usual optimal doses in clinical trials were 20 to 30 mg/day in divided doses

Buspirone Hydrochloride Dose Forms Available

- Tablets (scored): 5 mg, 7.5 mg, 10 mg.
- Dividose (scored for bisection or trisection): 15 mg, 30 mg.

Reports of Interest

Buspirone Hydrochloride in the Treatment of Adolescents with Various Diagnoses. Simeon (1991) reported the use of buspirone in 13 adolescents (age range, 12 to 20 years; mean age, 16 years) with various diagnoses who had shown unsatisfactory response to previous drug treatment. Diagnoses were anxiety and/or depressive disorder ($N = 5$), ADD, and/or conduct disorder ($N = 4$), obsessive-compulsive disorder ($N = 2$), and psychosis ($N = 2$). Daily dose of buspirone ranged from 10 to 40 mg (mean, 25 mg) and was given either alone or with other medications. Ratings 1 to 4 months after buspirone was administered initially showed clinical global improvement that was marked in seven cases, moderate in three cases, mild in two cases, and none in one case. Improvements were reported in mood ($N = 9$), anxiety ($N = 6$), social interaction ($N = 6$), sleep ($N = 4$), aggression ($N = 3$), concentration ($N = 3$), and irritability ($N = 1$). Correlations of improvement with diagnoses were not reported.

Buspirone Hydrochloride in the Treatment of Mixed Anxiety Disorders in Children and Adolescents. Simeon et al. (1994) treated 15 children (10 males, 5 females; age range, 6 to 14 years; mean age, 10 years) who were diagnosed with separation anxiety disorder (5); overanxious disorder (2); comorbid separation anxiety and overanxious disorders (4); separation, overanxious, and avoidant disorders (1); separation, overanxious, and obsessive-compulsive disorders (1), and overanxious disorder and attention-deficit/hyperactivity disorder (ADHD) (2). Subjects were rated moderately to severely impaired on the Clinical Global Impressions Scale (CGI). A single-blind placebo was administered for the initial 2 weeks. This was followed by 4 weeks of buspirone, which was administered initially at 5 mg daily and increased weekly by 5-mg increments, if clinically indicated, to a maximum of 20 mg/day. Optimal daily dose ranged from 5 mg twice daily to 10 mg twice daily; mean dose was 18.6 mg/day. No subjects improved significantly on placebo. After 4 weeks on buspirone, subjects' ratings on the CGI showed marked improvement (3), moderate improvement (10), and minimal improvement (2). Repeated measures of multivariate analysis of variance (MANOVA) showed a statistically significant treatment effect after 2 weeks on medication ($P < .016$), which increased in significance to $P < .001$ after both 3 and 4 weeks on medication. There were also significant improvements on several rating scales as reported by parents, teachers, and subjects themselves. Untoward effects included nausea or stomach pain (five), headache (four), and occasional sleepwalking, sleeptalking, or nightmares and daytime tiredness (eight), and seemed to occur following dosage increases. These were mild and transient, and none required cessation of therapy.

Buspirone Hydrochloride in the Treatment of Overanxious Disorder with School Phobia. Kranzler (1988) reported a single case study in which a 13-year-old adolescent diagnosed with overanxious disorder, school refusal, and intermittent enuresis was administered buspirone. A previous trial of desipramine yielded some improvement but was discontinued at the patient's request because of untoward effects. Buspirone was administered initially at 2.5 mg three times daily. At doses of 5 mg three times daily, some drowsiness occurred, particularly in the morning. Dosage was eventually stabilized at 5 mg twice daily. Scores on the Hamilton Anxiety Rating Scale dropped from 26 to 15 and stabilized, with improvement in phobic anxiety, insomnia, depressed mood, cardiovascular symptoms, and anxious behavior. The enuresis did not improve.

Buspirone Hydrochloride in the Treatment of Social Phobia and Mixed Personality Disorder. Zwier and Rao (1994) reported treating with buspirone a hospitalized 16-year-old male diagnosed with social phobia and schizotypal personality disorder. Buspirone was administered initially at 5 mg/day and increased to 20 mg in increments of 5 mg every 3 days. Scores on the Hamilton Anxiety Rating Scale fell from a predrug level of 5 to 0 at day 12 of treatment, at which time the patient was discharged. Over the subsequent year, buspirone was tapered to 5 mg/day. The patient maintained his gains, and his mild psychotic symptoms had resolved.

Buspirone Hydrochloride in the Treatment of Aggression. Quaison et al. (1991) treated a hospitalized 8-year-old boy, diagnosed with conduct and attention-deficit/hyperactivity disorders, with buspirone hydrochloride. Dosage was administered initially at 5 mg three times per day and titrated gradually to 15 mg three times a day. By day 10 there was a notable decrease in his aggressive and assaultive behavior, and the need for timeouts or seclusion ceased altogether.

Ratey et al. (1989, 1991) reported that buspirone hydrochloride in doses of 15 to 45 mg/day was useful in treating 20 developmentally disabled and mentally retarded adults (age range, 18 to 63 years) for symptoms of anxiety, aggression, and self-injurious behaviors. The decrease in aggressive behavior was independent of anxiety effects. The authors hypothesized that buspirone reduced aggression through its interaction with the serotonergic systems and that at low dosage levels (although not necessarily at the higher doses of 30 to 60 mg/day used for its anxiolytic-antidepressant effects) buspirone may act as a serotonin agonist, especially in brains with low serotonin activity. However, it remains to be seen if buspirone hydrochloride will be efficacious and safe when its use is extended downward in age.

Pfeffer et al. (1997) treated 25 prepubertal inpatients (19 males, 6 females; mean age, 8.0 ± 1.8 years; age range, 5 to 11 years) who had symptoms of anxiety and moderately aggressive behavior. (Approximately 25% of the hospitalized children, those with the most severely aggressive behaviors, required rapid treatment with mood stabilizers or neuroleptics and were excluded from the study.) Subjects' diagnoses by DSM-III-R (APA, 1987) criteria included 9 with mood disorder, 21 with a disruptive behavior disorder, 8 with anxiety disorders, and 9 with specific developmental disorders. The 11-week study consisted of a 2-week baseline evaluation followed by 3 weeks of dose titration during which buspirone was administered initially at 5 mg/day and increased by 5 to 10 mg every 3 days to a maximum of 50 mg/day. Subjects were then maintained at their optimal dose of buspirone for an additional 6 weeks. Efficacy was determined by analysis of ratings on the Child Depression Inventory (CDI); the Revised Children's Manifest Anxiety Scale (RCMAS); the Measure of Aggression, Violence, and Rage in Children (MAVRIC); the Suicidal and Assaultive Behavior Scales (SABS); the Overt Aggression Scale (OAS); the Children's Global Assessment Scale (CGAS); and the Udvalg for Kliniske Undersogelser (UKU) Side Effects Rating Scale (Lingjaerde et al. 1987).

During the second week of titration, four children developed behavioral toxicity (agitation and increased aggressivity) and were terminated from the study. Of the 21 subjects who entered the maintenance phase, 2 were terminated because they developed severe euphoric symptoms, increased impulsivity, and out-of-control behavior. Thus 19 (76%) completed the 11-week study. The mean dose for completers was 28 mg/day in two divided doses. For the 19 completers, there was a significant decrease ($P = .001$) in CDI scores from baseline (19 ± 8.2) to endpoint

(9.2 ± 7.5). This level of improvement was achieved during the sixth week on buspirone, and seven of the 10 completers with clinically significant depression at baseline (CDI score > 18) had a CDI score of < 12 (i.e., below the cutoff for non-clinically significant depression). There was a significant reduction in the number of restraints and/or seclusions ($P = .01$) and the duration of time children spent restrained and/or secluded ($P = .02$). Although there was a significant decrease ($P = .02$) in the MAVRIC at endpoint, subjects still remained with clinically significant levels of aggression. CGAS scores, reflecting clinical global functioning, improved from 40.68 ± 10.49 at baseline to 54.47 ± 14.18 at endpoint ($P = .01$). However, subjects remained with significant clinical impairments as reflected by the final score. Only three children improved sufficiently to continue on buspirone following completion of the study. Overall, although significant, the therapeutic efficacy on aggression and anxiety was limited, and clinically significant aggressivity, anxiety, and global impairment remained. Significant untoward effects required that six patients be terminated prematurely from the study. Overall results were not very promising (Pfeffer et al. 1997).

Buspirone Hydrochloride in the Treatment of Pervasive Developmental Disorder. Realmuto et al. (1989) treated four autistic children, 9 to 10 years of age, with buspirone 5 mg administered three times daily for 4 weeks, followed by a week-long washout period and 4 weeks of 10 mg twice daily of either fenfluramine or methylphenidate. Two of the four children showed decreased hyperactivity while on buspirone. None of the children experienced adverse untoward effects from buspirone.

Buitelaar et al. (1998) evaluated the efficacy and safety of buspirone in a 6- to 8-week, open-label study treating chronic manifest pervasive anxiety, irritability, and/or affect dysregulation in 22 inpatients (20 males, 2 females; age range, 6 to 16 years), 20 of whom were diagnosed with pervasive developmental disorder not otherwise specified (PDDNOS) and two of whom were diagnosed with autistic disorder by DSM-III-R criteria (APA. 1987). Target symptoms were anxiety in 14 patients, irritability in 1 , and both anxiety and irritability in 7 . Efficacy was determined by ratings on the Clinical Global Impressions (CGI) Scale, using subscales CGI-Anxiety and CGI-Irritability, and the CGI-Severity (CGI-S) and the CGI-Improvement (CGI-I) Scales. Buspirone was initiated at a dose of 5 mg three times daily and individually titrated based on clinical response; the maximum permitted dose of 45 mg/day could be achieved within 3 weeks. Eighteen subjects received buspirone only; four subjects continued to receive one additional drug. Twenty-one subjects completed 6 to 8 weeks on buspirone; one subject dropped out earlier because of lack of clinical response. Therapeutic improvement became apparent after 2 to 3 weeks of treatment in many subjects. The mean total daily dose of buspirone during the 6- to 8-week evaluation period was 29.3 mg/day (range, 15 to 45 mg/day). Overall on the CGI-I, 16 (76%) of 21 patients were responders (nine "marked" improvement, seven "moderate" improvement) with clinically significant reductions of overwhelming anxiety, irritability, and temper tantrums; six subjects did not experience therapeutic benefit. Of the 21 patients with targeted anxiety, 16 were responders (nine "marked" and seven "moderate"), and of the 8 patients with "irritability" 5 were responders (2 "marked" and 3 "moderate"). Untoward effects were reported in five subjects (two had initial sedation; two, slight agitation; one, initial nausea) and were mild. All 16 responders continued to receive buspirone and were followed for 2 to 12 months; therapeutic gains were maintained in all cases. One child, however, developed abnormal involuntary movement of the mouth, cheeks, and tongue after receiving 20 mg/day of buspirone for 10 months. The authors considered this a buspirone-associated orofacial-lingual dyskinesia and discontinued medication; the abnormal movements completely remitted within 2 weeks. The study suggests buspirone may be therapeutically useful in treating anxiety and irritability in some children and adolescents with pervasive developmental disorders.

Buspirone Hydrochloride in the Treatment of Attention-Deficit/Hyperactivity Disorder. McCormick et al. (1994) conducted a 4-week, double-blind, placebo-controlled, crossover study in which buspirone hydrochloride was administered to 10 males ranging in age from 11 years, 3 months to 16 years, 10 months (mean age, 13 years, 7 months) who were diagnosed with ADHD by DSM-III-R criteria (APA, 1987). The only comorbid diagnoses were learning disorders, which occurred in four (40%) of the subjects. Each subject was randomly assigned to buspirone or placebo for 2 weeks, and then the conditions were reversed for 2 weeks. Buspirone 5 mg at 8:00 AM and 11:00 AM or placebo was given only on school days, Mondays through Fridays. The 10-item Conners' Abbreviated Teacher Rating Scale was completed during weekly telephone interviews with families and subjects. Analysis showed no significant carryover effect between the two conditions. The mean Conners' baseline score of 20.2 decreased to 19.3 during the second week of placebo therapy and decreased to 14.8 during the second week of buspirone therapy. Nine of the 10 subjects improved on buspirone as compared with placebo with a significant treatment effect ($P < .025$). The only reported untoward effect for buspirone was by one subject who experienced nausea for 3 days.

Malhotra and Santosh (1998) treated, in a 6-week, open-label trial of buspirone, 12 outpatients (10 males, 2 females; mean age, 8.2 years; age range, 6 to 12 years) who were diagnosed with attention-deficit/hyperactivity disorder. Efficacy was rated on the Conners' Parent Abbreviated 10-item index (CPAI) and the Children's Global Assessment Scale (CGAS) at baseline, and 1, 2, 4, 6, and 8 weeks (i.e., after 2 weeks off medication). Subjects were administered an initial total dose of 0.5 mg/kg/day (dose range, 15 to 30 mg/day) of buspirone divided into two doses that was continued for 6 weeks; no other medication was administered during the study. The mean CPAI improvement at day 7 was significant at $P < .001$. Clinical improvement continued over the 6-week period, and at the end of the study, at day 42, was significant at $P < .0001$. All four domains of the CPAI, inattention, hyperactivity, impulsivity, and behavior, improved significantly ($P < .0001$ for each domain). Based on reduction of symptom severity by $> 50\%$ and significant clinical improvement, all 12 patients were responders. The CGAS scores improved significantly from baseline by day 7 ($P < .0001$) and by day 42 had improved significantly ($P < .0001$). All 12 subjects had reexacerbation of symptoms within 2 weeks after buspirone was discontinued (the mean CPAI score returned nearly to baseline). Following the period the subjects were off medication, all families elected to have their children again be medicated with buspirone. Only two subjects reported untoward effects; both experienced mild transient dizziness during the first week. The authors concluded that buspirone was safe and effective in reducing the symptoms of ADHD in this group of subjects.

CHAPTER 10

Other Drugs

ANTIHISTAMINES

Diphenhydramine (Benadryl) and hydroxyzine (Atarax, Vistaril) are the antihistamines most frequently used in treating children and adolescents with emotional disorders. Chronologically, they were also among the earliest drugs used in child and adolescent psychopharmacotherapy, and they remain among the safest medications yet employed.

Contraindications for Antihistamine Administration

Known hypersensitivity to antihistamines is a contraindication for their prescription.

Infants born prematurely and infants are especially sensitive to the stimulating effects of antihistamines, and overdose may cause hallucinations, convulsions, or death. Because antihistamines may be secreted in breast milk, nursing mothers should also avoid taking antihistamines.

Narrow-angle glaucoma, stenosing peptic ulcer, pyloroduodenal obstruction, and symptomatic prostatic hypertrophy or bladder-neck obstruction are relative contraindications. The anticholinergic effects of antihistamines and the additional atropine-like effect of diphenhydramine hydrochloride may cause drying and thickening of bronchial secretions; hence they should be used with caution in patients with clinical symptoms of asthma or poorly controlled asthma.

Interactions of Antihistamines with Other Drugs

Diphenhydramine and hydroxyzine have potentiating effects when used in conjunction with other central nervous system depressants, such as alcohol, narcotics, non-narcotic analgesics, barbiturates, hypnotics, antipsychotics, and anxiolytics.

Monoamine oxidase inhibitors prolong and intensify the drying effect (an anticholinergic action) of antihistamines.

Diphenhydramine Hydrochloride (Benadryl)

Diphenhydramine hydrochloride has been used for more than 50 years to treat psychiatrically disturbed children (Effron and Freedman, 1953). Although such use is still not approved for advertising by the U.S. Food and Drug Administration

(FDA), it is reviewed here because some child psychiatrists continue to find it clinically effective.

Fish (1960) reported that diphenhydramine is most effective in behavioral disorders associated with anxiety and hyperactivity but that it could also be useful in moderately (not severely) disturbed children with organic or schizophrenic (including autistic) disorders. A later study of 15 children, however, found no significant difference in behavioral improvement between diphenhydramine in doses of 200 to 800 mg/day and placebo (Korein et al. 1971).

Diphenhydramine is also effective as an anxiolytic, reducing anxiety before producing drowsiness or lethargy, in children up to approximately 10 years of age. However, it shows a marked decrease in efficacy when administered to older children; their response is similar to adults with untoward effects of malaise or drowsiness. Therefore, for older children diphenhydramine is useful primarily as a bedtime sedative for insomnia and/or nighttime anxiety (Fish, 1960).

Diphenhydramine has also been used to treat children with insomnia and/or children who wake up after falling asleep and have marked difficulty falling asleep again. Russo et al. (1976) compared diphenhydramine and placebo administered to 50 children, aged 2 to 12 years, who had difficulty falling asleep or problems with night awakenings. Diphenhydramine 1 mg/kg was significantly better than placebo in decreasing sleep-onset latency and decreasing the number of awakenings over a 7-day trial period. Total sleeping time, however, was not significantly increased. Side effects were minimal.

Contraindications for the Administration of Diphenhydramine Hydrochloride

The administration of diphenhydramine is contraindicated in premature infants and infants.

Untoward Effects of Diphenhydramine Hydrochloride

The most frequent untoward effects are anticholinergic effects and sedation. Children do seem more tolerant of the sedative effects of diphenhydramine, but the clinician should still be alert to any cognitive dulling that may interfere with learning. Young children may sometimes be excited rather than sedated by diphenhydramine. It is cautioned that overdose may cause hallucinations, convulsions, or death, particularly in infants and young children.

Diphenhydramine Hydrochloride Dosage Schedule for Treatment of Children and Adolescents

- Premature infants and infants under 20 pounds: The use of diphenhydramine is contraindicated.
- Infants > 20 pounds (9.1 kg) and older children: Administer initially a 12.5- or 25-mg dose and titrate upward with 12.5- or 25-mg increases for optimal response. A maximum dose of 300 mg/day or 5 mg/kg/day, whichever is less, is recommended. Maximum activity occurs in about 1 hour, and the effects last about 4 to 6 hours; therefore the drug is usually administered three to four times daily. Young children appear to tolerate a higher dose per unit of weight than do adolescents

(continued)

Diphenhydramine Hydrochloride Dosage Schedule for Treatment of Children and Adolescents *(Continued)*

and adults. Fish (1960) found a dose range of from 2 to 10 mg/kg/day, with an average daily dose of 4 mg/kg, to be most effective in treating behaviorally disturbed youngsters.

Diphenhydramine Hydrochloride Dose Forms Available

- Capsules: 25 mg, 50 mg
- Elixir: 12.5 mg/5 mL
- Injectable preparations: 10 mg/mL, 50 mg/mL

Hydroxyzine Hydrochloride (Atarax), Hydroxyzine Pamoate (Vistaril)

Hydroxyzine is an antihistamine that is absorbed rapidly from the gastrointestinal tract. Its clinical effects usually become evident within 15 to 30 minutes of oral administration. It has been used widely as a preanesthetic medication in children and adolescents because it produces significant sedation with minimal circulatory and respiratory depression. It also produces bronchodilation, decreases salivation, has antiemetic, antiarrhythmic, and analgesic effects, and produces a calming, tranquilizing effect (Smith and Wollman, 1985).

Use in Child and Adolescent Psychiatry

One manufacturer stated that "hydroxyzine has been shown clinically to be a rapid-acting, true ataraxic with a wide margin of safety. It induces a calming effect in anxious, tense, psychoneurotic adults, and also in anxious, hyperkinetic children without impairing mental alertness" (PDR, 1990, p. 1858); this statement has been deleted from the more recent PDRs (PDR, 1995, 2000, 2006). Hydroxyzine is approved for the symptomatic relief of anxiety and tension associated with psychoneurosis and as an adjunct in organic disease states in which anxiety is manifested. Its efficacy for periods longer than 4 months has not been demonstrated by systematic clinical studies.

Although not specifically indicated in the manufacturer's labeling, the sedation caused by hydroxyzine (as with diphenhydramine) has been utilized in the short-term treatment of insomnia and frequent night awakening in children.

Untoward Effects of Hydroxyzine

The most common untoward effects of hydroxyzine are sedation and dry mouth.

Hydroxyzine Hydrochloride Dosage Schedule for Treating Children and Adolescents

- *Children under 6 years old*: Medication should be titrated individually and administered four times daily to a maximum of 50 mg/day.

(continued)

Hydroxyzine Hydrochloride Dosage Schedule for Treating Children and Adolescents (Continued)

- *Children 6 years of age and older and adolescents*: Medication should be titrated individually and administered three to four times daily to a maximum of 100 mg/day.

Hydroxyzine Dose Forms Available

- *Tablets (hydroxyzine hydrochloride)*: 10 mg, 25 mg, 50 mg, 100 mg
- *Capsules (hydroxyzine pamoate)*: 25 mg, 50 mg, 100 mg
- *Syrup (hydroxyzine hydrochloride)*: 10 mg/5 mL
- *Oral suspension (hydroxyzine pamoate)*: 25 mg/5 mL
- *Intramuscular injection (hydroxyzine hydrochloride)*: 25 mg/mL, 50 mg/mL

OPIATE ANTAGONISTS

Opiate antagonists have been investigated in the treatment of mentally retarded persons with self-injurious behavior (for review see Sokol and Campbell, 1988) and in the treatment of autistic disorder. Deutsch (1986) has given a theoretical rationale for the use of opiate antagonists in the treatment of autistic disorder.

Naltrexone Hydrochloride (Trexan, Revia)

Naltrexone hydrochloride is a pure opioid antagonist. It is a synthetic congener of oxymorphone without any opioid agonist properties and completely blocks or markedly attenuates the subjective effects of intravenous opioids and precipitates withdrawal symptoms in subjects with physical tolerance to opioids.

Pharmacokinetics of Naltrexone Hydrochloride

Naltrexone is almost completely absorbed from the gastrointestinal tract and undergoes substantial first-pass metabolism by the liver to 6-beta-naltrexol. Peak plasma levels of naltrexone and 6-beta-naltrexol occur within 1 hour of an oral dose. Both compounds are biologically active and are excreted primarily by the kidneys. Serum half-life of naltrexone is approximately 4 hours and that of 6-beta-naltrexol is approximately 13 hours.

Contraindications for Naltrexone Hydrochloride Administration

The main contraindications are hypersensitivity, any liver abnormalities, and the concomitant use of any opiate-containing substances, legal or illegal.

Interactions of Naltrexone Hydrochloride with Other Drugs

Serious adverse effects (e.g., a severe, precipitous withdrawal syndrome) may occur if naltrexone is administered to individuals taking opioids.

Indications for Naltrexone Hydrochloride in Child and Adolescent Psychiatry

Naltrexone hydrochloride is approved for the treatment of alcoholism and for the blockade of the effects of exogenously administered opiates. It is not approved for any other psychiatric disorders.

Naltrexone Dosage Schedule

- Children and adolescents up to 17 years of age: Not recommended. Safety and efficacy have not been determined for this age group.
- Adolescents at least 18 years of age and adults: Usual recommended dose in the treatment of alcoholism or opioid dependency is 50 mg/day. (Read package insert carefully before using.)

Naltrexone Hydrochloride Dose Forms Available

- Tablets: 25 mg, 50 mg

Reports of Interest

Naltrexone in the Treatment of Autistic Disorder

Campbell et al. (1989) administered naltrexone on an open basis to 10 hospitalized children aged 3.42 to 6.5 years (mean age, 5.04 years). The study lasted 6 weeks. Following a 2-week baseline, single doses of 0.5, 1, and 2 mg/kg/day were administered at 1-week intervals. Ratings were made 1, 3, 5, 7, and 24 hours after each dose, and 1 week after the last dose. Subjects showed diminished withdrawal at all three dose levels. Verbal production increased at 0.5 mg/kg/day, and stereotypies decreased following the 2 mg/kg/day dose. Symptoms such as aggressiveness and "self-aggressiveness" showed little improvement. The major untoward effect was mild sedation, which occurred in 70% of the subjects. Laboratory measurements, including liver function tests and electrocardiograms (ECGs), showed no significant change from baseline. Overall, raters considered 80% of the children to be positive responders for some symptoms (Campbell et al. 1989).

Campbell et al. (1990) subsequently conducted a double-blind, placebo-controlled study of naltrexone in 18 children, aged 3 to 8 years, diagnosed with autistic disorder. The study consisted of a 2-week placebo baseline phase, random assignment to placebo or naltrexone for 3 weeks, and a posttreatment 1-week placebo phase. The initial naltrexone dose was 0.5 mg/kg/day; this was increased to 1 mg/kg/day, if no adverse effects occurred. Nine children received naltrexone; the optimal dose was 1 mg/kg/day. Six subjects receiving naltrexone were rated moderate (five) or marked (one) in improvement on Clinical Global Consensus Ratings, whereas only one child on placebo achieved a moderate rating and none was markedly improved. The difference was significant ($P = .026$). In contrast, no reduction in symptoms occurred on the Children's Psychiatric Rating Scale or Clinical Global Impressions. Naltrexone did not appear to affect discrimination learning in an automated laboratory. The authors also reported that overall symptom reduction seemed better in older autistic children than in younger ones.

Although there are case studies and open studies with some encouraging data, the 1993 report of Campbell et al.—an 8-week double-blind study in which 41 hospitalized children (2.9 to 7.8 years of age; mean, 4.9 years) diagnosed with autistic disorder were treated with naltrexone or placebo—did not support the efficacy of naltrexone in this population. All their subjects received placebo during the first 2 weeks while baseline data were obtained. Following this phase, subjects were randomly assigned to naltrexone or placebo for the next 3 weeks. During the final week all subjects again received placebo. Twenty-three patients were assigned to the naltrexone group and 18 to the placebo group. The initial dose was 0.5 mg/kg/day of either placebo or active drug given in the morning; dose was increased to 1.0 mg/kg/day after 1 week and maintained at that level because untoward effects were minimal and did not require a reduction in dose. Naltrexone did not improve the core symptoms of autism. The only significant finding was a modest decrease in hyperactivity on three different measures. It did not improve discrimination learning significantly more than placebo. Naltrexone was no better than placebo in reducing self-injurious behavior, but six of eight subjects who had a severity rating of mild or above on the Aggression Rating Scale who received naltrexone experienced rebound (increase) in symptoms during the final placebo period; only one child in the placebo group exhibited worsening of self-injurious behavior during that time. The authors concluded that it remains to be determined whether naltrexone is efficacious in treating moderate-to-severe self-injurious behavior and that its use cannot be recommended as a first-line treatment for patients diagnosed with either autistic disorder or self-injurious behavior (Campbell et al. 1993).

In a 7-week, double-blind, placebo-controlled, crossover study, Feldman et al. (1999) evaluated the efficacy of naltrexone in improving communication skills, a core deficit, in 24 children (mean age, 5.1 years; range, 3 to 8.3 years) diagnosed with autistic disorder by DSM-III-R criteria (APA, 1987) who had previously shown modest behavioral improvement on naltrexone in previous studies by the authors (Kolman et al. 1995; Kolman et al. 1997). Communication skills of the subjects at baseline ranged from preverbal to nearly normal for age. During the active drug phase, 1 mg/day of naltrexone was administered.

There was no significant improvement in communication skills with naltrexone treatment, including number of utterances, total number of words, number of different words, or reduction in echolalia in these subjects who had shown some behavioral improvement on naltrexone. Also, the authors reported that use of parental language with the patient did not change according to whether or the child was receiving naltrexone or not. The authors suggested that medications that improve core deficits and target symptoms of autistic disorder should be preferred over those that improve only associated symptoms.

BETA-ADRENERGIC BLOCKERS
Propranolol Hydrochloride (Inderal)

Although initially used primarily in controlling hypertension, angina pectoris, various cardiac arrhythmias, migraine prophylaxis, and other medical disorders, there has been considerable interest in the use of propranolol in general psychiatry.

Propranolol is a nonselective beta-adrenergic receptor-blocking agent with no other autonomic nervous system activity. Propranolol and other beta-adrenergic blocking agents reduce peripheral autonomic tone, thereby lessening somatic symptoms of anxiety such as palpitations, tremulousness, perspiration, and blushing. There is some evidence that the beta-adrenergic blocking agents significantly reduce these peripheral, autonomic, physical manifestations of anxiety but may not affect the psychological (emotional) symptoms of anxiety (Noyes, 1988). Noyes (1988) concludes from his review of the literature that beta-blockers are relatively weak anxiolytics compared with benzodiazepines and should be used for generalized anxiety disorder, primarily in patients for whom the use of benzodiazepines is contraindicated.

In adults, propranolol has been investigated in treating anxiety disorders, including generalized anxiety, performance anxiety (stage fright), social phobia, post-traumatic stress disorder, panic disorder and agoraphobia, and episodic dyscontrol and rage outbursts (Hayes and Schulz, 1987; Noyes, 1988). It has also been used in treating schizophrenia. Propranolol is effective in the treatment of some antipsychotic-induced akathisias (Adler et al. 1986).

Pharmacokinetics of Propranolol Hydrochloride

Propranolol is almost completely absorbed from the gastrointestinal tract. Peak serum values occur within 60 to 90 minutes; serum half-life is approximately 4 hours.

The manufacturer recommends using weight to determine propranolol doses for children, as this usually results in plasma levels comparable to those in the therapeutic range for adults.

The manufacturer notes that higher than expected serum levels of propranolol have occurred in patients diagnosed with Down syndrome (trisomy 21), suggesting that its bioavailability may be increased in such patients.

Contraindications for Propranolol Administration

Known hypersensitivity to propranolol is a contraindication.

Patients with bronchospastic diseases (bronchial asthma), cardiovascular conditions, diabetes, hyperthyroidism, or other medical disorders should have their medical status carefully reviewed (consultation with the physician providing care for the medical condition is recommended) before prescribing propranolol. Gualtieri et al. (1983) have cautioned that propranolol is contraindicated in children and adolescents with a history of cardiac or respiratory disease, those who have hypoglycemia, or those who are being medicated with a monoamine oxidase inhibitor. Because significant depression has been reported as an untoward effect, propranolol is not recommended for children and adolescents who are already depressed.

Interactions of Propranolol with Other Drugs

Propranolol may interact with many drugs. Three interactions among those most likely to be seen in child and adolescent psychiatric practice are: (a) if used concomitantly with chlorpromazine, plasma levels of both drugs are increased over what they would be if used separately; (b) alcohol slows the rate of absorption of propranolol; and (c) phenytoin, phenobarbital, and rifampin accelerate propranolol clearance.

Untoward Effects of Propranolol

There are few reports of untoward effects in children or adolescents who received propranolol for psychiatric indications. Of greatest concern have been cardiovascular effects, which are detailed in the subsequent text. Propranolol has also been reported to cause significant depression of mood, manifested by insomnia, lethargy, weakness, and fatigue. Vivid dreams, nightmares, and gastrointestinal symptoms have also been reported.

Indications for Propranolol Hydrochloride in Child and Adolescent Psychiatry

There are no approved uses of propranolol in psychiatrically disturbed children and adolescents.

Propranolol Dosage Schedule

- *Children and adolescents up to 17 years of age*: Manufacturer's recommendations for treating hypertension in this age group are an initial twice-daily dose of 0.5 mg/kg followed by individual titration based on clinical response. Usual dose range is 2 to 4 mg/kg/day in two divided doses. Doses of > 16 mg/kg/day should not be used.
- *Adolescents at least 18 years of age and adults*: Manufacturer's recommendations for treating hypertension are an initial dose of 80 mg daily in two divided doses followed by individual titration based on clinical response. The usual dose range is 120 to 240 mg/day. Some patients may require higher doses and some will need three-times-daily dosing.

Propranolol Discontinuation/Treatment Withdrawal

Because of the possibility of rebound in blood pressure, the dose of propranolol should be gradually tapered over 7 to 14 days when discontinued.

Propranolol Hydrochloride Dosage Forms Available

- *Tablets*: 10 mg, 20 mg, 40 mg, 60 mg, 80 mg
- *Long-acting capsules (Inderal LA)*: 60 mg, 80 mg, 120 mg, 160 mg

---

Reports of Interest

Propranolol in the Treatment of Children and Adolescents with Brain Dysfunction, Uncontrolled Rage Outbursts, and/or Aggressiveness. Williams et al. (1982) administered propranolol to 30 subjects (11 children, 15 adolescents, and 4 adults) with organic brain dysfunction and uncontrolled rage outbursts who had not responded to other treatments. The subjects had various psychiatric diagnoses, including 15 with diagnoses of both conduct disorder, unsocialized, aggressive type, and attention-deficit disorder with hyperactivity; 7 with comorbid diagnoses of conduct disorder, unsocialized, aggressive type, and attention-deficit disorder without hyperactivity; 3 with conduct disorder only; 3 with intermittent explosive disorders; and 2 with pervasive developmental disorders. Thirteen had IQs in the retarded range, and eight had borderline IQs. The authors reported that 80% of their subjects demonstrated moderate to marked improvement on follow-up examination between 2 and 30 months (mean, 8 months) later. Optimal dosages of propranolol ranged from 50 to 960 mg/day (mean, 160 mg/day). All untoward effects were transient and reversible with dosage reduction. Most of the patients were additionally treated with other medication: thirteen subjects received anticonvulsants; six, antipsychotics; and three, stimulants. Twenty-one had ongoing psychotherapy (Williams et al. 1982).

Kuperman and Stewart (1987) treated openly with propranolol 16 subjects whose mean age was 13.4 years (eight patients were 4 to 14 years old, four were between 14 and 17, and four were 18 to 24 years old). Seven subjects were diagnosed with conduct disorder, undersocialized aggressive type, five had infantile autism with varying degrees of mental retardation, two had moderate mental retardation only, one had borderline intellectual functioning, and one had attention-deficit disorder. All subjects exhibited significant physically aggressive behavior that had not responded adequately to behavior therapy and/or psychotropic medication. Propranolol was administered initially at 20 mg twice daily and increased by 40 mg every fourth day until symptom improvement occurred or standing systolic blood pressure fell below 90 mm Hg, diastolic blood pressure fell below 60 mm Hg, or resting pulse fell below 60 beats per minute. The average dose of propranolol was 164 ± 55 mg/day. Ten patients (62.5%) were rated moderately or much improved, based on concurrence of ratings by parents, teachers, and clinicians. Responders and nonresponders did not differ significantly regarding age, sex, IQ, vital signs, or dosage. The authors noted that, although not significant, six of their eight patients who were mentally retarded responded favorably, which is consistent with earlier findings in adults that suggests that aggressive patients with suspected central nervous system damage respond best. Nonresponders as a group tended to develop bradycardia, which may have prevented them from reaching potentially therapeutic doses of propranolol. The authors additionally noted that before considering propranolol a therapeutic failure, a patient should receive the maximum therapeutic dose tolerated for at least 1 month. When propranolol is discontinued, it should be tapered gradually over a 2-week period to avoid rebound tachycardia (Kuperman and Stewart, 1987).

Two 12-year-old boys treated with propranolol for episodic dyscontrol and aggressive behavior showed marked improvement (Grizenko and Vida, 1988). Dosage was initiated at 10 mg three times daily and was gradually increased to 50 mg three times daily.

Propranolol in the Treatment of Children Diagnosed with Posttraumatic Stress Disorder. Famularo et al. (1988) reported that 11 children (mean age, 8.5 years old) diagnosed with post-traumatic stress disorder (PTSD), acute type, had significantly lower scores on an inventory of PTSD symptoms during the period when they were receiving propranolol, compared with scores before and after the drug. Dosage was initiated at 0.8 mg/kg/day and administered in three divided doses; it was increased gradually over 2 weeks to approximately 2.5 mg/kg/day. Untoward effects prevented raising dosage to this level in only three cases. Propranolol was maintained at this level for 2 weeks and then tapered and discontinued over the fifth week. The authors emphasized that their subjects had presented in agitated, hyperaroused states, and that propranolol might be useful during this particular stage of the disorder (Famularo et al. 1988).

At present, although there are some encouraging initial data, the use of propranolol and the beta-blockers in children and adolescents must be further investigated. In particular, the use of propranolol in anxiety disorders remains to be elucidated.

Pindolol (Visken)

Pindolol is a synthetic, nonselective beta-adrenergic receptor-blocking agent that has sympathomimetic activity at therapeutic doses but does not possess quinidine-like membrane stabilizing activity (package insert).

It is approved for use in treating hypertension, but its safety and effectiveness have not been established in children.

Report of Interest

Buitelaar et al. (1994a) conducted a double-blind, placebo-controlled comparison of pindolol and methylphenidate in 52 subjects (age range, 6 to 13 years) diagnosed with Attention-deficit/Hyperactivity Disorder (ADHD). Treatment periods were of 4 weeks' duration. For the first 3 days, a morning dose of 10 mg of methylphenidate or 20 mg of pindolol or placebo was given. This was increased to 10 mg twice daily of methylphenidate or 20 mg twice daily of pindolol or placebo for the remainder of the period. Subjects were rated on various Conners Scales by parents and teachers. After 4 weeks, teachers rated students receiving methylphenidate as significantly better on impulsivity/hyperactivity, inattentiveness, and conduct than subjects receiving either pindolol or placebo. Parental ratings did not show a significant difference between pindolol and methylphenidate on improvements in impulsivity/hyperactivity or conduct, although both were better than placebo. The authors thought that the main effect of pindolol was to improve behavioral symptoms and conduct and that the drug was only modestly effective in treating ADHD.

Untoward effects of pindolol were of particular concern and limit the potential usefulness of this drug in children. Paresthesias was reported in 10% of children during treatment with pindolol and none while receiving placebo or methylphenidate ($P < .05$). Although hallucinations and nightmares were not significantly more frequent in children on pindolol, they were of significantly greater intensity ($P < .01$) and caused so much distress that the children's daily functioning was affected adversely. These adverse effects totally remitted within 1 day after discontinuation of pindolol. The authors note that some children may be particularly sensitive to these distressing untoward effects, further limiting the usefulness of pindolol in ADHD and requiring the clinician to be very cautious whenever prescribing pindolol to children (Buitelaar et al. 1994a, 1994b).

ALPHA-ADRENERGIC AGONISTS

Clonidine Hydrochloride (Catapres), Clonidine (Catapres-Transdermal Therapeutic System)

Clonidine is a centrally acting antihypertensive agent. The only therapeutic indication that has been approved by the FDA for advertising is treatment of hypertension in older adolescents and adults; its safety and efficacy in children have not been established.

Clonidine, an alpha-2-noradrenergic receptor agonist (stimulating agent), acts preferentially on presynaptic alpha-2 neurons to inhibit endogenous release of norepinephrine in the brain (Hunt et al. 1991). The authors note that the positive results in their studies with children diagnosed with ADHD suggest that the norepinephrine system may be important in causing behavioral and cognitive abnormalities, in at least some children with ADHD.

Pharmacokinetics of Clonidine Hydrochloride

Peak plasma levels of clonidine occur between 3 and 5 hours after ingestion, and plasma half-life is between 12 and 16 hours (package insert). Leckman et al. (1985), however, give different pharmacokinetic values for children and adolescents, stating that clonidine's half-life is approximately 8 to 12 hours in adolescents and adults, whereas in prepubertal children it is considerably shorter; approximately 4 to 6 hours. Between 40% and 60% of the drug is excreted unchanged by the kidneys within 24 hours after oral ingestion, and approximately 50% is metabolized by the liver (package insert).

Contraindications for Clonidine Hydrochloride Administration

Known hypersensitivity to clonidine hydrochloride is a contraindication. Significant cardiovascular disease is a relative contraindication; if clonidine is used in patients with such conditions, careful and frequent monitoring is required.

Children and adolescents with depressive symptomatology, past history of depression, or family history of mood disorder should not be given clonidine (Hunt et al. 1990).

Interactions of Clonidine Hydrochloride with Other Drugs

Tricyclic antidepressants may decrease the effects of clonidine, necessitating higher doses.

The central nervous system depressive effects of alcohol, barbiturates, and other drugs may be enhanced by simultaneous administration with clonidine. Interactions with additional drugs have been reported.

Clonidine and Methylphenidate

In the summer of 1995 (July 13th), a National Public Radio broadcast reported that sudden deaths had occurred in three children taking a combination of methylphenidate and clonidine, which caused alarm among parents and physicians of patients taking this combination of medications. Popper's editorial concerning this noted that the Food and Drug Administration (FDA) had not publicized the data or informed clinicians, as it considered the "link between the deaths and the medications highly dubious." Detailed reviews of the medications and the three cases by Popper (1995) and Fenichel (1995) concluded that there was no convincing evidence of an adverse methylphenidate–clonidine interaction in any of the cases. Popper (1995) and Swanson et al. (1995) concluded that combined clonidine–methylphenidate treatment of ADHD is usually safe and that the available evidence did not support discontinuation of such therapy in patients experiencing significant clinical benefit. All authors also noted the lack of systematic studies of the efficacy and safety of combined methylphenidate–clonidine treatment.

Swanson et al. (1995) noted in their review of untoward effects that when the combination of clonidine and a stimulant was given, sedation–hypotension–bradycardia would be most expected when the clonidine effect was at its peak and the stimulant's effect is decreasing and, conversely, that hypertension–tachycardia would be most expected when the stimulant is at its peak and clonidine's effect is waning.

In 1999, in a "Debate Forum" on "Combining Methylphenidate and Clonidine" published in the *Journal of the American Academy of Child and Adolescent Psychiatry*, Wilens and Spencer argued the affirmative ("A Clinically Sound Medication Option") and Swanson, Connor, and Cantwell argued the negative ("Ill-Advised").

Before prescribing this combination, it is recommended that the clinician reviews this literature and thoroughly discusses the risks and benefits with the parents/legal guardian and patient.

Untoward Effects of Clonidine Hydrochloride

Hunt et al. (1991) reported that sedation is the most frequent and troublesome untoward effect of clonidine in treating children. Cardiovascular untoward effects, including hypotension, were not usually clinically significant.

Clonidine worsened or induced depressive symptomatology in approximately 5% of children (Hunt et al. 1991). McCracken and Martin (1997) reported the case of an 8-year-old boy with autistic disorder who developed an apparent severe depressive reaction on a total daily dose of 0.2 mg of clonidine; there was rapid improvement following discontinuation of clonidine. They cautioned clinicians to monitor for depressive reactions secondary to clonidine that could be mistaken for worsening of the primary disorder.

Levin et al. (1993) reported the onset of precocious puberty in two 7-year-old girls with mild mental retardation who were being treated with clonidine for aggressivity; of note, discontinuation of clonidine halted the progression of puberty in both cases. Many other untoward effects have been reported in patients on clonidine (PDR, 1995).

Swanson et al. (1995) reviewed briefly 20 MedWatch adverse-event reports concerning subjects < 19 years of age who were taking clonidine and added three additional cases, one of which was fatal. Of the 23 patients, four were fatalities. Eleven cases were treated with clonidine only, 11 with combined clonidine–methylphenidate therapy, and one with combined clonidine–dexedrine therapy. In 12 cases the untoward effect occurred after a change in medication protocol (e.g., prescribed dose change, accidental change, or noncompliance. In 10 of the 19 nonfatal cases hypotension and/or bradycardia was reported, and in 5 cases hypertension and/or tachycardia was reported. (See also the preceding discussion on clonidine–methylphenidate under drug interactions.)

The Effects of Clonidine Hydrochloride on the Electrocardiograms of Children and Adolescents

Kofoed et al. (1999) reviewed relevant literature and conducted a retrospective study of the effects of clonidine alone ($N = 12$) and clonidine combined with stimulants (methylphenidate [$N = 14$], dextroamphetamine [$N = 13$], or magnesium pemoline [$N = 3$]) on 12-lead, electrocardiograms (ECGs) of 42 children and adolescents (36 males and 6 females; age range, 4 to 16 years). The mean clonidine dose was 0.16 ± 0.075 mg/day (dose range, 0.05 to 0.30 mg/day). The mean daily methylphenidate dose was 60 mg; the mean daily dextroamphetamine dose was 40 mg; and the mean daily magnesium pemoline dose was 112 mg. The authors stated that their data should be able to detect a difference of 0.012 second between baseline and postclonidine treatment PR intervals and of 0.015 second between pretreatment and postclonidine treatment for the QT_c interval. Their data should also detect differences between clonidine only and clonidine plus a stimulant of 0.020 second for the PR interval and 0.024 second for the QT_c interval. Two pediatric cardiologists, blinded to treatment condition, evaluated all ECGs.

The mean PR interval for all 42 subjects before clonidine was 0.140 ± 0.020 second versus 0.140 ± 0.022 second after clonidine treatment. The mean QT_c interval calculated by cardiologist A, before clonidine was 0.407 ± 0.025 second versus

0.407 ± 0.021 second after clonidine; for cardiologist B the QT_c interval before clonidine was 0.402 ± 0.027 second and after clonidine, 0.399 ± 0.023 second.

For the 12 subjects in the clonidine-only group, the mean pretreatment PR interval was 0.137 second and the posttreatment PR interval also 0.137 second. There was also no pretreatment to posttreatment change in the mean PR interval for the 30 subjects receiving a combination of clonidine and a stimulant (PR = 0.142 second for both); there was no statistically significant effect of treatment, drug group, or treatment–drug group interaction term on PR intervals.

For the 12 subjects in the clonidine-only group, cardiologist A calculated the mean QT_c pretreatment interval to be 0.409 second versus 0.405 second posttreatment. For the 30 subjects receiving a combination of clonidine and a stimulant, the mean QT_c pretreatment interval was calculated to be 0.406 second versus 0.408 second posttreatment; there was no statistically significant effect of treatment, drug group, or treatment–drug group interaction term on the QT_c interval.

For the 12 subjects in the clonidine-only group, cardiologist B calculated the mean QT_c pretreatment interval to be 0.412 second versus 0.398 second posttreatment. For the 30 subjects receiving a combination of clonidine and a stimulant, the mean QT_c pretreatment interval was calculated to be 0.398 second versus 0.400 second posttreatment; there was no statistically significant effect of treatment or drug group. However, treatment–drug group interaction term on the QT_c interval showed a significant difference (0.014 increase for clonidine only versus 0.002 increase for clonidine and stimulant, $P = 0.034$). The authors noted that the 0.014-second shortening calculated for the clonidine-only group was not consistent with known effects of clonidine and thought this value resulted from the combination of a small N with other confounding errors.

Six (14%) of the 42 subjects had ECG abnormalities before medication treatment (3 sinus bradycardia, 2 ectopic atrial rhythm, and 1 short PR interval), and 7 (17%) had ECG abnormalities after medication. The abnormal ECGs of two subjects normalized on medication and three subjects with normal pretreatment ECGs developed abnormal ECGs on medication ($P = .50$, not significant), suggesting spontaneous variability rather than drug effect. Except for a 10-year-old boy with a short PR interval that later required ablation of an accessory atrial pathway, all subjects had normal PR, QRS, and QT_c intervals, suggesting that clonidine alone or in combination with stimulants has no significant effect on these ECG parameters.

The authors emphasized the importance of pretreatment ECGs, as 14% of their subjects had abnormalities on their ECGs, some of which could have been attributed to clonidine if baseline data were not available. They also noted that spontaneous variations in ECGs over time occurred that were not caused by medication. Such variations in QT_c occur randomly with changes in the balance of sympathetic/parasympathetic input to the heart and possibly due to diurnal variations that have been reported in adults. The authors made the valuable suggestion that each subject's pre- and posttreatment ECGs should be recorded at the same time of day to minimize some of these possible confounding spontaneous variations. The authors concluded that clonidine alone or in combination with stimulants had no systematic cardiac effects on these behaviorally disturbed children but that rare idiosyncratic responses could occur.

Guidelines for the Administration of Clonidine Hydrochloride to Children and Adolescents

Hunt et al. (1990) recommend beginning clonidine administration with bedtime doses to utilize the usual initial sedative effect to facilitate sleep. Sedation is most severe during the first 2 to 4 weeks, after which tolerance usually develops (Hunt et al. 1991). Because of its short serum half-life, clonidine is usually administered three to four times daily and at bedtime. Hunt et al. (1990) have reported that some children have shown a loss of therapeutic effect or withdrawal symptoms when it is administered less frequently; transdermal patches eliminate this difficulty.

Cantwell et al. (1997) expressed additional concern about untoward effects and the lack of methodologically sound studies on using combined clonidine/stimulant treatment for behavioral disturbances in children. The following is a summary only of their suggested guidelines for clonidine.

- *Screening*: Preexisting cardiac or vascular disease is a contraindication for clonidine therapy for behavioral reasons. Sinus node and atrioventricular node disease and renal disease are relative contraindications.
- *Pulse and blood pressure*: Pulse rate and blood pressure should be obtained to provide a baseline, should be done weekly during titration, and should be repeated every 4 to 6 weeks on maintenance dosage. A thorough evaluation of "new-onset treatment-emergent" symptoms, especially if exercise related, is essential.
- *ECG*: Baseline bradycardia or impaired atrioventricular conduction indicating first-degree, second-degree, or complete heart block or QRS interval > 120 msec necessitates cardiac consultation for medical clearance. Baseline ECG should be compared with an ECG recorded on full dose of clonidine.
- *Dose titration*: Clonidine should be titrated gradually and not exceed a 0.05-mg increment every 3 days. Drug termination should be by gradual tapering of dose to minimize withdrawal effects.

Clonidine Administration with the Transdermal Therapeutic System

When transdermal patches were used in treating subjects diagnosed with ADHD, Hunt (1987) found that their efficacy wore off and that they had to be replaced in 50% of subjects after 5 days rather than the 7 days stated by the manufacturer. He also noted that, to achieve the same degree of symptom control, three of his eight subjects whose daily oral dose was 0.2 mg/day had to have their doses increased to 0.3 mg/day when clonidine was administered transdermally. Comings (1990), who has extensive clinical experience with patients with Tourette's syndrome, stated that he found that clonidine administered using a patch may work when oral clonidine is ineffective. Comings also found it convenient and useful to adjust the dose of clonidine by using scissors to cut the patch to the necessary size.

Indications for Clonidine Hydrochloride in Child and Adolescent Psychiatry

There are no FDA-approved uses of clonidine in the treatment of psychiatrically disturbed children and adolescents. However, clonidine has been investigated in

(continued)

Indications for Clonidine Hydrochloride in Child and Adolescent Psychiatry *(Continued)*

treating children and adolescents diagnosed with ADHD and/or Tourette disorder who have not responded to standard treatments for these disorders. Studies of these uses and the doses employed by the researchers are summarized later for each of these conditions.

Clonidine Discontinuation/Treatment Withdrawal

Clonidine should be gradually reduced over a period of 2 to 4 days to avoid a possible hypertensive reaction and other withdrawal symptomatology such as nervousness, agitation, and headache (package insert).

Clonidine Hydrochloride Dose Forms Available

- *Tablets (single scored)*: 0.1 mg, 0.2 mg, 0.3 mg
- *Transdermal therapeutic system (TTS)*: Programmed delivery by skin patch of 0.1 mg (Catapres-TTS 1), 0.2 mg (Catapres-TTS 2), or 0.3 mg daily (Catapres-TTS 3) for 1 week.

Reports of Interest

Clonidine in the Treatment of Attention-Deficit/Hyperactivity Disorder. Hunt et al. (1982) reported on an open pilot study in which clonidine 3 to 4 µg/kg/day was administered orally for 2 to 5 months to four children between 9 and 14 years of age diagnosed with ADDH. Improvement was noted by parents and teachers. The authors noted that distractibility often persisted but that the children were nevertheless more able to return to and complete tasks.

Hunt et al. (1985) conducted a double-blind, placebo-controlled crossover study of 12 children (mean age, 11.6 ± 0.54 years) who were diagnosed with ADDH. Ten children completed the study. Seven subjects had previously received stimulant medication; in four cases stimulants had been discontinued because of significant untoward effects. Clonidine was begun at 0.05 mg and increased every other day until a dose of 4 to 5 µg/kg/day (approximately 0.05 mg four times daily) was attained. Parents, teachers, and clinicians all noted statistically significant improvements on clonidine for the group as a whole. The best responders were children who had been overactive and who were uninhibited and impulsive, which, in turn, had impaired their opportunities to use their basically intact capacities for social relatedness and purposeful activity. During the placebo period, parents, teachers, and clinicians noted significant deterioration in overall behavior for the group, with symptoms usually returning between 2 and 4 days after discontinuing the medication (Hunt et al. 1985).

The most frequent untoward effect seen in this study was sedation, occurring approximately 1 hour after ingestion and lasting 30 to 60 minutes. In all cases but one, tolerance to this effect developed within 3 weeks. Mean blood pressure also decreased approximately 10%.

Hunt et al. (1990, 1991) have reported that children diagnosed with ADHD and treated with clonidine have been maintained on the same dose for up to 5 years without diminution of clinical efficacy. However, approximately 20% of such children require an increase in dose after several months of treatment, probably secondary to autoinduction of hepatic enzymes (Hunt et al. 1990).

Hunt (1987) compared the efficacies of clonidine (administered both orally and transdermally) and methylphenidate in an open study of 10 children diagnosed with ADDH, all of whom had ratings by both parents and teachers of > 1.5 SD above normal on Conners' Behavioral Rating Scales. Eight subjects (seven males, one female; mean age, 11.4 ± 0.6 years; range, 6.7 to 14.4 years) completed the protocol. Subjects received placebo, low-dose (0.3 mg/kg) methylphenidate, or high-dose (0.6 mg/kg) methylphenidate. Each of these conditions was randomized for a period of 1 week. All subjects then received an open trial of clonidine 5 µg/kg/day administered orally for 8 weeks. Eight subjects completed the open trial with positive results and were then switched from tablets to transdermal clonidine skin patch. Both clonidine and methylphenidate were significantly more effective than placebo, and clonidine in both dosage forms was as effective as methylphenidate (Hunt, 1987). Children reported that they felt more "normal" on clonidine than on methylphenidate. Transdermal administration was preferred to oral administration by 75% of the children and their families, partly because the embarrassment of taking pills at school was avoided but also because it was more convenient. Skin patches caused localized contact dermatitis, usually presenting with itching and erythema, in approximately 40% of children and at times limited their usefulness (Hunt et al. 1990).

Hunt (1987) noted that in contrast to the stimulants, clonidine appears to increase frustration tolerance but does not decrease distractibility. He noted that an additional small dose of methylphenidate may be safely added to help focus attention and that this combination frequently permits a much lower dose of methylphenidate than would be required if it were the only drug used (Hunt, 1987).

In a review of clonidine use in child and adolescent psychiatry, Hunt et al. (1990) explained more specifically the differences between clonidine and methylphenidate in treating ADHD and their possible synergistic use in treating ADHD and suggested the subgroups of ADHD children for whom each treatment would be most useful. Stimulants (methylphenidate) improve attentional focusing and decrease distractibility, whereas clonidine decreases hyperarousal and increases frustration tolerance and task orientation.

The authors found that children with ADHD who respond best to clonidine often have an early onset of symptoms, are extremely energetic or hyperactive (hyperaroused), and have a concomitant diagnosis of conduct disorder or opposi-tional disorder. Such children often respond to clonidine treatment with increased frustration tolerance and consequent improvement in task-orientated behavior; more effort, compliance, and cooperativeness; and better learning capacity and achievement. Clonidine was also efficacious in nonpsychotic inpatient adolescents with ADHD who were aggressive and hyperaroused (Hunt et al. 1990).

Unlike stimulants, clonidine does not directly improve distractibility; hence stimulants are preferable for mildly to moderately hyperactive children with significant deficits in distractibility and attentional focus. The combination of clonidine and methylphenidate was found to be helpful for children who were diagnosed with coexisting conduct or oppositional disorder and ADHD and who were both highly aroused and very distractible (Hunt et al. 1990). The combined use of these drugs may permit the effective dose of methylphenidate to be reduced by approximately 40%, making it potentially useful for ADHD patients in whom significant motor hyperactivity persists, or in whom rebound symptoms or dose-limiting side effects such as aggression, irritability, insomnia, or decrements in weight or height gain have occurred with stimulant treatment (Hunt et al. 1990).

Steingard et al. (1993) published a retrospective chart review of 54 patients (age range, 3 to 18 years; mean, 10.0 ± 0.5 years) who were diagnosed with ADHD only ($N = 30$) or ADHD and comorbid tic disorder ($N = 24$) and treated with clonidine. Of note, 17 subjects in the ADHD-only group had prior unsatisfactory responses to stimulant or tricyclic antidepressant medication. In the comorbid group, nine had developed tics when treated with stimulants and 10 had unsuccessful prior trials of tricyclic antidepressants. Clonidine was initiated at a low dose and titrated upward until a positive clinical result occurred or untoward effects prevented further increase. Mean optimal daily dose for all subjects was 0.19 ± 0.02 mg/day (range, 0.025 to 0.6 mg/day). There was no significant difference in mean daily dose between subjects with and without tics, responders and nonresponders, or subjects less and more than 12 years of age. Although 72% (39) of 54 subjects were rated as improved on the Clinical Global Improvement Scale subset of items for ADHD symptoms, a significantly greater proportion ($P = .0005$) of subjects with a comorbid tic disorder (23 [96%] of 24) improved than did subjects with ADHD only (16 [53%] of 30). On Clinical Global Improvement Scale items pertinent to tics, 75% (18 of 24) showed improvement. Sedation, the most frequent untoward effect, was reported in 22 (41%) patients. All seven patients whose untoward effects resulted in discontinuation of medication were in the ADHD-only group. Five were discontinued because of sedation; one, because of increased anxiety; and one, because of a depressive episode.

At present, clonidine may be regarded as a possible alternative treatment for ADHD. It may eventually prove useful in treating, in particular, a subgroup of ADHD children who do not respond well to stimulants. Clonidine may also be a useful alternative treatment for some ADHD children who have chronic tics or who develop side effects of sufficient severity as to preclude the use of stimulants (Hunt et al. 1985; Steingard et al. 1993).

Conners et al. (1999) reviewed the literature from 1980 to 1999 on the use of clonidine in the treatment of ADHD with and without comorbid diagnoses of conduct disorder, tic disorder, or developmental delay. Eleven of the 39 reports provided data sufficient to be used in a meta-analysis. The authors reported the overall effect size of clonidine for symptoms of ADHD to be moderate. It was similar to the effect size for tricyclic antidepressants but less than the large effect size for stimulants. The authors concluded that clonidine in doses of 0.1 to 0.3 mg/day was moderately effective in ameliorating common symptoms of ADHD and should be considered as a second-tier treatment. They also noted that clonidine's use is associated with many untoward effects, in particular sedation, irritability, and, when administered by transdermal patch, skin irritation, and rash.

Clonidine in the Treatment of Sleep Disturbances in Children and Adolescents Diagnosed with ADHD. Wilens et al. (1994) reported their experience in using the sedation that clonidine often produces to treat more than 100 patients diagnosed with ADHD who also had spontaneous or drug-induced sleep difficulties. The effect has allowed some children who responded very well to stimulants, but could not tolerate them because of significant insomnia to be treated successfully with them. Typically, an initial dose of 0.05 mg of clonidine for patients between 4 and 17 years of age was given about half an hour before bedtime and was increased by 0.05-mg increments to a maximum of 0.4 mg. A few very young or underweight children required only 0.025 mg, whereas a few other children required > 0.4 mg. Patients and parents reported better sleep, and there were decreased familial conflicts around sleep activities and fewer ADHD-like symptoms after treatment. Some of the latter improvement is likely to result from the fact that clonidine is also effective in treating ADHD independent of its sleep-enhancing qualities. Clonidine should be tapered gradually when it is discontinued, even if used only at night for insomnia.

Clonidine in the Treatment of Chronic Severe Aggressiveness. Kemph et al. (1993) treated openly with clonidine 17 outpatients (14 males and three females; age range, 5 to 15 years old; mean age, 10.1 years) diagnosed with conduct or oppositional defiant disorder. All subjects had a history of chronic and violent aggressiveness in multiple settings that had not responded to behavioral management. Clonidine was begun at an initial dose of 0.05 mg/day. After 2 days it was increased to 0.05 mg twice daily, and on day 5 it was increased to 0.05 mg three times daily, following which it was titrated as clinically indicated on an individual basis. The maximum effective dose was 0.4 mg daily administered in divided doses. A comparison of mean baseline and follow-up scores on the Rating of Aggression against People and/or Property Scale (RAAPP) showed significant improvement on drug ($P < .0001$). Drowsiness was the major untoward effect most frequently reported; it usually occurred during the first weeks of treatment, and most patients developed tolerance to it. There were no significant changes in blood pressure or cardiovascular parameters. The authors noted that plasma gamma-aminobutyric acid (GABA) levels increased significantly ($P < .01$) in five of the six children for whom it was available at follow-up, suggesting that GABA plasma levels may be correlated with childhood aggressiveness and may also be useful to verify compliance. Clonidine may be a useful agent in the control of aggression in children and adolescents and merits further study.

Clonidine in the Treatment of Autistic Disorder Accompanied by Inattention, Impulsivity, and Hyperactivity. Jaselskis et al. (1992) treated eight males (age range, 5.0 to 13.4 years; mean, 8.1 ± 2.8 years) diagnosed with autistic disorder who also had significant inattention, impulsivity, and hyperactivity that had not responded to prior psychopharmacotherapy (e.g., methylphenidate or desipramine); they received clonidine in a double-blind, placebo-controlled, crossover protocol. Clonidine or placebo was titrated over the initial 2 weeks to a daily total of 4 to 10 µg/kg/day (0.15 to 0.20 mg/day) divided into three doses; this regimen was maintained for the next 4 weeks. During the seventh week, subjects were tapered off clonidine or placebo. At week 8, subjects were crossed over to the other condition for 6 weeks. Parents' ratings on the Conners Abbreviated Parent-Teacher Questionnaire showed significant improvement while their children were on clonidine. Teachers' ratings on the Aberrant Behavior Checklist were significantly better during clonidine treatment for irritability ($P = .03$), hyperactivity ($P = .03$), stereotypy ($P = .05$), and inappropriate speech ($P = .05$). Attention-Deficit Disorder with Hyperactivity: Comprehensive Teacher's Rating Scale scores improved significantly only for oppositional behavior ($P = .05$). Although significant, improvement was modest. Clinician ratings at the end of each 6-week period showed no significant differences between clonidine and placebo. Untoward effects included significant drowsiness and hypotension requiring reduction of dosage in three subjects.

Clonidine in the Treatment of Tourette's Disorder. Cohen et al. (1980) reported that clonidine was clinically effective in at least 70% of 25 patients between 9 and 50 years of age diagnosed with Tourette's syndrome (TS) who either did not benefit from haloperidol or could not tolerate the untoward effects of that medication. Dosage was begun at 1 to 2 µg/kg/day (usually 0.05 mg/day) and gradually titrated up to a maximum of 0.60 mg/day. Most patients did best with small doses three to four times daily. Comings (1990) recommends a starting dose of 0.025 mg/day (one-fourth of a tablet) and sometimes found it necessary to administer as many as five divided doses daily for best results. He found it to be an excellent drug for the approximately 60% of his patients who responded and noted that it ameliorated oppositional, confrontational, and obsessive-compulsive behaviors and symptoms of ADHD when these were also present. In contrast, Shapiro and Shapiro (1989) noted that, in their experience, clonidine was only rarely effective in treating unselected patients with tics and Tourette's disorder.

Cohen et al. (1980) delineated five phases of treatment response to clonidine:

Phase I: Within hours or days, patients felt calmer, less angry, and more in control.
Phase II: Approximately 3 to 4 weeks after initiation of clonidine (usually coinciding with a therapeutic dose of 3 to 4 µg/kg/day [0.15 mg/day]), the patient recognized progressive benefits characterized by decreased compulsive behavior, further behavioral control, and decreased phonic and motor tics.
Phase III: A plateauing of improvement started at about the third month.
Phase IV: Five or more months after beginning, an increase in dosage up to 4 to 6 µg/kg/day (0.30 mg/day) of clonidine was needed to maintain clinical improvement.
Phase V: Further tolerance to clonidine may occur at a dose considered too high to increase further.

A review of the use of clonidine in Tourette's disorder (Leckman et al. 1982) noted discrepant results among studies. The reviewers estimated that approximately 50% of subjects improved meaningfully. Behavioral symptoms showed the most improvement and maximum benefit could take from 4 to 6 months. A minority of patients did not respond, and a few worsened.

Leckman et al. (1985) reported a 20-week, single-blind, placebo-controlled trial of clonidine in 13 patients, aged 9 to 16 years, diagnosed with Tourette's syndrome. This was followed by a 1-year open clinical trial. The mean dose of clonidine was 5.5 µg/kg/day (range, 3 to 8 µg/kg/day) (0.125 to 0.3 mg/day). There was significant improvement in motor and phonic tics and associated behavioral problems. Forty-six percent of subjects were unequivocal responders, and 46% responded equivocally. Of interest is the fact that nine of the 13 patients reported by Leckman et al. also had an additional diagnosis of ADDH. As noted earlier, some children with ADHD have symptoms that respond to clonidine.

Leckman et al. (1991) reported a 12-week, double-blind, placebo-controlled trial of clonidine completed by 40 subjects (age range, 7 to 48 years; mean, 15.6 ± 10.4 years; 31 of the subjects were younger than 18 years old) diagnosed with Tourette's syndrome. Clonidine was titrated gradually during the first 2 weeks to a total daily dose of 4 to 5 µg/kg/day (maximum, 0.25 mg/day) and administered in two to four divided doses per day, depending on the total dose. Mean clonidine dose at the end of the 12 weeks for the 21 subjects randomly

assigned to clonidine was 4.4 ± 0.7 µg/kg/day (range, 3.2 to 5.7 µg/kg/day); clonidine serum levels, available for 19 subjects, ranged from 0.24 to 1.0 ng/mL,
with a mean of 0.48 ± 0.23 ng/mL. Subjects receiving clonidine were rated as
significantly more improved than those receiving placebo on the Tourette Syndrome Global Scale for motor tics $(P = .008)$ and total score $(P = .05)$; on the
anchored Clinical Global Impressions Scale for Tourette syndrome (TS-CGI); on
the Shapiro Tourette Severity Symptom Scale for decrease in "tics noticeable to
others"; and on the Conners Parent Questionnaire for total score $(P = .02)$ and the
impulsive/hyperactive factor $(P = .01)$. Untoward effects most frequently reported
were sedation/fatigue (90%), dry mouth (57%), faintness/dizziness (43%), and
irritability (33%). Although clonidine is not as effective in controlling tic behavior as the D_2-dopamine receptor-blocking agents haloperidol and pimozide, its
more favorable untoward effect profile should prompt the clinician to consider
a trial of clonidine before using antipsychotic drugs in milder cases (Leckman
et al. 1991).

Bruun (1983) has provided useful guidelines for prescribing clonidine for
Tourette's disorder. She suggests initiating daily dosage at 0.025 mg twice daily
for small children and at 0.05 mg twice daily for older children and adolescents.
Medication is titrated upward gradually with increases of no > 0.05 mg/week; this
slow pace often prevents untoward effects from interfering with the treatment. The
usual optimal daily dose is between 0.25 and 0.45 mg. Doses above 0.5 mg/day may
be required, but untoward effects (e.g., drowsiness, fatigue, dizziness, headache,
insomnia, and increased irritability) become more troublesome. Bruun (1983) notes
that drowsiness may occur at very low doses and suggests that no further increases
in dosage be made until drowsiness subsides. Some patients note a decrease in
beneficial effects 4 to 5 hours after their last dose, and treatment is usually more
effective for all patients with total daily dosage administered in three or four
smaller doses (Bruun, 1983).

Although presently not an approved treatment, there is evidence that some
children and adolescents with Tourette's disorder respond favorably with significant symptom reduction when treated with clonidine. Clonidine may be regarded
as a possible treatment for those youngsters with Tourette's disorder who have
not responded satisfactorily or who have intolerable untoward effects to standard
treatments.

Clonidine in the Treatment of Children Who Stutter. Althaus et al. (1995)
reported that clonidine was *not effective* in the treatment of 25 children 6 to 13
years of age diagnosed with stuttering by DSM-III-R (APA, 1987) criteria. In a
28-week, double-blind, placebo-controlled crossover study. Medication or placebo
was gradually increased for 1 week, followed by maintenance for 8 weeks; dosage
was then tapered for 4 days followed by 4.5 weeks of washout before beginning
the other condition or at the end of the study before the final ratings. Clonidine
was given in a total dose of 4 µg/kg/day divided into three equal portions over the
day. Efficacy was determined by ratings of repetitions, prolongations, blockades,
and interjections at baseline, before first dose reduction, after first washout period,
before second dose reduction, and after the final washout. There was no significant
improvement in any of the measures used. Parents and teachers also rated no
significant difference between placebo and clonidine and improvement of children's
stuttering, but they did notice significant behavioral improvements in hyperactivity,
task orientation, and greater approachability. The authors concluded that clonidine
was not a useful drug for treating children diagnosed with stuttering.

Guanfacine Hydrochloride (Tenex)

Guanfacine hydrochloride is a centrally acting antihypertensive agent with alpha-2-adrenoreceptor agonist properties. The only FDA-approved indication for advertising for guanfacine hydrochloride is the treatment of hypertension. Its use is not recommended in children under the age of 12 years because its safety and efficacy have not been proved in this age range.

Pharmacokinetics of Guanfacine Hydrochloride

Peak plasma levels occur from 1 to 4 hours (mean, 2.6 hours) after ingestion. Average plasma half-life is approximately 17 hours; younger subjects tend to metabolize guanfacine more rapidly, however. Steady-state blood levels usually occur within 4 days. Guanfacine and its metabolites are excreted primarily by the kidneys.

Contraindications for Guanfacine Hydrochloride Administration

Known hypersensitivity to guanfacine hydrochloride is a contraindication.

Interactions of Guanfacine Hydrochloride with Other Drugs

The depressive effects of alcohol, barbiturates, and other drugs on the central nervous system may be enhanced by simultaneous administration of guanfacine.

Interactions with additional drugs have been reported.

Untoward Effects of Guanfacine Hydrochloride

Untoward effects include those typical of the central alpha-2 adrenoreceptor agonists such as dry mouth, sedation, fatigue, dizziness, constipation, weakness/asthenia, and impotence. Most are mild and transient if treatment is continued. Untoward effects are dose related and increase significantly with increasing dosage. This is noteworthy as most of guanfacine's clinical effects are usually apparent at a dose of 1 mg/day.

Horrigan and Barnhill (1998) reported five cases in which intense activation with a cluster of signs and symptoms resembling an acute-onset manic episode occurred within 3 days following the administration of guanfacine. These cases were from a series of 95 outpatients who were treated with guanfacine during a 12-month period. All five patients were reported to have personal and family risk factors for bipolar disorder.

Indications for Guanfacine Hydrochloride in Child and Adolescent Psychiatry

Guanfacine is approved only for the treatment of hypertension. There are no approved psychiatric uses.

Guanfacine Dosage Schedule

- *Children up to 11 years years of age*: Not recommended. Efficacy and safety have not been established in this age group. Hunt et al. (1995) begin guanfacine at a dose of 0.5 mg/day and, on the basis of clinical response, individually titrate

(continued)

Indications for Guanfacine Hydrochloride in Child and Adolescent Psychiatry *(Continued)*

guanfacine in 0.5-mg increments every 3 days to a maximum of 4 mg/day, which appears to be appropriate in the treatment of ADHD in this age group.
- *Adolescents > 12 years of age and adults*: For the treatment of hypertension, an initial dose of 1 mg at bedtime is recommended to minimize the impact of any initial sedation that may occur. If clinically indicated, higher doses may be administered.

Guanfacine Discontinuation/Treatment Withdrawal

Because of possible rebound phenomena, including nervousness and anxiety (from relative increases in catecholamines) and increases in blood pressure to over baseline, guanfacine should be tapered gradually when discontinued. Because of its relatively long half-life, rebound usually occurs 2 to 4 days after abrupt withdrawal. Although rebound hypertension can occur, it is infrequent and blood pressure usually returns to pretreatment levels over 2 to 4 days.

Guanfacine Hydrochloride Dose Forms Available

- *Tablets*: 1 mg, 2 mg

Reports of Interest

Guanfacine in the Treatment of Attention-Deficit/Hyperactivity Disorder. Guanfacine appears to have potential advantages over clonidine in the treatment of ADHD because it has a longer plasma half-life and appears to be less sedating (Hunt et al. 1995).

Hunt et al. (1995) treated, with guanfacine, 13 subjects (eleven males, two females; age range, 4 to 20 years; mean, 11.1 years) who were diagnosed with ADHD. Guanfacine was begun at a dose of 0.5 mg/day and individually titrated by 0.5-mg increments every 3 days to achieve optimal clinical response to a maximum of 4 mg/day. Mean therapeutic dose was 3.2 mg/day (0.091 mg/kg/day). Medication was usually administered in four divided doses with the morning, noon, and approximately 4:00 PM doses being somewhat less than the bedtime dose. Parental ratings on the Conners' 31-Item Parent Questionnaire at baseline and after 1 month of treatment with guanfacine showed a significant improvement on guanfacine in total average score ($P < .015$), Factor I (hyperactivity) ($P < .002$), Factor II (inattention) ($P < .004$), and Factor V (immaturity) ($P < .002$). In addition, scores on the following individual behavioral items of the Conners' questionnaire were significantly improved while on guanfacine: less fidgety ($P < .002$), less restless ($P < .01$), making fewer disruptive sounds ($P < .01$), less easily frustrated ($P < .005$), less anxious ($P < .005$), less excessive energy ($P < .01$), better able to finish projects ($P < .005$), more attentive ($P < .01$), functional with less supervision ($P < .025$), less rejected and unpopular in social groups ($P < .01$), less uncooperative ($P < .05$), and less constricted or rigid ($P < .01$). Untoward effects included significant initial tiredness on guanfacine compared with baseline ($P < .01$), which resolved within 2 weeks. Headaches and stomachaches were reported by approximately 25% of subjects but resolved within 2 weeks except in one patient. Decreased appetite occurred initially in 16% of the subjects but stabilized within 2 weeks. No subject had clinically significant changes in blood pressure.

Guanfacine in the Treatment of ADHD and Tics and/or Tourette's Disorder. Chappell et al. (1995) reported an open study of 10 subjects, aged 8 to 16 years, who were diagnosed with ADHD and Tourette's syndrome and treated with guanfacine. Two subjects received other psychoactive medications concurrently. An initial bedtime dose of 0.5 mg of guanfacine was titrated upward in 0.5-mg increments every 3 to 4 days and was given in two or three divided doses. Daily doses ranged from 0.75 to 3 mg; optimal daily dose was 1.5 mg for seven of the subjects. Although analysis of the group data did not show significant improvement in ADHD symptoms, three subjects had moderate and one had marked improvement based on ratings on the 48-item Conners' Parent Rating Scale. Group means measuring the severity of motor and phonic tics decreased in ratings by clinicians and patients themselves. The most common untoward effects were lethargy or fatigue (60%), headache (40%), insomnia (30%), and dizziness or lightheadedness (20%); these symptoms usually remitted over 3 to 4 days. No child experienced clinically significant exacerbation of tics. Guanfacine may be a useful drug for some children and adolescents who have comorbid ADHD and a chronic tic disorder.

Horrigan and Barnhill (1995) administered guanfacine to 15 treatment-resistant boys (age range, 7 to 17 years; mean, 13.3 years) diagnosed with ADHD. Most subjects also were diagnosed with comorbid psychiatric disorders, including Tourette's disorder $(N = 8)$ and specific developmental disorders $(N = 11)$. Overall, the subjects had a mean of 3.46 Axis I and Axis II diagnoses. Subjects failed to respond satisfactorily to a mean of 2.0 prior medications, including dextroamphetamine, methylphenidate, clonidine, imipramine, fluoxetine, carbamazepine, lithium, haloperidol, thyroid hormone, tryptophan, and biotin. Guanfacine was initiated with a 0.5-mg dose at bedtime and increased every 5 to 7 days by 0.25 to 0.5 mg increments as clinically indicated. Because the pediatric population metabolizes guanfacine more rapidly than adults, it was administered in two divided doses. After 10 weeks, the range of optimal doses was from 0.5 mg to 3 mg/day, with 0.5 mg twice daily being the most frequent optimal dose. Thirteen subjects received guanfacine only; one subject additionally received lithium carbonate 1,800 mg/day, and another received fluoxetine 10 mg/day.

Overall, guanfacine produced a significant clinical response. Parental ratings, made 4 to 8 weeks after the dose was stabilized on the 13 subjects who completed the study, showed decreases on the Conners' Parent-Teacher Scale (short form) of 11.1 points (from 19.9 to 8.8); on the Edelbrock CAP Inattention Subscale of 4.85 points; and on the Edelbrock CAP Overactivity Subscale of 3.23. The authors noted that the greater improvement in inattention compared with overactivity is the opposite of the pattern often seen with clonidine; they thought that this reversal might be explained by guanfacine's having a greater affinity for alpha-2 adrenoreceptors in the prefrontal areas compared with clonidine's having a greater affinity for the alpha-2 adrenoreceptors in more basal regions (Horrigan and Barnhill, 1995). One subject did not complete the trial because his mother discontinued the medication because of lack of improvement and another because he developed symptoms of overactivation/overarousal. The only other untoward effects noted were initial mild sedation in five boys. No patient experienced a significant change in blood pressure or pulse.

Scahill et al. (2000) conducted an 8-week, randomized, double-blind, placebo-controlled trial of guanfacine in the treatment of 34 subjects (31 males, three females; mean age, 10.4 ± 2.01 years; age range, 7 to 14 years) diagnosed with ADHD and comorbid Tourette's syndrome ($N = 20$), chronic motor tic disorder ($N = 12$), or stimulant-induced tic disorder ($N = 2$). Eleven subjects (32%) were medication naïve; 19 of the other 23 subjects who had previous trials on at least one stimulant medication had experienced worsening of tics on stimulants. Subjects were assigned randomly to guanfacine ($N = 14$) or placebo ($N = 14$). Efficacy was determined by ratings on the DuPaul ADHD Rating Scale (Teacher) and the Clinical Global Impressions-Improvement Scale (CGI-I), the Total Tic Score of the Yale Global Tic Severity Scale (YGTSS), and the Hyperactivity Index (HI) of the Parent Conners'. On the CGI-I, nine subjects receiving guanfacine were rated 1 ("very much improved") or 2 ("much improved") at endpoint compared with no such ratings on placebo ($P < .001$). Subjects on guanfacine improved by 38% on the ADHD Rating Scale versus only 8% improvement for subjects on placebo ($P < .001$). Total Tic Score on the YGTSS for subjects on guanfacine decreased by 30% versus no change in the placebo group ($P < .05$). There was no significant difference between placebo and guanfacine on HI Index scores. There were no clinically significant changes in pulse or blood pressure; one subject on guanfacine discontinued the study after 4 weeks because of sedation.

BARBITURATES AND HYPNOTICS

At the present time, the barbiturates and hypnotics have little, if any, place in treating psychiatric disorders in children and adolescents. Today barbiturates, especially phenobarbital, are used in children and adolescents primarily for their antiepileptic properties. Behaviorally disordered children frequently may worsen when given barbiturates. As long ago as 1939, Cutts and Jasper (1939) administered phenobarbital to 12 behavior-problem children with abnormal EEGs. Behavior worsened in nine (75%), with increased irritability, impulsivity, destructiveness, and temper tantrums. The authors concluded that phenobarbital was contraindicated in the treatment of such children. For sleep disorders, diphenhydramine and benzodiazepines, which are much safer to use, are now the drugs of choice.

Clinically, barbiturates have a disinhibiting and disorganizing effect on many psychiatrically disturbed children, including psychotic children. Cognitive dulling, an untoward effect of barbiturates, is also of major concern in children and adolescents. In adults, phenobarbital was found to decrease speed of access to information in short-term memory, and short-term memory itself was highly sensitive to phenobarbital levels (MacLeod et al. 1978). The authors noted that this effect could impair the ability of children and adolescents to maintain attention in the classroom and interfere with their learning new information.

Clinically, it is also important for the child and adolescent psychiatrist to remember that phenobarbital may contribute to disturbed behavior in some patients with seizure disorder in whom it is being used to control seizures. This is also the case in some younger children when phenobarbital is being used prophylactically (e.g., after febrile seizures). Some such children may show behavioral and cognitive improvement when they are switched to other antiepileptic medications or when they are gradually tapered off medication after a sufficiently long seizure-free period.

References

Adler L, Angrist B, Peselow E, Corwin J, Maslansky R, Rotrosen J. A controlled assessment of propranolol in the treatment of neuroleptic-induced akathisia. *Br J Psychiatry* 1986;149:42–45.

Adler LA, Peselow E, Rotrosen J, Duncan E, Lee M, Rosenthal M, Angrist B. Vitamin E treatment of tardive dyskinesia. *Am J Psychiatry* 1993;150:1405–1407.

Adler LA, Rotrosen J, Edson R, Lavori P, Lohr J, Hitzemann R, Raisch D, Caliguiri M, Tracy K. Vitamin E treatment for tardive dyskinesia. *Arch Gen Psychiatry* 1999;56:836–841.

Alderman J, Wolkow R, Chung M, Johnston HE. Sertraline treatment of children and adolescents with obsessive-compulsive disorder or depression: pharmacokinetics, tolerability, and efficacy. *J Am Acad Child Adolesc Psychiatry* 1998;37:386–394.

Alexandris A, Lundell FW. Effect of thioridazine, amphetamine and placebo on the hyperkinetic syndrome and cognitive area in mentally deficient children. *Can Med Assoc J* 1968;98:92–96.

Alfaro CL, Wudarsky M, Nicolson R, Gochman P, Sporn A. Lenane M, Rapoport JL. Correlation of antipsychotic and prolactin concentration in children and adolescents acutely treated with haloperidol, clozapine, or olanzapine. *J Child Adolesc Psychopharmacol* 2002;12:83–91.

Allen RP, Safer D, Covi L. Effects of psychostimulants on aggression. *J Nerv Ment Dis* 1975;160:138–145.

Altamura AC, Montgomery SA, Wernicke JF. The evidence for 20 mg a day of fluoxetine as the optimal dose in the treatment of depression. *Br J Psychiatry* 1988;153(suppl 3):109–112.

Althaus M, Vink HJF, Minderaa RB, Goorhuis-Brouwer SM, Oosterhoff MD. Lack of effect of clonidine on stuttering in children. *Am J Psychiatry* 1995;152:1087–1089.

Alvir JMJ, Lieberman JA, Safferman AZ, Schwimmer JL, Schaaf JA. Clozapine-induced agranulocytosis: incidence and risk factors in the United States. *N Engl J Med* 1993;329:162–167.

Aman MG, Arnold LE, McDougle CJ, Vitiello B, Scahill L, Davies M, McCracken JT, Tierney E., Nash PL, Posey DJ, Chuang S, Martin A, Shah B, Gonzalez NM, Swiezy NB, Ritz L, Koenig K, McGough J, Ghuman JS, Lindsay RL. Acute and long-term safety and tolerability of risperidone in children with autism. *J Child Adolesc Psychopharmcol* 2005;15:869–884.

Aman MG, Findling RL, Derivan A, Merriman U. Risperidone versus placebo for severe conduct disorder in children with mental retardation. (Abstract, 40th Annual NCDEU meeting). *J Child Adolesc Psychopharmacol* 2000;10:253.

Aman MG, Marks RE, Turbott SH, Wilsher CP, Merry SN. Clinical effects of methylphenidate and thioridazine in intellectually subaverage children. *J Am Acad Child Adolesc Psychiatry* 1991a;30:246–256.

Aman MG, Marks RE, Turbott SH, Wilsher CP, Merry SN. Methylphenidate and thioridazine in the treatment of intellectually subaverage children: effects on cognitive-motor performance. *J Am Acad Child Adolesc Psychiatry* 1991b;30:816–824.

Aman MG, Singh NN. Preface. In: Aman MG, Singh NN, eds. *Psychopharmacology of the developmental disabilities.* New York: Springer-Verlag; 1988:v–ix.

Ambrosini PJ. Pharmacotherapy in child and adolescent major depressive disorder. In: Meltzer HY, ed. *Psychopharmacology: the third generation of progress.* New York: Raven Press; 1987:1247–1254.

Ambrosini PJ, Bianchi MD, Rabinovich H, Elia J. Antidepressant treatments in children and adolescents I. Affective disorders. *J Am Acad Child Adolesc Psychiatry* 1993;32:1–6.

Ambrosini PJ, Sheikh RM. Increased plasma valproate concentrations when coadministered with guanfacine. *J Child Adolesc Psychopharmacol* 1998;8:143–147.

Ambrosini PJ, Wagner KD, Biederman J, Glick I, Tan C, Elia J, Hegeler JR, Rabinovich H, Lock J, Geller D. Multicenter open-label sertraline study in adolescent outpatients with major depression. *J Am Acad Child Adolesc Psychiatry* 1999;38:566–572.

American Academy of Child and Adolescent Psychiatry (AACAP). Desipramine and sudden death. Ad hoc committee on DMI [desipramine] and sudden death (J. Biederman, chair). Washington, DC; 1992 Member Forum, 1992 AACAP Program, p. 8.

American Diabetes Association and American Psychiatric Association. Consensus development conference on antipsychotic drugs and obesity and diabetes. *Diabetes Care* 2004;27:596–601.

American Medical Association. *Drug evaluations,* 6th ed. Chicago: American Medical Association; 1986.

American Medical Association. *Drug evaluations.* Chicago: American Medical Association; 1990.

American Medical Association. *Drug evaluations annual 1994.* Chicago: American Medical Association; 1993.

American Psychiatric Association. *Diagnostic and statistical manual of mental disorders,* 2nd ed. (DSM-II). Washington, DC: American Psychiatric Association; 1968.

American Psychiatric Association. *Diagnostic and statistical manual of mental disorders,* 3rd ed. (DSM-III). Washington, DC: American Psychiatric Association; 1980a.

American Psychiatric Association. *Diagnostic and statistical manual of mental disorders,* 3rd ed. rev. (DSM-III-R). Washington, DC: American Psychiatric Association; 1987.

American Psychiatric Association. *Diagnostic and statistical manual of mental disorders,* 4th ed. (DSM-IV). Washington, DC: American Psychiatric Association; 1994.

American Psychiatric Association. *Diagnostic and statistical manual of mental disorders,* 4th ed., Text Revision (DSM-IV-TR). Washington, DC: American Psychiatric Association; 2000.

American Psychiatric Association. *Tardive dyskinesia: task force report 18.* Washington, DC: American Psychiatric Association; 1980b.

American Psychiatric Association. Task Force on Tardive Dyskinesia. *Tardive dyskinesia: A task force report of the American Psychiatric Association.* Washington, DC: American Psychiatric Association; 1992.

Amery B, Minichiello MD, Brown GL. Aggression in hyperactive boys: response to d-amphetamine. *J Am Acad Child Psychiatry* 1984;23:291–294.

Amitai Y, Frischer H. Excess Fatality from Desipramine in Children and Adolescents *J Am Acad Child Adolesc Psychiatry;*2006:45:54–60.

Anderson LT, Campbell M, Grega DM, Perry R, Small AM, Green WH. Haloperidol in the treatment of infantile autism: effects on learning and behavioral symptoms. *Am J Psychiatry* 1984;141:1195–1202.

Apter A, Ratzone G, King RA, Weizman A, Iancu I, Binder M, Riddle MA. Fluvoxamine open-label treatment of adolescent inpatients with obsessive-compulsive disorder or depression. *J Am Acad Child Adolesc Psychiatry* 1994;33:342–348.

Armenteros JL, Whitaker AH, Welilson M, Stedge DJ, Gorman J. Risperidone in adolescents with schizophrenia: an open pilot study. *J Am Acad Child Adolesc Psychiatry* 1997;36:694–700.

Arnold LE, Huestis RD, Smeltzer DJ, Scheib J, Wemmer D, Colner G. Levoamphetamine vs. dextroamphetamine in minimal brain dysfunction. *Arch Gen Psychiatry* 1976;33:292–301.

Arnold LE, Lindsay RL, Conners K, Wigal SB, Levine AJ, Johnson DE, West SA, Sangal RB, Bohan TP, and Zeldis JB. A double-blind, placebo-controlled withdrawal trial of dexmethylphenidate hydrochloride in children with attention deficit hyperactivity disorder. *J Child Adolesc Psychopharmacol* 2004;14:542–554.

Axelson, DA, Perel JM, Birmaher B, Rudolph GR, Nuss S, Bridge J, and Brent DA. Sertraline Pharmacokinetics and Dynamics in Adolescents. *J Am Acad Child Adolesc Psychiatry* 2002;41:1037–1044.

Ayd FJ Jr. Social issues: misuse and abuse. In: Benzodiazepines 1980: Current update. *Psychosomatics* 1980;21(October suppl):21–25.

Ayd FJ Jr. *Lexicon of Psychiatry, Neurology and the Neurosciences.* Baltimore: Williams & Wilkins; 1995.

Ayd FJ Jr. *Lexicon of Psychiatry, Neurology, and the Neurosciences,* 2nd Ed. Baltimore: Lippincott Williams & Wilkins; 2000.

Baldessarini RJ. Drugs and the treatment of psychiatric disorders. In: Gilman AG, Rall TW, Nies AS, Taylor P, eds. *Goodman and Gilman's The pharmacological basis of therapeutics,* 8th ed. New York: Pergamon Press; 1990:383–435.

Baldessarini RJ, Stephens JH. Clinical pharmacology and toxicology of lithium salts. *Arch Gen Psychiatry* 1970;22:72–77.

Ballenger JC, Carek DJ, Steele JJ, Cornish-McTighe D. Three cases of panic disorder with agoraphobia in children. *Am J Psychiatry* 1989;146:922–924.

Bangs ME, Petti TA, Janus M-D. Fluoxetine-induced memory impairment in an adolescent. *J Am Acad Child Adolesc Psychiatry* 1994;33:1303–1306.

Barrickman L, Noyes R, Kuperman S, Schumacher E, Verda M. Treatment of ADHD with fluoxetine: a preliminary trial. *J Am Acad Child Adolesc Psychiatry* 1991;30:762–767.

Barrickman LL, Perry PJ, Allen AJ, Superman S, Arndt SV, Herrmann KJ, Schumacher E. Bupropion versus methylphenidate in the treatment of attention-deficit hyperactivity disorder. *J Am Acad Child Adolesc Psychiatry* 1995;34:649–657.

Benfield P, Heel RC, Lewis SP. Fluoxetine: a review of its pharmacodynamic and pharmacokinetic properties, and therapeutic efficacy in depressive illness. *Drugs* 1986;32:481–508.

Bennett WG, Korein J, Kalmijn M, Grega DM, Campbell M. Electroencephalogram and treatment of hospitalized aggressive children with haloperidol or lithium. *Biol Psychiatry* 1983;12:1427–1440.

Berard R, Fong, R, Carpenter DJ, Thomason C, Wilkinson C. An international, multicenter, placebo-controlled trial of paroxetine in adolescents with major depressive disorder. *J Child Adolescn Psychopharmacol* 2006; 16:59–75.

Berg I, Hullin R, Allsopp M, O'Brien P. MacDonald R. Bipolar manic-depressive psychosis in early adolescence, a case report. *Br J Psychiatry* 1974;125:416–417.

Bergstrom RF, Lemberger L, Farid NA, Wolen RL. Clinical pharmacology and pharmacokinetics of fluoxetine: a review. *Br J Psychiatry* 1988;153(suppl 3):47–50.

Berney T, Kolvin I, Bhate SR, Garside RF, Jeans J, Kay B, Scarth L. School phobia: a therapeutic trial with clomipramine and short-term outcome. *Br J Psychiatry* 1981;138:110–118.

Bernstein GA, Borchardt CM, Perwien AR, Crosby RD, Kushner MG, Thuras PD, Last CG. Imipramine plus cognitive-behavioral therapy in the treatment of school refusal. *J Am Acad Child Adolesc Psychiatry* 2000;39:276–283.

Bernstein GA, Carroll ME, Crosby RD, Perwien AR, Go FS, Benowitz NL. Caffeine effects on learning, performance, and anxiety in normal school-age children. *J Am Acad Child Adolesc Psychiatry* 1994;33:407–415.

Bernstein JG. *Handbook of drug therapy in psychiatry,* 2nd ed. Littleton, MA: PSG Publishing; 1988.

Bevan P, Cools AR, Archer T. *Behavioural pharmacology of 5-HT.* Hillsdale, NJ: Lawrence Erlbaum; 1989.

Bezchlibnyk-Butler KZ and Virani AS, Editors. *Clinical Handbook of Psychotropic Drugs for Children and Adolescents.* Cambridge, MA: Hogrefe & Huber Publishers; 2004.

Biederman J, Baldessarini RJ, Goldblatt A, Lapey KA, Doyle A, Hesslein PS. A naturalistic study of 24-hour electrocardiographic recordings and echocardiographic findings in children and adolescents treated with desipramine. *J Am Acad Child Adolesc Psychiatry* 1993;32:805–813.

Biederman J, Baldessarini RJ, Wright V, Knee D, Harmatz JS. A double-blind placebo controlled study of desipramine in the treatment of ADD: I. Efficacy. *J Am Acad Child Adolesc Psychiatry* 1989a;28:777–784.

Biederman J, Baldessarini RJ, Wright V, Knee D, Harmatz JS, Goldblatt A. A double-blind placebo controlled study of desipramine in the treatment of ADD: II. Serum drug levels and cardiovascular findings. *J Am Acad Child Adolesc Psychiatry* 1989b;28:903–911.

Biederman J, Gastfriend DR, Jellinek MS. Desipramine in the treatment of children with attention deficit disorder. *J Clin Psychopharmacol* 1986;6:359–363.

Biederman J, Lopez FA, Boellner SW, Chandler MC. A randomized, double-blind, placebo-controlled, parallel-group study of SLI381 (Adderall XR) in children with attention-deficit/hyperactivity disorder. *Pediatrics* 2002;110:258–266.

Biederman J, Mick E, Wozniak J, Aleardi M, Spencer T. Faraone SV. An open-label trial of risperidone in children and adolescents with bipolar disorder. *J Child Adolesc Psychopharmacol* 2005;15:311–317.

Birmaher B, Axelson DA, Monk K, Kalas C, Clark DB, Ehmann M, Bridge J, Heo J, Brent DA. Fluoxetine for the treatment of childhood anxiety disorders. *J Am Acad Child Adolesc Psychiatry* 2003;42:415–423.

Birmaher B, Baker R, Kapur S, Quintana H, Ganguli R. Clozapine for the treatment of adolescents with schizophrenia. *J Am Acad Child Adolesc Psychiatry* 1992;31:160–164.

Birmaher B, Greenhill LL, Cooper TB, Fried J, Maminski B. Sustained release methylphenidate: pharmacokinetic studies in ADDH males. *J Am Acad Child Adolesc Psychiatry* 1989;28:768–772.

Birmaher B, Quintana H, Greenhill LL. Methylphenidate treatment of hyperactive autistic children. *J Am Acad Child Adolesc Psychiatry* 1988;27:248–251.

Birmaher B, Waterman GS, Ryan N, Cully M, Balach L, Ingram J, Brodsky M. Fluoxetine for childhood anxiety disorders. *J Am Acad Child Adolesc Psychiatry* 1994;33:993–999.

Birmaher B, Waterman GS, Ryan ND, Perel J, McNabb J, Balach L, Beaudry MB, Nasr FN, Karambelkar J, Elterich G, Quintana H, Williamson DE, Rao U. Randomized, controlled trial of amitriptyline versus placebo for adolescents with "treatment resistant" major depression. *J Am Acad Child Adolesc Psychiatry* 1998;37:527–535.

Black B, Uhde TW. Treatment of elective mutism with fluoxetine: a double-blind, placebo-controlled study. *J Am Acad Child Adolesc Psychiatry* 1994;33:1000–1006.

Blanz B, Schmidt MH. Clozapine for schizophrenia [Letter]. *J Am Acad Child Adolesc Psychiatry* 1993;32:223–224.

Borison RL, Pathiraja AP, Diamond BI, Meibach RC. Risperidone: clinical safety and efficacy in schizophrenia. *Psychopharmacol Bull* 1992;28:213–218.

Boulos C, Kutcher S, Gardner D, Young E. An open naturalistic trial of fluoxetine in adolescents and young adults with treatment-resistant major depression. *J Child Adolesc Psychopharmacol* 1992;2:103–111.

Boulos C, Kutcher S, Marton P, Simeon J, Ferguson B, Roberts N. Response to desipramine treatment in adolescent major depression. *Psychopharmacol Bull* 1991;27:59–65.

Bowden CL, Sarabia F. Diagnosing manic-depressive illness in adolescents. *Compr Psychiatry* 1980;21:263–269.

Bradley C. The behavior of children receiving Benzedrine. *Am J Psychiatry* 1937;94:577–585.

Breitner C. An approach to the treatment of juvenile delinquency. *Ariz Med* 1962;19:82–87.

Brown S-LB, van Praag HM, eds. *The role of serotonin in psychiatric disorders.* New York: Brunner/Mazel; 1991.

Bruun R. TSA medical update: treatment with clonidine. *Tourette Syndrome Assoc Newsletter,* Spring 1983.

Buitelaar JK, van der Gaag RJ, Swaab-Barneveld, H, Kuipers M. A placebo-controlled comparison of methylphenidate and pindolol in ADHD. American Academy of Child and Adolescent Psychiatry: Scientific Proceedings of the 41st Annual Meeting, New York: NY, October 25–30, 1994, New Research NR-6, 1994a;X:43.

Buitelaar JK, van der Gaag RJ, Swaab-Barneveld H, Kuipers M. Side effects of pindolol, a beta-blocker, in ADHD. American Academy of Child and Adolescent Psychiatry: Scientific Proceedings of the 41st Annual Meeting, New York: NY, October 25–30, 1994, New Research NR-7, 1994b;X:43.

Buitelaar JK, van der Gaag RJ, van der Hoeven J. Buspirone in the management of anxiety and irritability in children with pervasive developmental disorders: results of an open-label study. *J Clin Psychiatry* 1998;59:56–59.

Burke P, Puig-Antich J. Psychobiology of childhood depression. In: Lewis M, Miller SM, eds. *Handbook of developmental psychopathology*. New York: Plenum Press; 1990:327–339.

Burke RE, Fahn S, Jankovic J, et al. Tardive dystonia: Late-onset and persistent dystonia caused by antipsychotic drugs. *Neurology* 1982;32:1335–1346.

Cameron OG, Thyer BA. Treatment of pavor nocturnus with alprazolam. *J Clin Psychiatry* 1985;46:504.

Campbell M, Adams PB, Small AM, Kafantaris V, Silva RR, Shell J, Perry R, Overall JE. Lithium in hospitalized aggressive children with conduct disorder: a double-blind and placebo-controlled study. *J Am Acad Child Adolesc Psychiatry* 1995: 34:445–453.

Campbell M, Anderson LT, Small AM, Adams P, Gonzalez NM, Ernst M. Naltrexone in autistic children: behavioral symptoms and attentional learning. *J Am Acad Child Adolesc Psychiatry* 1993;32:1283–1291.

Campbell M, Anderson LT, Small AM, Locascio JJ, Lynch NS, Choroco MC. Naltrexone in autistic children: a double-blind and placebo-controlled study. *Psychopharmacol Bull* 1990;26:130–135.

Campbell M, Green WH, Deutsch SI. *Child and adolescent psychopharmacology*. Beverly Hills, CA: Sage; 1985.

Campbell M, Overall JE, Small AM, Sokol MS, Spencer EK, Adams P, Foltz RL, Monti KM, Perry R, Nobler M, Roberts E. Naltrexone in autistic children: an acute open dose range tolerance trial. *J Am Acad Child Adolesc Psychiatry* 1989;28:200–206.

Campbell M, Perry R, Green WH. The use of lithium in children and adolescents. *Psychosomatics* 1984a;25:95–106.

Campbell M, Small AM, Green WH, Jennings SJ, Perry R, Bennett WG, Anderson L. Behavioral efficacy of haloperidol and lithium carbonate: a comparison in hospitalized aggressive children with conduct disorder. *Arch Gen Psychiatry* 1984b;41:650–656.

Cantwell DP, Swanson J, Connor DF. Case study: adverse response to clonidine. *J Am Acad Child Adolesc Psychiatry* 1997;36:539–544.

Carlson GA, Rapport MD, Pataki CS, Kelly KL. Lithium in hospitalized children at 4 and 8 weeks: mood, behavior and cognitive effects. *J Child Psychol Psychiatry* 1992;33:411–425.

Carlson GA, Strober M. Manic-depressive illness in early adolescence. *J Am Acad Child Psychiatry* 1978;17:138–153.

Carlson JS, Kratochwill TR, Johnston HF. Sertraline treatment of 5 children diagnosed with selective mutism: a single-case research trial. *J Child Adolesc Psychopharmacol* 1999;9:293–306.

Casat CD, Pleasants DZ, Schroeder DH, Parler DW. Bupropion in children with attention deficit disorder. *Psychopharmacol Bull* 1989;25:198–201.

Castellanos FX, Giedd JN, Elia J, March WL, Ritchie GF, Hamburger SD, Rapoport JL. Controlled stimulant treatment of ADHD and comorbid Tourette's syndrome: efficacy of stimulant and dose. *J Am Acad Child Adolesc Psychiatry* 1997;36:589–596.

Chappell PB, Riddle MA, Scahill L, Lynch KA, Schultz R, Arnsten A, Leckman JF, Cohen DJ. Guanfacine treatment of comorbid attention deficit hyperactivity disorder and Tourette's syndrome: preliminary clinical experience. *J Am Acad Child Adolesc Psychiatry* 1995;34:1140–1146.

Charach A, Figueroa M, Chen S, Ickowicz A, Schachar R. Stimulant treatment over 5 years: Effects on Growth. *J Am Acad Child Adolesc Psychiatry* 2006;45:415–421.

Chatoor I, Wells KC, Conners CK, Seidel WT, Shaw D. The effects of nocturnally administered stimulant medication on EEG sleep and behavior in hyperactive children. *J Am Acad Child Psychiatry* 1983;22:337–342.

Chez MG, Buchanan CP. Reply to B. Rimland's "Comments on 'Secretin and autism: a two-part clinical investigation.'" *J Autism Dev Disord* 2000;30:97

Chez MG, Buchanan CP, Bagan BT, Hammer MS, McCarthy KS, Ovrutskaya I, Nowinski CV, Cohen. Secretin and autism: a two-part clinical investigation. *J Autism Dev Disord* 2000;30:87–94.

Chouinard G, Jones B, Remington G, Bloom D, Addington D, MacEwan GW, Labelle A, Beauclair L, Arnott W. A Canadian multicenter placebo-controlled study of fixed doses of risperidone and haloperidol in the treatment of chronic schizophrenic patients. *J Clin Psychopharmacol* 1993;13:25–40.

Cioli V, Corradino C, Piccinelli D, Rocchi MG, Valeri P. A comparative pharmacological study of trazodone, etoperidone, and 1-(m-chlorophenyl)piperazine. *Pharmacol Res Commun* 1984;16:85–100.

Ciraulo DA, Shader RI, Greenblatt DJ, Creelman W., eds. *Drug interactions in psychiatry.* Baltimore: Williams & Wilkins; 1989.

Clark DB, Birmaher B, Axelson D, Monk K, Kalas C, Ehmann M, Bridge J, Wood DS, Muthen B, Brent D. Fluoxetine for the treatment of childhood anxiety disorders: Open-label, long-term extension to a controlled trial. *J Am Acad Child Adolesc Psychiatry* 2005;44:1263–1270.

Clay TH, Gualtieri CT, Evans RW, Gullion CM. Clinical and neuropsychological effects of the novel antidepressant bupropion. *Psychopharmacol Bull* 1988;24:143–148.

Clements SD. *Minimal brain dysfunction in children: terminology and identification, phase one of a three-phase project.* Washington, DC: US Department of Health, Education, and Welfare; 1966. (NINDB monograph no. 3.)

Coccaro EF, Murphy DL, eds. *Serotonin in psychiatric disorders.* Washington, DC: American Psychiatric Press; 1990.

Coffey BJ. Anxiolytics for children and adolescents: traditional and new drugs. *J Child Adolesc Psychopharmacol* 1990;1:57–83.

Coffey B, Shader RI, Greenblatt DJ. Pharmacokinetics of benzodiazepines and psychostimulants in children. *J Clin Psychopharmacol* 1983;3:217–225.

Cohen DJ, Detlor J, Young JG, Shaywitz BA. Clonidine ameliorates Gilles de la Tourette syndrome. *Arch Gen Psychiatry* 1980;37:1350–1357.

Comings DE. *Tourette syndrome and human behavior.* Duarte, CA: Hope Press; 1990.

Comings DE, Comings BG. Tourette's syndrome and attention deficit disorder with hyperactivity: Are they genetically related? *J Am Acad Child Psychiatry* 1984;23:138–146.

Conner DF, Fletcher KE, Swanson JM. A meta-analysis of clonidine for symptoms of attention-deficit hyperactivity disorder. *J Am Acad Child Adolesc Psychiatry* 1999;38:1551–1559.

Conners CK. Recent drug studies with hyperkinetic children. *J Learn Disabil* 1971;4:476–483.

Conners CK, Casat CD, Gualtieri CT, Weller E, Reader M, Reiss A, Weller RA, Khayrallah M, Ascher J. Bupropion hydrochloride in attention deficit disorder with hyperactivity. *J Am Acad Child Adolesc Psychiatry* 1996;34:1314–1321.

Conners CK, Kramer R, Rothschild GH, Schwartz L, Stone A. Treatment of young delinquent boys with diphenylhydantoin sodium and methylphenidate. *Arch Gen Psychiatry* 1971;24:156–160.

Cooper GL. The safety of fluoxetine: an update. *Br J Psychiatry* 1988;153(suppl 3):77–86.

Cooper TB, Bergner PE, Simpson GM. The 24-hour lithium level as a prognosticator of dosage requirements. *Am J. Psychiatry* 1973;130:601–603.

Correll CU, Carlson HE. Endocrine and metabolic adverse effects of psychotropic medications in children and adolescents. *J Am Acad Child Adolesc Psychiatry* 2006;45:771–791.

Cozza SJ, Edison DL. Risperidone in adolescents [Letter]. *J Am Acad Child Adolesc Psychiatry* 1994;33:1211.

Croonenberghs J, Fegert JM, Findling RL, De Smedt G, Van Dongen S, and the Risperidone Disruptive Behavior Study Group. Risperidone in children with disruptive behavior disorders and subaverage intelligence: A 1-year, open-label study of 504 patients. *J Am Acad Child and Adolesc Psychiatry* 2005;44:64–72.

Crumrine PK, Feldman HM, Teodori J, Handen BL, Alvin RM. The use of methylphenidate in children with seizures and attention deficit disorder. *Ann Neurol* 1987;22:441–442.

Cueva JE, Overall JE, Small AM, Armenteros JL, Perry R, Campbell M. Carbamazepine in aggressive children with conduct disorder: a double-blind and placebo-controlled study. *J Am Acad Child Adolesc Psychiatry* 1996;35:480–490.

Cutts KK, Jasper HH. Effect of benzedrine sulfate and phenobarbital on behavior problem children with abnormal electroencephalograms. *Arch Neurol Psychiatry* 1939;411:1138–1145.

D'Amato G. Chlordiazepoxide in management of school phobia. *Dis Nerv Sys* 1962;23:292–295.

Davis KL, Charney D, Coyle JT, Nemeroff C, Editors. *Neuropsychopharmacology: The fifth generation of progress.* Philadelphia: Lippincott Williams & Wilkins, 2002.

Daviss WB, Perel JM, Rudolph GR, Axelson DA, Gilchrist R, Nuss S, Birmahjer B, Brent DA. Steady-state pharmacokinetics of bupropion SR in juvenile patients. *J Am Acad Child Adolesc Psychiatry* 2005;44:349–357.

DeGatta MF, Garcia MJ, Acosta A, Rey F, Guiterrez JR, Dominiquea-Gil A. Monitoring of serum levels of imipramine and desipramine and individuation of dose in enuretic children. *Ther Drug Monit* 1984;6:438–443.

DelBello MP, Findling RL, Kushner S, Wang D, Olson WH, Capece JA, Fazzio L, Rosenthal NR. A pilot controlled study of topiramate for mania in children and adolescents with bipolar disorder. *J Am Acad Child Adolesc Psychiatry* 2005;44:539–547.

DeLong GR, Aldershof AL. Long-term experience with lithium treatment in childhood: Correlation with clinical diagnosis. *J Am Acad Child Adolesc Psychiatry* 1987;26:389–394.

Denckla MB, Bemporad JR, MacKay MC. Tics following methylphenidate administration: A report of 20 cases. *JAMA* 1976;235:1349–1351.

Deutsch SI. Rationale for the administration of opiate antagonists in treating infantile autism. *Am J Ment Deficiency* 1986;90:631–635.

DeVeaugh-Geiss MD, Moroz G, Biederman J, Cantwell D, Fontaine R, Greist JH, Reichler R, Katz R, Landau P. Clomipramine hydrochloride in childhood and adolescent obsessive-compulsive disorder-a multicenter trial. *J Am Acad Child Adolesc Psychiatry* 1992;31:45–49.

Donnelly M, Rapoport JL, Potter WZ, Oliver J, Keysor CS, Murphy DL. Fenfluramine and dextroamphetamine treatment of childhood hyperactivity. *Arch Gen Psychiatry* 1989;46:205–212.

Donnelly M, Zametkin AJ, Rapoport JL, Ismond DR, Weingartner H, Lane E, Oliver J, Linnoila M, Potter WZ. Treatment of childhood hyperactivity with desipramine: plasma drug concentration, cardiovascular effects, plasma and urinary catecholamine levels, and clinical response. *Clin Pharmacol Ther* 1986;39:72–81.

Donovan SJ, Stewart JW, Nunes EV, Quitkin FM, Parides M, Daniel W, Susser E, Klein DF. Divalproex treatment for youth with explosive temper and mood lability: a double-blind, placebo-controlled crossover design (Published errata appear in *Am J Psychiatry* 157:1038 and *Am J Psychiatry* 157:1192). *Am J Psychiatry* 2000;157:818–820.

Donovan SJ, Susser ES, Nunes Stewart JW, Quitkin FM, Klein DF. Divalproex treatment of disruptive adolescents: A report of 10 cases. *J Clin Psychiatry* 1997;58:12–15.

Dostal T. Antiaggressive effect of lithium salts in mentally retarded adolescents. In: Annell A-L, ed. *Depressive states in childhood and adolescence.* Stockholm: Almqvist & Wiksell; 1972:491–498.

Drug facts and comparisons, 49th ed. St. Louis: Facts and Comparisons; 1995.

Drug interactions and side effects index, Oradell, NJ: Medical Economics; 1995.

Dubovsky SL. Severe nortriptyline intoxication due to change from a generic to a trade preparation. *J Nerv Ment Dis* 1987;175:115–117.

Dugas M, Zarifian E, Leheuzey M-F, Rovei V, Durand G, Morselli PL. Preliminary observations of the significance of monitoring tricyclic antidepressant plasma levels in the pediatric patient. *Ther Drug Monit* 1980;2:307–314.

Dummit ES III,, Klein RG, Tancer NK, Asche G, Martin J. Fluoxetine treatment of children with selective mutism: an open trial. *J Am Acad Child Adolesc Psychiatry* 1996;35:615–621.

Duncan MK. Using psychostimulants to treat behavioral disorders of children and adolescents. *J Child Adolesc Psychopharmacol* 1990;1:7–20.

DuPaul GJ, Barkley RA, McMurray MB. Response of children with ADHD to methylphenidate: interaction with internalizing symptoms. *J Am Acad Child Adolesc Psychiatry* 1994;33:894–903.

Effron AS, Freedman AM. The treatment of behavioral disorders in children with Benadryl. *J Pediatr* 1953;42:261–266.

Elia J, Borcherding BG, Rapoport JL, Kaysor CS. Methylphenidate and dextroamphetamine treatments of hyperactivity: Are there true nonresponders? *Psychiatry Res* 1991;36:141–155.

Elliott GR, Popper CW. Tricyclic antidepressants: the QT interval and other cardiovascular parameters [editorial]. *J Child Adolesc Psychopharmacol* 1990/1991;1:187–189.

Emslie GJ, Rush AJ, Weinberg WA, Kowatch RA, Hughes CW, Carmody T, Rintelmann J. A double-blind, randomized, placebo-controlled trial of fluoxetine in children and adolescents with depression. *Arch Gen Psychiatry* 1997;54:1031–1037.

Esposito S, Prange AJ Jr, Golden RN. The thyroid axis and mood disorders: Overview and future prospects. *Psychopharmcol. Bull.* 1997;33:205–217.

Evans RW, Clay TH, Gualtieri CT. Carbamazepine in pediatric psychiatry. *J Am Acad Child Adolesc Psychiatry* 1987;26:2–8.

Famularo R, Kinscherff R, Fenton T. Propranolol treatment for childhood posttraumatic stress disorder, acute type. *Am J Dis Child* 1988;142:1244–1247.

Fairbanks JM, Pine DS, Tancer NK, Dummit III ES, Kenetgen LM, Martin J, Asche BK, Klein RG. Open fluoxetine treatment of mixed anxiety disorders in children and adolescents. *J Child Adolesc Psychopharmacol* 1997;7:17–29.

Faraone SV, Biederman J, Monuteaux M, Spencer T. Long-term effects of extended-release mixed amphetamine salts treatment of attention-deficit/hyperactivity disorder. *J Child Adolesc Psychopharmacol* 2005;15:191–202.

Feighner JP, Cohen JB. Analysis of individual symptoms in generalized anxiety: a pooled, multi-study double-blind evaluation of buspirone. *Neuropsychobiology* 1989;21:124–130.

Feldman HM, Kolman BK, Gonzaga AM. Naltrexone and communication skills in young children with autism. *J Am Acad Child Adolesc Psychiatry* 1999;38:587–593.

Fenichel RR. Combining methylphenidate and clonidine: the role of post-marketing surveillance. *J Child Adolesc Psychopharmacol* 1995;5:155–156.

Ferguson HB, Simeon JG. Evaluating drug effects on children's cognitive functioning. *Prog Neuro-psychopharmacol Biol Psychiatry* 1984;8:683–686.

Findling RL, McNamara NK, Branicky LA, Schluchter MD, Lemon E, Blumer JL. A double-blind pilot study of risperidone in the treatment of conduct disorder. *J Am Acad Child Adolesc Psychiatry* 1999;39:509–516.

Findling RL, McNamara NK, Gracious BL, O'Riordan MA, Reed MD, Demeter C, Blumer JL. Quetiapine in nine youths with autistic disorder. *J Child Adolesc PSychopharmacol* 2004;14:287–294.

Findling RL, McNamara NK, Youngstrom EA, Stanbrey R, Gracious BL. Reed MD, Calabrese JR. Double-blind 18-month Trial of Lithium Versus Divalproex Maintenance Treatment in Pediatric Bipolar Disorder.. *J Am Acad Child Adolesc Psychiatry* 2005;44:409–417.

Findling RL, Reed MD, Myers C, O'Riordan MA, Fiala S, Branicky L, Waldorf B, Blumer JL. Paroxetine pharmacokinetics in depressed children and adolescents. *J Am Acad Child Adolesc Psychiatry* 1999;38:952–959.

Fish B. Drug therapy in child psychiatry: pharmacological aspects. *Compr Psychiatry* 1960;1:212–227.

Fish B. The "one child, one drug" myth of stimulants in hyperkinesis. *Arch Gen Psychiatry* 1971;25:193–203.

Fisher S. *Child research in psychopharmacology*. Springfield, IL: Charles C Thomas; 1959.

Fisman S, Steele M. Use of risperidone in pervasive developmental disorders: a case series. *J Child Adolesc Psychopharmacol* 1996;6:177–190.

Fitzpatrick PA, Klorman R, Brumaghim JT, Borgstedt AD. Effects of sustained-release and standard preparations of methylphenidate on attention deficit disorder. *J Am Acad Child Adolesc Psychiatry* 1992;31:226–234.

Flament MF, Rapoport JL, Berg CJ, Sceery W, Kilts C, Mellström B, Linnoila M. Clomipramine treatment of childhood obsessive-compulsive disorder: a double blind controlled study. *Arch Gen Psychiatry* 1985;42:977–983.

Flament MF, Rapoport JL, Murphy DL, Berg CJ, Lake CR. Biochemical changes during clomipramine treatment of childhood obsessive-compulsive disorder. *Arch Gen Psychiatry* 1987;44:219–225.

Fleischhacker WW, Bergmann KJ, Perovich R, et al. The Hillside Akathisia Scale: a new rating instrument for neuroleptic-induced akathisia. *Psychopharmacol Bull* 1989;25:222–226.

Fras I. Trazodone and violence [Letter]. *J Am Acad Child Adolesc Psychiatry* 1987;26:453.

Frazier JA, Biederman J, Jacobs TG, Tohen MF, Toma V, Feldman PD, Rater MA, Tarazi RA, Kim GA, Garfield SB, Gonzalez-Heydrich J, Nowlin ZM. Olanzapine in the treatment of bipolar disorder in juveniles (Abstract 40th Annual NCDEU meeting). *J Child Adolesc Psychopharmacol* 2000;10:237–238.

Frazier JA, Gordon CT, McKenna K, Lenane MC, Jih D, Rapoport JL. An open trial of clozapine in 11 adolescents with child-onset schizophrenia. *J Am Acad Child Adolesc Psychiatry* 1994;33:658–663.

Frazier JA, Meyer MC, Biederman J, Wozniak J, Wilens TE, Spencer TJ, Kim GS, Shapiro S. Risperidone treatment for juvenile bipolar disorder: a retrospective chart review. *J Am Acad Child Adolesc Psychiatry* 1999;38:960–965.

Friedman JM, Polifka JE. *The effects of neurologic and psychiatric drugs on the fetus and nursing infant*. Baltimore, MD: Johns Hopkins University Press; 1998.

Fritz GK, Rockney RM, Yeung AS. Plasma levels and efficacy of imipramine treatment for enuresis. *J Am Acad Child Adolesc Psychiatry* 1994;33:60–64.

Gadow KD. *Children on medication*. Vol. I: Hyperactivity, learning disabilities, and mental retardation. San Diego: College-Hill Press; 1986a.

Gadow KD. *Children on medication: Vol. II*. Epilepsy, emotional disturbance, and adolescent disorders. San Diego: College-Hill Press; 1986b.

Gadow KD, Nolan EE, Sverd J. Methylphenidate in hyperactive boys with comorbid tic disorder. II: Short-term behavioral effects in school settings. *J Am Acad Child Adolesc Psychiatry* 1992;31:462–471.

Gadow KD, Poling AG. *Pharmacotherapy and mental retardation*. Boston: College-Hill Press; 1988.

Gadow KD, Sverd J, Sprafkin J, Nolan EE, Ezor SN. Efficacy of methylphenidate for attention-deficit hyperactivity disorder in children with tic disorder. *Arch Gen Psychiatry* 1995;52:444–455.

Gadow KD, Sverd J, Sprafkin J, Nolan EE, Grossman S. Long-term methylphenidate therapy in children with comorbid attention-deficit hyperactivity disorder and chronic multiple tic disorder. *Arch Gen Psychiatry* 1999;56:330–336.

Gammon GD, Brown TE. Fluoxetine and methylphenidate in combination for treatment of attention deficit disorder and comorbid depressive disorder. *J Child Adolesc Psychopharmacol* 1993;3:1–10.

Garfinkel BD, Wender PH, Sloman L, O'Neil I. Tricyclic antidepressant and methylphenidate treatment of attention deficit disorder in children *J Am Acad Child Psychiatry* 1983;22:343–348.

Gastfriend DR, Biederman J, Jellinek MS. Desipramine in the treatment of adolescents with attention deficit disorder. *Am J Psychiatry* 1984;141:906–908.

Geller, B. Commentary on unexplained deaths of children on Norpramin. *J Am Acad Child Adolesc Psychiatry* 1991;30:682–684.

Geller B, Carr LG. Similarities and differences between adult and pediatric major depressive disorders. In: Georgotas A, Cancro R, eds. *Depression and mania*. New York: Elsevier; 1988:565–580.

Geller B, Cooper TB, Carr LG, Warham JE, Rodriguez A. Prospective study of scheduled withdrawal from nortriptyline in children and adolescents. *J Clin Psychopharmacol* 1987a;7:252–254.

Geller B, Cooper TB, Chestnut EC, Anker JA, Price DT, Yates E. Child and adolescent nortriptyline single dose kinetics predict steady state plasma levels and suggested dose: preliminary data. *J Clin Psychopharmacol* 1985;5:154–158.

Geller B, Cooper TB, Chestnut EC, Anker JA, Schluchter MD. Preliminary data on the relationship between nortriptyline plasma level and response in depressed children. *Am J Psychiatry* 1986;143:1283–1286.

Geller B, Cooper TB, Graham DL, Fetner HH, Marsteller FA, Wells JM. Pharmacokinetically designed double-blind placebo-controlled study of nortriptyline in 6- to 12-year-olds with major depressive disorder. *J Am Acad Child Adolesc Psychiatry* 1992;31:34–44.

Geller B, Cooper TB, Graham DL, Marsteller FA, Bryant DM. Double-blind placebo-controlled study of nortriptyline in depressed adolescents using a "fixed plasma level" design. *Psychopharmacol Bull* 1990;26:85–90.

Geller B, Cooper TB, McCombs HG, Graham D, Wells J. Double-blind placebo-controlled study of nortriptyline in depressed children using a "fixed plasma level" design. *Psychopharmacol Bull* 1989;25:101–108.

Geller B, Cooper TB, Schluchter MD, Warham JE, Carr LG. Child and adolescent nortriptyline single dose pharmacokinetic parameters: final report. *J Clin Psychopharmacol* 1987b;7:321–323.

Geller B, Cooper TB, Sun K, Zimerman B, Frazier J, Williams M, Heath J. Double-blind and placebo-controlled study of lithium for adolescent bipolar disorders with secondary substance dependency. *J Am Acad Child Adolesc Psychiatry* 1998;37:171–178.

Geller B, Fox LW, Fletcher M. Effect of tricyclic antidepressants on switching to mania and on the onset of bipolarity in depressed 6- to 12-year-olds. *J Am Acad Child Adolesc Psychiatry* 1993;32:43–50.

Geller B, Guttmacher LB, Bleeg M. Coexistence of childhood onset pervasive developmental disorder and attention deficit disorder with hyperactivity. *Am J Psychiatry* 1981;138:388–389.

Geller, DA, Wagner, KD, Emslie G, Murphy, T, Carpenter DJ, Wetherhold, E, Perera, P, Machin A, Gardiner C. Paroxetine treatment in children and adolescents with obsessive-compulsive disorder: A randomized, multicenter, double-blind, placebo-controlled trial.. *J Am Acad Child Adolesc Psychiatry* 2004;43:1387–1396.

Gerbino-Rosen G, Roofeh, D, Tompkins DA, Feryo D, Nusser L, Kranzler H, Napolitano B, Frederickson A, Henderson I, Rhinewine J, Kumra S. Hematological adverse events in clozapine-treated children and adolescents. *J Am Acad Child Adolesc Psychiatry* 2005;44:1024–1031.

Ghaziuddin N, Alessi NE. An open clinical trial of trazodone in aggressive children. *J Child and Adolescent Psychopharmacology* 1992;2:291–297.

Gilbert AR, Moore GJ, Keshavan MS, Paulson LAD, Narula V, MacMaster FP, Stewart CM, Rosenberg DR. Decrease in thalamic volumes of pediatric patients with obsessive-compulsive disorder who are taking paroxetine. *Arch Gen Psychiatry* 2000;57:449–456.

Gilbert DL, Batterson JR, Sethuraman G, Sallee FR. Tic reduction with risperidone versus pimozide in a randomized, double-blind, crossover trial. *J AM Acad Child Adolesc Psychiatry* 2004;43:206–214.

Gillberg C, Melander H, von Knorring A-L, Janols L-O, Thernlund G, Hagglof B, Eidevall-Wallin L, Gustafsson P, Kopp S. Long-term stimulant treatment of children with attention-deficit hyperactivity disorder symptoms. *Arch Gen Psychiatry* 1997;54:857–864.

Gittelman-Klein R, Klein, D. Controlled imipramine treatment of school phobia. *Arch Gen Psychiatry* 1971;25:204–207.

Gittelman-Klein R, Klein DF, Katz S, Saraf KR, Pollack E. Comparative effects of methylphenidate and thioridazine in hyperkinetic children: I. Clinical results. *Arch Gen Psychiatry* 1976;33:1217–1231.

Glick BS, Schulman D, Turecki S. Diazepam (Valium) treatment in childhood sleep disorder. *Dis Nerv Sys* 1971;32:565–566.

Good CR, Feaster CS, Krecko VF. Tolerability of oral loading of divalproex sodium in child psychiatry inpatients. *J Child Adolescent Psychopharmacol* 2001;11:53–56.

Gordon CT, State RC, Nelson JE, Hamburger SD, Rapoport JL. A double-blind comparison of clomipramine, desipramine, and placebo in the treatment of autistic disorder. *Arch Gen Psychiatry* 1993;50:441–447.

Graae F, Milner J, Rizzotto L, Klein RG. Clonazepam in childhood anxiety disorders. *J Am Acad Child Adolesc Psychiatry* 1994;33:372–376.

Green WH. Pervasive developmental disorders. In: Kestenbaum CJ, Williams DT, eds. *Handbook of clinical assessment of children and adolescents.* Vol. 1. New York: New York University Press; 1988:469–498.

Green WH. Psychosocial dwarfism: psychological and etiological considerations. In: Lahey BB, Kazdin AE, eds. *Advances in clinical child psychology.* Vol. 9. New York: Plenum Press; 1986:245–278.

Green WH. Schizophrenia with childhood onset. In: Kaplan HI, Sadock BJ, eds. *Comprehensive textbook of psychiatry,* 5th ed. Baltimore: Williams & Wilkins; 1989:1975–1981.

Green WH. The treatment of attention-deficit hyperactivity disorder with nonstimulant medications. *Child Adolesc Psychiatr Clin N Am* 1995;4:169–195.

Green WH, Campbell M, Hardesty AS, Grega DM, Padron-Gayol M, Shell J, Erlenmeyer-Kimling L. A comparison of schizophrenic and autistic children. *J Am Acad Child Psychiatry* 1984;23:399–409.

Green WH, Deutsch SI. Biological studies of schizophrenia with childhood onset. In: Deutsch SI, Weizman A, Weizman R, eds. *Application of basic neuroscience to child psychiatry*. New York: Plenum Medical Book; 1990:217–229.

Green WH, Deutsch SI, Campbell M, Anderson LT. Neuropsychopharmacology of the childhood psychoses: a critical review. In: Morgan DW, ed. *Psychopharmacology: impact on clinical psychiatry*. St. Louis: Ishiyaku EuroAmerica; 1985:139–173.

Green WH, Padron-Gayol M, Hardesty AS, Bassiri M. Schizophrenia with childhood onset: a phenomenological study of 38 cases. *J Am Acad Child Adolesc Psychiatry* 1992;31:968–976.

Greenblatt DJ, Shader RI. *Benzodiazepines in clinical practice*. New York: Raven Press; 1974.

Greenblatt DJ, Shader RI, Abernethy DR. Current status of benzodiazepines (first of two parts). *N Engl J Med* 1983;309:354–358.

Greenhill LL. Attention-deficit hyperactivity disorder in children. In: Garfinkel BD, Carlson GA, Weller EB, eds. *Psychiatric disorders in children and adolescents*. Philadelphia: WB Saunders; 1990:149–182.

Greenhill LL, Pliszka S, Dulcan MK, and the Work Group on Quality Issues. Practice Parameters for the Use of Stimulant Medications in the Treatment of Children, Adolescents, and Adults. *J Am Acad Child Adolesc Psychiatry* 2002;41 (Suppl):26S–49S.

Greenhill LL, Rieder RO, Wender PH, Bushsbaum M, Zahn TP. Lithium carbonate in the treatment of hyperactive children. *Arch Gen Psychiatry* 1973;28:636–640.

Greenhill LL, Solomon M, Pleak R, Ambrosini P. Molindone hydrochloride treatment of hospitalized children with conduct disorder. *J Clin Psychiatry* 1985;46:20–25.

Grizenko N, Vida S. Propranolol treatment of episodic dyscontrol and aggressive behavior in children [Letter]. *Can J Psychiatry* 1988;33:776–778.

Groh C. The psychotropic effect of Tegretol in non-epileptic children, with particular reference to the drug's indications. In: Birkmayer W, ed. *Epileptic seizures-behaviour-pain*. Bern: Hans Huber Publishers; 1976:259–263.

Gross MD. Imipramine in the treatment of minimal brain dysfunction in children. *Psychosomatics* 1973;14:283–285.

Gross MD, Wilson WC. *Minimal brain dysfunction*. New York: Brunner/Mazel; 1974.

Grothe DR, Calis KA, Jacobsen L, Kumra S, DeVane CL, Rapoport JL, Bergstrom RF, Kkurtz DL. Olanzapine pharmacokinetics in pediatric and adolescent inpatients with childhood-onset schizophrenia. *J Clin Psychopharmacol* 2000;20:220–225.

Gualtieri CT, Golden R, Evans RW, Hicks RE. Blood level measurement of psychoactive drugs in pediatric psychiatry. *Ther Drug Monit* 1984a;6:127–141.

Gualtieri CT, Golden RN, Fahs JJ. New developments in pediatric psychopharmacology. *Dev Behav Pediatr* 1983;4:202–209.

Gualtieri CT, Keenan PA, Chandler M. Clinical and neuropsychological effect on desipramine in children with attention deficit hyperactivity disorder. *J Clin Psychopharmacol* 1991;11:155–159.

Gualtieri CT, Quade D, Hicks RE, Mayo JP, Schroeder SR. Tardive dyskinesia and other clinical consequences of neuroleptic treatment in children and adolescents. *Am J Psychiatry* 1984b;141:20–23.

Gualtieri CT, Wafgin W, Kanoy R, Patrick K, Shen D, Youngblood W, Mueller R, Breese G. Clinical studies of methylphenidate serum levels in children and adults. *J Am Acad Child Psychiatry* 1982;21:19–26.

Gutgesell H, Atkins D, Barst R, Buck M, Franklin W, Humes R, Ringel R, Shaddy R, members, Taubert KA, AHA staff. AHA scientific statement: cardiovascular monitoring of children and adolescents receiving psychotropic drugs. *J Am Acad Child Adolesc Psychiatry* 1999;38:1047–1050. (Reprinted from *Circulation* 1999;99:979–982.)

Guy, W. Dosage Record and Treatment Emergent Symptoms Scale (DOTES) in ECDEU Assessment Manual for Psychopharmacology—Revised (DHEW Publ No ADM 76–338). Rockville, MD, US Department of Health, Education, and Welfare, Public Health Service, Alcohol, Drug Abuse, and Mental Health Administration, NIMH Psychopharmacology Research Branch, Division of Extramural Research Programs, 1976, 223–244.

Hamill PVV, Drizd TA, Johnson CL, Reed RB, Roche AF. NCHS growth charts, 1976. *Monthly Vital Statistics Reports* 1976;25(suppl 3):1–22. (Health Examination Survey Data, National Center for Health Statistics Publication [HRA] 76–1120.)

Handen BJ, Feldman HM, Lurier A, Murray PJH. Efficacy of methylphenidate among preschool children with developmental disabilities and ADHD. *J Am Acad Child Adolesc Psychiatry* 1999;38:805–812.

Handen BJ, Johnson CR, Lubetsky M. Efficacy of methylphenidate among children with autism and symptoms of attention-deficit hyperactivity disorder. *J Autism Dev Disord* 2000;30:245–255.

Hayes PE, Schulz SC. Beta-blockers in anxiety disorders. *J Affect Disord* 1987;13:119–130.

Hayes TA, Logan Panitch M, Marker E. Imipramine dosage in children: a comment on "imipramine and electrocardiographic abnormalities in hyperactive children." *Am J Psychiatry* 1975;132:546–547.

Hellings JA, Weckbaugh M, Nickel EJ, Cain SE, Zarcone JR, Reese RM, Hall S, Ermer DJ, Tsai LY, Schroeder SR, and Cook EH. A double-blind, placebo-controlled study of valproate for aggression in youth with pervasive developmental disorders. *J Child Adolesce Psychopharmacol* 2005;15:682–692.

Hersh CB, Sokol MS, Pfeffer CR. Transient psychosis with fluoxetine [Letter]. *J Am Acad Child Adolesc Psychiatry* 1991;31; 851.

Herskowitz J. Developmental neurotoxicology. In: Popper C, ed. *Psychiatric pharmacosciences of children and adolescents.* Washington, DC: American Psychiatric Press; 1987:81–123.

Holzer JF. The process of informed consent. *Bull Am Coll Surgeons* 1989;74:10–14.

Horowitz HA. Lithium and the treatment of adolescent manic depressive illness. *Dis Nerv Sys* 1977;38:480–483.

Horrigan JP, Barnhill LJ. Does guanfacine trigger mania in children? [Letter]. *J Child Adolesc Psychopharmacol* 1998;8:149–150.

Horrigan JP, Barnhill LJ. Guanfacine for treatment of attention-deficit hyperactivity disorder in boys. *J Child Adolesc Psychopharmacol* 1995;5:215–223.

Horrigan JP, Barnhill LJ. Risperidone and explosive aggressive autism. *J Autism Develop Disorders* 1997;27:313–323.

Huessy HR, Wright AL. The use of imipramine in children's behavior disorders. *Acta Paedopsychiatrica* 1970;37:194–199.

Hughes CW, Emslie GJ, Crismon ML, Wagner KD, Birmaher B, Geller B, Plizka SR, Ryan ND, Strober M, Trivedi MH, Toprac MG, Sedillo A, Llana ME, Lopez M, Rush AJ, and the Texas consensus panel on medication treatment of childhood major depressive disorder. The Texas children's medication algorithm project: Report of the Texas consensus conference panel on medication treatment of childhood major depressive disorder. *J Am Acad Child Adolesc Psychiatry* 1999;38:1442–1454.

Hunt RD. Treatment effects of oral and transdermal clonidine in relation to methylphenidate: an open pilot study in ADD-H. *Psychopharmacol Bull* 1987;23:111–114.

Hunt RD, Arnsten AFT, Asbell MD. An open trial of guanfacine in the treatment of attention-deficit hyperactivity disorder. *J Am Acad Child Adolesc Psychiatry* 1995;34:50–54.

Hunt RD, Capper L, O'Connell P. Clonidine in child and adolescent psychiatry. *J Child Adolesc Psychopharmacol* 1990;1:87–102.

Hunt RD, Cohen DJ, Shaywitz SE, Shaywitz BA. Strategies for study of the neurochemistry of attention deficit disorder in children. *Schizophr Bull* 1982;8:236–252.

Hunt RD, Lau S, Ryu J. Alternative therapies for ADHD. In: Greenhill LL, Osman BB, eds. *Ritalin: theory and patient management.* New York: Mary Ann Liebert; 1991:75–95.

Hunt RD, Minderaa RB, Cohen DJ. Clonidine benefits children with attention deficit disorder and hyperactivity: report of a double-blind placebo-crossover therapeutic trial. *J Am Acad Child Psychiatry* 1985;24:617–629.

Isojarvi JIT, Laatikainen TJ, Pakarinen AJ, Juntunen KTS, Myllyla VV. Polycystic ovaries and hyperandrogenism in women taking valproate for epilepsy. *N Engl J Med.* 1993;329:1383–1388.

Jafri AB. Fluoxetine side effects [Letter]. *J Am Acad Child Adolesc Psychiatry* 1991;31:852.

Jain U, Birmaher B, Garcia M, Al-Shabbout M, Ryan N. Fluoxetine in children and adolescents with mood disorders: a chart review of efficacy and adverse effects. *J Child Adolesc Psychopharmacol* 1992;2:259–265.

Jann MW. Clozapine. *Pharmacotherapy* 1991;11:179–195.

Jaselskis CA, Cook EH, Fletcher KE, Leventhal BL. Clonidine treatment of hyperactive and impulsive children with autistic disorder. *J Clin Psychopharmacol* 1992;12:322–327.

Jatlow PI. Psychotropic drug disposition during development. In: Popper C, ed. *Psychiatric pharmacosciences of children and adolescents.* Washington, DC: American Psychiatric Press; 1987:27–44.

Jefferson JW, Greist JH, Ackerman DL, Carroll JA. *Lithium encyclopedia for clinical practice,* 2nd ed. Washington, DC: American Psychiatric Press; 1987.

Jefferson JW, Greist JH, Clagnaz PJ, Eischens RR, Marten WC, Evenson ME. Effect of strenuous exercise on serum lithium level in man. *Am J Psychiatry* 1982;139:1593–1595.

Jerome L. Hypomania with fluoxetine [Letter]. *J Am Acad Child Adolesc Psychiatry* 1991;30:850–851.

Jeste DV, Wyatt RJ. *Understanding and treating tardive dyskinesia.* New York: Guilford Press; 1982.

Johnston C, Pelham WE, Hoza J, Sturges J. Psychostimulant rebound in attention deficit disordered boys. *J Am Acad Child Adolesc Psychiatry* 1988;27:806–810.

Johnston HF. More on valproate and polycystic ovaries. [Letter]. *J Am Acad Child Adolesc Psychiatry* 1999;38:354.

Joshi PT, Capozzoli JA, Coyle JT. Low-dose neuroleptic therapy for children with childhood-onset pervasive developmental disorder. *Am J Psychiatry* 1988;145:335–338.

Joshi PT, Walkup JT, Capozzoli JA, Detrinis RB, Coyle JT. The use of fluoxetine in the treatment of major depressive disorder in children and adolescents. Paper presented at the 36th Annual Meeting of the American Academy of Child and Adolescent Psychiatry, October 11–15; 1989, New York.

Jou RJ, Handen BL, Hardan AY. Retrospective Assessment of Atomoxetine in Children and Adolescents with Pervasive Developmental Disorders. *J Child Adolesc Psychopharmacol* 2005;15:325–330.

Kafantaris V, Campbell M, Padron-Gayol MV, Small AM, Locascio JJ, Rosenberg CR. Carbamazepine in hospitalized aggressive conduct disorder children: An open pilot study. *Psychopharmacol Bull* 1992;28:193–199.

Kafantaris V, Colette D, Dicker R, Padula G, Kane JM. Lithium treatment of acute mania in adolescents: A large open trial. *J Am Acad Child Adolesc Psychiatry* 2003;42:1038–1045.

Kallen B, Tandberg A. Lithium and pregnancy. *Acta Psychiatr Scand* 1983;68:134–139.

Kane JM, Lieberman JA. *Adverse effects of psychotropic drugs.* New York: Guilford Press; 1992.

Kaplan SL, Simms RM, Busner J. Prescribing practices of outpatient child psychiatrists. *J Am Acad Child Adolesc Psychiatry* 1994;33:35–44.

Kashani JH, Shekim WO, Reid JC. Amitriptyline in children with major depressive disorder: a double-blind crossover pilot study. *J Am Acad Child Psychiatry* 1984;23:348–351.

Kastner T, Finesmith R, Walsh K. Long-term administration of valproic acid in the treatment of affective symptoms in people with mental retardation. *J Clin Psychopharmacol* 1993;13:448–451.

Kastner T, Friedman DL, Plummer AT, Ruiz MQ, Henning D. Valproic acid for the treatment of children with mental retardation and mood symptomatology. *Pediatrics* 1990;86:467–472.

Kaufmann CA, Wyatt RJ. Neuroleptic malignant syndrome. In: Meltzer HY, ed. *Psychopharmacology: the third generation of progress.* New York: Raven Press; 1987:1421–1430.

Kemner JE, Starr HL, Ciccone PE, Hooper-Wood CG, Crockett RS. Outcomes of OROS®methylphenidate compared with atomoxetine in children with ADHD: A multicenter, randomized prospective study. *Advances in Therapy* 2005;22:498–512.

Kemph JP, DeVane CL, Levin GM, Jarecke R, Miller RL. Treatment of aggressive children with clonidine: results of an open pilot study. *J Am Acad Child Adolesc Psychiatry* 1993;32:577–581.

Kessler AJ, Barklage NE, Jefferson JW. Mood disorders in the psychoneurological borderland: three cases of responsiveness to carbamazepine. *Am J Psychiatry* 1989;146:81–83.

King RA, Riddle MA, Chappell PB, Hardin MT, Anderson GM, Lombroso P, Scahill L. Emergence of self-destructive phenomena in children and adolescents during fluoxetine treatment. *J Am Acad Child Adolesc Psychiatry* 1991;30:179–186.

Klein DF, Gittelman R, Quitkin F, Rifkin A. *Diagnosis and drug treatment of psychiatric disorders: adults and children.* Baltimore: Williams & Wilkins; 1980.

Klein RG. Pharmacotherapy of childhood hyperactivity: an update. In:Meltzer HY, ed. *Psychopharmacology: the third generation of progress.* New York: Raven Press; 1987:1215–1224.

Klein RG. Thioridazine effects on the cognitive performance of children with attention-deficit hyperactivity disorder. *J Child Adolesc Psychopharmacol,* 1990–1991;1:263–270.

Klein RG, Abikoff H, Klass E, Ganeles D, Seese LM, Pollack S. Clinical efficacy of methylphenidate in conduct disorder with and without attention deficit hyperactivity disorder. *Arch Gen Psychiatry* 1997;54:1073–1080.

Klein RG, Koplewicz HS, Kanner A. Imipramine treatment of children with separation anxiety disorder. *Am J Acad Child Adolesc Psychiatry* 1992;31:21–28.

Klein RG, Landa B, Mattes JA, Klein DF. Methylphenidate and growth in hyperactive children: a controlled withdrawal study. *Arch Gen Psychiatry* 1988;45:1127–1130.

Klein RG, Last CG. *Anxiety disorders in children.* Newbury Park, CA: Sage; 1989.

Klein RG, Mannuzza S. Hyperactive boys almost grown up: III. Methylphenidate effects on ultimate height. *Arch Gen Psychiatry* 1988;45:1131–1134.

Kline AH. Diazepam and the management of nocturnal enuresis. *Clin Med* 1968;75:20–22.

Klorman R, Brumaghim JT, Salzman LF, Strauss J, Borgstedt AD, McBride MC, Loeb S. Effects of methylphenidate on attention-deficit hyperactivity disorder with and without aggressive/noncompliant features. *J Abnorm Psychol* 1988a;97:413–422.

Klorman R, Coons HW, Brumaghim JT, Borgstedt AD, Fitzpatrick P. Stimulant treatment for adolescents with attention deficit disorder. *Psychopharmacol Bull* 1988b;24:88–92.

Kofoed L, Tadepalli G, Oesterheld JR, Awadallah S, Shapiro S. Case series: clonidine has no systematic effects on PR or QT_c intervals in children. *J Am Acad Child Adolesc Psychiatry* 1999;38:1193–1196.

Kolman BK, Feldman HM, Handen BL, Janosky JE. Naltrexone in young autistic children: a double-blind, placebo-controlled crossover study. *J Am Acad Child Adolesc Psychiatry* 1995;34:223–231.

Kolman BK, Feldman HM, Handen BJ, Janosky JE. Naltrexone in young autistic children: replication study and learning measures. *J Am Acad Child Adolesc Psychiatry* 1997;36:1570–1578.

Korein J, Fish B, Shapiro T, Gehner EW, Levidon L. EEG and behavioral effects of drug therapy in children: chlorpromazine and diphenhydramine. *Arch Gen Psychiatry* 1971;24:552–563.

Kraft IA, Ardall C, Duffy JH, Hart JT, Pearce P. A clinical study of chlordiazepoxide used in psychiatric disorders of children. *Int J Neuropsychiatry* 1965;1:433–437.

Krakowski AJ. Chlordiazepoxide in treatment of children with emotional disturbances. *N Y State J Med* 1963;63:3388–3392.

Krakowski AJ. Amitriptyline in treatment of hyperkinetic children. *Psychosomatics* 1965;6:355–360.

Kramer AD, Feiguine RJ. Clinical effects of amitriptyline in adolescent depression: a pilot study. *J Am Acad Child Psychiatry* 1981;20:636–644.

Kranzler H, Roofeh D, Gerbino-Rosen G, Dombrowiski C, McMeniman M, DeThomas C, Frederickson A, Nusser L, Bienstock MD, Fisch GS, and Kumra S. Clozapine: Its impact on aggressive behavior among children and adolescents with schizophrenia. *J Am Acad child Adolesc Psychiatry* 2005;44:55–63.

Kranzler HR. Use of buspirone in an adolescent with overanxious disorder. *J Am Acad Child Adolesc Psychiatry* 1988;27:789–790.

Kuhn-Gebhart V. Behavioural disorders in non-epileptic children and their treatment with carbamazepine. In: Birkmayer W, ed. *Epileptic seizures-behaviour-pain.* Bern: Hans Huber Publishers; 1976:264–267.

Kumra S, Frazier JA, Jacobson LK, McKenna K, Gordon CT, Lenane MC, Hamburger SD, Smith AK, Allbus KE, Alaghband-Rad J, Rapoport JL. Childhood-onset schizophrenia: a double-blind clozapine-haloperidol comparison. *Arch Gen Psychiatry* 1996;53:1090–1097.

Kumra S, Herion D, Jacobsen LK, Briguglia C, Grothe D. Case study: risperidone-induced hepatotoxicity in pediatric patients. *J Am Acad Child Adolesc Psychiatry* 1997;36:701–705.

Kumra S, Jacobson LK, Lenane M, Karp BI, Frazier JA, Smith AK, Bedwell J, Lee P, Malanga CJ, Hamburger S, Rapoport JL. Childhood-onset schizophrenia: an open-label study of olanzapine in adolescents. *J Am Acad Child Adolesc Psychiatry* 1998;37:377–385.

Kuperman S, Stewart MA. Use of propranolol to decrease aggressive outbursts in younger patients. *Psychosomatics* 1987;28:315–319.

Kutcher, S, Editor. *Practical child and adolescent psychopharmacology.* Cambridge, UK: Cambridge University Press; 2002.

Kutcher SP. *Child and adolescent psychopharmacology.* Philadelphia: WB Saunders; 1997.

Kutcher S, Boulos C, Ward B, Marton P, Simeon J, Ferguson HB, Szalai J, Katic M, Roberts N, Dubois C, Reed K. Response to desipramine treatment in adolescent depression: a fixed-dose, placebo-controlled trial. *J Am Acad Child Adolesc Psychiatry* 1994;33:686–694.

Kutcher SP, MacKenzie S. Successful clonazepam treatment of adolescents with panic disorder [Letter]. *J Clin Psychopharmacol* 1988;8:299–301.

Kutcher SP, MacKenzie S, Galarraga W, Szalai J. Clonazepam treatment of adolescents with neuroleptic-induced akathisia. *Am J Psychiatry* 1987;144:823–824.

Kutcher SP, Marton P, Korenblum M. Adolescent bipolar illness and personality disorder. *J Am Acad Child Adolesc Psychiatry* 1990;29:355–358.

Labellarte M, Biederman J, Emslie G, Ferguson J, Khan A, Ruckle J, Sallee R, Riddle M. Multiple-dose pharmacokinetics of fluvoxamine in children and adolescents. *J AM Acad Child Adolesc Psychiatry* 2004;43:1497–1505.

Lader M. Fluoxetine efficacy vs comparative drugs: an overview. *Br J Psychiatry* 1988:153(suppl 3):51–58.

Law SF, Schachar RJ. Do typical clinical doses of methylphenidate cause tics in children treated for attention-deficit hyperactivity disorder? *J Am Acad Child Adolesc Psychiatry* 1999;38:944–951.

Latz SR, McCracken JT. Neuroleptic malignant syndrome in children and adolescents: two case reports and a warning. *J Child Adolesc Psychopharmacol* 1992;2:123–129.

Leckman JF, Cohen DJ, Detlor J, Ort S, Shaywitz BA, Cohen DJ. Clonidine in the treatment of Tourette syndrome: a review of data. In: Friedhoff AJ, Chase TN, eds. *Gilles de la Tourette syndrome.* New York: Raven Press; 1982:391–401.

Leckman JF, Detlor J, Harcherik DF, Stevenson J, Ort SI, Cohen DJ. Short- and long-term treatment of Tourette's syndrome with clonidine: a clinical perspective. *Neurology* 1985;35:343–351.

Leckman JF, Hardin MT, Riddle MA, Stevenson J, Ort SI, Cohen DJ. Clonidine treatment of Gilles de la Tourette's syndrome. *Arch Gen Psychiatry* 1991;48:324–328.

Lefkowitz MM. Effects of diphenylhydantoin on disruptive behavior. *Arch Gen Psychiatry* 1969;20:643–651.

Lena B, Surtees SJ, Maggs R. The efficacy of lithium in the treatment of emotional disturbance in children and adolescents. In: Johnson FN, Johnson S, eds. *Lithium in medical practice.* Baltimore: University Park Press; 1978:79–83.

Leonard HL, Swedo SE, Lenane MC, Rettew DC, Cheslow DL, Hamburger SD, Rapoport JL. A double-blind desipramine substitution during long-term clomipramine treatment in children and adolescents with obsessive-compulsive disorder. *Arch Gen Psychiatry* 1991;48:922–927.

Leonard HL, Swedo SE, Rapoport JL, Koby EV, Lenane MC, Cheslow DL, Hamburger SD. Treatment of obsessive-compulsive disorder with clomipramine and desipramine in children and adolescents: a double-blind crossover comparison. *Arch Gen Psychiatry* 1989;46:1088–1092.

Leonard HL, Topol D, Bukstein O, Hindmarsh D, Allen AJ, Swedo SE. Clonazepam as an augmenting agent in the treatment of childhood-onset obsessive-compulsive disorder. *J Am Acad Child Adolesc Psychiatry* 1994;33:692–694.

Levin GM, Burton-Teston K, Murphy T. Development of precocious puberty in two children treated with clonidine for aggressive behavior. *J Child Adolesc Psychopharmacol* 1993;3:127–131.

Levkovitch Y, Kaysar N, Kronnenberg Y, Hagai H, Gaoni B. Clozapine for schizophrenia [Letter]. *J Am Acad Child Adolesc Psychiatry* 1994;33:431.

Levy RH. Psychopharmacological interventions. In: Katz SE, Nardacci D, Sabatini A, eds. *Intensive treatment of the homeless mentally ill.* Washington, DC: American Psychiatric Press; 1993:129–165.

Lingjaerde O, Ahlfors UG, Bech P, et al. The UKU side effect rating scale: a new comprehensive rating scale for psychotropic drugs, and a cross sectional study of side effects in neuroleptic-treated patients. *Acta Psychiatr Scand Suppl* 1987;76:1–100.

Linnoila M, Dejong J, Virkkunen M. Monoamines, glucose metabolism, and impulse control. *Psychopharmacol Bull* 1989;25:404–406.

Linnoila M, Gualtieri CT, Jobson K, Staye J. Characteristics of the therapeutic response to imipramine in hyperactive children. *Am J Psychiatry* 1979;136:1201–1203.

Looker A, Conners CK. Diphenylhydantoin in children with severe temper tantrums. *Arch Gen Psychiatry* 1970;23:80–89.

Lowe TL, Cohen DJ, Detlor J, Kremenitzer MW, Shaywitz BA. Stimulant medications precipitate Tourette's syndrome. *JAMA* 1982;247:1729–1931.

Lucas AR, Pasley FC. Psychoactive drugs in the treatment of emotionally disturbed children: haloperidol and diazepam. *Compr Psychiatry* 1969;10:376–386.

MacLeod CM, Dekaban AS, Hunt E. Memory impairment in epileptic patients: selective effects of phenobarbital concentration. *Science* 1978;202:1102–1104.

Malhotra S, Santosh PR. An open clinical trial of buspirone in children with attention-deficit/hyperactivity disorder. *J Am Acad Child Adolesc Psychiatry* 1998;37:364–371.

Malone RP, Delaney MA, Luebbert JF, Cater J, Campbell M. A double-blind placebo-controlled study of lithium in hospitalized aggressive children and adolescents with conduct disorder. *Arch Gen Psychiatry* 2000;57:649–654.

Mandoki M. Clozapine for adolescents with psychosis: literature review and two case reports. *J Child Adolesc Psychopharmacol* 1993;3:213–221.

Mann JJ, Marzuk PM, Arango V, McBride PA, Leon AC, Tierney H. Neurochemical studies of violent and nonviolent suicide. *Psychopharmacol Bull* 1989;25:407–413.

Manos MJ, Short EJ, Findling RL. Differential effectiveness of methylphenidate and Adderall in school-age youth with attention-deficit/hyperactivity disorder. *J Am Acad Child Adolesc Psychiatry* 1999;38:813–819.

March JS, Biederman J, Wolkow R, Safferman A, Mardekian J, Cook EH, Cutler NR, Cominguez R, Ferguson J, Muller B, Riesenberg R, Rosenthal M, Sallee FR, Wagner KD. Sertraline in children and adolescents with obsessive-compulsive disorder: a multicenter randomized controlled trial. *JAMA* 1998;280:1752–1756.

Mattes JA, Gittelman R. Growth of hyperactive children on maintenance regimen of methylphenidate. *Arch Gen Psychiatry* 1983;40:317–321.

Martin A, Landau J, Leebens P, Ulizio K, Cicchetti D, Scahill L, Leckman JF. Risperidone-associated with gain in children and adolescents: a retrospective chart review. *J Child Adolesc Psychopharmacol* 2000;10:259–268.

Martin A, Koenign K, Scahill L, Bregman J. Open-label quetiapine in the treatment of children and adolescents with autistic disorder. *J Child Adolesc Psychopharmacol* 1999;9:99–107.

Martin A, Scahill L, Charney DS, Leckman JF, Editors. *Pediatric psychopharmacology: principles and practice.* New York: Oxford University Press; 2003.

McBride MC, Wang DD, Torres C. Methylphenidate in therapeutic doses does not lower seizure threshold. *Ann Neurol* 1986;20:428.

McConville BJ, Minnery KL, Sorter MT, West SA, Friedman LM, Christian K. An open study of the effects of sertraline on adolescent major depression. *J Child Adolesc Psychopharmacol* 1996;6:41–51.

McCormick LH, Rizzuto GT, Knuckles HB. A pilot study of buspirone in attention-deficit hyperactivity disorder. *Arch Fam Med* 1994;3:68–70.

McCracken JT, Biederman J, Greenhill LL, Swanson JM, McGough JJ, Spencer TJ, Posner K, Wigal S, Patake C, Zhang Y, Tulloch S. Analog classroom assessment of a once-daily mixed amphetamine formulations, SLI381 (Adderall XR) in children with ADHD. *J Am Acad Child Adolesc Psychiatry* 2003;42:673–683.

McCracken JT, Martin W. Clonidine side effect [Letter]. *J Am Acad Child Adolesc Psychiatry* 1997;36:160–161.

McCracken JT, McGough J, Shah B, Cronin P, Hong D, Aman MG, Arnold LE, Lindsay R, Nash P, Hollway J, McDougle CJ, Posey D, Swiezy N, Kohn A, Scahill L, Martin A, Koenig, K, Volkmar F, Carroll D, Lancor A, Tierney E, Ghuman J, Gonzalez NM, Grados, M, Vitiello B, Ritz L, Davies M, Robinson J, McMahon D. [Research Units on Pediatric Psychopharmacology Autism Network]. Risperidone in children with autism and serious behavioral problems. *NEJM* 2002;347:314–321.

McDougle CJ, Holmes JP, Bronson MR, Anderson GM, Volkmar FR, Price LH, Cohen DJ. Risperidone treatment of children and adolescents with pervasive developmental disorders: a prospective open-label study. *J Am Acad Child Adolesc Psychiatry* 1997;36:685–693.

McDougle CJ, Kem DL, Posey DJ. Case series: Use of ziprasidone for maladaptive symptoms in youths with autism. *J Am Acad Child Adolesc Psychiatry* 2002;41:921–927.

McGough JJ, Biederman J, Wigal SB, Lopez FA, McCracken JT, Spencer T, Zhang Y, Tulloch SJ. Long-term tolerability and effectiveness of once-daily mixed amphetamine salts (Adderall XR) in children with ADHD. *J Am Acad Child Adolesc Psychiatry* 2005;44:539–547.

Meyers B, Tune LE, Coyle JT. Clinical response and serum neuroleptic levels in childhood schizophrenia. *Am J Psychiatry* 1980;137:1459–1460.

Michelson D, Allen AJ, Busner J, Casat C, Dunn D, Kratochvil C, Newcorn J, Sallee FR, Sangal RB, Saylor K, West S. Once-daily atomoxetine treatment for children and adolescents with attention deficit hyperactivity disorder: A randomized, placebo-controlled study. *Am J Psychiatry* 2002;159:1896–1901.

Michelson D, Faries DE, Wernicke J, Kelsey DK, Kendrick KL, Sallee FR, Spencer T. (Atomoxetine ADHD Study Group). Atomoxetine in the treatment of children and adolescents with ADHD: A randomized, placebo-controlled dose-response study. *Pediatrics* 2001;108:e83.

Molitch M, Eccles AK. The effect of benzedrine sulfate on the intelligence scores of children. *Am J Psychiatry* 1937;94:587–590.

Molitch M, Poliakoff S. The effect of benzedrine sulfate on enuresis. *Arch Pediatr* 1937;54:499–501.

Molitch M, Sullivan JP. The effect of benzedrine sulfate on children taking the New Stanford Achievement Test. *Am J Orthopsychiatry* 1937;7:519–522.

Morselli PL, Bianchetti G, Dugas M. Therapeutic drug monitoring of psychotropic drugs in children. *Pediatr Pharmacol* 1983;3:149–156.

Mozes T, Toren P, Chernauzan N, Mester R, Yoran-Hegesh R, Blumensohn R, Weizman A. Clozapine treatment in very early onset schizophrenia. *J Am Acad Child Adolesc Psychiatry* 1994;33:65–70.

MTA Cooperative Group. A 14-month randomized clinical trial of treatment strategies for attention-deficit/hyperactivity disorder. *Arch Gen Psychiatry* 1999a;56:1073–1986.

MTA Cooperative Group. Moderators and mediators of treatment response for children with attention-deficit/hyperactivity disorder. *Arch Gen Psychiatry* 1999b;56:1088–1096.

Musten LM, Firestone P, Pisterman S, Bennett S, Mercer J. Effects of methylphenidate on preschool children with ADHD: cognitive and behavioral functions. *J Am Acad Child Adolesc Psychiatry* 1997;36:1407–1415.

Myers WC, Carrera F III. Carbamazepine-induced mania with hypersexuality in a 9-year-old boy. *Am J Psychiatry* 1989;146:400.

Naruse H, Nagahata M, Nakane Y, Shirahashi K, Takesada M, Yamazaki K. A multi-center double-blind trial of pimozide (Orap), haloperidol and placebo in children with behavioral disorders, using crossover design. *Acta Paedopsychiatr* 1982;48:173–184.

National Institute of Mental Health/National Institutes of Health Consensus Development Panel. Mood disorders: pharmacologic prevention of recurrences. *Am J Psychiatry* 1985;142:469–476.

National Medical Association (102nd Annual Convention and Scientific Assembly of the National Medical Association, San Diego, CA, August 3, 2004) Summary downloaded from: http://

www.jnj.com/news/jnj_news/20040802_151359.htm?pageTemplate+printer_friendly   on   4/1/ 2006.)

Neppe VM, Ward NG. The evaluation and management of neuroleptic-induced acute extrapyra-midal syndromes. In: Neppe VM, ed. *Innovative psychopharmacology.* New York: Raven Press; 1989:152–176.

New York State Department of Health. *Safe, effective and therapeutically equivalent prescription drugs,* 7th ed. Albany, NY: New York State Department of Health Office of Health Systems Management; 1988.

Newcorn JH, Spencer TJ, Biederman J, Milton DR, Michelson D. Atomoxetine treatment in children and adolescents with attention-deficit/hyperactivity disorder and comorbid oppositional defiant disorder. *J Am Acad Child Adolesc Psychiatry* 2005;44:240–248.

Newton JEO, Cannon DJ, Couch L, Fody EP, McMillan DE, Metzer WS, Paige SR, Reid GM, Summers BN. Effects of repeated drug holidays on serum haloperidol concentration, psy-chiatric symptoms, and movement disorders in schizophrenic patients. *J Clin Psychiatry* 1989;50:132–135.

Nicolson R, Awad G, Sloman L. An open trial of risperidone in young autistic children. *J Am Acad Child Adolesc Psychiatry* 1998;37:372–376.

Nobile M, Bellotti B, Marino C, Molteni M, Battaglia M. An open trial of paroxetine in the treat-ment of children and adolescents diagnosed with dysthymia. *J Child Adolesc Psychopharmacol* 2000;10:103–109.

Noyes R. Beta-adrenergic blockers. In: Last CG, Hersen M, eds. *Handbook of anxiety disorders.* New York: Pergamon Press; 1988:445–459.

Nurcombe B. Malpractice. In: Lewis M, ed. *Child and adolescent psychiatry: a comprehensive textbook.* Baltimore: Williams & Wilkins; 1991:1127–1139.

Nurcombe B, Partlett DF. *Child mental health and the law.* New York: Free Press; 1994:220–272.

Olvera RL, Pliszka SR, Luh J, Tatum R. An open trial of venlafaxine in the treatment of attention-deficit/hyperactivity disorder in children and adolescents. *J Child Adolesc Psychopharmacol* 1996;6:241–250.

Owley, T, Walton L, Salt J, Guter SJ, Winnega M, Leventhal BL, Cook Jr, EH. An open-label trial of escitalopram in pervasive developmental disorders. *J Am Acad Child Adolesc Psychiatry* 2005:343–348.

Oxford English Dictionary, Second Edition. Oxford: Oxford University Press; 1989.

Pangalila-Ratulangi EA. Pilot evaluation of Orap (Pimozide, R 6238) in child psychiatry. *Psychiatr Neurol Neurochir* 1973;76:17–27.

Papatheodorou G, Kutcher SP, Katic M, Szalai JP. The efficacy and safety of divalproex sodium in the treatment of acute mania in adolescents and young adults: an open clinical trial. *J Clin Psychopharmacol* 1995;15:110–116.

Pappagallo M, Silva R. The effect of atypical antipsychotic agents on prolactin levels in children and adolescents. *J Child Adolesc Psychopharmacol* 2004;14:359–371.

Pare CMB, Kline N, Hallstrom C, Cooper T. Will amitriptyline prevent the "cheese" reaction of monoamine oxidase inhibitors? *Lancet* 1982;2:183–186.

Pataki CS, Carlson GA, Kelly KL, Rapport MD, Biancaniello TM. Side effects of methylphenidate and desipramine alone and in combination in children. *J Am Acad Child Adolesc Psychiatry* 1993;32:1065–1072.

Patrick KS, Mueller RA, Gualtieri CT, Breese GR. Pharmacokinetics and actions of methylphenidate. In: Meltzer HY, ed. *Psychopharmacology: the third generation of progress.* New York: Raven Press; 1987:1387–1395.

Pearson DA, Lane DM, Santos, CW, Casat CD, Jerger SW, Loveland KA, Faria LP, Mansour R, Henderson JA, Payne CD, Roache JD, Lachar D, Cleveland LA. Effects of methylphenidate treatment in children with mental retardation and ADHD: Individual variation in medication response. *J Am Acad Child Adolesc Psychiatry* 2004a;43:686–698.

Pearson DA, Santos CW, Casat CD, Lane DM, Jerger SW, Roache JD, Loveland KA, Lachar D, Faria LP, Payne CD, Cleveland LA. Treatment effects of methylphenidate on cognitive func-tioning in children with mental retardation and ADHD. *J Am Acad Child Adolesc Psychiatry* 2004b;43:677–685.

Pearson DA, Santos CW, Roache JD, Casat CD, Loveland KA, Lachar D, Lane DM, Faria LP, Cleveland LA. Treatment effects of methylphenidate on behavioral adjustment in children with mental retardation and AHDH. *J Am Acad Child Adolesc Psychiatry* 2003;42:209–216.

Pelham WE, Bender ME, Caddell J, Booth S, Moorer SH. Methylphenidate and children with attention deficit disorder. *Arch Gen Psychiatry* 1985;42:948–952.

Pelham WE, Sturges J, Hoza JA, Schmidt C, Bijlsma JJ, Milich R, Moorer S. Sustained release and standard methylphenidate effects on cognitive and social behavior in children with attention deficit disorder. *Pediatrics* 1987;80:491–501.

Pelham WE, Greenslade KE, Vodde-Hamilton M, Murphy DA, Greenstein JJ, Gnagy EM, Guthrie KJ, Hoover MD, Dahl RE. Relative efficacy of long-acting stimulants on children with attention deficit-hyperactivity disorder: a comparison of standard methylphenidate, sustained-release methylphenidate, sustained-release dextroamphetamine, and pemoline. *Pediatrics* 1990;86:226–237.

Perry R, Bangaru BS. Secretin in autism. (Letter). *J Child Adolesc Psychopharmacol* 1998;8:247–248.

Perry R, Campbell M, Adams P, Lynch N, Spencer EK, Curren EL, Overall JE. Long-term efficacy of haloperidol in autistic children: continuous versus discontinuous drug administration. *J Am Acad Child Adolesc Psychiatry* 1989;28:87–92.

Perry R, Campbell M, Green WH, Small AM, DieTrill ML, Meiselas K, Golden RR, Deutsch SI. Neuroleptic-related dyskinesias in autistic children: a prospective study. *Psychopharmacol Bull* 1985;21:140–143.

Perry R, Campbell M, Grega DM, Anderson L. Saliva lithium levels in children: their use in monitoring serum lithium levels and lithium side effects. *J Clin Psychopharmacol* 1984;4:199–202.

Perry R, Pataki C, Munoz-Silva DM, Armenteros J, Silva RR. Risperidone in children and adolescents with pervasive developmental disorder: pilot trial and follow-up. *J Child Adolesc Psychopharmacol* 1997;7:167–179.

Pesikoff RB, Davis PC. Treatment of pavor nocturnus and somnambulism in children. *Am J Psychiatry* 1971;128:778–781.

Petti, TA, Fish B, Shapiro T, Cohen IL, Campbell M. Effects of chlordiazepoxide in disturbed children: a pilot study. *J Clin Psychopharmacol* 1982;2:270–273.

Pfeffer CR, Jiang H, Domeshek LJ. Buspirone treatment of psychiatrically hospitalized children with symptoms of anxiety and moderately severe aggression. *J Child Adolesc Psychopharmacol* 1997;7:145–155.

Pfefferbaum G, Overall JE, Boren HA, Frankel LS, Sullivan MR, Johnson K. Alprazolam in the treatment of anticipatory and acute situational anxiety in children with cancer. *J Am Acad Child Adolesc Psychiatry* 1987;26:532–535.

Physicians' desk reference (PDR), 44th ed. Oradell, NJ: Medical Economics; 1990.

Physicians' desk reference (PDR), 49th ed. Oradell, NJ: Medical Economics; 1995.

Physicians' desk reference (PDR), 54th ed. Oradell, NJ: Medical Economics; 2000.

Physician's desk reference (PDR), 58th ed. Montvale, NJ: Thomson PDR; 2005.

Physicians' desk reference (PDR), 59th ed. Montvale, NJ: Thomson PDR; 2006.

Piontek CM, Wisner KL. Appropriate clinical management of women taking valproate. *J Clin Psychiatry* 2000;61:161–163.

Platt JE, Campbell M, Green WH, Grega DM. Cognitive effect of lithium carbonate and haloperidol in treatment resistant aggressive children. *Arch Gen Psychiatry* 1984;41:657–662.

Pleak RR, Birmaher B, Gavrilescu A, Abichandani C, Williams DT. Mania and neuropsychiatric excitation following carbamazepine. *J Am Acad Child Adolesc Psychiatry* 1988;27:500–503.

Pliszka SR. Tricyclic antidepressants in the treatment of children with attention deficit disorder. *J Am Acad Child Adolesc Psychiatry* 1987;26:127–132.

Pliszka SR, Browne RG, Olvera RL, Wynne SK. A double-blind, placebo-controlled study of Adderall and methylphenidate in the treatment of attention-deficit/hyperactivity disorder. *J Am Acad Child Adolesc Psychiatry* 2000;39:619–626.

Pliszka SR, Greenhill LL, Crismon ML, Sedillo A, Carlson C, Conners CK, McCracken JT, Swanson JM, Hughes CW, Llana ME, Lopez M, Toprac MG, and the Texas Consensus Conference Panel on Medication Treatment of Childhood Attention-Deficit/Hyperactivity Disorder. The

Texas children's medication algorithm project: report of the Texas consensus conference panel on medication treatment of childhood attention-deficit/hyperactivity disorder. Part I. *J Am Acad Child Adolesc Psychiatry* 2000a; 39:908–919.

Plisza SR, Greenhill LL, Crismon ML, Sedillo A, Carlson C, Conners CK, McCracken JT, Swanson JM, Hughes CW, Llana ME, Lopez M, Toprac MG, and the Texas Consensus Conference Panel on Medication Treatment of Childhood Attention-Deficit/Hyperactivity Disorder. The Texas children's medication algorithm project: Report of the Texas consensus conference panel on medication treatment of childhood attention-deficit/hyperactivity disorder. Part II: Tactics. *J Am Acad Child Adolesc Psychiatry* 2000b;39:920–927.

Pool D, Bloom W, Mielke DH, Roniger JJ, Gallant DM. A controlled evaluation of loxitane in seventy-five adolescent schizophrenic patients. *Curr Ther Res* 1976;19:99–104.

Popper C. Medical unknown and ethical consent: prescribing psychotropic medications for children in the face of uncertainty. In: Popper C, ed. *Psychiatric pharmacosciences of children and adolescents*. Washington, DC: American Psychiatric Press; 1987a.

Popper C, ed. *Psychiatric pharmacosciences of children and adolescents*. Washington, DC: American Psychiatric Press; 1987b.

Popper CW. Combining methylphenidate and clonidine: pharmacologic questions and news reports about sudden death. *J Child Adolesc Psychopharmacol* 1995;5:157–166.

Popper CW, Zimnitzky B. Sudden death putatively related to desipramine treatment in youth: a fifth case and a review of speculative mechanisms. *J Child Adolesc Psychopharmacol* 1995;5:283–300.

Post RM. Mechanisms of action of carbamazepine and related anticonvulsants in affective illness. In: Meltzer HY, ed. *Psychopharmacology: the third generation of progress*. New York: Raven Press; 1987:567–576.

Potenza MN, Holmes JP, Kanes SJ, McDougle CJ. Olanzapine treatment of children, adolescents, and adults with pervasive developmental disorders: an open-label pilot study. *J Clin Psychopharmacol* 1999;19:37–44.

Potter WZ, Calil HM, Sutfin TA, Zavadil III AP, Jusko WJ, Rapoport J, Goodwin FK. Active metabolites of imipramine and desipramine in man. *Clin Pharmacol Ther* 1982;31:393–401.

Poussaint AF, Ditman KS. A controlled study of imipramine (Tofranil) in the treatment of childhood enuresis. *J Pediatr* 1965;67:283–290.

Preskorn SH, Bupp SJ, Weller EB, Weller RA. Plasma levels of imipramine and metabolites in 68 hospitalized children. *J Am Acad Child Adolesc Psychiatry* 1989a;28:373–375.

Preskorn SH, Jerkovich GS, Beber JH, Widener P. Therapeutic drug monitoring of tricyclic antidepressants: a standard of care issue. *Psychopharmacol Bull* 1989b:25:281–284.

Preskorn SH, Weller EB, Hughes CW, Weller RA, Bolte K. Depression in prepubertal children: dexamethasone nonsuppression predicts differential response to imipramine vs. placebo. *Psychopharmacol Bull* 1987;23:128–133.

Preskorn SH, Weller E, Jerkovich G, Hughes CW, Weller R. Depression in children: concentration dependent CNS toxicity of tricyclic antidepressants. *Psychopharmacol Bull* 1988;24:275–279.

Prien RF. Methods and models for placebo use in pharmacotherapeutic trials. *Psychopharmacol Bull* 1988;24:4–8.

Prince JB, Wilens TE, Biederman J, Spencer TJ, Millstein R, Polisner DA, Bostic JQ. A controlled study of nortriptyline in children and adolescents with attention deficit hyperactivity disorder. *J Child Adolesc Psychopharmacol* 2000;10:193–204.

Psychopharmacology Bulletin. Special issue: *Pharmacotherapy of children*. US Department of Health, Education, and Welfare; 1973. (Publication. no. [HSM] 73–9002.)

Puente RM. The use of carbamazepine in the treatment of behavioural disorders in children. In: Birkmayer W, ed. *Epileptic seizures-behaviour-pain*. Bern: Hans Huber Publishers; 1976:243–252.

Puig-Antich J. Major depression and conduct disorder in prepuberty. *J Am Acad Child Adolesc Psychiatry* 1982;21:118–128.

Puig-Antich J. Affective disorders in children and adolescents: diagnostic validity and psychobiology. In: Meltzer HY, ed. *Psychopharmacology: the third generation of progress*. New York: Raven Press; 1987:843–859.

Puig-Antich J, Perel JM, Lupatkin W, Chambers WJ, Tabrizi MA, King J, Goetz R, Davies M, Stiller RL. Imipramine in prepubertal major depressive disorders. *Arch Gen Psychiatry* 1987;44: 81–89.

Quiason H, Ward D, Kitchen T. Buspirone for aggression [Letter]. *J Am Acad Child Adolesc Psychiatry* 1991;30:1026.

Quinn PO, Rapoport JL. One-year follow-up of hyperactive boys treated with imipramine or methylphenidate. *Am J Psychiatry* 1975;132:241–245.

Quintana H, Birmaher B, Stedge D, Lennon S, Freed J, Bridge J, Greenhill L. Use of methylphenidate in the treatment of children with autistic disorder. *J Autism Dev Disord* 1995;25:283–294.

Rall TW. Hypnotics and sedatives; ethanol. In: Gilman AF, Rall TW, Nies AS, et al., eds. *Goodman and Gilman's The pharmacological basis of therapeutics*, 8th ed. New York: Pergamon Press; 1990:345–382.

Rapoport JL. Clozapine and child psychiatry [editorial]. *J Child Adolesc Psychopharmacol* 1994;4:1–3.

Rapoport JL, Buchsbaum MS, Weingartner H, Zahn TP, Ludlow C, Mikkelsen EJ. Dextroamphetamine: Its cognitive and behavioral effects in normal and hyperactive boys and normal men. *Arch Gen Psychiatry* 1980a;37:933–943.

Rapoport JL, Buchsbaum MS, Zahn TP, Weingartner H, Ludlow C, Mikkelsen EJ. Dextroamphetamine: cognitive and behavioral effects in normal prepubertal boys. *Science* 1978a;199:560–563.

Rapoport JL, Mikkelsen EJ. Antidepressants. In: Werry JS, ed. *Pediatric psychopharmacology: The use of behavior modifying drugs in children*. New York: Brunner/Mazel; 1978b:208–233.

Rapoport JL, Mikkelsen EJ, Werry JS. Antimanic, antianxiety, hallucinogenic and miscellaneous drugs. In: Werry JS, ed. *Pediatric psychopharmacology: the use of behavior modifying drugs in children*. New York: Brunner/Mazel; 1978c:316–355.

Rapoport JL, Mikkelsen EJ, Zavadil A, Nee L, Gruenau C, Mendelson W, Gillin JC. Childhood enuresis: psychopathology, plasma tricyclic concentration and antienuretic effect. *Arch Gen Psychiatry* 1980b; 37:1146–1152.

Rapoport JL, Quinn PO, Bradbard G, Riddle D, Brooks E. Imipramine and methylphenidate treatment of hyperactive boys. *Arch Gen Psychiatry* 1974;30:789–798.

Rapport MD, Carlson GA, Kelly KL, Pataki C. Methylphenidate and desipramine in hospitalized children: I. Separate and combined effects on cognitive function. *J Am Acad Child Adolesc Psychiatry* 1993;32:333–342.

Rapport MD, Denney C, DuPaul GJ, Gardner MJ. Attention deficit disorder and methylphenidate: normalization rates, clinical effectiveness, and response prediction in 76 children. *J Am Acad Child Adolesc Psychiatry* 1994;33:882–893.

Ratey JJ, Sovner R, Mikkelsen E, et al. Buspirone therapy for maladaptive behavior and anxiety in developmentally disabled persons. *J Clin Psychiatry* 1989:50:382–384.

Ratey J, Sovner R, Parks A, Rogentine K. Buspirone treatment of aggression and anxiety in mentally retarded patients: a multiple-baseline, placebo lead-in study. *J Clin Psychiatry* 1991;52:159–162.

Rating scales and assessment instruments for use in pediatric psychopharmacology research. *Psychopharmacol Bull* 1985;21:713–1124.

Realmuto GM, August GJ, Garfinkel BD. Clinical effect of buspirone in autistic children. *J Clin Psychopharmacol* 1989;9:122–125.

Realmuto GM, Erickson WD, Yellin AM, Hopwood JH, Greenberg LM. Clinical comparison of thiothixene and thioridazine in schizophrenic adolescents. *Am J Psychiatry* 1984;141:440–442.

Reisberg B, Gershon S. Side effects associated with lithium therapy. *Arch Gen Psychiatry* 1979;36:879–887.

Reiss AL, O'Donnell DJ. Carbamazepine-induced mania in two children: case report. *J Clin Psychiatry* 1984;45:272–274.

Reite ML, Nagel KE, Ruddy JR. *Concise guide to evaluation and management of sleep disorders*. Washington, DC: American Psychiatric Press; 1990.

Remschmidt H. The psychotropic effect of carbamazepine in non-epileptic patients, with particular reference to problems posed by clinical studies in children with behavioural disorders. In:

Birkmayer W, ed. *Epileptic seizures-behaviour-pain.* Bern: Hans Huber Publishers; 1976:253–258.

Remschmidt H, Schulz E, Martin PDM. An open trial of clozapine in thirty-six adolescents with schizophrenia. *J Child Adolesc Psychopharmacol* 1994;4:31–41.

Rey-Sanchez F, Gutierrez-Casares JR. Paroxetine in children with major depressive disorder: an open trial. *J Am Acad Child Adolesc Psychiatry* 1997;36:1443–1447.

Richardson MA, Haugland G, Craig TJ. Neuroleptic use, parkinsonian symptoms, tardive dyskinesia and associated factors in child and adolescent psychiatric patients. *Am J Psychiatry* 1991;148:1322–1328.

Riddle MA, ed. Pediatric psychopharmacology I. *Child Adolesc Psychiatr Clin N Am* 1995a;4:1–260 (Entire issue).

Riddle MA, ed. Pediatric psychopharmacology II. *Child Adolesc Psychiatr Clin N Am* 1995b;4:261–520 (Entire issue).

Riddle MA, Geller B, Ryan N. Another sudden death in a child treated with desipramine. *J Am Acad Child Adolesc Psychiatry* 1993;32:792–797.

Riddle MA, Geller B, Ryan ND. The safety of desipramine: reply [Letter]. *J Am Acad Child Adolesc Psychiatry* 1994;33; 589–590.

Riddle MA, Hardin MT, Cho SC, Woolston JL, Leckman JF. Desipramine treatment of boys with attention-deficit hyperactivity disorder and tics: preliminary clinical experiences. *J Am Acad Child Adolesc Psychiatry* 1988;27:811–814.

Riddle MA, Hardin MT, King R, Scahill L, Woolston JL. Fluoxetine treatment of children and adolescents with Tourette's and obsessive compulsive disorders: Preliminary clinical experience. *J Am Acad Child Adolesc Psychiatry* 1990;29:45–48.

Riddle MA, King RA, Hardin MT, Scahill L, Ort SI, Chappell P, Rasmusson A, Leckman JF. Behavioral side effects of fluoxetine in children and adolescents. *J Child Adolesc Psychopharmacol* 1990/1991;1:193–198.

Riddle MA, Nelson JC, Kleinman CS, Rasmusson A, Leckman JF, King RA, Cohen DJ. Sudden death in children receiving Norpramin: A review of three reported cases and commentary. *J Am Acad Child Adolesc Psychiatry* 1991;30:104–108.

Riddle MA, Scahill L, King RA, Hardin MT, Anderson GM, Ort SI, Smith JC, Leckman JF, Cohen DJ. Double-blind, crossover trial of fluoxetine and placebo in children and adolescents with obsessive-compulsive disorder. *J Am Acad Child Adolesc Psychiatry* 1992:31:1062–1069.

Rifkin A, Quitkin F, Klein DF. Akinesia: a poorly recognized drug-induced extrapyramidal behavior disorder. *Arch Gen Psychiatry* 1975;32:672–674.

Riggs PD, Leon SL, Mikulich SK, Pottle LC. An open trial of bupropion for ADHD in adolescents with substance use disorders and conduct disorder. *J Am Acad Child Adolesc Psychiatry* 1998;37:1271–1278.

Rimland B. Comments on "Secretin and autism: a two-art clinical investigation" by M.G.Chez et al. *J Autism Dev Disord* 2000;30:95.

Rivera-Calimlim L, Griesbach PH, Perlmutter R. Plasma chlorpromazine concentrations in children with behavioral disorders and mental illness. *Clin Pharmacol Ther* 1979;26:114–121.

Rivera-Calimlim L, Nasrallah H, Strauss J, Lasagna L. Clinical response and plasma levels: effect of dose, dosage schedules, and drug interactions on plasma chlorpromazine levels. *Am J Psychiatry* 1976;133:646–652.

Rosack J. New data show declines in antidepressant prescribing. *Psychiatric News* 40:1, 2005.

Rosenbaum JF, Fava M, Hoog SL, Ascroft RC, Krebs WB. Selective serotonin reuptake inhibitor discontinuation syndrome: a randomized clinical trial. *Biol. Psychiatry* 1998;44:77–87.

Rosenberg DR, Holttum J, Gershon S. *Textbook of pharmacotherapy for child and adolescent psychiatric disorders.* New York: Brunner/Mazel; 1994

Rosenberg DR, Davanzo PA, Gershon S. *Pharmacotherapy for child and adolescent psychiatric disorders.* Second Edition. New York: Marcel Dekker, Inc; 2002.

Rosenberg DR, Johnson K, Sahl R. Evolving mania in an adolescent treated with low-dose fluoxetine. *J Child Adolesc Psychopharmacol* 1992;2:299–306.

Rosenberg, DR, Stewart CM, Fitzgerald KD, Tawile V, Carroll E. Paroxetine open-label treatment of pediatric outpatients with obsessive-compulsive disorder. *J Am Acad Child Adolesc Psychiatry* 1999;38:1180–1185.

Ross DC, Piggott LR. Clonazepam for OCD [Letter]. *J Am Acad Child Adolesc Psychiatry* 1993;32:470–471.

Rosse RB, Giese AA, Deutsch SI, Morihisa JM. *Laboratory diagnostic testing in psychiatry.* Washington, DC: American Psychiatric Press; 1989.

Rudorfer MV, Potter WZ. Pharmacokinetics of antidepressants. In: Meltzer HY, ed. *Psychopharmacology: the third generation of progress.* New York: Raven Press; 1987:1353–1363.

Russo RM, Gururaj VJ, Allen JE. The effectiveness of diphenhydramine HCl in pediatric sleep disorders. *J Clin Pharmacol* 1976;4:284–288.

Ryan ND. Heterocyclic antidepressants in children and adolescents. *J Child Adolesc Psychopharmacol* 1990;1:21–31.

Ryan ND, Meyer V, Dachille S, Mazzie D, Puig-Antich J. Lithium antidepressant augmentation in TCA-refractory depression in adolescents. *J Acad Child Adolesc Psychiatry* 1988a;27:371–376.

Ryan ND, Puig-Antich J, Cooper T, Rabinovich H, Ambrosini P, Davies M, King J, Torres D, Fried, J. Imipramine in adolescent major depression: plasma level and clinical response. *Acta Psychiatr Scand* 1986;73:275–288.

Ryan ND, Puig-Antich J, Cooper TB, Rabinovich H, Ambrosini P, Fried J, Davies M, Torres D, Suckow RF. Relative safety of single versus divided dose imipramine in adolescent major depression. *J Am Acad Child Adolesc Psychiatry* 1987;26:400–406.

Ryan ND, Puig-Antich J, Rabinovich H, Fried J, Ambrosini P, Meyer V, Torres D, Dachille S, Mazzie R. MAOIs in adolescent major depression unresponsive to tricyclic antidepressants. *J Am Acad Child Adolesc Psychiatry* 1988b;27:755–758.

Safer D, Allen RP, Barr E. Depression of growth in hyperactive children on stimulant drugs. *N Engl J Med* 1972;287:217–220.

Safer DJ, Krager M. A survey of medication treatment for hyperactive/inattentive students. *JAMA* 1988;260:2256–2258.

Saito E, Correll CU, Gallelli K, McMeniman M, Parikh UH, Malhotra AK, Kafantaris V. A prospective study of hyperprolactinemia in children and adolescents treated with atypical antipsychotic agents. *J Child Adolesc Psychopharmacol*;2004:14:350–358.

Sakkas P, Davis JM, Han J, Wang Z. Pharmacotherapy of NMS. *Psychiatr Ann* 1991;21:157–164.

Sallee FR, DeVane CL, Ferrell RE. Fluoxetine-related death in a child with cytochrome P-450 2D6 genetic deficiency. *J Child Adolesc Psychopharmacol* 2000;10:27–34.

Sallee FR, Nesbitt L, Jackson C, Sine L, Sethuraman G. Relative efficacy of haloperidol and pimozide in children and adolescents with Tourette's disorder. *Am J Psychiatry* 1997;154:1057–1062.

Salzman C. Benzodiazepine dependency: Summary of the APA task force on benzodiazepines. *Psychopharmacol Bull* 1990;26:61–62.

Saraf KR, Klein DF, Gittelman-Klein R, Groff S. Imipramine side effects in children. *Psychopharmacologia (Berlin)* 1974;37:265–274.

Saul RC. Nortriptyline in attention deficit disorder. *Clin Neuropharmacol* 1985;8:382–384.

Scahill L, Chappell PB, Kim YS, Schultz RT, Katsovich L, Arnsten AFT, Leckman JF. Guanfacine in the treatment of children with tic disorders and ADHD: a placebo-controlled study. (Abstract, 40th Annual NCDEU meeting.) *J Child Adolesc Psychopharmacol* 2000;10:250.

Scahill L, McCracken J, Mcdougle CJ, Aman M, Arnold LE, Tierney E, Cronin P, Davies M:, Ghuman J, Gonzalez J, Koenig K, Lindsay R, Martin A, McGough J, Posey DJ, Swiezy N:, Volkmar F, Ritz, L, Vitiello B. Methodological issues in designing a multisite trial of risperidone in children and adolescents with autism. *J Child Adolesc Psychopharmacol* 2001;11:377–388.

Sharko, AM. Selective serotonin reuptake inhibitor-induced sexual dysfunction in adolescents: A review. *Jam Assn Child Adolesc Psychiatry* 2004;43:1071–1079.

Schmidt MH, Trott, G-E, Blanz B, Nissen G. Clozapine medication in adolescents. In: Stefania CN, Rabavilas AD, Soldatos CR, eds. *Psychiatry: a world perspective.* Proceedings of the Eighth World Congress of Psychiatry. Amsterdam: Excerpta Medica; 1990;1:1100–1104.

Schooler NR, Kane JM. Research diagnoses for tardive dyskinesia. *Arch Gen Psychiatry* 1982;38:486–487.

Schou M. Lithium: elimination rate, dosage, control, poisoning, goiter, mode of action. *Acta Psychiatr Scand* 1969;207(suppl):49–59.

Schroeder JS, Mullin AV, Elliott GR, Steiner H, Nichols M, Gordon A, Paulow M. Cardiovascular effects of desipramine in children. *J Am Acad Child Adolesc Psychiatry* 1989;28:376–379.

Shapiro AK, Shapiro E. Controlled study of pimozide vs. placebo in Tourette's syndrome. *J Am Acad Child Psychiatry* 1984;23:161–173.

Shapiro AK, Shapiro E. Do stimulants provoke, cause, or exacerbate tics and Tourette syndrome? *Compr Psychiatry* 1981;22:265–273.

Shapiro AK, Shapiro E. Tic disorders. In: Kaplan HI, Sadock BJ, eds. *Comprehensive textbook of psychiatry*, 5th ed. Baltimore: Williams & Wilkins; 1989:1865–1878.

Shapiro AK, Shapiro E, Eisenkraft GJ. Treatment of Gilles de la Tourette syndrome with pimozide. *Am J Psychiatry* 1983;140:1183–1186.

Sheard MH. Lithium in the treatment of aggression. *J Nerv Ment Dis* 1975;160:108–118.

Sheitman BB, Bird PM, Binz W, Akinli L, Sanchez C. Olanzapine-induced elevation of plasma triglyceride leverls. *Am J Psychiatry* 1999;156:1471–1472.

Sholevar EH, Baron DA, Hardie TL. Treatment of childhood-onset schizophrenia with olanzapine. *J Child Adolesc Psychopharmacol* 2000;10:69–78.

Siefen G, Remschmidt H. Behandlungsergebnisse mit clozapin bei schizophrenen jugendlichen [Clozapine in the treatment of adolescents with schizophrenia: Treatment outcome]. *Zeitschrift fur Kinder-und-Jugendpsychiatrie* 1986;14:245–257. (English translation by the Ralph McElroy Co., provided by the manufacturer.)

Silva RR, Munoz DM, Alpert M. Carbamazepine use in children and adolescents with features of attention-deficit hyperactivity disorder: A meta-analysis. *J Am Acad Child Adolesc Psychiatry* 1996;35:352–358.

Silva RR, Muniz R, Pestreich L, Childress A, Brams M, Lopez FA, and Wang J. Efficacy and duration of effect of extended-release dexmethylphenidate versus placebo in schoolchildren with attention-deficit/hyperactivity disorder. *J Child Adolesc Psychopharmacol* 2006;16:239–251.

Simeon JG. Buspirone effects in adolescent psychiatric disorders. *Eur Neuropsychopharmacol* 1991;1:421.

Simeon JG, Carrey NJ, Wiggins DM, Milin RP, Hosenbocus SN. Risperidone effects in treatment-resistant adolescents: preliminary case reports. *J Child Adolesc Psychopharmacol* 1995;5:69–79.

Simeon JG, Dinicola VF, Ferguson HB, Copping W. Adolescent depression: a placebo-controlled fluoxetine treatment study and follow-up. *Prog Neuro-psychopharmacol Biol Psychiatry* 1990; 14:791–795.

Simeon JG, Ferguson HB. Alprazolam effects in children with anxiety disorders. *Can J Psychiatry* 1987;32:570–574.

Simeon JG, Ferguson HB. Recent developments in the use of antidepressant and anxiolytic medications. *Psychiatr Clin North Am* 1985;8:893–907.

Simeon JG, Ferguson HB, Fleet JVW. Bupropion effects in attention deficit and conduct disorder. *Can J Psychiatry* 1986;31:581–585.

Simeon JG, Ferguson HB, Knott V, Roberts N, Gauthier B, Dubois C, Wiggins D. Clinical, cognitive, and neurophysiological effects of alprazolam in children and adolescents with overanxious and avoidant disorders. *J Am Acad Child Adolesc Psychiatry* 1992;31:29–33.

Simeon JG, Knott VJ, DuBois C, Wiggins D, Geraets I, Thatte S, Miller W. Buspirone therapy of mixed anxiety disorders in childhood and adolescence: a pilot study. *J Child Adolesc Psychopharmacol* 1994;4:159–170.

Simon GE, Savarino J, Operskalski B, Wang PS. Suicidal Risk During Antidepressant Treatment. *Am J Psychiatry* 2006;163:41–47.

Sleator EK. Diagnosis. In: Sleator EK, Pelham WE Jr, eds. *Attention deficit disorder: dialogues in pediatric management.* Vol. 1, No. 3. Norwalk, CT: Appleton-Century-Crofts; 1986:11–42.

Sleator EK, von Neumann A, Sprague RL. Hyperactive children: a continuous long-term placebo-controlled follow-up. *JAMA* 1974;229:316–317.

Small JG, Milstein V, Marhenke JD, Hall DD, Kellams JJ. Treatment outcome with clozapine in tardive dyskinesis, neuroleptic sensitivity, and treatment resistant psychosis. *J Clin Psychiatry* 1987;48:263–267.

Smith TC, Wollman H. History and principles of anaesthesiology. In: Gilman AF, Goodman LS, Rall TW, et al, eds. *Goodman and Gilman's The pharmacological basis of therapeutics*, 7th ed. New York: Macmillan; 1985:260–275.

Snyder R, Turgay A, Aman M, Binder C, Fisman S, Carroll A, and The Risperidone Conduct Study Group. Effects of risperidone on conduct and disruptive behavior disorders in children with subaverage IQs. *J Am Acad Child Adolesc Psychiatry* 2002;41:1026–1036.

Sokol MS, Campbell M. Novel psychoactive agents in the treatment of developmental disorders. In: Aman MG, Singh NN, eds. *Psychopharmacology of the developmental disabilities*. New York: Springer-Verlag; 1988:147–167.

Spencer EK, Kafantaris V, Padron-Gayol MV, Rosenberg CR, Campbell M. Haloperidol in schizophrenic children: early findings from a study in progress. *Psychopharmacol Bull* 1992;28:183–186.

Spencer T, Biederman J, Kerman K, Steingard R, Wilens T. Desipramine treatment of children with attention-deficit hyperactivity disorder and tic disorder or Tourette's syndrome. *J Am Acad Child Adolesc Psychiatry* 1993a;32:354–360.

Spencer T, Biederman J, Steingard R, Wilens T. Bupropion exacerbates tics in children with attention-deficit hyperactivity disorder and Tourette's syndrome. *J Am Acad Child Adolesc Psychiatry* 1993b;32:211–214.

Spencer T, Biederman J, Wilens T, Steingard R, Geist D. Nortriptyline treatment of children with attention-deficit hyperactivity disorder and tic disorder or Tourette's syndrome. *J Am Acad Child Adolesc Psychiatry* 1993c;32:201–210.

Spencer T, Biederman J, Wilens T, Prince J, Hatch M, Jones J, Harding M, Faraone SV, Seidman L. Effectiveness and tolerability of tomoxetine in adults with attention deficit hyperactivity disorder. *Am J Psychiatry* 1998;155:693–695.

Spitzer RL, Endicott J, Robins E. Research diagnostic criteria. *Arch Gen Psychiatry* 1978;35:773–782.

Sprague RL, Sleator EK. Methylphenidate in hyperkinetic children: differences in dose effects on learning and social behavior. *Science* 1977;198:1274–1276.

Stahl SM. *Essential psychopharmacology: neuroscientific basis and practical applications*, 2nd ed. Cambridge, England: Cambridge; 2000.

Staller JA. Intramuscular ziprasidone in youth: a retrospective chart review. *J Child Adolesc Psychopharmacol* 2004;14:590–592.

Staller JA, Kunwar A, Simionescu M. Oxcarbazepine in the treatment of child psychiatric disorders: a retrospective review. *J Child Adolesc Psychopharmacol* 2005;15:964–969.

Stanley B. An integration of ethical and clinical considerations in the use of placebos. *Psychopharmacol Bull* 1988;24:18–20.

Starr HL, Kemner J. Multicenter, randomized, open-label study of OROS methylphenidate versus atomoxetine: treatment outcomes in African-American children with ADHD. *J Natl Med. Assoc* 2005;97(10 Suppl):11S–16S.

Steingard R, Biederman J, Spencer T, Wilens T, Gonzalez A. Comparison of clonidine response in the treatment of attention-deficit hyperactivity disorder with and without comorbid tic disorders. *J Am Acad Child Adolesc Psychiatry* 1993;32:350–353.

Steingard R, Khan A, Gonzales A, Herzog DB. Neuroleptic malignant syndrome: review of experience with children and adolescents. *J Child Adolesc Psychopharmacol* 1992;2:183–198.

Stores G. Antiepileptics (anticonvulsants). In: Werry JS, ed. *Pediatric psychopharmacology: the use of behavior modifying drugs in children*. New York: Brunner/Mazel; 1978:274–315.

Strayhorn JM, Rapp N, Donina W, Strain PS. Randomized trial of methylphenidate for an autistic child. *J Am Acad Child Adolesc Psychiatry* 1988;27:244–247.

Strober M, Freeman R, Rigali J. The pharmacotherapy of depressive illness in adolescents: I. An open label trial of imipramine. *Psychopharmacol Bull* 1990;26:80–84.

Strober M, Freeman R, Rigali J, Schmidt S, Diamond R. The pharmacotherapy of depressive illness in adolescents: II. Effects of lithium augmentation in nonresponders to imipramine. *J Am Acad Child Adolesc Psychiatry* 1992;31:16–20.

Sudden death in children treated with a tricyclic antidepressant. *Med Lett* 1990(June 1);32:53.

Sussman N. The potential benefits of serotonin receptor-specific agents. *J Clin Psychiatry* 1994a;55(suppl 1):45–51.

Sussman N. The uses of buspirone in psychiatry. *J Clin Psychiatry Monograph* 1994b;12:3–19.

Sussman N, Ginsberg D. Valproate and risk of polycystic ovary syndrome. *Prim Psychiatry* 1998;5:42–48.

Sverd J. Methylphenidate treatment for children with attention deficit hyperactivity disorder and tic disorder: Inadvisable or indispensable? In: Greenhill LL, Osman BB, eds., *Ritalin: theory and practice,* 2nd ed. Larchmont, NY: Mary Ann Liebert, Inc, 2000:301–319.

Swanson J, Greenhill L, Pelham W, Wilens T, Wolraich M, Abikoff H, Atkins M, August G, Biederman J, Bukstein O, Conners CK, Efron L, Friebelkorn K, Fried J, Hoffman J, Lambrech L, Lerner M, Leventhal B, McBurnett K, Morse E, Palumbo D, Pfiffner L, Stein M, Wigal S, Winans E. Initiating Concerta (OROS methylphenidate HCl) qd in children with attention-deficit hyperactivity disorder. *J Clin Res* 2000;3:59–76.

Swanson JM, Connor DF, Cantwell D. Combining methylphenidate and clonidine: ill-advised/and negative rebuttal (debate forum). *J Am Acad Child Adolesc Psychiatry* 1999;38:614–622.

Swanson JM, Flockhart D, Udrea D, Cantwell D, Connor D, Williams L. Clonidine in the treatment of ADHD: questions about safety and efficacy (Letter). *J Child Adolesc Psychopharmacol* 1995;5:301–304.

Swanson JM, Lerner M, Cantwell D. Blood levels and tolerance to stimulants in ADDH children. *Clin Neuropharmacol* 1986;9(suppl 4):523–525.

Swanson JM, Lerner MA, Gupta S, Shoulson I., Wigal S. Development of a new once-a-day formulation of methylphenidate for the treatment of ADHD. *Arch Gen Psychiatry* 2003;60:204–211.

Swanson JM, Wigal S, Greenhill LL, Browne R, Waslik B, Lerner M, Williams L, Flynn D, Agler D, Crowley K, Fineberg E, Baren M, Cantwell DP. Analog classroom assessment of Adderall in children with ADHD. *J Am Acad Child Adolesc Psychiatry* 1998;37:519–526.

Szigethy E, Wiznitzer M, Branicky LA, Maxwell K, Findling RL. Risperidone-induced hepatotoxicity in children and adolescents? A chart review study. *J Child Adolesc Psychopharmacol* 1999;9:93–98.

Taylor E, Schachar R, Thorley G, Wieselberg HM, Everitt B, Rutter M. Which boys respond to stimulant medication? A controlled trial of methylphenidate in boys with disruptive behavior. *Psychol Med* 1987;17:121–143.

Teicher MH, Baldessarini RJ. Developmental pharmacodynamics. In: Popper C, ed. *Psychiatric pharmacosciences of children and adolescents*. Washington, DC: American Psychiatric Press; 1987:45–80.

Teitelbaum M. Oxcarbazepine in bipolar disorder [letter]. *J Am Acad Child Adolesc Psychiatry* 2001;40:993–994.

Thase ME, Kupfer DJ, Frank E, Jarrett DB. Treatment of imipramine-resistant recurrent depression: II. An open clinical trial of lithium augmentation. *J Clin Psychiatry* 1989;50:413–417.

Thomsen PH. Child and adolescent obsessive-compulsive disorder treated with citalopram: findings from an open trial of 23 cases. *J Child Adolesc Psychopharmacol* 1997;7:157–166.

Tierney E, Joshi PT, Llinas JF, Rosenberg LLA, Riddle MA. Sertraline for major depression in children and adolescents: preliminary clinical experience. *J Child Adolesc Psychopharmacol* 1995;5:13–27.

Treatment for Adolescents With Depression Study (TADS) Team [March JS, Silva S, Petrycki S, Curry J, Wells K, Fairbank J, Burns B, Domino M, McNulty, Vitiello B, Severe J.] : Fluoxetine, cognitive-behavioral therapy, and their combination for adolescents with depression: Treatment for adolescents with depression study (TADS) randomized controlled trial. *JAMA* 2004;292:807–820.

United States Pharmacopeial Dispensing Information (USPDI). *Drug information for the health care professional.* Rockville, MD: United States Pharmacopeial Convention; 1990.

United States Pharmacopeial Dispensing Information (USPDI). Thompson Healthcare (eds.), *Drug information for the health care professional*, 25th Edition, *Volume 1*, Greenwood Village, Colorado. Thomson MICROMEDEX, 2005.

Upadhyaya, HP, Brady, KT, Wang, W. Bupropion SR in adolescents with comorbid ADHD and nicotine dependence: A pilot study. *J Am Acad Child Adolesc Psychiatry* 2004;43:199–205.

Van Putten T, Marder SR. Behavioral toxicity of antipsychotic drugs. *J Clin Psychiatry* 1987;48(suppl 9):13–19.

Van Putten T, May PRA, Marder SR. Akathisia with haloperidol and thiothixene. *Arch Gen Psychiatry* 1984;41:1036–1039.

Varanka TM, Weller RA, Weller EB, Fristad MA. Lithium treatment of manic episodes with psychotic features in prepubertal children. *Am J Psychiatry* 1988;145:1557–1559.

Varley CK, McClellan J. Case study: two additional sudden deaths with tricyclic antidepressants. *J Am Acad Child Adolesc Psychiatry* 1997;36:390–394.

Venkataraman S, Naylor MW, King CA. Mania associated with fluoxetine treatment in adolescents. *J Am Acad Child Adolesc Psychiatry* 1992;31:276–281.

Vetro A, Szentistvanyi I, Pallag L, Vargha M, Szilard J. Therapeutic experience with lithium in childhood aggressivity. *Pharmacopsychiatry* 1985;14:121–127.

Villeneuve A. The rabbit syndrome: a peculiar extrapyramidal reaction. *Can Psychiatr Assoc J* 1972;17:69–72.

Vincent J, Varley CK, Leger P. Effects of methylphenidate on early adolescent growth. *Am J Psychiatry* 1990;147:501–502.

Vitiello B. A multi-site double-blind placebo-controlled trial of fluvoxamine for children and adolescents with anxiety disorders. (Abstract, 40th Annual NCDEU meeting.) *J Child Adolesc Psychopharmacol* 2000;10:257–258.

Vitiello B, Behar D, Malone R, Delaney MA, Ryan PJ, Simpson GM. Pharmacokinetics of lithium carbonate in children. *J Clin Psychopharmacol* 1988;8:355–359.

Volavka J. The effects of clozapine on aggression and substance abuse in schizophrenic patients. *J Clin Psychiatry* 60 (suppl 12):43–46, 1999.

Wagner KD, Berard R, Stein MB, Wetherhold E, Carpenter DJ, Perera P, Gee M, Davy K, Machin A. A multicenter, randomized, double-blind, placebo-controlled trial of paroxetine in children and adolescents with social anxiety disorder. *Arch Gen Psychiatry* 2004;61:1153–1162.

Waizer J, Hoffman SP, Polizos P, Engelhardt DM. Outpatient treatment of hyperactive school children with imipramine. *Am J Psychiatry* 1974;131:587–591.

Walkup JT. Clinical decision making in child and adolescent psychopharmacology. *Child Adolesc Psychiatr Clin N Am* 1995;4:23–40.

Walsh BT, ed. *Child psychopharmacology*. Washington, DC: American Psychiatric Press; 1998.

Walsh BT, Giardina E-GV, Sloan RP, Greenhill L, Goldfein J. Effects of desipramine on autonomic control of the heart. *J Am Acad Child Adolesc Psychiatry* 1994;33:191–197.

Walsh BT, Greenhill LL, Giardina E-GV, Bigger JT, Waslick BD, Sloan RP, Bilich K, Wolk S, Bagiella E. Effects of desipramine on autonomic input to the heart. *J Am Acad Child Adolesc Psychiatry* 1999;38:1186–1192.

Weiner JM, ed. *Diagnosis and psychopharmacology of childhood and adolescent disorders*. New York: John Wiley; 1985.

Weiner JM, Jaffe SL. Historical overview of childhood and adolescent psychopharmacology. In: Weiner JM, ed. *Diagnosis and psychopharmacology of childhood and adolescent disorders*. New York: John Wiley; 1985:3–50.

Weiner N. Norepinephrine, epinephrine, and the sympathomimetic amines. In: Gilman AG, Goodman LS, Gilman A, eds. *Goodman and Gilman's The pharmacological basis of therapeutics*, 6th ed. New York: Macmillan; 1980:138–175.

Weiss G, Hechtman LT. *Hyperactive children grown up: empirical findings and theoretical considerations*. New York: Guilford Press; 1986.

Weiss G, Kruger E, Danielson U, Elman M. Effect of long-term treatment of hyperactive children with methylphenidate. *Can Med Assoc J* 1975;112:159–165

Weiss M, Tannock R, Kratochvil C, Dunn D, Velez-Borras J, Thomason C, Tamura R, Kelsey D, Stevens L, Allen AJ. A randomized, placebo-controlled study of once-daily atomoxetine in the school setting in children with ADHD. *J Am Acad Child Psychiatry* 2005;44:647–655.

Weizman A, Weitz R, Szekely GA, Tyano S, Belmaker RH. Combination of neuroleptic and stimulant treatment in attention deficit disorder with hyperactivity. *J Am Acad Child Psychiatry* 1984;23:295–298.

Weller EB, Weller RA, Fristad MA. Lithium dosage guide for prepubertal children: a preliminary report. *J Am Acad Child Psychiatry* 1986;25:92–95.

Weller EB, Weller RA, Fristad MA, Cantwell M, Tucker S. Saliva lithium monitoring in prepubertal children. *J Am Acad Child Adolesc Psychiatry* 1987;26:173–175.

Weller EB, Weller RA, Preskorn SH, Glotzbach R. Steady-state plasma imipramine levels in prepubertal depressed children. *Am J Psychiatry* 1982;139:506–508.

Wender PH. Attention deficit hyperactivity disorder. In: Howells JG, ed. *Modern perspectives in clinical psychiatry.* New York: Brunner/Mazel; 1988:149–169.

Wernicke JF. The side effect profile and safety of fluoxetine. *J Clin Psychiatry* 1985;46:59–67.

Werry JS. The safety of desipramine [Letter]. *J Am Acad Child Adolesc Psychiatry* 1994;33:588–589.

Werry J, Aman M. Methylphenidate and haloperidol in children: effects on attention, memory, and activity. *Arch Gen Psychiatry* 1975;32:790–795.

Werry J, Aman MG, Diamond E. Imipramine and methylphenidate in hyperactive children. *J Child Psychol Psychiatry* 1980;21:27–35.

Werry J, Weiss G, Douglas V, Martin J. Studies on the hyperactive child III: the effects of chlorpromazine upon behavior and learning ability. *J Am Acad Child Psychiatry* 1966;5:292–312.

Werry JS, ed. *Pediatric psychopharmacology: the use of behavior modifying drugs in children.* New York: Brunner/Mazel; 1978.

Werry JS, Aman MG, eds. *Practitioner's guide to psychoactive drugs for children and adolescents,* 2nd ed. New York: Plenum Medical Book; 1999.

Werry JS, McClellan, Chard L. Childhood and adolescent schizophrenia, bipolar, and schizoaffective disorders: a clinical outcome study. *J Am Acad Child Adolesc Psychiatry* 1991;30:457–465.

West SA, Keck PE, McElroy SL, Strakowski SM, Minnery KL, McConville BJ, Sorter MT. Open trial of valproate in the treatment of adolescent mania. *J Child Adolesc Psychopharmacol* 1994;4:263–267.

Whalen CK, Henker B, Swanson JM, Granger D, Kliewer W, Spencer J. Natural social behaviors in hyperactive children: dose effects of methylphenidate. *J Consult Clin Psychol* 1987;55:187–193.

White L, Tursky B, Schwartz GE, eds. *Placebo: theory, research, and mechanisms.* New York: Guilford Press; 1985.

Wigal S, Swanson JM, Feifel D, Sangal B, Elia J, Casat CD. Zeldis JB, Conners CK. A double-blind, placebo-controlled trial of dexmethylphenidate hydrochloride and *d,l-threo*-methylphenidate hydrochloride in children with attention-deficit/hyperactivity disorder. *J Am Acad Child Adolesc Psychiatry* 2004;43:1406–1414.

Wigal SB, McGough JJ, McCracken JT, Biederman J, Spencer TJ, Posner KL, Wigal TL, Kollins SH, Clark, TM, Mays DA, Zhang Y, Tulloch SJ. A laboratory school comparison of mixed amphetamine salts extended release (Adderall XR) and atomoxetine (Strattera) in school-aged children with attention deficit/hyperactivity disorder. *J Atten Disorder* 2005;9:275–289.

Wilens T, McBurnett K, Stein M, Lerner M, Spencer T, Wolraich M. ADHD treatment with once-daily OROS methylphenidate: final results from a long-term open-label study. *J Am Acad Child Adolesc Psychiatry* 2005;44:1015–1023.

Wilens TE, Biederman J, Baldessarini RJ, Puopolo PR, Flood JG. Developmental changes in serum concentrations of desipramine and 2-hydroxydesipramine during treatment with desipramine. *J Am Acad Child Adolesc Psychiatry* 1992;31:691–698.

Wilens TE, Biederman J, Baldessarini RJ, Puopolo PR, Flood JG. Electrocardiographic effects of desipramine and 2-hydroxydesipramine in children, adolescents, and adults treated with desipramine. *J Am Acad Child Adolesc Psychiatry* 1993a;32:798–804.

Wilens TE, Biederman J, Geist DE, Steingard R, Spencer T. Nortriptyline in the treatment of ADHD: a chart review of 58 cases. *J Am Acad Child Adolesc Psychiatry* 1993b;32:343–349.

Wilens TE, Biederman J, March JS, Wolkow R, Fine CS, Millstein RB, Faraone SV, Geller D, Spencer TJ. Absence of cardiovascular adverse effects of sertraline in children and adolescents. *J Am Acad Child Adolesc Psychiatry* 1999;38:573–577.

Wilens TE, Biederman J, Spencer T. Clonidine for sleep disturbances associated with attention-deficit hyperactivity disorder. *J Am Acad Child Adolesc Psychiatry* 1994;33:424–426.

Wilens TE, Spencer TJ. Combining methylphenidate and clonidine: a clinically sound medication option/and Affirmative rebuttal (Debate Forum). *J Am Acad Child Adolesc Psychiatry* 1999;38:614–622.

Wilens TE, Spencer TJ. The stimulants revisited. *Child Adolesc Psychiatr Clin N Am* 2000;9:573–603.

Wilens TE, Spencer T, Biederman J, Wozniak J, Conner D. Combined pharmacotherapy: an emerging trend in pediatric psychopharmacology. *J Am Acad Child Adolesc Psychiatry* 1995;34:110–112.

Williams DT, Mehl R, Yudofsky S, Adams D, Roseman B. The effect of propranolol on uncontrolled rage outbursts in children and adolescents with organic brain dysfunction. *J Am Acad Child Psychiatry* 1982;21:129–135.

Winsberg BG, Kupietz SS, Sverd J, Hungund BL, Young NL. Methylphenidate oral dose plasma concentrations and behavioral response in children. *Psychopharmacology* 1982;76:329–332.

Wolf DV, Wagner KD. Tardive dyskinesia, tardive dystonia, and tardive Tourette's syndrome in children and adolescents. *J Child Adolesc Psychopharmacol* 1993;3:175–198.

Woolston J. Case study: carbamazepine treatment of juvenile-onset bipolar disorder. *J Am Acad Child Adolesc Psychiatry* 1999;38:335–338.

Wudarsky M, Nicolson R, Hamburger SD, Spechler L, Gochman P, Bedwell J, Lenane MC, Rapoport JL. Elevated prolactin in pediatric patients on typical and atypical antipsychotics. *J Child Adolesc Psychopharmacol* 1999;9:239–245.

Wysowski DK, Barash D. Adverse behavioral reactions attributed to triazolam in the Food and Drug Administration's spontaneous reporting system. *Arch Intern Med* 1991;151:2003–2008.

Yepes LE, Balka EB, Winsberg BG, Bialer I. Amitriptyline and methylphenidate treatment of behaviorally disordered children. *J Child Psychol Psychiatry* 1977;18:39–52.

Zametkin AJ, Rapoport JL. Noradrenergic hypothesis of attention deficit disorder with hyperactivity: a critical review. In: Meltzer HY, ed. *Psychopharmacology: the third generation of progress.* New York: Raven Press; 1987:837–842.

Zametkin A, Rapoport JL, Murphy DL, Linnoila M, Ismond D. Treatment of hyperactive children with monoamine oxidase inhibitors. I. Clinical efficacy. *Arch Gen Psychiatry* 1985;42:962–966.

Zickler, P. NIDA initiative targets increasing teen use of anabolic steroids. *NIDA [National Institute on Drug Abuse] Notes* 2000;15 (3):1, 6–7. (NIH Publication No. 00–3478.)

Zito JM, Craig TJ, Wanderling J. Pharmacoepidemiology of 330 child/adolescent psychiatric patients. *J Pharmacoepidemiol* 1994;3:47–62.

Zrull JP, Westman JC, Arthur B, Bell WA. A comparison of chlordiazepoxide, d-amphetamine, and placebo in the treatment of the hyperkinetic syndrome in children. *Am J Psychiatry* 1963;120:590–591.

Zrull JP, Westman JC, Arthur B, Rice DL. A comparison of diazepam, d-amphetamine, and placebo in the treatment of the hyperkinetic syndrome in children. *Am J Psychiatry* 1964;121:388–389.

Zubieta JK, Alessi NE. Acute and chronic administration of trazodone in the treatment of disruptive behavior disorders in children. *J Clin Psychopharmacol* 1992;12:346–351.

Zuddas A, DiMartino A, Muglia P, Cianchetti C. Long-term risperidone treatment for pervasive developmental disorder: efficacy, tolerability, and discontinuation. *J Child Adolesc Psychopharmacol* 2000;10:79–90.

Zwier KJ, Rao U. Buspirone use in an adolescent with social phobia and mixed personality disorder (cluster A type). *J Am Acad Child Adolesc Psychiatry* 1994;33:1007–1011.

Index

Note: Page numbers followed by *t* indicate tables.

DSM-IV Diagnoses in Childhood and Adolescence for Which Psychopharmacotherapy May Be Therapeutically Indicated

Diagnosis	Page references
Major Depressive Disorder	
Fluoxetine	pp. 206–209
Fluvoxamine	p. 232
Other SSRIs	pp. 169, 237
Other Antidepressants	pp. 160–258
Lithium augmentation	pp. 176–177
Lithium for prophylaxis	pp. 176–177
Manic Episode	
Lithium	pp. 265–269
Valproic acid	pp. 274–277
Atypical Antipsychotics	pp. 122–159
Mental Retardation (with Severe Behavioral Disorder and/or Self-injurious Behavior)	
Atypical Antipsychotics	pp. 122–159
Chlorpromazine	pp. 92, 107
Haloperidol	pp. 92, 111–114
Lithium	pp. 259–272
Propranolol	pp. 318–321
Naltrexone	pp. 316–318
Obsessive-Compulsive Disorder	
Sertraline	pp. 217–219
Fluoxetine	pp. 209–210
Fluvoxamine	pp. 231–232
Paroxetine	pp. 226–229
Fluvoxamine	p. 232
Clomipramine	pp. 195–196
Clonazepam	p. 307
Panic Disorder	
Fluoxetine	pp. 202–214
Sertraline	pp. 217–222
Paroxetine	pp. 224–229
Alprazolam	p. 180
Clonazepam	p. 306
Tricyclic Antidepressants	p. 180
Pervasive Developmental Disorders	
Risperidone	pp. 136–142
Other Atypical Antipsychotics	pp. 122–159
Haloperidol	p. 113
Fluphenazine	pp. 117–118
Naltrexone	pp. 316–318
Methylphenidate	pp. 72–78
Amphetamines	pp. 86–87
Clomipramine	pp. 196–197
Buspirone	pp. 310–311
Clonidine	p. 330
Posttraumatic Stress Disorder	
Sertraline	p. 321
Paroxetine	p. 224
Propranolol	p. 321

(continued on inside back cover)